THE INTERVENTIONAL CARDIAC CATHETERIZATION HANDBOOK

4th edition

4TH EDITION

THE INTERVENTIONAL CARDIAC CATHETERIZATION HANDBOOK

Edited by

Morton J. Kern, MD, FSCAI, FACC, FAHA
Chief
Department of Medicine
Veterans Administration Long Beach Health Care System
Long Beach, California
Associate Chief and Professor of Medicine
Department of Cardiology
University of California, Irvine
Orange, California

Paul Sorajja, MD
Director
Center for Valve and Structural Heart Disease
Minneapolis Heart Institute Abbott Northwestern Hospital
Minneapolis, Minnesota

Michael J. Lim, MD
Jack Ford Shelby Endowed Professor of Cardiology
Center for Comprehensive Cardiovascular Care
St. Louis University
St. Louis, Missouri

ELSEVIER

ELSEVIER

1600 John F. Kennedy Blvd.
Ste 1800
Philadelphia, PA 19103-2899

THE INTERVENTIONAL CARDIAC
CATHETERIZATION HANDBOOK, ed. 4   ISBN: 978-0-323-47671-3

Notices

Knowledge and best practice in this field are constantly changing. As new
research and experience broaden our understanding, changes in research
methods, professional practices, or medical treatment may become necessary.

Practitioners and researchers must always rely on their own experience and
knowledge in evaluating and using any information, methods, compounds, or
experiments described herein. In using such information or methods they should
be mindful of their own safety and the safety of others, including parties for whom
they have a professional responsibility.

With respect to any drug or pharmaceutical products identified, readers are
advised to check the most current information provided (i) on procedures
featured or (ii) by the manufacturer of each product to be administered, to verify
the recommended dose or formula, the method and duration of administration,
and contraindications. It is the responsibility of practitioners, relying on their own
experience and knowledge of their patients, to make diagnoses, to determine
dosages and the best treatment for each individual patient, and to take all
appropriate safety precautions.

To the fullest extent of the law, neither the Publisher nor the authors,
contributors, or editors assume any liability for any injury and/or damage to
persons or property as a matter of products liability, negligence or otherwise, or
from any use or operation of any methods, products, instructions, or ideas
contained in the material herein.

Library of Congress Cataloging-in-Publication Data

Names: Kern, Morton J., Lim, Michael J., Sorajja, Paul, editors.
Title: The interventional cardiac catheterization handbook / edited by Morton J. Kern.
Description: 4th edition. | Philadelphia, PA : Elsevier, [2018] | Includes index.
Identifiers: LCCN 2016058714 | ISBN 9780323476713 (pbk. : alk. paper)
Subjects: | MESH: Cardiac Catheterization–methods | Handbooks
Classification: LCC RC683.5.C25 | NLM WG 39 | DDC 616.1/20754–dc23 LC record
available at https://lccn.loc.gov/2016058714

Content Strategist: Maureen Iannuzzi/Robin Carter
Content Development Specialist: Lisa Barnes
Publishing Services Manager: Patricia Tannian
Project Manager: Ted Rodgers
Design Direction: Brian Salisbury

Working together
to grow libraries in
developing countries

www.elsevier.com • www.bookaid.org

Printed in China

Last digit is the print number: 9   8   7   6   5   4   3

I thank my wife, Margaret, and daughter, Anna Rose, for giving me purpose beyond measure. They are the true systole of my life.

Morton Kern

I dedicate this to my loving parents, Kent and Mon Sorajja, and my two incredible daughters, Natali and Amalin.

Paul Sorajja

To those in my life who have supported me and helped along the way: My parents, Dorothy and Jess Lim; my beautiful children, Parker and Taylor; and my love – Kerri.

Michael J. Lim

Contributors

Anoop Agrawal, MD, FAAC
Interventional Cardiology fellow
St. Vincent's Heart Center of Indiana
Indianapolis, Indiana

Wail Alkashkari, MD
Consultant, Adult Congenital and Structural Intervention
King Faisal Cardiac Center
King Abdulaziz Medical City
Ministry of National Guard
Jeddah, Saudi Arabia

Subhash Banerjee, MD, FACC, FSCAI
Chief, Division of Cardiology
Co-director Cardiac Catheterization Laboratories
Veterans Administration North Texas Health Care System
Associate Professor
University of Texas Southwestern Medical Center
Dallas, Texas

Ryan Berg, MD
Chief of Cardiology
Veteran's Administration Central California Healthcare System
Associate Clinical Professor of Medicine
University of California, San Francisco
Fresno, California

Emmanouil S. Brilakis, MD, PhD
Veterans Administration North Texas Healthcare System
University of Texas Southwestern Medical Center
Dallas, Texas

Qi Ling Cao, MD
Director, Echocardiography Research Laboratory
Sidra Medical and Research Center
Doha, Qatar

Mauro Carlino, MD
Department of Interventional Cardiology
San Raffaele Hospital Milano
Milan, Italy

Cheng-Han Chen, MD, PhD, FACC
Clinical Instructor in Medicine
Division of Cardiology
Columbia University Medical Center/New York-Presbyterian Hospital
New York, New York

Michael Forsberg, MD
Assistant Professor of Medicine
St. Louis University School of Medicine
Staff Physician
John Cochran Veteran's Administration Medical Center
St. Louis, Missouri

Philippe Genereux, MD
Cardiovascular Research Foundation
New York-Presbyterian/Columbia University Medical Center
New York, New York
Hôpital du Sacré-Coeur de Montréal
Montréal, Québec, Canada

Tarek Helmy, MD
Center for Comprehensive Cardiovascular Care
St. Louis University School of Medicine
St. Louis, Missouri

James Hermiller, MD, FACC, FSCAI
Director of Interventional Cardiology
St. Vincent's Heart Center of Indiana
Indianapolis, Indiana

Ziyad M. Hijazi, MD, MPH, MSCAI, FACC
Chairman, Department of Pediatrics
Director, Cardiac Program
Sidra Medical and Research Center
Doha, Qatar

Morton J. Kern, MD, MSCAI, FAHA, FACC
Chief
Department of Medicine
Long Beach Veterans Health Care System
Long Beach, California
Associate Chief and Professor
Department of Cardiology
University of California, Irvine
Orange, California

Ajay J. Kirtane, MD, SM, FACC, FSCAI
Associate Professor at Columbia University Medical Center
Chief Academic Officer, Center for Interventional Vascular Therapy
Director, New York-Presbyterian/Columbia Cardiac Catheterization
    Laboratories
New York, New York

Andrew J. Klein, MD, FACC, FSCAI
Staff Interventional Cardiologist
Piedmont Heart Institute
Piedmont Atlanta
Atlanta, Georgia
Associate Professor of Medicine
Division of Cardiology
St. Louis University School of Medicine
St. Louis, Missouri

Michael J. Lim, MD
Jack Ford Shelby Endowed Professor of Cardiology
Center for Comprehensive Cardiovascular Care
St. Louis University
St. Louis, Missouri

Yves Louvard, MD
Institut Cardiovasculaire Paris Sud
Massy, France

Ammar Nasir, MD
Assistant Professor of Medicine
Center for Comprehensive Cardiovascular Care Staff
St. Louis University School of Medicine
Staff Interventional Cardiologist
St. Louis VA Medical Center
St. Louis, Missouri

Keval K. Patel, MD
Department of Internal Medicine
St. Louis University School of Medicine
St. Louis, Missouri

Pranav M. Patel
Chief of Cardiology and Associate Professor of Medicine
University of California, Irvine
Orange, California

Matthew J. Price, MD
Director, Cardiac Catheterization Laboratory
Division of Cardiovascular Diseases
Scripps Clinic
La Jolla, California

Rahil Rafeedheen, MD
Chief Cardiology Fellow
St. Louis University School of Medicine
St. Louis, Missouri

Stephane Rinfret, MD, SM
Chief
Interventional Cardiology
McGill University Medical Center
Montréal, Québec, Canada

Jason H. Rogers, MD
Professor of Cardiovascular Medicine
University of California, Davis, Medical Center
Sacramento, California

Arang Samim, MD
Cardiovascular Division
University of California, San Francisco, Fresno
Fresno, California

Arnold J. Seto, MD, MPA
Chief of Cardiology
Long Beach Veterans Affairs Medical Center
Long Beach, California
Director of Interventional Cardiology Research
University of California, Irvine
Orange, California

Gagan D. Singh, MD
Assistant Professor of Cardiovascular Medicine
University of California, Davis, Medical Center
Sacramento, California

Paul Sorajja, MD
Director
Center for Valve and Structural Heart Disease
Minneapolis Heart Institute Abbott Northwestern Hospital
Minneapolis, Minnesota

Jose D. Tafur, MD
Department of Cardiology
Ochsner Clinic Foundation
New Orleans, Louisiana

Barry F. Uretsky, MD
Director, Interventional Cardiology
University of Arkansas for Medical Sciences
Director, Cardiac Catheterization Laboratory
Central Arkansas Veterans Health System
Little Rock, Arkansas

Christopher J. White, MD
Chairman and Professor of Medicine
Department of Cardiovascular Diseases
Ochsner Clinical School of the University of Queensland
Ochsner Medical Institutions
New Orleans, Louisiana

Preface

It is a pleasure to provide to those working in the field of interventional cardiology a practical and yet detailed handbook to guide both the novice and the advanced practitioner toward best practices. Since the American Board of Internal Medicine certified the subspecialty almost 20 years ago, it is common knowledge that an operator needs an in-depth understanding of the extensive array of techniques to apply them appropriately and solidify the unique skill sets that will make cardiovascular interventions successful. It is our fervent wish that this book will help the interventional cardiologist and his or her team in their mastery and acquisition of both the complex skills and knowledge base.

This edition is noted for addressing the most recent, advanced techniques used to implant coronary and peripheral stents, repair injured vessels, and treat structural heart defects. It highlights the management of the critically ill patients in the cath lab before and during their interventions. *Percutaneous coronary intervention (PCI)* is in part a team sport; that is, the entire lab team members should all have a thorough understanding of the indications, contraindications, and guidelines for percutaneous coronary and structural interventions, coronary bypass graft, and valve surgery, and concomitant medical therapy for an individual patient coming into the lab. The patient's conditions and findings must also be integrated into tailored decisions for a specific patient, given a large variety of clinical factors and comorbidities.

The 4th edition of *The Interventional Cardiac Catheterization Handbook* continues to provide the critical information to those beginning their journey into interventional cardiology. It is understood that the practice of interventions cannot proceed without the prior mastery of techniques and methods employed for diagnostic catheterization and specially described in *The Cardiac Catheterization Handbook*, 6th edition. Excellence in intervention begins with excellence in diagnostic catheterization. As with all "handbooks," the material covered here cannot include every aspect of interventional cardiology. For those interested in more detailed information and studies supporting the approaches for treatment we discuss, we refer you to the larger textbooks in the field.

The contents of the *ICCH*, 4th edition, have been brought up to date as much as possible. The basic chapters on understanding what PCI does, how to achieve best access, and useful approaches to angiography now reflect current thinking regarding radial access, drug-eluting stents, and lesion assessment before, during, and after the procedure, always emphasizing the methods that increase safety whenever possible. Angiographic views for intervention, use of different contrast media, and identification of patients at high risk are fundamental reading for all students and physicians embarking on this path.

The *ICCH*, 4th edition, presents more focused and specific chapters emphasizing the unique nature of several well-recognized and well-studied angiographic subsets undergoing complex PCI, such as bifurcation lesions, left main stenosis, chronic total occlusions, saphenous vein graft interventions, complications, and peripheral vascular disease.

Each chapter concentrates on the topic in a concise and practical presentation by one of the experts in the field.

The chapter on complications, Chapter 10, highlights the fact that no area of cardiology has a greater need for the latest in information than PCI. To minimize the unanticipated complications, the planning and execution of PCI require an in-depth understanding of the options, limitations, and alternative methods of proceeding if the initial approach fails.

Students know that it is impossible for reading alone to substitute for experience. But the hands-on exposure to the different types of guiding catheters, guidewires, balloon catheters, stents, intravascular ultrasound imaging, and other non-balloon interventional devices is greatly facilitated by reviewing the descriptions, pitfalls, and anticipated technical problems that may occur.

The most critical step in performing an intervention begins well before introducing a stent. That step is ensuring that the correct procedure will be performed for the correct indications. The use of intravascular ultrasound imaging and translesional physiology, specifically fractional flow reserve (FFR), is critical in selecting which lesions do and do not require treatment and must be part of the complete interventional cardiologist's practice.

We thank our colleagues and cardiology fellows in training who contributed their valuable time, knowledge, and effort to make this book possible. Finally, this book would have no value were it not for our belief that the knowledge gained will aid the overwhelming desire of the cath lab physicians, nurses, techs, and fellows to help their patients through what may be a life or death procedure. We am humbled and at the same buoyed by our mutual goals to care for our patients through better knowledge in the cath lab.

Morton J. Kern

Paul Sorajja

Michael J. Lim

Acknowledgment

The editors sincerely thank Dr. Khalil Ahmad Ahrari, of Herat, Afghanistan, a Fellow in Interventional Cardiology at Artemis Hospital, Gurgaon, Haryana, India, for his dedicated reading of our work and the very thoughtful comments.

Contents

Video Contents

Case Studies

To access this material, which includes 205 videos, go to ExpertConsult.com.

1

The Basics of Percutaneous Coronary Interventions

MORTON J. KERN

Introduction

On September 16, 1977, Andreas Grüentzig performed the first human percutaneous transluminal coronary angioplasty (PTCA) in Zurich, Switzerland. Until then, coronary artery bypass surgery was the only alternative to medicine for the treatment of coronary artery disease. Over the past four decades, PTCA evolved into more sophisticated techniques involving predominantly stenting and other nonballoon devices and is now called *percutaneous coronary intervention (PCI)*. PCI is a highly successful method of coronary revascularization with more than 1,500,000 procedures done in the United States annually. PCI has been undertaking more complex lesions than discrete single- and double-vessel coronary lesions and routinely takes on complex multivessel coronary artery disease including significant left main stenosis. High-risk PCI in patients with depressed left ventricular function requires specialized support team work and techniques. PCI methodology now extends into the treatment of peripheral arterial disease and, most recently, structural heart disease (valves, septal defects, etc.) as an emerging separate discipline within interventional cardiology.

PCI encompasses various coronary techniques, such as balloons, stents, cutters, lasers, grinders, suckers, filters, and other tools. The term *percutaneous transluminal coronary angioplasty* or PTCA may be used when describing techniques and older study outcomes related to use of the original balloon inflation technique first employed by Grüentzig.

This chapter is an extension of the PCI chapter from *The Cardiac Catheterization Handbook,* 6e (2015), and will present the basic method and mechanisms of balloon angioplasty and stenting as an introduction to the practice of interventional cardiology. The various techniques of PCI can be placed into niche applications for specific devices (Table 1.1).

Overview

Percutaneous coronary intervention technique is an extension of the basic procedures used for diagnostic cardiac catheterization and coronary angiography. After appropriate clinical evaluation and the establishment of suitable indications for revascularization, PCI can be performed as a procedure separate from the diagnostic angiography or as an add-on or ad hoc procedure following the diagnostic study.

To begin the PCI, it is critical to recall that vascular access remains one of the most important decision points. The same techniques for the placement of an arterial sheath through the arm (radial artery) or leg (femoral artery) are used (see Chapter 2, Vascular Access), but, in contrast

1

Table 1.1

Niche Applications of Percutaneous Coronary Intervention (PCI) Devices

Lesion Type	Stent	Cutting balloon	Rotoblator	Clot Aspiration	Special Devices
Type A	+++	+	±	−	−
Complex	++	++	+	−	Guideliners
Ostial	++	++	+	−	−
Diffuse	+	+	++	−	−
Chronic total occ	++	+	−	−	Special equip*
Calcified bifurcation	±	++	+++	−	(orbital ath)
SVG focal	+++	±	±	−	Filters, prox occ
SVG diffuse	+	±	−	−	−
SVG thrombotic	±	−	−	++	Filters, prox occ
Complication	+++	−	±	±	Snares
Acute occlusion	++	−	−	±	−
Thrombosis	+	−	−	+++	−
Perforation	±	−	−	−	Covered stent

+++, highly applicable; ++, somewhat helpful; +, applicable; ±, marginal depending on status; −, not applicable. *specialized equipment includes uniques guidewires, balloons with reentry ports, and transport catheters for antegrade or retrograde access. Occ, Occlusion. Prox occ, Proximal occlusion. Roto, rotational atherectomy. SVG, saphenous vein graft.

to diagnostic catheters, PCI often requires larger lumen, specialized "guiding" catheters and hence larger sheaths. The potential for access site bleeding must be carefully considered. Technique also varies when engaging the coronary artery. Although the method is generally the same as for a diagnostic catheter, the stiffer construction needed to provide stabilization or backup for delivery of PCI equipment adds some difficulty. Nonetheless, good guide support is the next most critical aspect to a successful procedure.

Steps in the PCI Procedure

The steps in the PCI procedure are shown in Fig. 1.1. First, a guiding catheter is seated in the coronary ostium. Next a thin, steerable guidewire is introduced into the guide catheter and then advanced into the coronary artery and positioned across the stenosis into the distal coronary artery. A very small angioplasty balloon catheter is placed on the guidewire, advanced through the guiding catheter, and positioned in the stenotic area by tracking the balloon over the guidewire. Once correctly placed within the narrowed area to be treated, the PCI balloon is inflated several times for brief periods (10–60 seconds) expanding the stenosis and restoring blood flow to the area of the heart previously deprived by the stenosed artery.

After the balloon expands the stenosis, the balloon catheter is exchanged for a stent catheter. The stent is a metal scaffold, mounted and compressed on another balloon catheter and delivered exactly as the first balloon. The stent is positioned in the dilated stenosis and deployed by inflation of the balloon, again exactly as for dilating the balloon. It is inflated with the same pressure gauge syringe (8–16 atm pressure) for 10–20 seconds. A full stent opening (expansion) with complete strut apposition to the vessel wall is important for best short- and long-term results.

After the stent is well implanted into the artery wall, the balloon is deflated and the delivery catheter is removed. Intravascular imaging is often performed using a specialized catheter (intravascular ultrasound [IVUS] or optical coherence tomography [OCT]) to confirm appropriate vessel/stent matching and full stent strut expansion and strut apposition

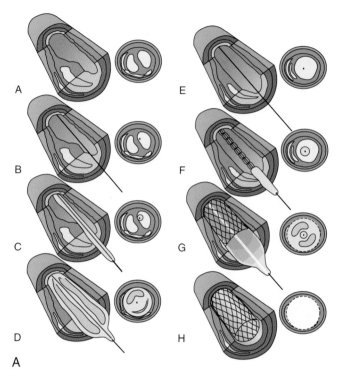

A

Figure 1.1A How angioplasty and stenting works. (A) The artery is filled with atherosclerotic material, compromising the lumen. A cross-section of the artery is shown on the right side. (B) A guidewire is positioned past the stenoses through the lumen. (C) A balloon catheter is advanced over the guidewire. (D) The balloon is inflated. (E) The balloon is deflated and withdrawn. (F) The balloon catheter is exchanged for a stent (on a balloon). (G) The stent is expanded. (H) The expanded stent remains in place after the deflated balloon is withdrawn. *(From American Heart Association,* Your PTCA, Our Guide to Percutaneous Transluminal Coronary Angioplasty, *2001.)*

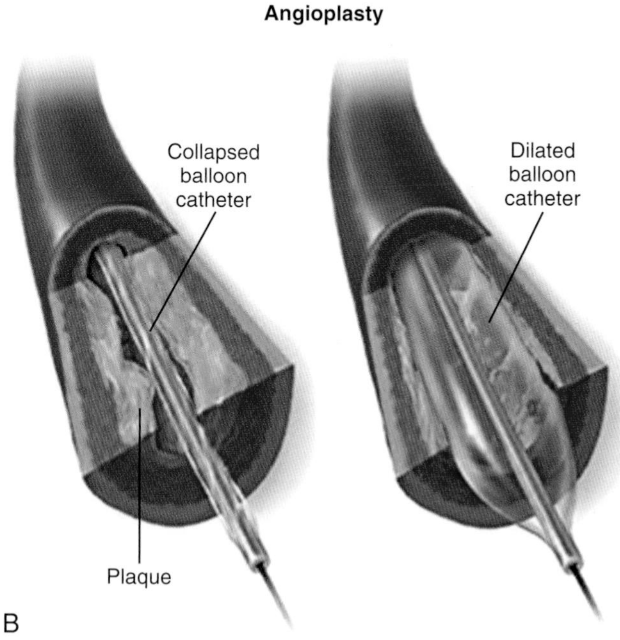

Angioplasty

Collapsed balloon catheter

Dilated balloon catheter

Plaque

B

Figure 1.1B Drawing of angioplasty balloon before *(left)* and during inflation *(right)*. *(Courtesy of Guidant Corp.)*

(contact without space against the wall). After IVUS/OCT and final angiography, the guide catheter is removed, and arterial hemostasis after sheath removal is obtained. The patient is then transferred to a recovery area and then to his or her room. If no complications occur, the patient is discharged depending on the lab's habits: later that day for radial access patients, the next morning for femoral procedures. The patient commonly returns to work shortly (<2 days) thereafter. The definitions of a successful PCI procedure are summarized in Box 1.1.

Mechanisms of Angioplasty and Stenting

1. Disruption of plaque and the arterial wall

   The inflated balloon exerts pressure against the plaque and the arterial wall, causing fracturing and splitting. Concentric (round or circumferential) lesions fracture and split at the thinnest and weakest points. Eccentric lesions split at the junction of the plaque and the normal arterial wall. Dissection or separation of the plaque from the vessel wall releases the restraining effect caused by the lesion and results in a larger lumen. This is the major mechanism of balloon angioplasty.

2. Loss of elastic recoil

   Balloon dilatation causes stretching and thinning of the medial musculature of the vessel wall. Stretching causes the vessel wall to temporarily lose its elastic (recoil) properties. The degree of elastic recoil is affected by the balloon-to-artery size ratio. Almost all vessels have some elastic recoil and, over time, will recoil, which is a contributing mechanism to restenosis. The major initial benefit of stenting is the elimination of elastic recoil, which maintains a large lumen over time.

3. Redistribution and compression of plaque components

   During angioplasty, balloon pressure causes denudation of the vessel wall lining (endothelial) cells and the extrusion or pushing out of plaque components. There may be some extrusion longitudinally of the softer lipid material, but this effect accounts for a very small part of the overall effect.

Box 1.1   Definitions of Percutaneous Coronary Intervention (PCI)

Success: PCI success may be defined by angiographic, procedural, and clinical criteria.

Angiographic Success
- Final minimum stenosis diameter reduction to <10%.

Procedural Success
- Angiographic success without in-hospital major clinical complications (e.g., death, myocardial infarction [MI], emergency coronary artery bypass surgery). MI is often defined as the development of Q-waves in addition to elevation of troponins three times the upper limits of laboratory's normal value. Cardiac troponin T and I as measurements of myocardial necrosis are more sensitive and specific than CK-MB. Enzyme elevations in the absence of new Q-waves is counted as MI, peri-procedural. There is no consensus on what level of troponin alone is clinically important enough to change major management following the interventional procedure.

Clinical Success
- A clinically successful PCI is an anatomic and procedural success with relief of signs and/or symptoms of myocardial ischemia after recovery from the procedure. The long-term clinical success requires that the patient has continued relief of signs and symptoms of myocardial ischemia for more than 6 months. Restenosis is the principal cause of lack of long-term clinical success when short-term clinical success has been achieved.

Indications for PCI

Guidelines and recommendations for the performance of PCI are provided in extensive detail in the American Heart Association, American College of Cardiology, and Society for Cardiac Angiography and Interventions (AHA/ACC/SCAI) PCI updated Guidelines of 2015. Specific anatomic and clinical features for each patient should be considered for the likelihood of success, failure and risk of complications, morbidity, mortality, and restenosis. Restenosis and incomplete revascularization must also be weighed against the outcome anticipated for coronary artery bypass grafting (CABG).

In general, PCI is indicated for patients with

- Stable angina pectoris unrelieved by optimal medical therapy with objective evidence of ischemia (abnormal stress testing or ECG changes with pain) and a coronary lesion in a vessel supplying a large area of myocardium
- Unstable angina
- Acute myocardial infarction (MI)
- Angina pectoris after CABG surgery
- Symptomatic restenosis after PCI

Relative Contraindications to PCI

- Unsuitable coronary anatomy (e.g., multiple severe complex lesions or diffuse distal disease)
- High-risk coronary anatomy in which closure of vessel would result in death
- Inability to take antiplatelet agents

Absolute contraindications to PCI are relatively few. However, it should be noted that some patients with contraindications may have no options regarding coronary revascularization, and PCI becomes their only alternative to medical therapy. Contraindications include:

- Bleeding diathesis (low platelet count, peptic ulcer disease, coagulopathy, and so on)
- Patient noncompliance with procedure and post-PCI instructions and inability to take dual antiplatelet therapy (acetylsalicylic acid [ASA], clopidogrel [Plavix], etc.)
- Multiple PCI restenoses

Complications of PCI (see also Chapter 10)

For most elective procedures:

1. Death (0.1%)
2. MI (1–3%)
3. Emergency coronary artery bypass grafting (0.5–2%)

Of course, any complications that can occur during diagnostic cardiac catheterizations can also occur during PCI, such as femoral access site bleeding, especially with larger sheaths and prolonged anticoagulation (1 : 250 patients), contrast-medium reactions, cerebral vascular accident, MI, and vascular injury (e.g., pseudoaneurysm of femoral artery, radial artery occlusion).

4. Restenosis (5–10% for drug-eluting stents, 10–20% for bare metal stents; see also Chapter 7)

Restenosis within the stent at the edges of the stent occurs in approximately 10% of patients and may lead to recurrence of anginal symptoms. Typically, restenosis occurs most frequently within the initial 12 months

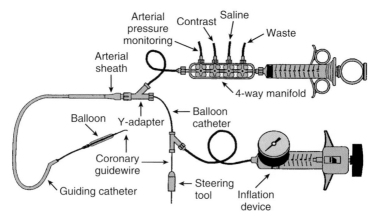

Figure 1.2 Diagram of components of percutaneous coronary intervention equipment. *(From Safian R, Freed M, eds.* The Manual of Interventional Cardiology, *3rd ed. Birmingham, MI: Physicians' Press, 2001.)*

after PCI. This biological effect is not considered a complication but rather a clinical response to angioplasty.

PCI Equipment

The most commonly used PCI equipment include a guiding catheter, a coronary guidewire, a balloon catheter, and a stent (Fig. 1.2). PCI equipment is designed to overcome or facilitate three major operational challenges: (1) stable guide catheter positioning and support, (2) guidewire and balloon catheter navigation of tortuous vessel segments, (3) and delivery of the stent through tortuous vessel segments. A successful PCI requires the operator to control the three principal movable components (guide catheter, balloon catheter, and guidewire) simultaneously.

The Guiding Catheter

A special large-lumen catheter (5–8F) is used to deliver the coronary balloon catheter and other interventional devices to the target lesion. There are three major guide catheter functions during angioplasty:

1. Balloon/stent catheter delivery
2. Backup support for balloon/stent advancement
3. Coronary pressure monitoring and contrast injections

Fig. 1.3 shows guide catheter features that differentiate it from diagnostic catheters.

Balloon Catheter Delivery

To effectively deliver and position the balloon/stent catheter over the guidewire across the stenosis, the guiding catheter must be well seated. This position is best achieved when the catheter tip is parallel or coaxial to the long axis of the proximal or ostial part of the artery. Coaxial alignment permits safer transmission of the force needed to advance the balloon across a stenosis. Alignment may require guide catheter repositioning or occasionally deep seating into the artery. A specialized guide-within-a-guide or secondary catheter (e.g., *guideliner*, also called *mother-and-child guides*) may be required for suitable backup support in some difficult situations.

Adequate contrast visualization during the procedure is critical to positioning the balloon/stent and is, in part, a function of the guide

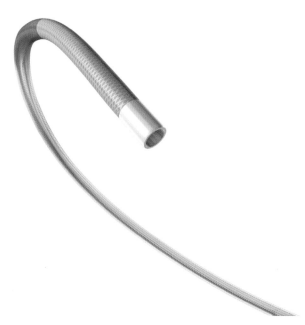

Figure 1.3 Illustration of a guiding catheter shows stiffer body; variable softer primary curve; wire braiding; atraumatic tip; large lumen (optional radio-opaque marker); lubricous coating. *(Courtesy of Boston Scientific, Inc., Boston, MA.)*

catheter lumen when occupied by the angioplasty device in place. Sufficient x-ray contrast with the PCI catheter in place must be delivered to see the target vessel and lesion. Large, non-balloon PCI devices (e.g., rotoblator, thrombus aspiration catheters, etc.) in small guide catheters may not allow adequate vessel visualization. This problem has been overcome with larger lumen catheters and contrast media power injectors used in some labs.

While balloon and PCI catheters have become smaller, the size of internal diameter of the guiding catheter has become larger thus achieving the goal of adequate visualization through small catheters. However, a large guide catheter (>7F) may be critical when using double balloon/stent systems for complex or bifurcated lesions.

Backup Support for Balloon/Stent Advancement

Support or "backup" for stent advancement is achieved after seating (cannulation) the guide catheter in the coronary ostium. The guiding catheter provides a platform from which one can push the stent over the guidewire through the artery and across the stenosis.

Inadequate backup support will result in failure to cross a lesion and an unsuccessful procedure. Backup support requires a combination of correct coaxial (in line with the artery ostium) alignment, as well as the ability to carefully control advancement (deep seating; also see the section on guideliner systems) of the guiding catheter into the coronary ostium.

For more complex and technically difficult lesions, the choice of an appropriate guiding catheter for extra support and lesion visualization remains essential. When there is insufficient backup, attempts to cross a very tight stenosis will cause the guiding catheter to disengage from the coronary ostium and back out into the aortic root. When pressure is applied to the stent catheter during attempts to cross the lesion, repositioning the guide catheter after forward stent motion in a stepwise fashion may overcome the loss of support. However, aggressive intubation of the coronary ostium may damage the vessel, stopping the procedure prematurely, or may require additional stenting to repair an ostial dissection.

Historically, deep seating of the guide catheter is achieved by manipulating the guide catheter over the balloon catheter shaft, past the aortocoronary ostium, and farther into the vessel. This maneuver is used to obtain increased backup support for crossing difficult lesions and is typically a last resort maneuver because of the increased chance of guide catheter–induced dissection of the left main or proximal vessel. The use of guide-within-a-guide system (e.g., guideliner) has obviated the need for such deep intubation of a larger guide catheter and its potential for vessel damage. However, inserting even the guideliner guide extension is not without risk of vessel injury.

Pressure Monitoring

The guiding catheter measures aortic pressure during the procedure. Pressure wave damping may occur if the guide catheter blocks the ostium, if there is non-coaxial seating, or if plaque obstructs flow through the coronary ostium. In addition, translesional pressure using proximal pressure measured through the guide catheter and distal post-stenotic pressure measured with a pressure sensor guidewire is used for determining the hemodynamic significance of the lesion before and after PCI.

Some catheters have side holes near the tip to permit perfusion into the artery when the catheter is deeply seated and obstructing flow. These catheters should be used with caution and are not suitable for hemodynamic lesion assessment (i.e., fractional flow reserve [FFR]) due to the creation of a pseudo-stenosis through the side holes.

Guide Catheter Characteristics

Compared to the diagnostic catheters, the guiding catheters do not have tapered tips. They have thinner walls, larger lumens, and stiffer shafts (Fig. 1.3). A large catheter lumen is achieved at the expense of catheter wall thickness and thus may result in decreased catheter wall strength, increased catheter kinking, or less torque control. Guiding catheters are generally stiffer to provide backup support for the balloon/stent catheter advancement into the coronary artery and therefore respond differently to manipulation than do diagnostic catheters. Pressure wave damping upon engaging the coronary ostium is seen more often than with similar-size diagnostic angiographic catheters. Some guide catheters have relatively shorter and more flexible tips to decrease catheter-induced trauma.

Guide catheter coronary occlusion is noted by the change in the arterial pressure waveform to one of "damping," which shows a flattened diastolic portion or ventricular-like pattern (Fig. 1.4). Guiding catheters with small side holes near the tip permit blood to enter the coronary artery when the ostium is blocked by the guide catheter and can reduce ischemia. Side holes are used when the guide catheter either partially or totally occludes blood flow into the coronary artery. However, side holes may lead to inadequate artery visualization from loss of contrast

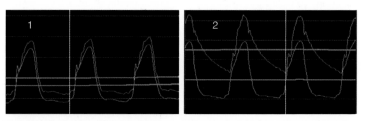

Figure 1.4 Pressure tracings demonstrating guide catheter pressure damping (*left*) and after withdrawal of guide from ostium (*right*). Guide catheter pressure is red, pressure wire inside coronary artery is green.

media exiting the catheter before entering the artery. Although side holes may provide reliable aortic pressure, coronary flow can still be compromised during the angioplasty procedure. The guide catheter and side holes act as a "second stenosis" at the coronary ostium.

Small shaft diameter guide catheters (e.g., ≤6F) are the most frequently used size of guiding catheter. 6F guide catheters are associated with fewer femoral vascular complications than 8F catheters. Smaller (<5F) guide catheters may not permit adequate visualization with some stent systems. 7F or 8F guide catheters are used for complex procedures requiring larger PCI devices (e.g., rotoblator) or simultaneous positioning of two stents for treatment of bifurcation lesions. Use of 6F (or, in some patients, 7F) guide catheters from the radial artery approach is now common practice for most routine PCI because of the markedly reduced vascular complications associated with radial PCI procedures.

Balloon Dilatation Catheter Systems

There are two types of PCI balloon catheters: over-the-wire (OTW) (Fig. 1.5) and monorail (Fig. 1.6).

OTW Angioplasty Balloon Catheters

A standard OTW angioplasty balloon catheter has two lumens that run throughout the length of the catheter; one for the guidewire and another for balloon inflation (Fig. 1.5). These balloons are approximately 145–155 cm long and are designed to be used with guidewires of various dimensions (0.010–0.014 in). The major OTW advantage is the ability to maintain distal artery access with the balloon beyond the lesion while exchanging one guidewire for another. The OTW system tracks very well since the whole balloon length has a wire lumen. It permits long guidewire exchanges. In addition, one can deliver contrast and drugs distally in an artery through the guidewire lumen (after the guidewire is removed, of course).

To exchange PCI catheters, the balloon is advanced over the wire to a distal position. The standard short (145 cm) wire is then removed from the balloon. A longer guidewire (300 cm) is then inserted, and, while maintaining distal wire position, the balloon catheter is completely withdrawn over the guidewire and another balloon catheter is introduced over the same long guidewire and repositioned for additional dilatations. OTW catheters can accept multiple guidewires, which allows for exchanging additional devices that may require stronger, stiffer, or specialized guidewires.

OTW balloon catheters have several limitations that include a slightly larger diameter than the rapid-exchange (monorail) catheters and the need for additional personnel to help with long guidewire catheter exchanges.

Inflation port

Wire port   Strain relief band   Balloon with 2 markers

Figure 1.5 Typical over-the-wire balloon catheter. Quantum Maverick OTW. OTW "Quantum" Maverick Balloon. *(Courtesy of Boston Scientific, Boston, MA.)*

            Strain relief support   Beginning of distal   Balloon with 2
Inflation port and hub   guidewire lumen   markers

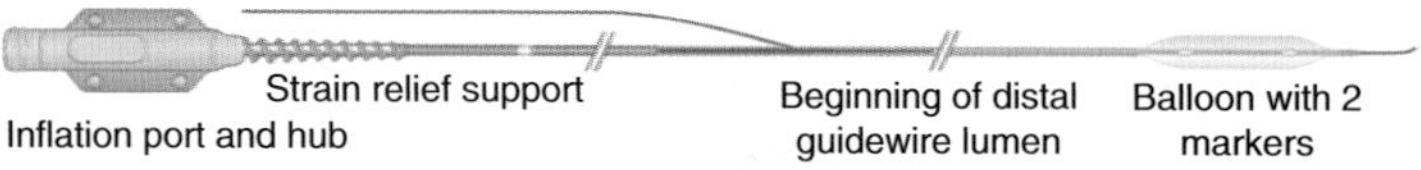

Figure 1.6 Typical rapid exchange or monorail balloon catheter. *(Courtesy of Boston Scientific, Boston, MA.)*

Rapid-Exchange (Monorail) Balloon Catheters

Rapid-exchange or monorail catheters were developed to permit the exchange of angioplasty balloon catheters by a single operator. Rapid-exchange catheters have one complete long lumen to inflate the balloon, and only a short (30–40 cm) length of the distal catheter shaft contains two lumens (Fig. 1.6), the second to let the catheter travel on a guidewire. Because only a limited portion of the catheter requires two lumens, rapid-exchange catheters are smaller in diameter than OTW balloon catheters.

Rapid-exchange balloon catheters address certain inherent limitations of OTW catheters. First, OTW balloon exchanges require a long (or extension) guidewire, which is unnecessary for the rapid-exchange balloon. Second, a single operator can use rapid-exchange balloon catheters without the aid of other assistants to maintain distal guidewire position.

Limitations of monorail catheters include the need for more care in manipulation of the guidewire, balloon catheter, and guiding catheter. Extra caution when moving the balloon is needed. If the monorail balloon is advanced beyond the distal end of the guidewire, the wire may come out of its short lumen, necessitating catheter withdrawal and reassembly of the balloon and guidewire. This is especially true when catheters with relatively short (<2 cm) "rail" segments are used. Additionally, if the balloon catheter requires excess force during advancement, a loop of guidewire may sometimes form outside the guide catheter in the aorta. This loop is nearly invisible but should be considered if the operator advances the catheter without seeing motion at the balloon tip.

Characteristics of Balloon Catheters

The plastic material of the balloon determines its compliance (defined as the amount of expansion or diameter size for given amount of pressure) and strength. Compliance is the main differentiating feature among balloon catheters. Inflation of a compliant balloon above factory-determined average mean pressure (also called nominal pressure for a known balloon size) will lead to further expansion of the balloon size approximately 10–20% over the predicted diameter. Noncompliant balloons, on the other hand, remain very close to their rated diameter even when inflated several atmospheres above nominal pressure.

A compliant balloon may result in oversizing, particularly on second and third high-pressure inflations, possibly resulting in dissections. After stent deployment, high-pressure inflations are performed with noncompliant balloons to firmly and completely implant the stent struts into the vessel wall.

Understanding the mechanical aspects of balloon inflation influences the approach to stent implantation. Several fundamental principles apply broadly to balloon inflation:

1. There is balloon overinflation at balloon ends.

   According to Laplace's law, wall stress increases with radius. At a given pressure, a larger balloon undergoes more wall stress than a smaller balloon, promoting balloon rupture. Artery sites adjacent to the lesion may be traumatized by inflations at high pressures. When inflating a balloon above the rated burst pressure, consider limiting the number and duration of inflations.

2. Balloon diameters always increase with increasing pressure.

   Even noncompliant balloons will grow in diameter (usually by <10% over nominal) with high pressure. Compliant balloons may increase by more than 20%. The balloon diameter–pressure relation is usually linear, reflecting the compliance characteristics. Fig. 1.7 shows the balloon during inflation and a graph for pressure versus diameter. Balloons do not return to their original dimensions after deflation. At any given pressure, the balloon diameter during a subsequent inflation will be larger than during the first inflation. When dilating

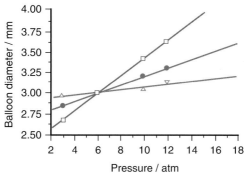

Figure 1.7 Three hypothetical compliance curves of angioplasty balloons. Triangles, non-compliant; circle, intermediate compliance; square, high compliance. For each type of balloon, the change in diameter may differ with increasing pressure. Parts of the balloon outside of a stent may expand in excess of rated size for pressure.

Table 1.2

Conversion of French Size to Millimeters

1 French = 0.33 mm
2 French = 0.67
3 French = 1
4 French = 1.33
5 French = 1.67
6 French = 2
7 French = 2.33
8 French = 2.67

Note: Each increment of French sizing equals 0.33 mm; for example, a 3F catheter equals 1 mm outer diameter. The disadvantage of the French scale is that it does not specify the inner diameter of the catheter or tubing.

two lesions with a compliant balloon, consider approaching the narrower lesion first.

Selection of Balloon Catheters

The selection of a balloon catheter is highly subjective and less critical in the current era of stents. The balloon size is selected to achieve a 1:1 size match with the vessel. Balloon-to-artery ratios of more than 1.2:1 are associated with increased complications. Longer balloons (30–40 mm) are useful for dilating long and diffuse narrowings. Short (10–15 mm) balloons are used for stent re-expansion to avoid stretching the vessel wall outside the stent.

The balloon/stent size is determined using the distal arterial reference segment diameter compared to the size of the guiding catheter (Table 1.2 provides conversion of French size to mm). Visual estimation of artery diameter is less accurate than quantitative angiographic and intravascular imaging (IVUS or OCT) approaches, but it is the method used by nearly all interventionalists during the procedure. From IVUS studies, most stents selected by visual sizing are 0.5 mm smaller than true vessel dimensions.

Important technical considerations for selecting stent systems include device profile, ease of delivery, and restenosis and acute thrombosis rates. There appears to be no practical difference among balloon catheters used for stent delivery. Stent profile alone is not the only factor in facilitating a stent to cross a lesion. Resistance to balloon/stent catheter forward motion may occur as a result of guidewire friction, guide catheter friction, or tortuous artery friction.

Balloon Inflation Strategies

Stenosis resolution occurs when the balloon pressure eliminates the balloon indentation caused by the stenosis (called the *waist*). Unstable or thrombotic lesions are generally soft and are associated with a lower balloon inflation pressure than are chronic, stable lesions. Most coronary lesions respond to inflation pressures of less than 10 atm. Calcific or fibrotic lesions may require higher inflation pressure (12–17 atm) to eliminate the balloon waist. Because stenting is now routine, issues regarding optimal balloon inflation strategies are relatively unimportant. Balloon inflations are generally brief (<60 sec) but should be inflated long enough to permit elastic tissue to relax and stretch. However, in the uncommon event that some lesions may not receive a stent, high pressures in compliant balloons may produce an oversized balloon-to-artery ratio associated with an increased incidence of dissection and complications. Low-pressure inflations may reduce complications. Most procedures start with low pressures, but operators often feel compelled to use higher pressures to achieve satisfactory angiographic results.

PCI Guidewires

PCI guidewires are small-caliber (0.010–0.018 in) steerable wires advanced into the coronary artery or its branches beyond the lesion to be dilated. A J-tip of varying degree, usually shaped by the operator, allows steering across side branches and through tortuous artery curves.

Guidewires are made with an inner core wire and an outer spring tip. The shorter the distance between the end of the central core and the spring tip, the stiffer and more maneuverable the wire. Differences in core construction affect guidewire handling. Important considerations when selecting a guidewire include diameter, coating, torque control, flexibility, malleability, radio-opacity, and trackability. The diameter for the most commonly used coronary guidewires is 0.014 in. Custom tip shaping will help steer the guidewire for specific anatomy.

Guidewire Characteristics

The selection and successful placement of a guidewire distal to the stenosis depend on the clinical situation and the operator's experience and skills. Several guidewire characteristics should be considered in selection.

Stiffness of the guidewire determines specific performance. Soft wires may be easier to advance through tortuous artery branches. Stiff wires torque better and are often useful for crossing difficult or total chronic occlusions. Extra-stiff guidewires provide better support for difficult stent placement in highly tortuous arteries.

"Steerability," "flexibility," and "malleability" are terms used to differentiate various guidewires. One feature that helps position the guidewire is tip shaping. The specific shape is made by bending the wire by rolling the guidewire tip over a needle or bending the wire tip at the end of an introducer tool. In general, the length of the distal bend in a large vessel should approximate half the usual diameter of the vessel (about 2 mm). A larger bend may be needed to reach a takeoff. When steering the wire into an abruptly angled branch, a double 45-degree bend is often helpful.

Radio-Opacity, Marker Bands, and Special Coatings

Visualization of the guidewire is provided by a radio-opaque coating usually applied only to the distal part of the wire. The limited radio-opaque segment permits lesion visualization without obscuring useful angiographic detail, such as small dissections. Calibrated radio-opaque marker bands are used to gauge lesion length. Stent/balloon catheters usually have two markers, one at each end of the balloon. Small balloons (e.g., 1.5 mm diameter) have one central marker. These markers may be confused for the markers on some guidewires.

A variety of different wire coatings increase ease of wire movement within the balloon catheter and artery. Some coated plastic-tipped wires, especially those with hydrophilic tips, have a higher likelihood of perforating the arterial wall. With the emergence of the special approaches to chronic total occlusions (CTO), families of specialized guidewires have been developed that increase procedure success (see Chapter 8 on CTO).

An exchange guidewire is available and is similar to those just mentioned except that its length is 280–300 cm. This long wire replaces the initial 140-cm wire when an exchange of the balloon catheter is necessary (e.g., upsizing balloon or insertion of stent). Alternatively, a 120–145-cm extension wire can be connected to a companion 145-cm guidewire thus creating a long exchange guidewire to allow balloon catheter exchanges. Some guidewires have the ability to accept an extension and thus become an exchange wire.

Accessory Equipment (Fig. 1.8)

Adjustable Hemostasis and Rotating Y-Connector Valve

The Y-connector is attached to the guide catheter to permit introduction of a PCI catheter into the guide while allowing contrast injection through the guide catheter. The end of the Y-connector has a rotating hub and a valve. The valve minimizes back bleeding from the guide catheter while the PCI catheter is inserted or removed. The Y-connector also permits pressure monitoring through the guiding catheter regardless of PCI catheter position.

Balloon Inflation Devices

A disposable syringe device is used to inflate the PCI balloon. A pressure gauge or digital display indicates the precise inflation pressure in atmospheres (atm or torr) or pounds/square inch (psi). Typically, the balloon is inflated with sufficient pressure (4–12 atm) to fully expand the stenosis indentation ("dumbbell" or "waist") of the partially inflated balloon. Occasionally, some calcified or highly fibrotic lesions require very high inflation pressures (>14 atm) to expand and eliminate the "dumbbell" appearance of the balloon.

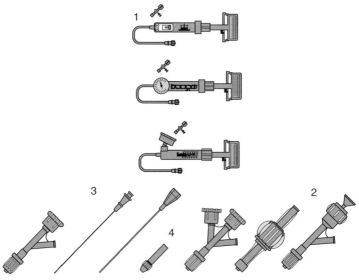

Figure 1.8 Ancillary equipment, Y-connectors, inflation devices. (1) Indeflators, (2) Y connectors, (3) needle wire introducers, (4) torque tool. *(Courtesy Merit Medical Inc. South Jordan, UT)*

Guidewire Torque (Tool) Device and Guidewire Introducer

A small, cylindrical pin vise clamp slides over the end of a guidewire and permits the operator to perform fine steering manipulations of the guidewire. A guidewire introducer is a very thin, needlelike tube with a tapered conical opening on one end that helps the operator insert the guidewire through a Y-connector valve or into a balloon catheter.

Stents

Stents prevent abrupt vessel closure from dissections and reduce vascular smooth muscle recoil. In reducing recoil and minimizing regrowth of neointima (aka, hyperplasia) through the use of antiproliferative coatings, stents reduce coronary restenosis. Numerous stent designs are available to overcome patent issues, improve vascular scaffolding mechanisms, provide unique antiproliferative coatings, and, most recently, become resorbable over time. Stents are composed of metal mesh, wire coil, slotted tube, multicellular designs, or unique bioabsorbable materials of custom design. Currently, uncoated stents (called bare metal) and drug-eluting stents are the most commonly used, with bioresorbable (BV) scaffolds soon to be in widespread use. Box 1.2 lists several ideal stent characteristics.

There are two mechanisms of stent expansion: balloon expandable and self-expanding. Nearly all coronary stents are balloon-expandable. They are premounted on a balloon catheter, delivered to the lesion, and then the inflated balloon deploys the stent. Self-expanding stents often are used for peripheral vascular disease interventions. They are compressed on a delivery catheter and covered with a sheath to prevent premature deployment. Once the stent/cover is delivered to the lesion, the cover is withdrawn, permitting the stent to expand on its own. Often nitinol is the memory metal used in these stents.

Stent metals may be made of stainless steel, cobalt-based alloy, tantalum, titanium, or nitinol. Drug-eluting stents have drug-impregnated coatings, biodegradable drug carrier coatings, and/or other types of drug delivery systems. Biodegradable and bioabsorbable stents are currently in clinical trials.

Stent Dimensions and Specialized Designs

For native coronary arteries, expanded stent diameters range from 2.25 to 5 mm. Stent lengths vary from 8 to 33 mm. For saphenous vein grafts and peripheral vessels, larger stent diameters (>5 mm) are available. Specialized stents are specifically designed for particular problems. For example, a unique covered stent with a polytetrafluoroethylene (PTFE) coating is designed for coronary perforation or rupture and can be used to cover aneurysms. Dedicated bifurcated stents are in development.

Fig. 1.9 shows several currently available stents. Fig. 1.10 lists stent types, characteristics, and specialized features of material and cell configuration. Fig. 1.11 is an example of stent placement in right coronary angioplasty (RCA). (See Chapter 6, Stents, Restenosis, and Stent Thrombosis, for a full discussion.)

Box 1.2   Ideal Stent Characteristics

- Biocompatible and bioabsorbable
- Conformity to tortuosity
- Flexibility
- High radial strength
- Low metallic surface area
- Low profile
- Radio-opaque
- Secure delivery system
- Side branch access
- Thromboresistant
- Trackability

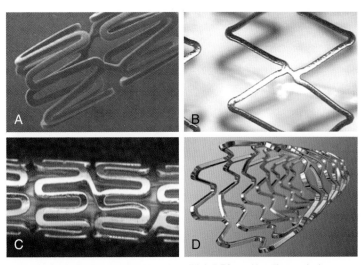

Figure 1.9 (A, B) The cobalt chromium Elixir DESyne Novolimus-eluting stent crimped (A) and expanded (B). A is reproduced with permission from Costa et al. (C, D) The platinum chromium everolimus-eluting Element stent crimped (C) and expanded (D). Images C and D are courtesy of Boston Scientific. *(From Garg S, Serruys PW. Coronary stents: looking forward.* J Am Coll Cardiol. *August 31, 2010;56:S43–S78.)*

US FDA approval	Stent	Manufacturer	Generation	Type of stent: Platform	Drug eluted
2000	Bx Velocity	*Cordis, Bridgewater, NJ*	*First*	*BMS: 316L Stainless steel*	*N/A*
2002	Liberté→ VeriFLEX*	*Boston Scientific, Natick, MA*	*First*	*BMS: 316L Stainless steel*	*N/A*
2003	Vision	*Guidant/Abbott, Indianapolis, IN*	*Second*	*BMS: Cobalt chromium*	*N/A*
2003	Driver/ Integrity	*Medtronic, Minneapolis, MN*	*Second*	*BMS: Cobalt chromium*	*N/A*
Trials under way	Omega	*Boston Scientific, Natick, MA*	*Third*	*BMS: Platinum chromium*	*N/A*
2003†	Cypher	*Cordis, Bridgewater, NJ*	*First*	*DES: 316L Stainless steel*	*Sirolimus*
2004	Taxus express	*Boston Scientific, Natick, MA*	*First*	*DES: 316L Stainless steel*	*Paclitaxel*
2008	Taxus liberté	*Boston Scientific, Natick, MA*	*First*	*DES: 316L Stainless steel*	*Paclitaxel*
2008	Endeavor	*Medtronic, Minneapolis, MN*	*Second*	*DES: Cobalt chromium*	*Zotarolimus*
2008	Xience V/ Prime	*Guidant/Abbott, Indianapolis, IN*	*Second*	*DES: Cobalt chromium*	*Everolimus*
2008	Promus	*Boston Scientific, Natick, MA*	*Second*	*DES: Cobalt chromium*	*Everolimus*
2011	Promus element	*Boston Scientific, Natick, MA*	*Third*	*DES: Platinum chromium*	*Everolimus*
2012	Taxus element	*Boston Scientific, Natick, MA*	*Third*	*DES: Platinum chromium*	*Paclitaxel*
2013	Resolute integrity	*Medtronic, Minneapolis, MN*	*Third*	*DES: Cobalt chromium*	*Zotarolimus*

Figure 1.10 Table of US Food and Drug Administration (FDA) approved stents to 2013. *(From Vette TR, Short RT, Hawn MT, Marques MB. Perioperative management of the patient with a coronary artery stent.* Anesthesiology. *2014;121(5):1093–1098.)*

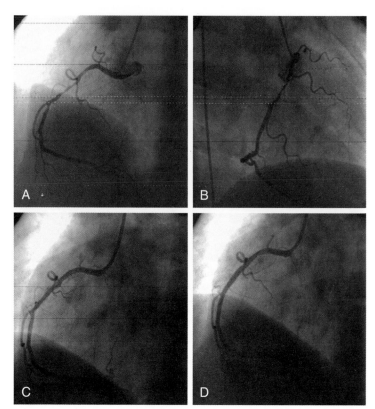

Figure 1.11 Stent placement in right coronary angioplasty. (A) Cineangio-graphic frames of right coronary artery before percutaneous coronary intervention (PCI) with a stenosis in the proximal segment (left anterior oblique view). (B) Right coronary artery (RCA) in right anterior oblique view. (C) RCA after balloon angioplasty. (D) RCA after stent placement. Note compression of plaque into ostium of right ventricular marginal branch.

Contraindications to Stenting

Relative contraindications to stenting are based on patient and anatomic factors. Patient factors are those related to performing elective invasive procedures in suitably stable patients as described for elective diagnostic catheterization. There are no contraindications to emergency life-saving interventions except for patient refusal and malfunctioning equipment.

There are several anatomic factors that are associated with poor stent outcomes and may be considered relative contraindications. These include:

- Small vessels of less than 2.5 mm
- Vessels with poor distal runoff or severe diffuse disease
- Vessels supplying poorly functional or nonfunctional myocardium
- Extensive and heavily calcified vessels

Complex or High-Risk PCI

Stenting for patients with complex and high-risk anatomy or clinical presentations should be carefully considered. PCI for patients considered at higher risk for complications will be discussed in detail in Chapter 9. Anatomic concerns include the following:

- Long lesions requiring more than one stent per lesion
- Small coronary artery reference vessel diameters (<2.5 mm)

- Significant thrombus at the lesion site
- Lesions in saphenous vein grafts, the left main coronary artery, ostial locations, or bifurcated lesions
- Restenotic lesions
- Diffuse disease or poor outflow distal to the identified lesion
- Very tortuous vessels in the region of the obstruction or proximal to the lesion
- Unprotected left main stenosis
- Complex CAD with significant impairment of left ventricular function

Considerations for Stent Delivery

Delivery of a stent to the lesion is usually performed after initial balloon angioplasty of the lesion or can be performed without predilation (direct stenting). A preliminary balloon dilation informs the operator about the difficulty of negotiating the artery, crossing the lesion, and selecting the correct stent size. After the initial expansion of the stenosis, the increased blood flow produces flow-mediated vasodilation and, on second-look angiography, the vessel diameter is often larger than when seen before dilation, thus altering stent sizing.

Stenting without predilation is called "direct" stenting. Although this method saves a small amount of time, the advantage is minimal.

Stent implantation technique differs from balloon angioplasty technique in two respects: (1) selecting the correct stent diameter and length is more critical than balloon sizing since a stent becomes a permanent implant and undersized stents are associated with poor long-term results; and (2) stent delivery to the stenosis can be more difficult than advancing a balloon catheter due to vessel calcification, tortuosity, angulation, and lesion length. These conditions are not generally problems for balloon catheters but can be significant problems for stents and must be considered beforehand. Stent delivery can be performed equally well from the femoral or radial approach with 6F sheaths and guide catheters; 7F or 8F systems should be used if double balloons or stents are anticipated for bifurcation lesions or for rotoblator use.

Prior to stent implantation, predilation with a balloon that is slightly undersized relative to the reference vessel diameter is a safe strategy that gives the operator useful information such as the pressure needed to expand the lesion. Using a slightly undersized balloon also leaves an indication of the lesion so the stent can be optimally positioned. Predilation also allows for the vessel to be repressurized with restored flow, which often produces vasodilation. It is not uncommon to find a vessel enlarged after balloon dilation. This enlargement results in the operator selecting a larger stent than would have been chosen initially.

Alternatively, an operator may choose to go directly to stenting without balloon predilation. While commonly very successful, stents cannot always be delivered to the lesion site because of tortuosity or calcifications. In these cases, exchange for a balloon catheter, predilation, and/or exchange for a stiff guidewire may be needed. It is not only disconcerting to the operator but potentially dangerous to place a stent directly in a lesion only to find that the stent cannot be fully expanded because of heavy calcification.

Guiding Catheter and Guidewire Selection

Coaxial guiding catheter support is critically important for effective stent delivery. Correct guide catheter selection is especially important for stenting in an angulated circumflex or traversing the vertical orientation of a "shepherd's crook" right coronary artery, tortuous vessels, distal lesions, or vessels with long complex dissections. These types of lesions or vessels often require use of stronger backup guides than standard right and left Judkins. Many operators prefer EBU, Q, Voda, or Amplatz radial guides or similar wide-curve configurations or guide-in-guide assistance. Stent delivery into some saphenous vein graft conduits, especially to the circumflex or left anterior descending (LAD) artery, may require a multipurpose guiding catheter support. No matter what the catheter size, contrast power injection facilitates visualization and can therefore reduce procedure time and contrast load.

Routine stent procedures can be easily performed with regular support guidewires. Extra-support or stiff guidewires (0.014 in) provide a stronger, stiffer "rail" on the stent catheter to cross lesions with extreme angulation, calcification, or tortuosity and for lesions with long dissections. The extra-support guidewire assists both guiding catheter stability and stent delivery. Although often helpful, extra-support guidewires can sometimes create difficulties by straightening the vessel and folding the intima causing "pseudo" lesions or vessel spasm. Exchanging back to a softer, floppy-tipped wire after stent delivery may prevent these effects. Using two wires, one to straighten the vessel and help the balloon/stent catheter running over the second wire, is called the "buddy" wire technique and is also helpful in tortuous, calcified vessels.

Stent Implantation

After positioning the stent, it is important to confirm that it covers the lesion by its position relative to side branches and landmarks around the target lesion. Remember that the stent is a permanent implant, and time should be taken to place it correctly, thus avoiding additional and unnecessary stents. It is also important that the stent covers the entire length of the lesion (or dissection) without leaving any inflow and outflow obstruction.

Stent expansion should be performed under fluoroscopy to see whether it is fully expanded and to ensure that its inflated diameter matches the proximal and distal reference coronary artery diameter(s). Optimal implantation requires that the stent be fully and symmetrically expanded. Struts should be in full contact (i.e., apposed) with the arterial wall. If the stent is not symmetrically expanded, a larger balloon (up to 4 mm) or high inflation pressures (>14 atm) may be used. Ideally, the final stent diameter should match that of the referenced vessel segment. All efforts should be taken to ensure that the stent is not underexpanded. Intravascular imaging with IVUS or OCT is the only method of guaranteeing this.

Cautionary Notes for Stent Deployment

1. When stenting multiple lesions, stent the distal lesion first, followed by the proximal lesion. Stenting in this order obviates the need to recross the proximal stent with another stent and reduces the chances of stent delivery failure or loss of stent when pulling back an undeployed stent for whatever reason.

2. When recrossing a recently implanted stent, use a large J-wire tip curve or even loop to ensure that the guidewire does not go under the stent or between the stent and the vessel wall, which may result in inadvertent stent damage or dislodgement and failure to advance equipment beyond the stent.

3. If there is stent inflow or outflow obstruction or residual distal vessel narrowing, a freshly prepared balloon catheter can be advanced through the stented area for further dilatations.

4. Eliminate any inflow or outflow narrowing by additional high-pressure balloon inflations or additional stent implantations (especially if the stent margin has a dissection).

5. An acceptable angiographic result is a residual narrowing of less than 10% by visual estimate, but a truly optimal stent result can only be confirmed by IVUS or OCT.

6. Vasospasm may occur during the procedure when high inflation pressures are used for stent optimization. Vasospasm is often self-limiting, nearly always resolves with time or intracoronary nitroglycerin, and has not been associated with any unfavorable clinical events. Extraordinarily high-pressure inflations (>16 atm) are generally unnecessary and have been associated with stent overexpansion, vasospasm, and higher in-stent restenosis rates.

7. Crossing a proximally implanted stent to deliver a stent more distally may be difficult because of the friction of stent-on-stent contact. Excess stent catheter force or deep guide seating may deform the implanted stent. Consider repeated high-pressure proximal stent expansion, balloon-assisted guide catheter advancement (advance guide over deflated balloon catheter inside the stent), a stiff buddy wire, or a guideliner to facilitate stent-through-stent advancement.

Optimizing Stent Implantation

Stent optimization is the expansion of the stent to the maximal safe extent without vessel injury. Optimal stent expansion is determined by the ratio of the stent lumen cross-sectional area (CSA) relative to the vessel CSA at the stent site and also relative to the reference lumen CSA. The essential features of the stent optimization technique are:

1. Evaluation of the dimensions of reference vessel and implanted stent by IVUS/OCT

2. Selection of an appropriately sized, noncompliant balloon based on IVUS/OCT target vessel diameter at the stent site

3. Performance of high-pressure balloon dilatation of the stent (usually >12 atm) or dilation with a larger balloon

Optimization Based on the Reference Lumen

Successful stent expansion is achieved when (1) there is no significant difference between the lumen diameters of the stent and the reference site (particularly the distal reference), and (2) there is complete apposition of the stent to the vessel wall. For small vessels, the IVUS criterion of achieving a final stent lumen CSA larger than the distal reference lumen CSA is strongly recommended. In larger (>2.5 mm) vessels, a final stent lumen CSA greater than the distal reference CSA is accepted with optimal stent apposition. This is accepted because the reference sites in large vessels commonly have less disease in the reference segments than do the small vessels. This also makes the achievement of a final stent lumen larger than the distal CSA more difficult to achieve in large vessels than in small vessels. Typically, a final stent lumen CSA of 80% of the distal reference vessel is also acceptable.

IVUS Optimization Based on the Reference Vessel Area

Using criteria based only on IVUS vessel area has the inherent flaw of not incorporating stent expansion relative to the reference lumen CSA. The use of a criterion of 50% of the average vessel area would leave a significant number of patients with a stent that was underexpanded compared to the distal reference lumen. The use of a criterion of 60% of the average would position the final stent lumen between the CSAs of the proximal and distal reference lumen (Fig. 1.12A,B). The use of reference vessel criteria has the disadvantage of requiring multiple additional measurements, in contrast to using the reference lumen criterion, which requires only a few.

Stent Expansion Strategies

There are two methods of improving the CSA of the stent lumen: (1) high pressure and (2) a larger diameter balloon. When an oversized balloon is used, there is an increased likelihood of coronary vessel rupture or dissection. Using high pressure with a balloon that is

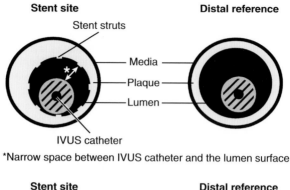

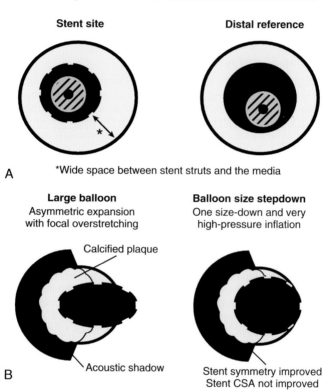

Figure 1.12 (A) Diagrams of an intravascular image for measurements after stent deployment. Top: The proximal and stent segments are compared to the distal reference site. Bottom: Comparison of area of deployed stent relative to distal reference area and amount of plaque in each segment. (B) Balloon inflation strategy based on intravascular ultrasound imaging after stent placement. (A) Asymmetric stent expansion may require larger balloon. (B) Stent symmetry is improved but cross-sectional area is not increased; use smaller balloon at very high inflation pressure.

appropriately sized to the vessel allows stent expansion to occur within the natural confines of the vessel. To avoid complications, the balloon-to-reference vessel ratio should be approximately 1.0. If a balloon-to-vessel ratio is greater than 1.0, a short, noncompliant balloon with medium pressure (12–16 atm) should be used. Use of a balloon larger than the distal IVUS minimum vessel diameter (MLD, measured media to media) should be avoided. When there is a large diameter difference between the proximal and distal vessels (e.g., LAD before and after a diagonal branch), use a lower inflation pressure when treating the distal part of the stent segment and a higher pressure for the proximal. Care should be taken not to overexpand the distal stent edge with an oversized balloon. Occasionally, for significant vessel tapering, two balloons of different diameters are used.

Noncompliant balloons are preferable to compliant balloons for final stent inflations for several reasons. Noncompliant balloons will expand and dilate uniformly, even in focal areas of resistant lesions, and they are more likely to maintain a uniform diameter even at high pressures, without balloon overexpansion vessel injury in the adjacent unstented segments. Additionally, IVUS has shown that 25% of stents will improve stent expansion with an increase in pressure from 15 to 18 atm or more.

Asymmetric Stent Expansion

Stent expansion should be symmetric, which is easily accomplished in soft plaques. Hard fibrotic or calcified plaques, seen in approximately 20–30% of lesions, are not easily compressed and result in asymmetric stent expansion into the normal arc of the vessel. In lesions with a significant arc ($\geq$270 degrees) of hard fibrocalcific disease, stent expansion has a low symmetry index of less than 0.7 minimum-to-maximum lumen diameter ratio. Further balloon inflation produces focal overstretching, especially if an oversized balloon is used (Fig. 1.12B). Using a balloon that is 0.25–0.5 mm smaller than the size of the vessel at high pressure may safely improve the symmetry index but will not necessarily increase the CSA of the lumen at the stent site.

Asymmetric overexpansion is associated with a risk of vessel rupture. If the stent lumen CSA is acceptable relative to the distal lumen CSA and the stent is well apposed, avoid efforts to make stent symmetry perfect.

Incomplete Stent Expansion

Full stent expansion is related to the plaque burden and composition. Optimal stent expansion in lesions with 50–70% diameter stenosis or lesions with a spiral dissection can be easily accomplished because there is not much atheroma. In lesions of greater than 90% diameter stenosis, full stent expansion is more difficult to achieve with a higher asymmetry. Incomplete stent expansion (i.e., when the stent struts do not contact the intimal surface) can occur, particularly in ectatic vessels (e.g., aneurysm sites) and in the ostial LAD artery, near the left main trunk (Fig. 1.13A,B). In the latter case, dilation of the ostial lesion with only the shoulder of the balloon does not provide sufficient expansion force to implant the stent fully.

Dissection at the Stent Margin

Stent implantations sometimes cause dissection at the edge of the stent and diseased vessel, and this may require additional stents to stabilize the newly produced injury (Fig. 1.14A,B). Misplacement of the postdilation balloon at the edge of the stent, especially if the balloon is clearly oversized, can cause stent margin dissection. Stent margin dissections for elastic or soft lesions may also be seen when the stents are deployed on highly angulated bend points.

Plaque Prolapse

Plaque prolapse through stent struts may occur in 5% of coil-type stent implantation. Although the coiled stents have advantages in flexibility, the stent structure provides less complete radial support to the vessel wall. Further dilation does not improve the stent lumen CSA. An additional stent within the primary stent is necessary.

Working Through Stent Problems

The complex nature of the stent procedure predisposes to unique complications and technical challenges. Problems of stenting can be broken into six major categories.

Incomplete stent expansion

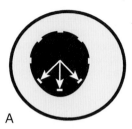

Stent struts are not attached to the intima

This can occur in the ostial LAD lesion or in the ectatic vessel (poststenotic dilation site)

A

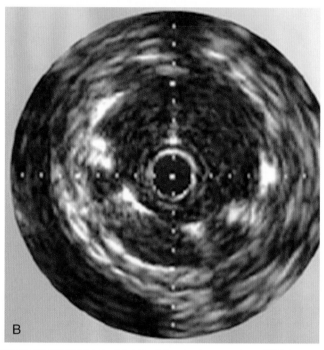

B

Figure 1.13 (A) Diagram of incomplete stent expansion. (B) Intravascular ultrasound image of incomplete stent expansion.

A. Delivery Failure: Failure to deliver the stent is most often due to:
1. Suboptimal guide support
2. Failure to cross lesion (e.g., failure to predilate a significant stenosis or calcific segment)
3. Failure to negotiate proximal tortuosity or calcific segment (e.g., unanticipated vessel rigidity or acute angulation).

To manage these problems, predilatation rather than direct stenting is recommended and has the advantage of identifying factors associated with delivery failure. A predeployment balloon that tracks easily to the lesion, dilates the lesion simply, and provides evidence of good guide catheter support bodes well for the easy delivery of the stent to the lesion. Difficulties with advancing the balloon, guide catheter instability, and difficulty in dilating through tortuous segments, on the other hand, herald stent delivery problems.

In highly tortuous arteries with multiple bends, guidewire selection is an important factor in stent delivery success. Extra-support guidewires may not be ideal for initially crossing lesions because of vessel straightening, producing intimal folds and pseudostenoses. Conventional softer guidewires may permit stent delivery while creation of pseudostenoses. Box 1.3 lists several technical manipulations that may help when a stent fails to advance.

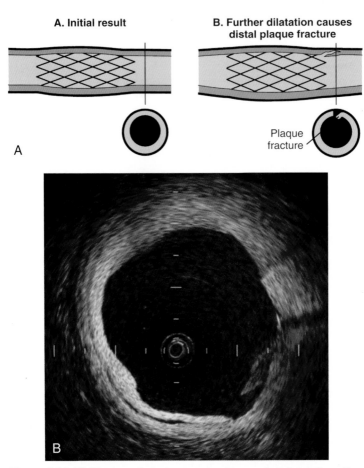

Figure 1.14 (A) Diagram of stent overexpansion causing distal dissection. (B) Optical coherence tomographic image of coronary dissection.

B. Underexpanded Stent: The inability to fully expand the stent with persistent narrowing after implantation may be due to calcification or rigid vessels. Images that may be confused for underexpansion of a stent include dissection around the stent originating at stent margins or unsuspected thrombus formation within or adjacent to the stent, which may appear as narrowings related to stent implantation.

During the balloon inflation, if an indentation persists, higher balloon inflation pressures or a larger, short balloon should be used. Failure of full stent expansion is usually the result of an inadequate predilatation approach. In cases where stent deployment appears suboptimal, intravascular imaging (IVUS/OCT) will confirm the mechanism of persistent narrowing due to tissue prolapse, incomplete apposition, heavy calcification, or, in some cases, thrombus. Failure to adequately expand the stent is associated with increased restenosis rates and/or acute thrombosis. Caution is needed when extracting the balloon from the underexpanded stent so that the guide catheter is not drawn into the vessel and causes proximal vessel dissection.

C. Loss of Access to the Stent

1. Loss of guidewire access may prevent successful recrossing for postdilation balloon inflations. Failure to recross through the central lumen and not under a strut may result in stent deformation. Recrossing a recently deployed stent is facilitated by using a soft guidewire with an exaggerated tip loop to prolapse through the

Box 1.3   Technical Manipulations When a Stent Fails to Advance

General

- Best technical manipulation: Secure a more stable guide position or, if possible, the guide can be deep-seated safely. A potential late complication is ostial stenosis due to endothelial trauma. The use of a guide extension such as a guideline can obviate dangerous deep seating of the guide catheter.
- Place constant forward pressure on the stent catheter while pulling the wire back to decrease friction inside the stent catheter lumen and to straighten the stent catheter.
- Use additional proximal segment dilation or plaque modification (e.g., rotoblator) to facilitate stent advancement.

Wire Manipulations

- Advance a second stiffer wire to straighten the artery (the buddy wire technique). This stiff wire can cause wire bias and misdirect the stent if not carefully maneuvered.
- Advance the stent on the second, stiffer buddy wire. Occasionally stents may actually advance more easily over a softer wire.
- Shape the wire along the curve of the artery to lessen wire bias so there is less friction or resistance at the outer curve of the vessel and the path of the wire is more coaxial with the path of the vessel.
- Use a "wiggle" wire.

Stent Manipulations

- If the problem is due to tortuosity of the proximal segment, change to shorter stent.
- Select a stent with better flexibility.
- Gently bend the stent to conform it along the curve of the artery (rarely done).

Guide Manipulations

- Change to a different curve to achieve better backup, and more coaxial to allow less friction at the ostium.
- Use a larger or smaller guide to achieve better backup.
- Use guideliner extension.

Techniques Facilitating Recrossing of a Stented Area by a Balloon or Another Stent

General

- Best technical manipulation: Steer the wire into a different direction or to a different branch to lessen wire bias and increase wire centering.
- Rotate the balloon catheter while advancing it and let the catheter enter the stent by itself through its rotational energy (like torquing the Judkins Right catheter).

Guidewire Manipulations

- Bend the wire and place the bent segment near the ostium of the stent to be crossed to position the wire more at the center of the entrance of the stented segment and to decrease wire bias.
- Insert a second, stiffer wire to straighten the vessel.
- Change the current wire to a stiffer one.

Balloon/Stent Manipulations

- Use a shorter balloon or stent.
- Use a more flexible balloon or stent.
- Use partial tip inflation to deflect the nose of stent away from struts.
- If only the balloon needs to enter the stented segment, inflate the balloon with 1–2 atm so the balloon centers the wire in the lumen and facilitates the crossing of the wire and balloon.

Modified from Nguyen T, et al. *J Interventional Cardiol.* 2002;15:237–241.

stent. All efforts should be made to prevent the guidewire entering between the strut and the arterial wall.

2. Recrossing stents with balloons may be difficult when the proximal border of the stent is on a tortuous vessel segment, thus forcing the tip of the dilatation balloon into the vessel wall where it is blocked by the stent struts. Stent-on-stent friction also makes distal stent positioning difficult. Several approaches can be used to overcome this problem:

   a. The guide catheter can be repositioned in a more coaxial manner.

   b. A stiffer guidewire or buddy wire can be advanced to reshape the curve of the artery. Several operators have recommended putting a curve into a stiff part of the guidewire and using it to advance across a tortuous segment proximal to a stent and placing a curve on the balloon by using a technique similar to that of putting a gentle curve on a guidewire. Box 1.3 summarizes several technical manipulations that may be employed to recross a deployed stent.

D. Embolized Stent: Several techniques for recovery of embolized stents have been proposed and include loop snares, basket retrieval devices, biliary forceps, biopsy forceps, and other specifically designed retrieval systems.

E. Artery Perforation: Consider using a covered stent (see Chapter 10, Complications of Percutaneous Coronary Interventions).

F. Stent-Related Dissection, Thrombosis, and Ischemia: The following factors are associated with an increased risk of stent thrombosis and ischemia:

   1. Inadequate stent expansion (e.g., highly calcified lesion which did not undergo rotoblator)

   2. Dissection, not covered by the stent

   3. Poor distal runoff or infarct in related vessel

   4. Presence of thrombus

   5. Subtherapeutic anticoagulation

   6. Vessels less than 2.5 mm in diameter.

      Subacute thrombotic occlusion is rare within the first week after implantation but may happen during the week following discharge if dual antiplatelet therapy is not maintained. Risk factors for subacute occlusion were noted earlier. The risk of subacute thrombosis is increased when multiple overlapping stents are used. Subacute occlusion is treated with repeat balloon dilatations, confirmation of adequate implantation by IVUS/OCT, and continuation antiplatelet agents.

   7. Ruptured inflation balloon: Although uncommon, loss of inflation pressure during expansion of the stent can indicate balloon rupture or perforation. The ruptured balloon must be exchanged for a new one. If balloon rupture occurs after the ends of the stent are flared and anchored in the artery wall, the balloon can be deflated, rotated two or three times inside the stent, and gently pulled back inside the sheath and removed.

Safety of Magnetic Resonance Imaging After Stent Implantation

A magnetic resonance imaging (MRI) scan should not be performed until the implanted stent has begun to be endothelialized (>4 weeks). The risk of migration of the stent under a strong magnetic field is small, given the implant method, but the stent may cause artifacts in MRI scans due to distortion of the magnetic field. In most patients, MRI scanning is not an issue since many stents may be nonferromagnetic.

Stent Implantation Before Noncardiac Surgery

Catastrophic outcomes have been reported for recently stented patients early after noncardiac surgery. Kaluza et al. noted that patients who underwent coronary stent placement less than 6 weeks before noncardiac surgery requiring general anesthesia had a high incidence of MI, bleeding, and death. It is recommended that elective noncardiac surgery be postponed for more than 1 month after bare metal stenting and more than 3 months after drug-eluting stenting, which should permit satisfactory stent endothelialization and reduce the risk of stent thrombosis. Cessation of the dual antiplatelet regimen will reduce surgically related bleeding complications.

The Pre-PCI Workup

Noninvasive testing for ischemia provides the objective basis and support to proceed with PCI in stable patients The most common ischemic tests are (1) exercise stress with/without perfusion imaging or echo left ventricular (LV) wall motion, as indicated; (2) pharmacologic stress study (e.g., dipyridamole); and (3) two-dimensional echocardiogram (as indicated for assessment of LV function or valvular heart disease).

In the absence of objective evidence of noninvasive ischemia testing, invasive assessment of the ischemic potential of a stenosis can be obtained during coronary angiography measuring translesional pressure-derived FFR determination.

Pre-PCI Preparation: Holding Area

- Patient preparation (intravenous access, meds, consent)
- Patient and family teaching (procedure, results, complications)
- Cardiothoracic surgeon consultation, particularly for high-risk, multivessel disease or decreased LV function
- Appropriate laboratory data (type and cross-match, complete blood cell and platelet counts, prothrombin time [PT], partial thromboplastin time [PTT], electrolytes, blood urea nitrogen [BUN], creatinine)

Patient Preparation in Catheterization Suite

- ECG (inferior and anterior wall leads): 12-lead (radiolucent) ECG
- 1 or 2 IV lines
- Sterile preparation for both inguinal areas or wrist for radial artery
- Venous access for temporary pacing if anticipated need during high-risk PCI for acute MI, left bundle branch block requiring RCA PCI, and rotoblator or thrombus aspiration device
- Aspirin (325 mg PO): Failure to administer aspirin before PCI is associated with a two to three times higher acute complication rate.
- P2Y12 oral antagonist agent (e.g., clopidogrel 600 mg PO, best 24 hours beforehand). Best outcomes are associated with antiplatelet preloading.
- Continue routine antihypertensive and other medications
- Heparin 40–70 u/kg bolus (or 40 u/kg bolus if glycoprotein IIb/IIIa blockers used). Target activated clotting time (ACT) >200 sec. Heparin is critical for PCI, despite controversies regarding dosing and unpredictable therapeutic responses. Higher levels of anticoagulation are roughly correlated with reduced complications during coronary angioplasty, albeit at the expense of increased bleeding complications at higher heparin doses. Weight-adjusted

heparin provides a clinically superior anticoagulation method over fixed heparin dosing. Bivalirudin can be substituted for heparin (see Chapter 3, Interventional Pharmacology).

- Consider GPIIb/IIIa blockers for some acute coronary syndrome patients or clot formation during the PCI.
- Premedication is helpful (e.g., fentanyl 25–50 mg IV and midazolam [Versed] 1–2 mg IV).

Postprocedure Angiograms and Hemostasis

- Final angiography should be made with the guidewire removed (the guidewire hides dissection flaps) and after intracoronary nitroglycerin (relieves vasospasm).
- Femoral angiography is needed before vascular closure device insertion. Perform a right anterior oblique (RAO) view for right femoral artery (FA) and left anterior oblique (LAO) for left FA. If artery is not suitable for closure device, secure arterial and venous sheaths in place. Remove with manual compression hemostasis in 4 hours when ACT is less than 150 sec.
- Apply radial artery compression band for hemostasis after final coronary angiography.
- Do not give routine postprocedure heparin unless there are clinical indications beyond the stent procedure (e.g., deep vein thrombosis [DVT], pulmonary embolism [PE]; also see Chapter 10, Complications of Percutaneous Coronary Interventions).

Postprocedure Care: Recovery Area

Nurses should begin patient teaching on hospital course, potential bleeding problems, late complications, and restenosis. After the PCI, the cath lab team notifies the recovery area, the ICU if needed, and any standby surgical team. Postprocedure labs and ECG are obtained.

Postprocedure Care: Step-Down Area

After PCI, chest pain may occur in about 10% of patients. ECG evidence of ischemia identifies those at significant risk of acute vessel closure. When angina pectoris with ischemic ECG changes occurs within the first 24 hours, a return to the cath lab for diagnosis and possible thrombolysis and/or restenting is often needed. The decision to proceed with further interventional procedures, CABG surgery, or medical therapy must be individualized based on factors such as hemodynamic stability, amount of myocardium at risk, and the likelihood that the treatment will be successful. Following PCI, the hospital care team should monitor the patient for recurrent myocardial ischemia, puncture site hemostasis, and contrast-induced renal failure.

Post-PCI Care: Medications

- Aspirin (325 mg/day PO), continued for 30 days before reducing to 81 mg/day PO.
- P2Y12 oral platelet inhibitor agents (clopidogrel 600-mg loading dose and 75 mg/day, prasugrel 60-mg loading with 10 mg/day, or ticagrelor 180 mg PO with 90 mg PO b.i.d., for at least 6 months after stenting with a bare metal stent and 12 months with a drug-eluting stent)
- Initiate statin drugs, if not already prescribed.
- Restart or initiate antihypertensive or antianginal medications depending on the patient's clinical needs.
- Resume prior medications for other conditions (e.g., GERD, etc.).

Appropriate secondary atherosclerosis prevention programs should be started involving adherence to recommended medical therapies and behavior modifications to reduce morbidity and mortality from coronary heart disease.

Patients with renal dysfunction and diabetes should be monitored for contrast-induced nephropathy. In addition, those patients receiving higher contrast loads (>5 mL/kg) or a second contrast load within 72 hours should have their renal function assessed over several days. Whenever possible, nephrotoxic drugs (certain antibiotics, nonsteroidal anti-inflammatory agents, and cyclosporin) and metformin (especially in those with pre-existing renal dysfunction) should be withheld for 24–48 hours after PCI.

After discharge, the patient then returns to activities of daily living within 1–2 days. Factors preventing rapid return to work include access site complications and persistent symptoms. A functional (ischemic testing) evaluation for patients with multivessel coronary angioplasty or incomplete revascularization after angioplasty will identify cardiac limitations, if any, on work status.

CAD Risk-Factor Modification

All patients should be instructed about risk-factor modification and medical therapies for secondary atherosclerosis prevention before leaving the hospital. The interventional cardiologist should emphasize these measures directly to the patient and family. Failure to do so suggests that secondary prevention therapies are not important. The interventional cardiologist should contact the primary care physician regarding the secondary prevention therapies initiated and those to be maintained, including aspirin therapy, hypertensive control, diabetic management, aggressive control of serum lipids to a target LDL goal of less than 100 mg/dL following AHA guidelines, abstinence from tobacco use, weight control, regular exercise, and angiotensin-converting enzyme (ACE) inhibitor therapy as recommended in the AHA/ACC consensus statement on secondary prevention.

Follow-Up Schedule and Stress Testing

- Access site check on first office visit, 2–4 weeks
- Routine stress testing is not performed after PCI. Annual stress testing is not recommended by guidelines unless symptoms appear. There is no indication for annual exercise testing in asymptomatic patients. The AHA/ACC practice guidelines recommend selective evaluation in patients considered to be at particularly high risk (e.g., patients with decreased LV function, multivessel coronary artery disease, proximal LAD disease, previous sudden death, diabetes mellitus, hazardous occupations, and suboptimal PCI results). For many reasons, stress imaging is preferred to evaluate symptomatic patients after PCI. If the patient's exertional capacity is significantly limited, coronary angiography may be more expeditious to evaluate symptoms of typical angina. Exercise testing after discharge is helpful for activity counseling and/or exercise training as part of cardiac rehabilitation. Neither exercise testing nor radionuclide imaging is indicated for the routine, periodic monitoring of asymptomatic patients after PCI without specific indications.
- If symptoms or signs of ischemia are present early after PCI, coronary angiography is repeated.

PCI Programs Without Surgical Backup

PCI is performed in laboratories without on-site surgical backup. Criteria for the performance of PCI at hospitals without on-site cardiac surgery have been summarized as follows:

1. The operators must be experienced interventionalists who regularly perform elective intervention at a surgical center (75 cases/year). The institution must perform a minimum of 36 primary PCI procedures per year.

2. The nursing and technical catheterization laboratory staff must be experienced in handling acutely ill patients and comfortable with interventional equipment. They must have acquired experience in dedicated interventional laboratories at a surgical center. They participate in a 24-hour, 365-day call schedule.

3. The catheterization laboratory itself must be well equipped, with optimal imaging systems, resuscitative equipment, and LV support devices (e.g., intra-aortic balloon pump [IABP], Impella, Tandem Heart) and must be well stocked with a broad array of interventional equipment to handle any emergency.

4. The cardiac care unit nurses must be adept in hemodynamic monitoring and LV support device management.

5. The hospital administration must fully support the program and enable the fulfillment of the preceding institutional requirements.

6. There must be formalized written protocols in place for immediate (within 1 hour) and efficient transfer of patients to the nearest cardiac surgical facility that are reviewed/tested on a regular (quarterly) basis.

7. Primary intervention must be performed routinely as the treatment of choice around the clock for a large proportion of patients with acute MI to ensure streamlined care paths and increased case volumes.

8. Case selection for the performance of primary angioplasty must be rigorous. Criteria for the types of lesion appropriate for primary angioplasty and for the selection for transfer for emergency aortocoronary bypass surgery are shown in Box 1.4.

9. There must be an ongoing program of outcomes analysis and formalized periodic case review.

10. Institutions should participate in a 3- to 6-month period of implementation, during which time the development of a formalized primary PCI program is instituted that includes establishing standards, training staff, detailed logistic development, and creation of a quality assessment and error management system. (Levine G, et al. *Circulation*. 2011;124:e574–e576)

Box 1.4 Patient Selection for Percutaneous Coronary Intervention (PCI) at Hospitals Without On-Site Cardiac Surgery

Avoid intervention in hemodynamically stable patients with:

1. Significant unprotected left main coronary artery narrowing upstream from an acute occlusion in the left coronary system that might be disrupted by the angioplasty catheter
2. Extremely long or angulated infarct-related lesions with thrombolysis in myocardial infarction (TIMI) grade 3 flow
3. Infarct-related lesions with TIMI grade 3 flow in stable patients with three-vessel disease
4. Infarct-related lesions of small or secondary vessels
5. Lesions in other than the infarct artery
6. Patients with high-grade residual left main or multivessel coronary disease and clinical or hemodynamic instability should be transferred to a coronary artery bypass graft-capable center by prearrangement ambulance agreement.

Adapted from Wharton TJ Jr, McNamara NS, Fedele FA, et al. Primary angioplasty for the treatment of acute myocardial infarction: experience at two community hospitals without cardiac surgery. *J Am Coll Cardiol*. 1999;33:1257–1265.

Training for Coronary Angioplasty

Advances in interventional procedures have maintained high and durable success rates despite increasingly complex procedures. The need for appropriate training and guidelines for the procedure is obvious. Recent guidelines for the assessment and proficiencies of coronary interventional procedures have been summarized in a report from a joint task force from the AHA/ACC (Box 1.5). American Board of Internal Medicine (ABIM) board certification in interventional cardiology requires documentation of training in an accredited fellowship program during which a minimum of 125 coronary angioplasty procedures must be performed, including 75 performed with the trainee as primary operator (Table 1.3).

Box 1.5 American Heart Association (AHA) Proficiencies

Considerations for the Assessment and Maintenance of Proficiency in Coronary Interventional Procedures

Institutions

- Quality assessment monitoring of privileges and risk-stratified outcomes
- Provide support for a quality assurance staff person (e.g., nurse) to monitor complications
- Minimal institutional performance activity of 200 interventions per year with the ideal minimum of 400 interventions per year
- Interventional program director who has a career experience of more than 500 percutaneous coronary intervention (PCI) procedures and is board certified by the American Board of Internal Medicine (ABIM) in interventional cardiology
- Facility and equipment requirements to provide high-resolution fluoroscopy and digital video processing
- Experienced support staff to respond to emergencies
- Establishment of a mentoring program for operators who perform fewer than 75 procedures per year by individuals who perform 150 procedures per year.

Physicians

- Procedural volume of 75 per year
- Continuation of privileges based on outcome benchmark rates with consideration of not granting privileges to operators who exceed adjusted case-mix benchmark complication rates for a 2-year -period
- Ongoing quality assessment comparing results with current benchmarks, with risk stratification of complication rates
- Board certification by ABIM in interventional cardiology

From Hirshfeld JW, Elllis SG, Faxon DP, et al. *J Am Coll Cardiol* 1998;31:722–743. See Naidu SS, Aronow HD, Box LC, et al. SCAI Expert Consensus Statement: 2016 Best Practices in the Cardiac Catheterization Laboratory: Endorsed by the Cardiological Society of India, and Sociedad Latino Americana de Cardiologia Intervencionista; Affirmation of Value by the Canadian Association of Interventional Cardiology–Association Canadienne de Cardiologie d'intervention. *Cath Cardiovasc Interv.* 2016;88(3):407–423.

Table 1.3

Recommendations for Clinical Competence in Percutaneous Transluminal Coronary Interventions	
Angiography: Minimum Recommended	**Number of Cases per Year**
Total number of cases	125
Cases as primary operator	75
Practicing, Number of cases per year	50–75 to maintain competency

Angiography for PCI

Angiography for PCI expands on the fundamentals of diagnostic angiography and requires establishing details regarding the best method of stent delivery and deployment. Before PCI, the angiographer should acquire the following additional angiographic detail:

1. Establish the relationship of coronary ostium to aorta for guide catheter selection.
2. Verify target vessel, pathway, and angle of entry.
3. Confirm lesion length and morphology using additional angulated views eliminating vessel overlap.
4. Separate associated side branches and degree of ostial atherosclerosis.
5. Visualize distribution of collateral supply.
6. Determine the true (maximally vasodilated) diameter of the coronary artery at the target site.

Optimal definition of the ostial and proximal coronary segments is critical to plan the procedure and select an appropriate PCI guide catheter. Assessment of calcium from angiography is less reliable than IVUS but is still useful in assessing the need for rotational atherectomy and its associated risks.

Classical terminology for angiographic projections with regard to left and right anterior oblique, cranial and caudal angulation, and lateral projections remains as defined in previous discussions of diagnostic coronary angiography (see *The Cardiac Catheterization Handbook,* 6e, 2015, Chapter 3).

Visualization of vessel bifurcations, origin of side branches, the portion of the vessel proximal to a significant lesion, and previously "unimportant" lesion characteristics (length, eccentricity, calcium, and the like) will assist in device selection and identifying potential procedural risk. For total chronic vessel occlusions, the distal vessel should be visualized as clearly as possible by injecting the coronary arteries that supply collaterals and taking cineangiograms with panning long enough to visualize late collateral vessel filling and the length of the occluded segment.

Optimal radiographic imaging technique is also critical to a successful intervention by enhancing accurate interpretation of procedure results. Modification of panning technique to reduce motion artifact, optimal use of beam restrictors (collimation) to reduce scatter, and improved contrast media delivery all can enhance clinical results. A working knowledge of the principles of radiographic imaging permits the interventionalist to improve his or her imaging outcomes.

Radiation exposure is higher in PCI than in diagnostic procedures. Continued awareness of the inverse square law of radiation propagation will reduce the exposure to patient, operators, and the cath lab team. Obtaining quality images should not necessitate increasing the ordinary procedural radiation exposure to either the patient or catheterization personnel.

Common Angiographic Views for Angioplasty

The routine coronary angiographic views described here should include those that best visualize the origin and course of the major vessels and their branches in at least two different (preferably orthogonal) projections. Naturally, there is a wide variation in coronary anatomy, and appropriately modified views will need to be individualized. The nomenclature for angiographic views is described in Chapter 3 of *The Cardiac Catheterization Handbook,* 6e, but will be reviewed briefly here, emphasizing the interventionalist's thinking.

Position for Anteroposterior Imaging

The image intensifier positioned is directly over the patient, with the beam perpendicular to the patient lying flat on the x-ray table (Figs. 1.15 and 1.16). The anteroposterior (AP) view or shallow RAO displays the left main coronary artery in its entire perpendicular length. In this view, the branches of the LAD and left circumflex coronary arteries branches overlap. Slight RAO or LAO angulation may be necessary to clear the density of the vertebrae and the catheter shaft in the thoracic descending aorta. In patients with acute coronary syndromes, this view will exclude left main stenosis, which can preclude or complicate PCI. The AP cranial view is excellent for visualizing the LAD with septals moving to the left (on screen) and diagonals to the right, thus helping wire placement.

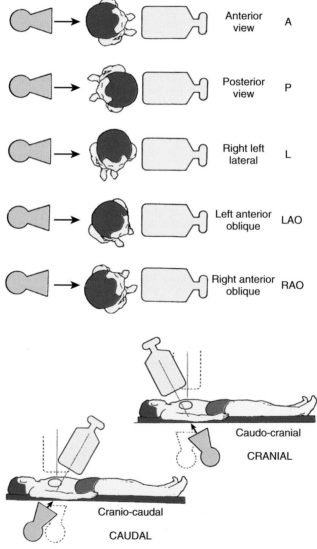

Figure 1.15 Nomenclature for angiographic views. *(Modified from Paulin S. Terminology for radiographic projections in cardiac angiography.* Cathet Cardiovasc Diagn. *1981;7:341.)*

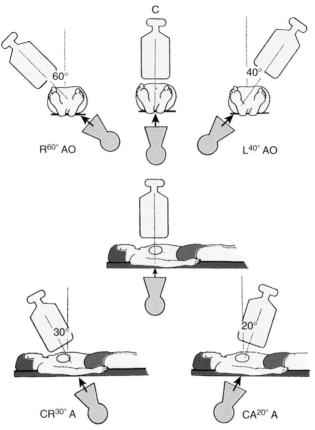

Figure 1.16 Nomenclature for angiographic views. *(Modified from Paulin S. Terminology for radiographic projections in cardiac angiography.* Cathet Cardiovasc Diagn. *1981;7:341.)*

Position for Right Anterior Oblique Imaging

The image intensifier is to the right side of the patient. The RAO caudal view shows the left main coronary artery bifurcation with the origin and course of the circumflex/obtuse marginals, intermediate branch, and proximal left anterior descending segment well seen. The RAO, caudal view is one of the best two views for visualization of the circumflex artery. The LAD beyond the proximal segment is often obscured by overlapped diagonals.

The RAO or AP cranial view is used to open the diagonals along the mid and distal LAD. Diagonal branch bifurcations are well visualized. The diagonal branches are projected upward. The proximal LAD and circumflex usually are overlapped. Marginals may overlap, and the circumflex is foreshortened.

For the right coronary artery (RCA), the RAO view shows the mid RCA and the length of the posterior descending artery and posterolateral branches. Septals supplying an occluded LAD via collaterals may be clearly identified. The posterolateral branches overlap and may need the addition of the cranial view.

Position for Left Anterior Oblique Imaging

In the LAO position, the image intensifier is to the left side of the patient. The LAO/cranial view also shows the left main coronary artery (slightly foreshortened), LAD, and diagonal branches. Septal and diagonal branches are separated clearly. The circumflex and marginals are foreshortened and overlapped. Deep inspiration will move the density of the diaphragm out of the field. The LAO angle should be set so that the course of the LAD is parallel to the spine and stays in the "lucent wedge" bordered by the spine and the curve of the diaphragm. Cranial angulation tilts the left main coronary artery down and permits a view of the LAD/circumflex bifurcation (Fig. 1.17). Too steep a LAO/cranial angulation or shallow inspiration produces considerable overlapping with the diaphragm and liver, thus degrading the image.

For the RCA, the LAO/cranial view shows the origin of the artery, its entire length, and the posterior descending artery bifurcation (crux). Cranial angulation tilts the posterior descending artery down to show vessel contour and reduces foreshortening. Deep inspiration clears the diaphragm. The posterior descending artery and posterolateral branches are foreshortened.

The LAO/caudal view ("spider" view; Fig. 1.17) shows a foreshortened left main coronary artery and the bifurcation of the circumflex and LAD. Proximal and midportions of the circumflex and the origins of obtuse marginal branches are usually seen excellently. Poor image quality may be due to overlapping of diaphragm and spine. The LAD is considerably foreshortened in this view.

A left lateral view shows the mid and distal LAD best. The LAD and circumflex are well separated. Diagonals usually overlap. The course of the (ramus) intermediate branch is well visualized. This view is best to see CABG conduit anastomosis to the LAD. For the RCA, the lateral view

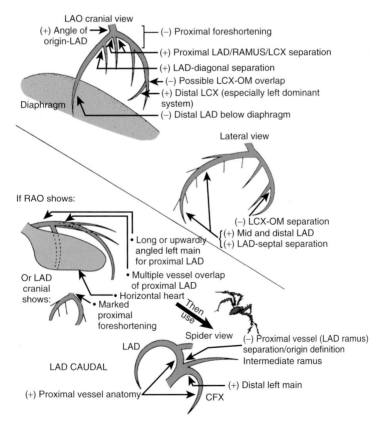

Figure 1.17 Diagrammatic view of left coronary artery demonstrating special positioning to best observe branch segments. *(From Boucher RA, Myler RK, Clark DA, Stertzer SH. Coronary angiography and angioplasty.* Cathet Cardiovasc Diagn. *1988;14:269–285.)*

also shows the origin (especially in those with more anteriorly oriented orifices) and the mid RCA well. The posterior descending artery and posterolateral branches are foreshortened.

Angulations for Saphenous Bypass Grafts

Coronary artery saphenous vein grafts are visualized in at least two views (LAO and RAO). It is important to show the aortic anastomosis, the body of the graft, and the distal anastomosis. The distal runoff and continued flow or collateral channels are also critical. The graft vessel anastomosis is best seen in the view that depicts the native vessel best. A general strategy for graft angiography is to perform the standard views while assessing the vessel key views for specific coronary artery segments (Table 1.4) to determine the need for contingency views or an alteration/addition of special views. Therefore, the graft views can be summarized as follows:

1. RCA graft: LAO cranial/RAO and lateral
2. LAD graft (or internal mammary artery): Lateral, RAO cranial, LAO cranial, and AP (the lateral view is especially useful to visualize the anastomosis to the LAD)
3. Circumflex (and obtuse marginals) grafts: LAO and RAO caudal

Table 1.4

Recommended "Key" Angiographic View for Specific Coronary Artery Segments		
Coronary Segment	**Origin/Bifurcation**	**Course/Body**
Left main	AP	AP
	LAO cranial	LAO cranial
	LAO caudal*	
Proximal LAD	LAO cranial	LAO cranial
	RAO caudal	RAO caudal
Mid LAD	LAD cranial	
	RAO cranial	
	Lateral	
Distal LAD	AP	
	RAO cranial	
	Lateral	
Diagonal	LAO cranial	RAO cranial, caudal, or straight
	RAO cranial	
Proximal circumflex	RAO caudal	LAO caudal
	LAO caudal	
Intermediate	RAO caudal	RAO caudal
	LAO caudal	Lateral
Obtuse marginal	RAO caudal	RAO caudal
	LAO caudal	
	RAO cranial	(distal marginals)
Proximal RCA	LAO	
	Lateral	
Mid RCA	LAO	LAO
	Lateral	Lateral
	RAO	RAO
Distal RCA	LAO cranial	LAO cranial
	Lateral	Lateral
PDA	LAO cranial	RAO
Posterolateral	LAO cranial	RAO cranial
	RAO cranial	RAO cranial

*Horizontal hearts
AP, anteroposterior; *LAD*, left anterior descending artery; *LAO*, left anterior oblique; *PDA*, posterior descending artery (from RCA); *RAO*, right anterior oblique; *RCA*, right coronary artery.
From Kern MJ, ed. *The Cardiac Catheterization Handbook*. St. Louis, MO: Mosby, 1995:286.

Techniques for Coronary Arteriography

Imaging During Respiration

During diagnostic angiography, deep inspiration moves the diaphram away from the heart to visualize the vessels without density overlap. However, when working with PCI equipment, deep inspiration may change the proximal course of the artery and the spatial relation of the lesion to anatomic landmarks. Knowing where the lesion is relative to these landmarks is important. Guiding angiograms should be taken in such a way that frequent inspiratory effort leading to patient fatigue during manipulation is not necessary. Select a view requiring minimal inspiratory breath holding while providing an optimum presentation of the lesion.

Power Injection Versus Hand Injection for Coronary Arteriography

Power injection of the coronary arteries has been used in thousands of cases in many laboratories and is equal in safety to hand injection. A power injector at a fixed setting may require several injections to find the optimal contrast delivery flow rate. Power injectors now incorporate hand controls, permitting precise operator touch-sensitive variable volume injection (Acist, Bracco Diagnostics, Milan, Italy), as well as a computer touch screen for precise contrast delivery settings. Typical settings for power injections are:

- Right coronary artery: 6 mL at 2–3 mL/sec; maximum pressure 450 psi
- Left coronary artery: 10 mL at 4–6 10 mL/sec; maximum pressure 450 psi.

Panning Techniques

Many laboratories use x-ray image mode sizes of greater than 7 inch diameter, which precludes having the entire coronary artery course visualized without panning over the heart to include late filling of the distal arterial or collateralized segments. In addition, in most views, some degree of panning will be necessary to identify regions that are not seen in the initial setup positioning. Some branches may unexpectedly appear later from collateral filling or other unusual anatomic sources.

Angiographic TIMI Classification of Blood Flow

Thrombolysis in myocardial infarction (TIMI) flow grading has been used to qualitatively assess the degree of restored perfusion achieved after thrombolysis or angioplasty in patients with acute MI. Table 1.5 provides descriptions used to assign TIMI flow grades. The distal angiographic contrast runoff is classified into four stages (also known as *TIMI grade*):

- Normal distal runoff (TIMI 3)
- Good distal runoff (TIMI 2)
- Poor distal runoff (TIMI 1)
- Absence of distal runoff (TIMI 0)

TIMI Frame Count

Contrast runoff is now performed quantitatively by using cine frame counts from the first frame of the filled catheter tip to the frame where

Table 1.5

Thrombolysis in Myocardial Infarction (TIMI) Flow: Grade and Blush Scores

TIMI Flow Grade	Description
Grade 3 (complete reperfusion)	Anterograde flow into the terminal coronary artery segment through a stenosis is as prompt as anterograde flow into a comparable segment proximal to the stenosis. Contrast material clears as rapidly from the distal segment as from an uninvolved, more proximal segment.
Grade 2 (partial reperfusion)	Contrast material flows through the stenosis to opacify the terminal artery segment. However, contrast enters the terminal segment perceptibly more slowly than more proximal segments. Alternatively, contrast material clears from a segment distal to a stenosis noticeably more slowly than from a comparable segment not preceded by a significant stenosis.
Grade 1 (penetration/ with minimal perfusion)	A small amount of contrast flows through the stenosis but fails to fully opacify the artery beyond.
Grade 0 (no perfusion)	There is no contrast flow through the stenosis.

Modified from Sheehan F, Braunwald E, Canner P, et al. The effect of intravenous thrombolytic therapy on left ventricular function: a report on tissue-type plasminogen activator and streptokinase from the Thrombolysis in Myocardial Infarction (TIMI) Phase I Trial. *Circulation.* 1987;72:817–829.

Myocardial Blush Grade

0 No myocardial blush or contrast density; or myocardial blush persisted ("staining")
1 Minimal myocardial blush or contrast density
2 Moderate myocardial blush or contrast density but less than that obtained during angiography of a contralateral or ipsilateral noninfarct-related coronary artery
3 Normal myocardial blush or contrast density, comparable with that obtained during angiography of a contralateral or ipsilateral noninfarct-related coronary artery

contrast is seen filling a predetermined distal arterial end point. Myocardial blood flow has been assessed angiographically using the TIMI score for qualitative grading of coronary flow. TIMI flow grades 0–3 have become a standard description of coronary blood flow in clinical trials. TIMI grade 3 flows have been associated with improved clinical outcomes.

The method uses cineangiography with 6F catheters and filming at 30 frames per second. The number of cine frames from the introduction of dye in the coronary artery to a predetermined distal landmark is counted. The TIMI frame count (TFC) for each major vessel is thus standardized according to specific distal landmarks. The first frame used for TIMI frame counting is that in which the dye fully opacifies the origin of the artery and in which the dye extends across the width of the artery, touching both borders and with antegrade motion of the dye. The last frame counted is when dye enters the first distal landmark branch. Full opacification of the distal branch segment is not required. Distal landmarks used commonly in analysis are:

1. For the LAD, the distal bifurcation of the LAD artery
2. For the circumflex system, the distal bifurcation of the branch segments with the longest total distance
3. For the RCA, the first branch of the posterolateral artery.

Typically a normal contrast frame count reflecting normal flow is 24 ± 10 frames.

The TFC can further be corrected for the length of the LAD. The TFC in the LAD requires normalization or correction for comparison to the two other major arteries. This is called the *corrected TFC (CTFC)*. The average LAD is 14.7 cm long, the right is 9.8 cm, and the circumflex is 9.3 cm, according to Gibson et al. The CTFC accounts for the distance the dye has to travel in the LAD relative to the other arteries. The CTFC divides the absolute frame count in the LAD by 1.7 to standardize the distance of dye travel in all three arteries. Normal TFC for the LAD is 36 ± 3, and CTFC 21 ± 2; for the circumflex artery, TFC is 22 ± 4; for the RCA, TFC is 20 ± 3. TIMI flow grades do not correspond to measured Doppler flow velocity or CTFC. High TFC may be associated with microvascular dysfunction despite an open artery. A CTFC of less than 20 frames was associated with low risk for adverse events in patients following MI. A contrast injection rate increase of more than 1 mL/sec by hand injection can decrease the TFC by two frames. The TFC method provides valuable information relative to clinical response after coronary intervention.

TIMI Myocardial Blush Grades (MBG)

Washout of contrast from the microvasculature in the acute infarction patient is coupled to prognosis. Better blush scores indicate better myocardial salvage. Myocardial blush grade (MBG) scoring is shown in Table 1.5.

Angiographic Classification of Collateral Flow

Collateral flow can be seen and classified angiographically. The late opacification of a totally or subtotally (99%) occluded vessel through antegrade or retrograde channels will assist in correct guidewire place- ment, lesion localization, and a successful procedure. The collateral circulation is graded angiographically as follows:

- Grade 0: No collateral branches seen
- Grade 1: Very weak (ghostlike) opacification
- Grade 2: Opacified segment is less dense than the source vessel and filling slowly
- Grade 3: Opacified segment is as dense as the source vessel and filling rapidly.

Collateral visualization will help establish the size of the recipient vessel for the purposes of selecting an appropriately sized balloon. Determining whether the collateral circulation is ipsilateral (e.g., proximal RCA to distal RCA collateral supply) or contralateral (e.g., circumflex to distal RCA collateral supply) and exactly which region will be affected should collateral supply be disrupted is important in order to gauge procedural risk. The evaluation of collaterals must be included when making decisions on which vessels should be protected or lost during coronary angioplasty.

Assessment of Coronary Stenoses

The degree of an angiographic narrowing (stenosis) is reported as the estimated percentage lumen reduction of the most severely narrowed segment compared to the adjacent angiographically normal vessel segment, seen in the worst x-ray projection. Because the operator uses visual estimations, an exact evaluation is impossible. There is a ±20% variation between readings of two or more experienced angiographers. Stenosis severity alone should not always be assumed to be associated with abnormal physiology (flow) and ischemia. Moreover, CAD is a diffuse process and thus minimal luminal irregularities on angiography may represent significant albeit nonobstructive CAD at the time of angiography. The stenotic segment lumen is compared with a nearby lumen that does not appear to be obstructed but that may have diffuse atherosclerotic disease. This explains why postmortem examinations as well as IVUS describe much more plaque than is seen on angiography. The percent diameter is estimated from the angiographically normal adjacent segment. Because coronary arteries normally taper as they travel to the apex, proximal segments are always larger than distal segments, often explaining the large disparity between several observers' estimates of stenosis severity. *Area stenosis* is always greater than *diameter stenosis* and assumes the lumen is circular, whereas the lumen is usually eccentric. In general, four categories of lesion severity can be assigned:

1. Minimal or mild CAD; narrowings <50%
2. Moderate; stenosis between 50% and 75%
3. Severe; stenosis between 75% and 95%
4. Total occlusion

Technical note: Stenosis anatomy should not be confused with abnormal physiology (flow) and ischemia, especially for lesions 40–70% narrowed. For nonquantitative reports, the length of a stenosis is simply mentioned (e.g., LAD proximal segment stenosis diameter 25%, long or short). Other features of the coronary lesion may not be appreciated by angiography and require IVUS imaging. Anatomic factors producing resistance to coronary flow across a coronary stenosis include entrance angle, length of disease, length of stenosis, minimal lumen diameter, minimal lumen area, eccentricity of lumen, area of reference vessel segment, and viscosity (Fig. 1.18).

Quantitative Coronary Angiography

The degree of coronary stenosis is quantitated from the cineangiogram and, in clinical practice, is usually a visual estimation of the percentage of diameter narrowing using the presumed proximal normal arterial

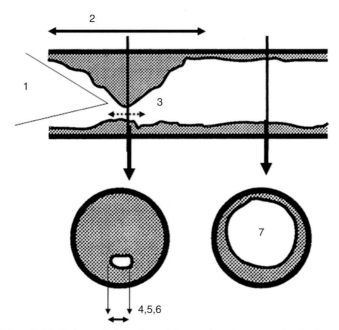

Figure 1.18 Factors of stenosis resistance. 1, entrance angle; 2, disease length; 3, stenosis length; 4, 5, 6, shape and size of lumen; 7, area of normal reference vessel. These factors determine the hemodynamic significance of a lesion and explain the visual function mismatch between angiography and ischemic testing.

segment and the ratio of the stenosis diameter to the normal reference diameter. This technique is widely applicable in clinical practice but is inadequate for the quantitative methodology done in most research studies. The intraobserver variability may range between 40% and 80%, and there is frequently as wide as a 20% range of interobserver differences. Quantitative methodology uses digital calipers or automated or manual edge detection systems. Densitometric analysis with digital angiography also provides quantitative lesion measurements. Quantitative coronary angiography (QCA) is best used for research where variability of image interpretation should be minimized.

Coronary Lesion Descriptions for Angioplasty

There are at least three different major classifications of lesion severity (Table 1.6). These classifications were derived from large studies in which the characteristics of the lesions were associated with different clinical outcomes of the techniques and times of the study. These are helpful to assess risk for adverse cardiac events in the performance of PCI.

General characteristics of the artery proximal to the lesion dilated are as follows:

1. Tortuosity: None/mild, straight proximal segment or only one bend of 60 degrees or more; Moderate, two bends of 60 degrees or more proximal to the lesion; Severe, three or more bends of 60 degrees or more proximal to the lesion

2. Arterial calcification: Light, proximal artery wall calcification (not necessarily the lesion) seen as thin line(s); Heavy, easily seen calcification

Angiographic characteristics of the dilated target lesion are as follows:

1. Arrangement of the lesion(s). Tandem, two lesions located within one balloon length (i.e., both lesions can be covered during a single balloon inflation); Sequential, two lesions located at a distance longer than the balloon.

2. Length. Discrete, 5 mm or more in length; Tubular 5–10 mm in length; Diffuse, greater than 10 mm in length

3. Eccentricity: Concentric, lumen axis is located along the long axis of the artery or on either side of it but by no more than 25% of the normal arterial diameter.

4. Ostial: Lesion is located at the aorto-ostial or bifurcation points.

5. Side branch: Bypassable side branch 1.5 mm or larger

6. Contour: Smooth, irregular, or ulcerated

7. Thrombus: Definite, intraluminal, round filling defect, visible in two views, largely separated from the vessel wall and/or documentation of embolization of this material; Possible, other filling defects not associated with calcification, lesion haziness, irregularity with ill-defined borders, intraluminal staining at the total occlusion site

8. Stenosis calcification: Calcification at the actual lesion site

9. Angulation: None/mild, lesion located on a straight segment or a bend of less than 45 degrees; Moderate, 45- to 90-degree bend; Severe, bend of greater than 90 degrees; bend should be evaluated in end-diastolic frame.

Use of the SYNTAX Score to Describe PCI Risk Versus CABG

In 2009, the SYNTAX trial compared multivessel PCI (including patients with left main narrowings) to CABG. The angiograms of the patients were analyzed and given SYNTAX scores. The SYNTAX score is an angiographic grading tool to determine the complexity of CAD. The results of this randomized study demonstrated that patients who had high SYNTAX scores (>34) did better with CABG compared to PCI than did those with lower SYNTAX scores, in whom PCI had similar major adverse cardiac events with lower stroke rates.

The SYNTAX score was derived from pre-existing lesion classifications, which included the AHA classification of coronary artery tree segments modified for the ARTS study, the Leaman score, the ACC/AHA lesion classification system, the total occlusion classification system, the Duke and International Classification for Patient Safety (ICPS) classification

Table 1.6

Classifications of Lesion Severity

ACC/AHA Lesion-Specific Characteristics

Type A Low Risk	Type B Medium Risk	Type C High Risk
Discrete (<10 mm length)	Tubular (10–20 mm length)	Diffuse (length >2 cm)
Concentric	Eccentric	Excessive tortuosity of proximal segment
Readily accessible	Moderate tortuosity of proximal segment	Extremely angulated segments >90 degrees
Nonangulated segment <45 degrees	Moderately angulated segment, 45–90 degrees	Total occlusions >3 mos. old ± bridging collaterals
Smooth contour	Irregular contour	Inability to protect major side branches
Little or no calcification	Moderate to heavy calcification	Degenerated vein grafts with friable lesions
Less than totally occlusive	Ostial in location	
Not ostial in location	Bifurcation lesions requiring double guidewires	
No major branch involvement	Some thrombus present	
Absence of thrombus	Total occlusion <3 months old	
Procedure success rate 92%	Procedure success rate 76%	Procedure success rate 61%
Complication rate 2%	Complication rate 10%	Complication rate 21%

Note: If more than two medium risk factors are present, lesion is classified as Type B2 and is considered complex.
National Cardiovascular Disease Registry, Cath PCI Registry v4.3.1 Coder's Data Dictionary, 2008.

SCAI Lesion-Specific Characteristics

Type I	Type II	Type III	Type IV
Patent and does not meet criteria for ACC/AHA type C lesion	Patent and meets any criteria for type C lesion	Occluded and does not meet any criteria for type C lesion	Occluded and meets any criteria for type C lesion
Procedure success rate 98%	Procedure success rate 94%	Procedure success rate 91%	Procedure success rate 80%
Complication rate 2.4%	Complication rate 5.1%	Complication rate 9.8%	Complication rate 10.1%

Note: Major complications were the composite of in-hospital death, acute myocardial infarction, emergency angioplasty, or emergency coronary artery bypass surgery. Lesion success was defined as a greater than 20% decrease in stenosis with a residual stenosis of less than 50%.
From Krone RJ, Shaw RE, Klein LW, et al. Evaluation of the American College of Cardiology/American Heart Association and the Society for Coronary Angiography and Interventions lesion classification system in the current stent era of coronary interventions (from the ACC-National Cardiovascular Data Registry). *Am J Cardiol.* 2003;92:389–394.

Continued

Table 1.6

Classifications of Lesion Severity (Continued)

Ellis Lesion-Specific Classification

Class I Low Risk	Class II Moderate Risk	Class III High Risk	Class IV Highest Risk
No risk factors	1.2 moderate correlates and the absence of strong correlates	≥3 moderate correlates and the absence of strong correlates	Either of the strongest correlates
Complication rate 2.1%	Complication rate 3.4%	Complication rate 8.2%	Complication rate 12.7%

Moderately strong correlates:
Length ≥10 mm
Lumen irregularity
Large filling defect
Calcium + angle ≥45 degrees
Eccentric
Severe calcification
SVG age ≥10 years

Strongest correlates:
Nonchronic total occlusion
Degenerated SVG

Note: Complication defined as death, myocardial infarction, or emergent coronary artery bypass grafting.

From Ellis SG, Guetta S, Miller D, et al. Relation between lesion characteristics and risk with percutaneous intervention in the stent and glycoprotein IIb/IIIa era - an analysis of results from 10907 lesions and proposal for new classification scheme. *Circulation*. 1999;100:1971–1976.

system for bifurcation lesions, and a consensus opinion from among the world's experts.

The SYNTAX score is the sum of the points assigned to each individual lesion identified in the coronary tree with greater than 50% diameter narrowing in vessels of greater than 1.5 mm diameter. The coronary tree is divided into 16 segments according to the AHA classification (Fig. 1.19A). Each segment is given a score of 1 or 2 based on the presence of disease, and this score is then weighted, based on a chart, with values ranging from 3.5 for the proximal LAD to 5.0 for left main and 0.5 for smaller branches. Branches of less than 1.5 mm in diameter, despite having severe lesions, are not included in the SYNTAX score. The percent diameter stenosis is not a consideration in the SYNTAX score, only the presence of a stenosis of from 50–99% diameter, less than 50% diameter narrowing, or total occlusion. A multiplication factor of 2 is used for nonocclusive lesions, and 5 is used for occlusive lesions, reflecting the difficulty of PCI.

Further characterization of the lesions adds points. For example, a total occlusion duration of more than 3 months, a blunt stump, a bridging collateral image, the first segment visible beyond the total occlusion, and a side branch of larger than 1.5 diameter all receive one point. For trifurcations, one diseased segment gets three points, two diseased segments get four points, three diseased segments get five points, and four disease segments get six points. For bifurcation lesions, one point is given for simple types; two points are given for complex types; and one point is given for an angulation of greater than 70 degrees. Additionally, an aorto-ostial lesion is worth one point, severe tortuosity of vessel is worth two points, lesion length greater than 20 mm is worth one point, heavy calcification is worth two points, thrombus is worth one point, and diffuse disease or small-vessel disease is worth one point per segment involvement. Multiple lesions less than three reference vessel diameters apart are scored as a single lesion. However, at a distance greater than three vessel diameters, these are considered separate lesions. The types of bifurcations are shown in Fig. 1.19B. Segments in which bifurcations are evaluated are those involving the proximal LAD and left main, the mid LAD, the proximal circumflex, mid-circumflex, and crux of the right

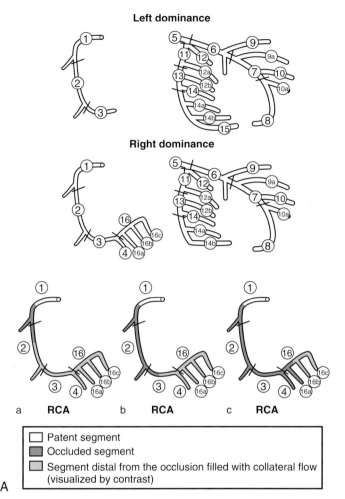

Figure 1.19

(A) The SYNTAX diagram. Definition of the coronary tree segments: 1, RCA proximal: From the ostium to one-half the distance to the acute margin of the heart; 2, RCA mid: From the end of first segment to acute margin of heart; 3, RCA distal: From the acute margin of the heart to the origin of the posterior descending artery; 4, Posterior descending artery: Running in the posterior interventricular groove; 16, Posterolateral branch from RCA: Posterolateral branch originating from the distal coronary artery distal to the crux; **16a**, Posterolateral branch from RCA: First posterolateral branch from segment 16; **16b**, Posterolateral branch from RCA: Second posterolateral branch from segment 16; **16c**, Posterolateral branch from RCA: Third posterolateral branch from segment 16; 5, Left main: From the ostium of the LCA through bifurcation into left anterior descending and left circumflex branches; 6, LAD proximal: Proximal to and including first major septal branch; 7, LAD mid: LAD immediately distal to origin of first septal branch and extending to the point where LAD forms an angle (RAO view). If this angle is not identifiable this segment ends at one half the distance from the first septal to the apex of the heart. 8, LAD apical: Terminal portion of LAD, beginning at the end of previous segment and extending to or beyond the apex; 9, First diagonal: The first diagonal originating from segment 6 or 7; **9a**, First diagonal a: Additional first diagonal originating from segment 6 or 7, before segment 8; 10, Second diagonal: Originating from segment 8 or the transition between segment 7 and 8; **10a**, Second diagonal a: Additional second diagonal originating from segment 8; 11, Proximal circumflex artery: Main stem of circumflex from its origin of left main and including origin of first obtuse marginal branch; 12, Intermediate/anterolateral artery: Branch from trifurcating left main other than proximal LAD or LCX. It belongs to the circumflex territory; **12a**, Obtuse marginal a: First side branch of circumflex running in general to the area of obtuse margin of the heart; **12b**, Obtuse marginal b: Second additional branch of circumflex

Continued

Figure 1.19, cont'd
running in the same direction as 12; **13**, Distal circumflex artery: The stem of the circumflex distal to the origin of the most distal obtuse marginal branch, and running along the posterior left atrioventricular groove. Caliber may be small or artery absent; **14**, Left posterolateral: Running to the posterolateral surface of the left ventricle. May be absent or a division of obtuse marginal branch; **14a**, Left posterolateral a: Distal from 14 and running in the same direction; **14b**, Left posterolateral b: Distal from 14 and 14a and running in the same direction; **15**, Posterior descending: Most distal part of dominant left circumflex when present. It gives origin to septal branches. When this artery is present, segment 4 is usually absent. *(From Sianos G, Morel M., Kappetein Ap, et al. The SYNTAX Score: an angiographic tool grading the complexity of CAD. Eurointerv. 2005;1:219–227.)* (B) Example of SYNTAX Score and specific angiographic anatomy.

Table 1.7

The SYNTAX Score Algorithm

1. Dominance
2. Number of lesions
3. Segments involved per lesion, with lesion characteristics
4. Total occlusions with subtotal occlusions:
   a. Number of segments
   b. Age of total occlusions
   c. Blunt stumps
   d. Bridging collaterals
   e. First segment beyond occlusion visible by antegrade or retrograde filling
   f. Side branch involvement
5. Trifurcation, number of segments diseased
6. Bifurcation type and angulation
7. Aorto-ostial lesion
8. Severe tortuosity
9. Lesion length
10. Heavy calcification
11. Thrombus
12. Diffuse disease, with number of segments

coronary artery. With regard to trifurcation lesions, these also are additive in the number of segments involved. The SYNTAX score algorithm then sums each of these features for a total SYNTAX score. Table 1.7 summarizes the SYNTAX grade categories. A computer algorithm is then queried, and a summed value is produced.

The SYNTAX score was validated using a series of patients undergoing three-vessel PCI, such as the ARTS II trial. The variables were then associated with outcome events in the PCI studies. Low SYNTAX scores are less than 18, intermediate SYNTAX scores range from 18 to 27, and high SYNTAX scores are greater than 27. High scores are associated with increasing cardiac mortality, major adverse cardiac events, and a specific, predefined combination of end points. The SYNTAX angiographic grading system was used alone to identify potential risk for revascularization. When comparing all clinical and angiographic factors, it was evident that the SYNTAX score, in addition to age, gender, smoking, diabetes, and acute coronary syndromes, is one of the highest predictors of cardiac mortality and major adverse cardiac events in patients undergoing multivessel and, specifically, unprotected left main PCI. A SYNTAX score of higher than 34 also identifies a subgroup with a particularly high risk of cardiac death independent of age, gender, acute coronary syndrome, ejection fraction, Euro score, and degree of revascularization.

The SYNTAX score is a useful differentiator for the outcome of patients undergoing three-vessel PCI. Examples of the types of SYNTAX score are provided in figures from the original paper (Fig. 1.20). Those patients with the highest scores have the highest risk; those with the lowest scores have the lowest risk. The SYNTAX scores can be divided into three tertiles. The high scores indicate complex conditions and represent greatest risks to patients undergoing PCI. High scores have the worst prognosis for revascularization with PCI compared to CABG. Equivalent or superior outcomes for percutaneous intervention were noted in comparison to CABG surgery for patients in the lowest two tertiles (Fig. 1.20). The best discriminating feature of the SYNTAX score was between the lowest and highest tertiles of grading.

Angiographic Problems and Artifacts

The basic issues regarding angiography are described in detail in Chapter 3 of *The Cardiac Catheterization Handbook,* 6e. The following brief discussion directs our attention to problem issues specifically for the PCI procedure.

Vessel/lesion overlap: Coronary target lesions may be obscured by overlapping images of contrast-filled vessels, which impairs one's ability to accurately assess true lesion length, especially for the proximal vessel segments. Without a clear view of the target vessel and its stenosis, the size, extent, and characteristics of the lesion for best technique selection will not be optimal.

Poor contrast opacification of the vessel may lead to a false impression of an angiographically significant lesion or lucency that could be considered a clot. Inadequate mixing of contrast and blood presents as a luminal irregularity. A satisfactory bolus injection of contrast must be delivered. Large intravascular equipment may not permit this to occur, and the operator must consider whether a larger guide catheter is needed to see the lesion better. Enhanced contrast delivery can be achieved by obtaining better coaxial engagement of the guiding catheter or using a larger catheter, injecting during Valsalva maneuver phase III, or using a power injector.

Catheter-induced spasm may appear as a fixed stenotic lesion and be confused with a true organic lesion. This has been observed in both right and left (and left main) coronary arteries. These spastic segments may be single and proximal or may be multiple and located some distance from the ostium. Nitroglycerin should be administered in every case prior to initiating intervention, especially if there is any possibility of catheter-induced spasm. Repositioning of the catheter and administration of nitroglycerin (100–200 mcg through the catheter) may clarify if the presumed lesion is structural and not spastic. Often a change to a smaller-diameter (6 or 5F) catheter or to catheters that do not seat deeply may help.

Syntax Study Event Rates by Syntax Score

Syntax Score	0–22	23–32	>33
PCI MACE (%)	13.6	16.7	23.4
CABG MACE (%)	14.7	12.0	10.9

Figure 1.20 (A-C), Outcomes of percutaneous coronary intervention (PCI) vs. coronary artery bypass graft (CABG) by SYNTAX scores. *(Data from Serruys PW, et al. Percutaneous coronary intervention versus coronary artery bypass grafting for severe coronary artery disease. The SYNTAX Trial. N Engl J Med. 2009:360.)*

Aorto-ostial lesion assessment: Because of the eccentric nature of ostial lesions, optimal views to identify the left main coronary artery will need to be individually determined. In general, the standard views remain the same as for those during diagnostic studies, with a shallow RAO with cranial or caudal angulation often providing the best starting point. In addition, among the best views is the LAO caudal view (spider view) to display the left main artery and its distal bifurcation with the LAD and circumflex. An additional problem is the appreciation of the visual–functional mismatch between angiographic stenosis and the corresponding hemodynamic significance of the left main stenoses, especially when the angiographic narrowing is of questionable severity. For this situation, FFR measurement can provide the hemodynamic severity, with a value of greater than 0.80 having a low 5-year major adverse cardiac event rate. Some operators prefer IVUS before performing revascularization to better appreciate the size and composition of the left main (see Chapter 4, Intravascular Lesion Assessment Physiology and Imaging).

Delineation of the tortuous proximal left circumflex coronary artery is important to plan for a successful if not difficult PCI. The origin of the circumflex and its angle of departure from the left main should be shown in several projections to demonstrate whether it is steeply angled cranially or caudally. Guide catheter selection for the circumflex artery often requires left Amplatz, Q, Voda, or guideliners for good backup support.

A discussion of the angiography of anomalous coronary arteries is provided in Chapter 3 of *The Cardiac Catheterization Handbook,* 6e. PCI for these arteries is performed in a routine fashion once stable guide catheter position is achieved.

Radiographic Contrast Media for PCI

The contrast material is selected from several commercially available solutions with varying features of osmolarity, viscosity, and sodium content found to be appropriate for the specific procedure to be conducted. The most common contrast media for PCI is nonionic or low-osmolar contrast agents because of safety, patient tolerance, and cost. Selection of a nonionic or low osmolar contrast agent for the particular interventional procedure is, to a large extent, a matter of personal preference.

Radiation Exposure During PCI

Coronary angioplasty will deliver greater x-ray exposure than diagnostic studies because of the more complicated and time-consuming nature of the procedure. Previous studies have demonstrated that operator exposure is 93% greater for angioplasty than for routine diagnostic coronary angiography. This increase is due to longer fluoroscopy times in angioplasty without correspondingly longer cineradiography times. Because of the angled projections used in coronary angioplasty, increased x-ray exposure may be present. The scattered x-ray dose has been reported to be four times higher with angioplasty than with diagnostic cardiac catheterization (Fig. 1.21).

Fluoroscopy Times

A study by Pattee et al. (1993) of radiation risk to patients from coronary angioplasty indicated that radiation doses varied considerably during the procedure because of large differences in exposure times. Skin exposures estimated for PCI are, on average, higher than for other x-ray procedures, and the cancer mortality risk does not exceed the mortality risk of bypass surgery. Good professional practice requires maximal benefit-to-risk ratio for angioplasty procedures employing high-dose fluoroscopy or cineradiography. Device-specific procedure times may be longer than routine stent placement (Table 1.8).

Angulated views increase radiation exposure. LAO views produce 2.6–6.1 times the dose of radiation for the operator of equivalently angled RAO views (Table 1.9). Steeper LAO views also increased operator dose. An LAO of 90 degrees produces eight times the dose of an LAO of 60 degrees and three times the dose of an LAO of 30 degrees. Fluoroscopy produced more radiation than cine during angioplasty, by a factor of 6:1. Reducing the steepness of angulation reduces operator radiation dosage.

Pacemakers During PCI

The routine use of pacemakers for PCI is not required. Cardiac pacemakers may be used prophylactically during PCI to reduce the hemodynamic compromise of heart block and are needed to rescue patients after the development of conduction abnormalities associated with hypotension. External pacing patches are useful for emergency pacing when a temporary pacing wire cannot be immediately positioned. When using pacing patches, the patient must be sedated because each electrical

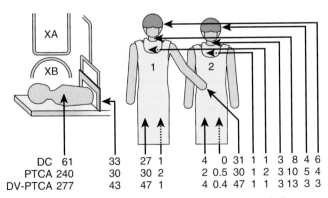

Figure 1.21 Radiation exposure rates for two operators during coronary angioplasty. DC, Diagnostic catheterization; DV-PTCA, double-vessel percutaneous transluminal coronary angioplasty; XA, x-ray amplifier in plane A; XB, x-ray amplifier in plane B. (*Modified from Finci L, Meier B, Steffenino G, et al. Radiation exposure during diagnostic catheterization and single- and double-vessel percutaneous transluminal coronary angioplasty. Am J Cardiol. 1987;60:1401–1403.*)

Table 1.8

Estimated Radiation Entrance Exposure of Patients Using Phantom Model Data		
Procedure	Fluoroscopy (R)	Cine (R)
Isolated balloon angioplasty	43	25
Isolated directional coronary atherectomy	32	23
Directional coronary atherectomy + balloon angioplasty	66	29
Isolated laser coronary angioplasty	45	18
Laser coronary angioplasty + balloon angioplasty	57	27
Elective stenting	52	27
Emergency stenting	96	41

From Federman J, Bell MR, Wondrow MA, et al. Does the use of new intracoronary interventional devices prolong radiation exposure in the cardiac catheterization laboratory? *J Am Coll Cardiol.* 1994;23:347–357.

Table 1.9

Radiation Dose and Angulation	
View	Dose (Relative Increase)
Image intensifier position	
RAO 30–60 degrees	1
LAO 30–60 degrees	2.6–6.1
Increasing angulation	
LAO 30 degrees	1
LAO 60 degrees	3
LAO 90 degrees	9

LAO, left anterior oblique; *RAO*, right anterior oblique.

stimulation causes contraction of chest muscles as well as heart muscle and may be painful.

Indications

1. Previously demonstrated high-degree conduction block
2. Symptomatic bradycardia (after contrast or angiography of RCA)
3. Acute MI with trifascicular block
4. Prophylactic use for rotational atherectomy and thrombectomy procedures, especially involving the RCA
5. Transluminal alcohol septal artery ablation in hypertrophic obstructive cardiomyopathy (HOCM) patients.

Atropine may be used to prevent bradycardia, but a pacemaker should be on standby for patients who experience severe bradycardia during coronary injections.

Temporary transvenous pacemaker placement can be achieved through the internal jugular, subclavian, brachial, or femoral vein route. The easiest access is usually the vein next to the arterial entry site. Right ventricular pacing is best accomplished with a 5F balloon-tipped pacing catheter because there is a reduced incidence of perforation of the thin free wall or apex of the right ventricle when the balloon is inflated.

Cutaneous patch pacemakers are also effective until secured pacing routes can be established. Muscle contractions induced by the cutaneous pacing patches are uncomfortable, so the patient should be well sedated.

Suggested Readings

Anderson HV, Shaw RE, Brindis RG, et al. Relationship between procedure indications and outcomes of percutaneous coronary interventions by American College of Cardiology/American Heart Association Task Force Guidelines. *Circulation*. 2005;112:2786-2791.

Bakalyar DM, Castellani MD, Safian RD. Radiation exposure to patients undergoing diagnostic and interventional cardiac catheterization procedures. *Cathet Cardiovasc Diagn*. 1997;42:121-125.

Balter S, Moses J. Managing patient dose in interventional cardiology. *Catheter Cardiovasc Interv*. 2007;70:244-249.

Bashore TM, Balter S, Barac A, et al. 2012 American College of Cardiology Foundation/Society for Cardiovascular Angiography and Interventions expert consensus document on cardiac catheterization laboratory standards update: American College of Cardiology Foundation Task Force on expert consensus documents Society of Thoracic Surgeons Society for Vascular Medicine. *Catheter Cardiovasc Interv*. 2012;80:E37-E49.

Blankenship JC, Gigliotti OS, Feldman DN, et al. Ad hoc percutaneous coronary intervention: a consensus statement from the Society for Cardiovascular Angiography and Interventions. *Catheter Cardiovasc Interv*. 2013;81:748-758.

Boden WE. Optimal medical therapy with or without PCI for stable coronary artery disease. *N Engl J Med*. 2007;356:1503-1516.

Brilakis ES, Banerjee S, Berger PB. Perioperative management of patients with coronary stents. *J Am Coll Cardiol*. 2007;49:2145-2150.

Chida K, et al. Patient skin dose in cardiac interventional procedures: conventional fluoroscopy versus pulsed fluoroscopy. *Catheter Cardiovasc Interv*. 2007;69:115-121.

Garg S, Serruys PW. Coronary stents: current status. *J Am Coll Cardiol*. 2010;56:S1-S42.

Garg S, Serruys PW. Coronary stents: looking forward. *J Am Coll Cardiol*. 2010;56:S43-S78.

Gibson CM, Cannon CP, Daley WL, et al. TIMI frame count: a quantitative method of assessing coronary artery flow. *Circulation*. 1996;93:879-888.

Green NE, Chen SYJ, Hansgen AR, et al. Angiographic views used for percutaneous coronary interventions: a three-dimensional analysis of physician-determined vs. computer-generated views. *Catheter Cardiovasc Interv*. 2005;64:451-459.

Hirshfeld JW Jr, Balter S, Brinker JA, et al. ACCF/AHA/HRS/SCAI Clinical competence statement on physician knowledge to optimize patient safety and image quality in fluoroscopically guided invasive cardiovascular procedures: a report of the American College of Cardiology Foundation/American Heart Association/American College of Physicians Task Force on Clinical Competence and Training. *J Am Coll Cardiol*. 2004;44:2259-2282.

Hirshfeld JW Jr, Balter S, Brinker JA, et al. ACCF/AHA/HRS/SCAI Clinical competence statement on physician knowledge to optimize patient safety and image quality in fluoroscopically guided invasive cardiovascular procedures: a report of the American College of Cardiology Foundation/American Heart Association/American College of Physicians Task Force on Clinical Competence and Training. *Circulation*. 2005;111:511-532.

Holmes DR Jr, Kereiakes D, Garg S, et al. Stent thrombosis. *J Am Coll Cardiol*. 2010;56:1357-1365.

Jacobs AK, Babb JD, Hirshfeld JW Jr, et al. Task Force 3: training in diagnostic and interventional cardiac catheterization: endorsed by the Society for Cardiovascular Angiography and Interventions. *J Am Coll Cardiol*. 2008;51:355-361.

Katritsis D, Efstathopoulos E, Betsou S, et al. Radiation exposure of patients and coronary arteries in the stent era: a prospective study. *Catheter Cardiovasc Interv*. 2000;51:259-264.

Kaul P, Medvedev S, Hohmann SF, et al. Ionizing radiation exposure to patients admitted with acute myocardial infarction in the United States. *Circulation*. 2010;122:2160-2169.

Kern MJ, ed. *Hemodynamic Rounds: Interpretation of Cardiac Pathophysiology from Pressure Waveform Analysis*. 3rd ed. New York: Wiley-Liss; 2009.

Kern MJ, ed. *Interventional Cardiac Catheterization Handbook*. 3rd ed. St Louis: Mosby; 2012.

Kern MJ, ed. *The Interventional Cardiac Catheterization Handbook*. 3rd ed. Philadelphia: Elsevier; 2012.

Kern MJ, ed. *The Cardiac Catheterization Handbook*. 6th ed. Philadelphia: Elsevier; 2015.

Koenig TR, Wolff D, Metter FA, et al. Skin injuries from fluoroscopically guided procedures: part I, characteristics of radiation injury. *AJR*. 2001;177:3-11.

Mahesh M. Fluoroscopy: patient radiation exposure issues. *Radiographics*. 2001;21:1033-1045.

Moscucci M. *Baim's Cardiac Catheterization, Angiography, and Intervention*. 8th ed. Philadelphia: Wolters/Kluwer/Lippincott Williams; 2014.

Naidu SS, Aronow HD, Box LC, et al. SCAI Expert Consensus Statement: 2016 best practices in the cardiac catheterization laboratory: Endorsed by the Cardiological Society of India, and Sociedad Latino Americana de Cardiologia Intervencionista; Affirmation of Value by the Canadian Association of Interventional Cardiology–Association Canadienne de Cardiologie d'intervention. *Catheter Cardiovasc Interv*. 2016;doi:10.1002/ccd.26551.

Patel MR, Dehme G Jr, Hirshfeld JW, et al. ACCF/SCAI/STS/AATS/AHA/ASNC 2009 Appropriateness Criteria for Coronary Revascularization: a report by the American College of Cardiology Foundation Appropriateness Criteria Task Force, Society for Cardiovascular Angiography and Interventions, Society of Thoracic Surgeons, American Association for Thoracic Surgery, American Heart Association, and the American Society of Nuclear Cardiology; endorsed by the American Society of Echocardiography, the Heart Failure Society of America, and the Society of Cardiovascular Computed Tomography. *J Am Coll Cardiol*. 2009;53:530-553.

Rao SV, Tremmel JA, Gilchrist IC, et al. Best practices for transradial angiography and intervention: a consensus statement from the Society for Cardiovascular Angiography and Intervention's Transradial Working Group. *Catheter Cardiovasc Interv*. 2013.

Serruys PW, et al. Percutaneous coronary intervention versus coronary artery bypass grafting for severe coronary artery disease. The SYNTAX Trial. *N Engl J Med*. 2009;360.

Sianos G, Morel M, Kappetein AP, et al. The SYNTAX Score: an angiographic tool grading the complexity of CAD. *Eurointerv.* 2005;1:219-227.

Urestky B, ed. *Cardiac Catheterization: Concepts, Techniques and Applications.* Malden, MA: Blackwell Science; 1997.

Valgimigli M, Serruys PW, Tsuchida K, et al. Cyphering the complexity of coronary artery disease using the SYNTAX score to predict clinical outcome in patients with three vessel lumen obstruction undergoing percutaneous coronary intervention. *Am J Cardiol.* 2007;99(8):1072-1081.

White CJ, Jaff MR, Haskal ZJ, et al. Indications for renal arteriography at the time of coronary arteriography: a science advisory from the American Heart Association Committee on Diagnostic and Interventional Cardiac Catheterization, Council on Clinical Cardiology, and the Councils on Cardiovascular Radiology and Intervention and on Kidney in Cardiovascular Disease. *Circulation.* 2006;114:1892-1895.

2

Vascular Access ▶

MORTON J. KERN · ARNOLD H. SETO ·
MICHAEL FORSBERG

Vascular access techniques for interventional procedures are the same as those used for diagnostic catheterization but require greater precision due to the increased risk of bleeding with most interventions and their associated anticoagulation regimens. For both diagnostic and interventional procedures, vascular access is the most frequent cause of procedural morbidity. The site and size of the access and sheath are determined by the anatomic and clinico-pathologic conditions (e.g., peripheral vascular disease) and the anticipated interventional techniques required.

To avoid known pitfalls and potential complications, operators should review previous procedure notes and any difficulties encountered during prior procedures. At the minimum, assessment of all arterial pulses before and after the procedure is mandatory. Additional information from ultrasound studies or computed tomographic (CT) imaging (especially for transcatheter aortic valve replacement [TAVR] procedures) may be required for appropriate access site selection in higher risk subjects.

Percutaneous Radial and Femoral Artery Access

In the United States, the femoral artery approach has been standard for decades. However in recent years many laboratories have adopted the radial approach for both the diagnostic and interventional procedures. For large-bore devices, the femoral artery is larger than the radial and thus preferred. The radial approach has significantly fewer access-related complications and, in most comparative studies, better late outcomes including bleeding and mortality. Many operators familiar with current clinical data advocate a "radial first" approach when possible. Conditions in which radial artery access should be favored are listed in Box 2.1.

Femoral Artery Puncture Technique

The basic access techniques for both the femoral and radial arteries are presented in detail in the *Cardiac Catheterization Handbook*, 6e, Chapter 2. This section will highlight issues and advanced techniques pertinent to vascular access for the interventional procedures.

The proper entry site for femoral artery puncture is the common femoral artery (CFA), defined as that segment above the femoral artery bifurcation and below the inferior epigastric artery (Figs. 2.1 and 2.2). Because the CFA generally has a consistent position over the femoral head, this target zone is located by visualizing the head of the femur with a metal marker (e.g., hemostat) indicating the planned path of the

---

Sections of this chapter are retained from third edition chapter by Connie N. Hess, Sunil V. Rao, Kimberly A. Skelding, Morton J. Kern, and Mitchell W. Krucoff.

Box 2.1 Conditions in Which Radial Artery Access Should Be Favored

1. Claudication
2. Absent leg pulses
3. Femoral bruits
4. Prior femoral artery graft surgery
5. Extensive inguinal scarring from previous procedures
6. Surgery or radiation treatment near inguinal area
7. Excessively tortuous iliac system and lower abdominal aorta
8. Abdominal aortic aneurysm
9. Severe back pain or inability to lie flat
10. Downward origin of renal arteries (for renal artery stenting)
11. Patient request

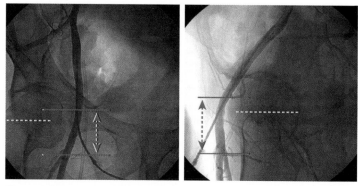

Figure 2.1 Femoral angiogram: (*left*) AP view, (*right*) lateral view. The common femoral artery (CFA) has the inferior epigastic artery and bifurcation of the superficial and profunda femoral arteries as the top and bottom markers. Yellow dotted line is middle of femoral head. Lower red line is bifurcation of superficial and profunda femoral arteries, top red line is lower border of inferior epigastic artery. The arrow shows the target zone for proper puncture in the CFA over the femoral head, with the center third of the femoral head being the optimal location.

needle by fluoroscopy. The operator palpates the femoral pulse 2 cm below the center of the femoral head and administers local anesthesia. The inguinal crease is generally inferior to the center of the femoral head (especially in the obese patient) but should not be used as a marker for insertion. Using standard Seldinger technique with an 18- or 21-gauge micropuncture needle, a single front wall puncture is best for two reasons:

1. Reduced chance of bleeding from multiple punctures in the artery in the setting of potent anticoagulation and antiplatelet agents.

2. Reduced bleeding after successful vascular closure device placement since a second arterial puncture on the back wall would not be controlled. Multiple punctures may be a source of bleeding complications, including retroperitoneal hematoma, femoral pseudoaneurysms, or arteriovenous fistula (AVF).

When a staged interventional procedure is planned for a separate day, contralateral femoral access should be considered. Ipsilateral radial access is acceptable when the radial pulse is intact. Repeat ipsilateral femoral punctures soon after a prior procedure may be associated with a higher incidence of bleeding or infection. Repeat femoral puncture after placement of a vascular closure device may be relatively contra-indicated. Although access through a vascular closure device site can be performed, repuncture in a femoral artery closed with an Angio Seal is not recommended before 90 days. Those sites closed with StarClose, Perclose, or Mynx may be reaccessed immediately, although there is a remote chance of reentering the central opening of the StarClose clip.

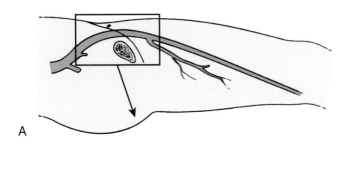

A

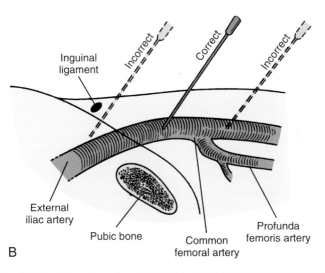

B

Figure 2.2 Technique of single-wall arterial puncture. Parasagittal cross-sectional diagram of inguinal region at level of femoral artery. Correct needle entry position is below inguinal ligament and above femoral artery bifurcation. Correct access is particularly critical for procedures. *(From* The Interventional Cardiac Catheterization Handbook, *3e, Philadelphia: Elsevier; 2012. Originally from Kulick DL, Rahimtoola SH, eds.* Techniques and Applications in Interventional Cardiology. *St. Louis, MO: Mosby, 1991:3.)*

Micropuncture Technique

Fluoroscopy-assisted micropuncture access has the potential to improve the safety and accuracy of femoral access, which is particularly useful for large bore sheath placement.

The key elements of fluoroscopic guidance include (1) identification of the mid-third of the femoral head, (2) femoral artery puncture, (3) wire navigation with fluoroscopy, and (4) contrast angiographic confirmation of the arterial entry site. Micropuncture access packs consist of a low-profile needle or needle (21 vs. 18 gauge), a 0.018-inch nitinol or hydrophilic guidewire, and a 4F or 5F tapered micropuncture sheath with an inner dilator. When access is achieved and the inner dilator and wire are removed, a standard 0.035- or 0.038-inch guidewire can be inserted to facilitate final sheath placement.

Advantages of the micropuncture access technique include a smaller initial puncture with less arterial trauma (particularly important if multiple attempts are needed to access the vessel) and contrast angiography through the 4F or 5F micropuncture catheter or inner dilator to confirm an optimal location of the arteriotomy before large sheath placement. If the operator is not satisfied with the position of entry, the small catheter can be removed and access reattempted after

5 minutes of manual compression. The micropuncture needle also has a lower crossing profile, which can be helpful in highly resistant (calcified) arteries.

Despite the potential advantages of the micropuncture technique, its use is still controversial. A more recent but small, prospective, randomized trial demonstrated a reduction in vascular complications with micropuncture compared to standard 18-gauge femoral access. Larger scale studies are necessary to settle the issue.

Stepwise Micropuncture Access

Fig. 2.3 provides the basic steps of micropuncture arterial access.

1. Review any available angiograms or CT imaging of the iliofemoral system.
2. In contrast to larger 18-gauge needles, micropuncture needle flow on entry into the femoral artery be brisk but generally nonpulsatile.
3. After needle placement, limited femoral angiography is performed with a 3-mL syringe through the micropuncture needle. Alternatively, one can place the sheath/cannula over the wire since it is easier to inject contrast through the inner cannula of the micropuncture catheter.
4. Introduce the 0.018-inch micropuncture wire into the artery through the micropuncture needle under fluoroscopy. The wire tip should move freely in the artery. For aberrant wire movement, withdraw the wire and readvance in another direction.
5. Advance the micropuncture catheter and inner dilator over the wire into the femoral artery. Perform femoral angiography using a 3-mL syringe with full strength or diluted contrast.
6. If femoral artery puncture location is acceptable, advance a 0.035-inch wire into the micropuncture catheter, followed by a 6–8F sheath.
7. If the femoral artery puncture site is unacceptable, remove the micropuncture catheter, apply manual compression for 3–5 minutes, and repeat the sequence of access.
8. Once successful access is achieved, as needed, a large-bore 14–26F TAVR sheath can be placed using a stiff guidewire and progressively larger dilators.

Note: For hemostasis after vascular access for large-bore catheters, consider two methods: (1) *pre-closure;* pre-close suture placement for access control at the end of the case, and (2) a *retrograde crossover method* (see later discussion) to provide better safety and manageability should a complication occur.

Use of Ultrasound Imaging for Femoral Access

Over the past two decades, there has been a shift in practice toward ultrasound image-guided access, particularly in the fields of anesthesia, critical care medicine, vascular surgery, and interventional radiology. Numerous publications and reviews across multiple specialties and in almost every anatomic area have demonstrated that ultrasound guidance provides vascular access with greater accuracy and speed and with a decrease in complications. For central venous access, ultrasound guidance is a standard of care according to national guidelines.

The anatomy of the CFA at times varies from its predicted location, with the CFA bifurcation occurring over the femoral head one-third of the time and the inferior epigastric artery encroaching on the middle third of the femoral head 10% of the time. Ultrasound imaging can

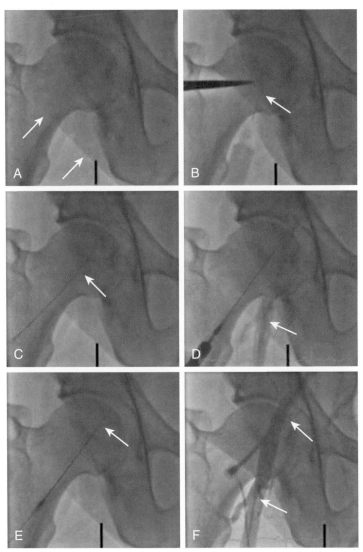

Figure 2.3 Micropuncture arterial access technique. (A) Using fluoroscopy, the mid-femoral head is identified. The arrows show the femoral skin crease. (B) A hemostat marks the mid-femoral head, and the local anesthesia needle is just below the skin surface (*arrow*). This provides some idea of where the micropuncture needle should be introduced into the skin. (C) Repeat fluoroscopy once the needle is deep in the subcutaneous tissue, but not yet into the femoral artery, is required to achieve an ideal location of femoral puncture at the level of the mid-femoral head. The arrow shows the tip of the micropuncture needle. (D) Contrast injection through the micropuncture needle shows the level of needle entry in the common femoral artery (CFA) (*arrow* shows the level of CFA bifurcation). (E) A 0.018-inch guidewire is advanced into the femoral artery. The arrow shows the guidewire exit point from the needle tip, which is the site of needle entry into the CFA lumen. (F) Angiography via a 6F sheath confirms the arterial entry site. The arrows show the takeoff of the inferior epigastric artery and the CFA. The sheath entry is above the mid-femoral head, but clearly inferior to the inferior sweep of the inferior epigastric artery (*upper arrow*) and above the bifurcation (*lower arrow*). *(From Cilingiroglu M, Feldman T, Salinger MH, Levisay J, Turi ZG. Fluoroscopically-guided micropuncture femoral artery access for large-caliber sheath insertion. J Invasive Cardiol. 2011;23(4):157–161.)*

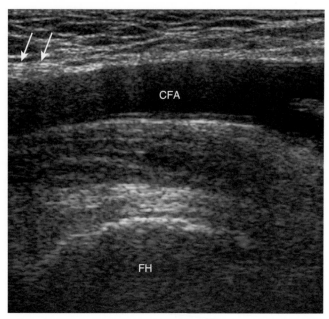

Figure 2.4 Longitudinal ultrasound of common femoral artery. Ultrasound image shows the inguinal ligament (*arrows*) and femoral head (FH) along the longitudinal plane and common femoral artery (CFA) with its bifurcation. *(From Yun SJ, Nam DH, Ryu JK. Femoral artery access using the US-determined inguinal ligament and femoral head as reliable landmarks: prospective study of usefulness and safety. J Vasc Interv Radiol. 2015;26(4):552–559.)*

identify the CFA bifurcation consistently and ensure the access is above it. In the longitudinal view, ultrasound can also identify the femoral head, the posterior course of the external iliac artery, and the soft-tissue inguinal ligament (which appears as an echodense triangle; Fig. 2.4). These landmarks may protect against an overly superior insertion.

In the large Femoral Arterial Access with Ultrasound Trial (FAUST), ultrasound guidance reduced the number of attempts required to successfully cannulate the femoral artery (1.3 vs. 3.0; $p < 0.001$), increased the first-pass success rate (82.7% vs. 46.4%; $p < 0.001$), and reduced the risk of accidental venipuncture (2.4% vs. 15.8%; $p < 0.001$). As a result, the incidence of any vascular complications was reduced with ultrasound (1.4% vs. 3.4%; $p = 0.041$). The average time to access was reduced with ultrasound guidance from 213 to 185 seconds ($p = 0.016$). In the trial, ultrasound guidance was associated with a learning curve requiring approximately 10 procedures before proficiency was achieved.

Stepwise Ultrasound Access

Step 1: Prepare the ultrasound probe by placing transducer gel in the base of the probe cover. Cover the probe with the sterile sheath cover and place gel on the front. The image display settings should be set at a minimum of depth penetration needed (i.e., 3–4 cm) and high gain. Turn on the centerline guide markers.

Step 2: Image the vessel in the axial plane by holding the ultrasound probe perpendicular to the course of the vessel. Gently compress the vessels by applying downward pressure on the probe. An artery will be an echolucent circle that pulsates on gentle compression. A vein will often be larger, easily compressible or collapsing with respiration, and without visible pulsation. Ultrasound is able to image the CFA bifurcation (Fig. 2.5) and guard against an overly low or inferior cannulation.

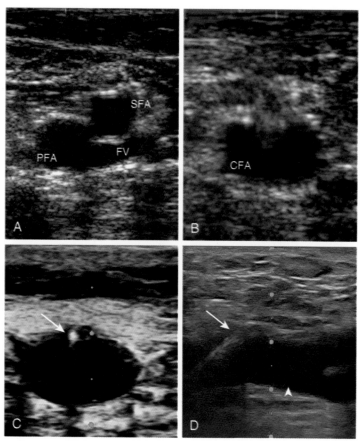

Figure 2.5 Axial ultrasound of common femoral artery. (A) The right common femoral bifurcation is imaged in the axial plane, demonstrating the profunda femoral artery and superficial femoral artery. Compression is used to differentiate arteries from the femoral vein. (B) The probe is moved or angled superiorly to the common femoral artery (CFA). During needle advancement, the anterior wall of the vessel is indented by the needle tip. (C) The guidewire insertion point (*arrow*) can be imaged in the axial plane after cannulation to confirm that the insertion is above the CFA bifurcation. (D) Longitudinal view shows the guidewire entry (*arrow*) is superior to the CFA bifurcation (*arrowhead*).

Step 3: Align the target vessel with the centerline guide on the display by moving the probe. This ensures that the target vessel is directly beneath the center of the probe.

Step 4: Inject lidocaine subcutaneously under the center of the probe.

Step 5: Insert the needle into the skin underneath the center marking of the probe at about a 45- to 60-degree angle (Fig. 2.6). For a deep vessel, the needle can be inserted some distance (a) from the probe to match the depth (b) of the vessel, so that a 45-degree angled needle intersects the ultrasound plane at the depth of the vessel.

Step 6: Use short jabs (short in-and-out movements of the needle) to see the approximate course of the needle. Adjust the probe position distance from the needle or angulation (f) (fanning) if the tip of the needle is not seen. Adjust the needle angle or puncture location to move the needle toward the vessel. Eventually, you should see the needle tip compress and puncture the vessel wall.

With a needle guide, the needle is preloaded into a guide attached to the transducer, and the needle angle is fixed to intersect the ultrasound plane at a specified depth. This provides superior control, such that the needle is guaranteed to insert at the specified depth.

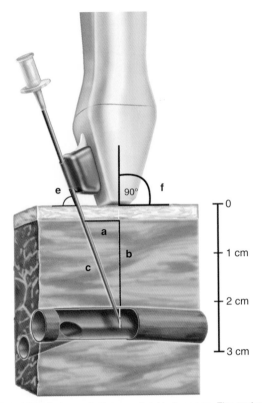

Figure 2.6 Axial technique of ultrasound guided access. The probe is aligned perpendicular (f) to the vessel creating a circular image of the vessel. Without a needle guide, the needle is inserted at an angle (e) and at a distance (a) from beneath the center of the probe. The needle is not visible until it crosses the imaging plane of the probe at a depth (b). Changes to (a), (b), (e), and (f) are interrelated, such that the success of this technique depends on experience, repeated jabbing motions of the needle, and adjustment to probe angle (f) to visualize the course of the needle. With a needle guide selected based on the depth (b) of the vessel, the needle angle (e) is fixed to intersect the ultrasound plane at the set distance below the ultrasound plane, guaranteeing needle puncture at the location imaged. The probe angle (f) can and should be adjusted to allow for a more shallow entry of the needle. *(Modified from Seto AH, Abu-Fadel MS, Sparling JM, et al. Real-time ultrasound guidance facilitates femoral arterial access and reduces vascular complications: FAUST (Femoral Arterial Access With Ultrasound Trial). JACC Cardiovasc Interv. 2010;3:751–758.)*

Step 7: When appropriate blood flashback is seen, the guidewire is inserted through the needle and into the vessel. The ultrasound image can be used to confirm appropriate intravascular placement of the guidewire and that the arteriotomy does not involve the CFA bifurcation.

Tips for ultrasound femoral arterial access:

1. Attempting to cannulate just above the bifurcation will generally avoid a high stick and can be performed consistently with some practice.

2. Combining axial ultrasound with manual palpation of landmarks, fluoroscopic guidance, or longitudinal views of the femoral head can help avoid arteriotomies that are superior to the desired location.

3. Avoid puncturing locations that are heavily calcified on ultrasound to ensure successful access and closure.

4. If a single artery and vein are not well separated laterally and the vein is often located posterior to the artery, and likely represents the superficial femoral artery. Puncture here should be avoided.

5. A needle guide is of particular utility in the femoral artery because it helps control the superior course of the needle.

6. Tilting the probe and needle guide together is a good way of inserting the needle at a flatter/shallower angle (reduced risk of wire/sheath kinking). However doing so will make the point of insertion more superior. Anytime you tilt the transducer, you change the cranial–caudal site of cannulation.

7. The most common cause of a high stick is *tilting the probe cranially* after successfully imaging the CFA bifurcation in a perpendicular angle. Instead, one should image the needle insertion and bifurcation at the same angle and translocate the probe at the fixed, desired angle rather than tilting the probe.

Percutaneous Femoral Vein Puncture

Indications for femoral venous sheath placement in patients undergoing percutaneous coronary intervention (PCI) include the need for transseptal access, intracardiac imaging, temporary pacemaker, or pulmonary artery pressure monitoring. Avoid unnecessary or "routine" venous access since bleeding complications are more frequent in combined arterial–venous procedures. Safety indicates avoiding an inadvertent arterial puncture. Common practice accesses the vein first then the artery. If the artery is accidentally punctured, check the location and, if acceptable, place the arterial sheath. Then with an angle slightly more medial try another puncture. Ultrasound guidance is particularly helpful for cannulation of decompressed veins.

Radial Artery Access for PCI

In 1996, to reduce bleeding complications associated with early stent procedures, Kiemeneij of the Netherlands pioneered the radial approach for coronary interventions, increasing the success rate, improving patient comfort, and providing a method for excellent hemostasis in the fully anticoagulated patient. Rates of major bleeding are significantly lower for transradial procedures, even in populations at high risk for arterial access complications, such as women and the elderly. Data from patients of all ages suggest that reduced bleeding may translate into reduced rates of death and ischemic events. In addition, patient comfort and satisfaction are enhanced by the transradial procedure because patients can sit up immediately and ambulate as soon as their sedation has worn off.

Patient Selection for Transradial Intervention

Transradial intervention (TRI) presents an important first-line option for many patients undergoing coronary intervention. Proper patient selection remains central to achieving optimal outcomes. In general, TRI is *avoided* in patients in whom:

1. The radial artery is being considered for use in coronary artery bypass graft (CABG) surgery or in whom hemodialysis via AVF may be necessary, as well as in patients with an existing AVF.

2. There is known upper extremity vascular disease (severe athero-sclerosis, active carotid disease, extreme tortuosity), vascular anomalies, or vasospastic disorders (Raynaud's disease, Buerger's disease, or systemic sclerosis).

3. The procedure will likely require guide catheters of 7F or larger.

Prior CABG is not a contraindication to the radial approach since right or left internal mammary artery graft conduits may be approached from the ipsilateral or even contralateral wrist. Although one small randomized study suggested that CABG patients require more time and guide catheters from the radial approach, most TRI for CABG patients can be successfully performed from the left radial artery with sufficient experience.

Transradial catheterization for ST-elevation acute myocardial infarction (STEMI) can be performed without significant delays in door-to-balloon time and without increasing procedure duration, radiation exposure, or contrast if used in experienced labs with experienced operators. STEMI patients have demonstrated a reduction in mortality with transradial access, likely because of an ability to apply the maximal antithrombotic regimen necessary with less concern for bleeding.

TRI is an especially good option for patients on systemic anticoagulation with elevated international normalized ratio (INR), especially those with mechanical heart valves. The ability to perform angiography without interrupting or bridging anticoagulation is a major logistical advantage. For patients with suspicion of descending aortic dissection or peripheral vascular disease (which preferentially affects the lower extremities), TRI overcomes these potential barriers. In all cases, TRI patient selection should balance the risks and benefits of radial versus femoral access.

Radial Access Technique

Operators should familiarize themselves with the relevant anatomy of the arm and wrist (Fig. 2.7) to avoid cannulation of the radial artery too distally and appreciate anatomic variants that may make moving through the radial artery to ascending aorta challenging.

Use of the Allen's Test

Some labs continue to test the adequacy of the palmar arch collaterals before radial cath, with a concern for hand ischemia during or after transradial access. A full description of the Allen's test is provided in Chapter 2 of *The Cardiac Catheterization Handbook,* 6e (Fig. 2.8). While the Allen test effectively demonstrates the presence of collaterals, its usefulness in predicting hand ischemia has not been demonstrated in prospective studies, and it has issues of subjectivity.

A more objective measurement of satisfactory ulnar flow can also be documented by pulse oximetry. Using oximetry from the ipsilateral thumb (which is primarily fed by the radial artery), the pulse wave is displayed with both arteries open (Fig. 2.9A). The radial artery is then compressed and the pulse wave of ulnar flow observed (Fig. 2.9B and C). The results of the oximetric Allen's test are divided into four grades of waveforms: type A, no change in pulse wave; type B, damping of waveform that returns to normal within 2 minutes; type C, loss of phasic pulse waveform that returns within 2 minutes; type D, loss of pulse waveform without recovery within 2 minutes. Radial artery cannulation is recommended with type A or B results, can be considered with type C results, and may be relatively contraindicated with type D results.

Based on the clinical and physiologic studies to date, although the Allen's and Barbeau's tests can reassure the operators of the adequacy of the palmar arch and ulnar flow, neither is required to proceed with TRI. Many higher volume TRI labs have abandoned the practice of checking the palmar circulation, and, to date, fewer than five cases of major and permanent hand ischemic complications have been reported in the literature from TRI.

Room and Patient Setup

Transradial coronary angiography can be performed from either the right or left arm. In general, the right arm is more convenient because

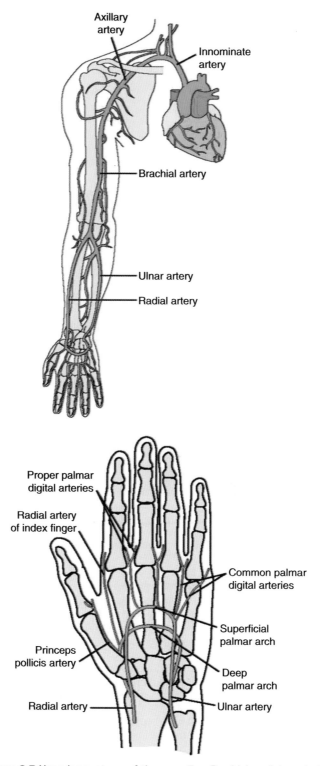

Figure 2.7 Vascular anatomy of the arm. *Top*: Brachial, radial, and ulnar arteries and their connections. *Bottom*: Radial and ulnar arteries as they join the palmar arch. Note that the thumb has its own arterial supply.

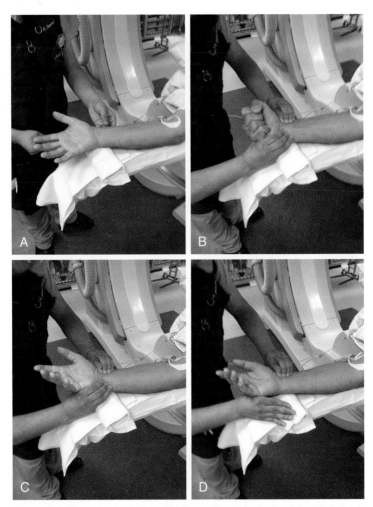

Figure 2.8 Manual Allen's test. (A) Normally, the palm is pink. (B) A fist is made and the radial and ulnar arteries are compressed. (C) The hand is opened and blanches after compression of both ulnar and radial artery. (D) The palm is pink after release of ulnar artery with radial artery occluded.

most catheterization labs are set up with the operator on the right side of the patient and the video screens on the left. Use of the right arm obviates the need to reach over the patient. Recent comparisons have suggested that left radial access and catheter manipulation is similar to that of femoral angiography and may take less time and use less contrast than the right radial approach. During catheterization via the left radial artery, the left arm should be comfortably adducted over the patient's belly toward the operator (standing on the right side) after access has been obtained.

For either the right or left radial approach, correct positioning and preparation of the patient's arm are important for successful arterial access (Fig. 2.10). Preparation and placement of the arm and hand are the same as for the diagnostic procedure. Some operators may employ additional radiation-protective drapes. An optional short (elbow to hand) cushioned arm board typically used for arterial pressure lines can also help to secure the wrist in an optimal position. An innovative way to keep the patient's hand both sterile and free of blood during the procedure is to place a sterile glove on the patient's hand prior to the top drape (Fig. 2.11).

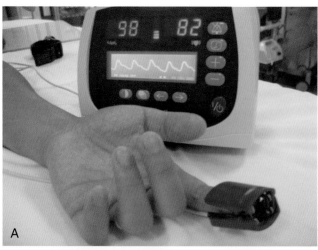

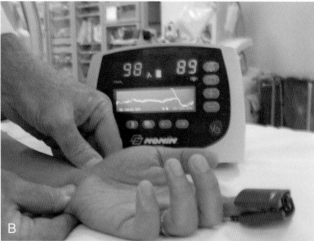

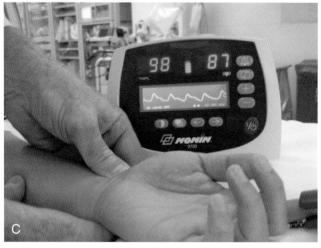

Figure 2.9 (A) Oximetric Allen's test. Before radial or ulnar artery compression, pulse oximeter waveform is normal. (B) Waveform is flat when both radial and ulnar arteries are compressed. (C) Pulse waveform is normal when only ulnar is released. Radial artery is still compressed. This is a type A response. Type B is blunted waveform, and type C is a flattened wave.

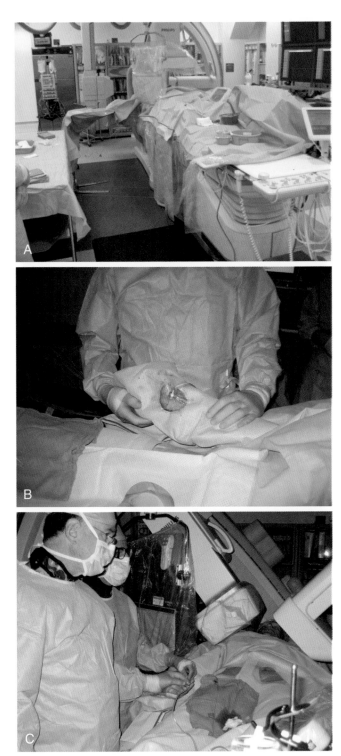

Figure 2.10 (A) Right arm is positioned extended on arm board. (B) After radial sheath insertion, the arm is moved to the patient's hip for introduction of catheters and (C) performance of angiography and intervention.

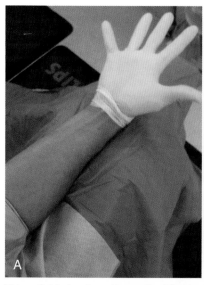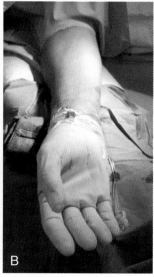

Figure 2.11 An alternative method for draping the hand is to cover the hand with a sterile glove. (A) Arm is prepared with betadine, put through a drape with elastic hole. The glove is then put on hand. (B) Radial access with sheath in artery and tegaderm dressing securing the sheath to the skin and part of the glove.

Whether the groin should also be prepped for a transradial case depends on the comfort and experience of the operator and lab and the type of intervention needed. Access-site crossover rates range from 5% to 10% in most studies. For elective cases, converting to the contralateral radial site is preferable to femoral access.

Ultrasound Imaging for Radial Artery Access

Multiple small trials and one large multicenter trial have demonstrated that ultrasound guidance facilitates radial access by improving the first-pass success rate, decreasing the total number of attempts, and reducing time to access. Ultrasound can also help rescue a failed access by manual palpation, reducing the need for crossover to another access site. However clinical events such as spasm and bleeding are not changed with ultrasound.

Some operators would prefer to utilize ultrasound guidance up front, while others may only turn to it when initial palpation attempts have failed. Absent any benefit in clinical outcomes, either approach is reasonable, though not necessarily as efficient. However the transradial operator should become comfortable with the technique because failure of palpation guidance is ultimately unavoidable. An operator can become proficient after only 25 ultrasound-guided cases.

The following characteristics should lead the operator to consider up front or very early use of ultrasound guidance:

1. Significant hypotension (e.g., shock)
2. Weak pulses (hypotension, peripheral vascular disease [PVD], or obesity)
3. Prior transradial catheterization to rule out radial occlusion
4. Patients at risk of spasm or transradial failure (women, PVD, prior coronary bypass patients)
5. ST-elevation myocardial infarction

The size of the radial artery can be assessed with ultrasound prior to the procedure, which may affect the likelihood of spasm or radial artery occlusion. A very small artery might suggest that smaller sheath sizes, sheathless approaches, or alternative access sites (i.e., ulnar) may be helpful. Preprocedure ultrasound screening may also detect calcified

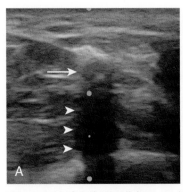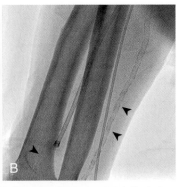

Figure 2.12 Calcified radial artery. (A) Ultrasound image of calcified ulnar artery. Note the prominent posterior shadowing (*white arrowheads*) below the artery (*arrow*). (B) Fluoroscopy demonstrating extensive calcification of ulnar artery (*black arrowheads*) and, to a lesser extent, the radial artery. Ultrasound located a segment of radial artery that was less calcified and successfully cannulated.

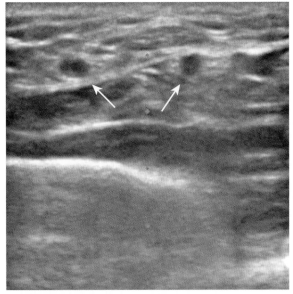

Figure 2.13 Dual radial systems or high radial bifurcations (*arrows*) are evident on ultrasound, where one branch may be small or have a radial loop that can make navigation difficult.

radial arteries (Fig. 2.12), dual radial artery systems (Fig. 2.13), and radial artery loops (Fig. 2.14) in up to 10% of patients, which can make the transradial procedure difficult or unfeasible.

Duplex ultrasonography is the gold standard for detection of radial artery occlusion and may be useful for confirming patent hemostasis. Other complications such as dissections and pseudoaneurysms (Fig. 2.15) are easily detected with ultrasound.

Stepwise Approach to Ultrasound Guided Radial Access

Step 1: Prepare the ultrasound probe with sterile cover. Place sterile gel inside and on the front of the covered probe. The image display settings should be set at a minimum of depth penetration (i.e., 2 cm) and high gain. Turn on the centerline guide markers (see ultrasound setup for femoral access above).

Step 2: Image the radial artery in the axial plane by holding the ultrasound probe perpendicular to the course of the artery (Fig. 2.16).

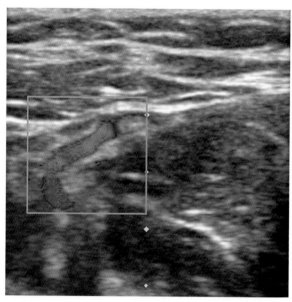

Figure 2.14 Radial artery loop. Preprocedure Doppler ultrasound in axial plane.

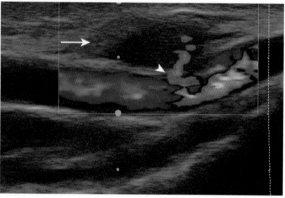

Figure 2.15 Radial pseudoaneurysm (*arrow*) following transradial catheterization. Color Doppler shows the pseudoaneurysm neck with active flow (*arrowhead*).

The artery will be an echolucent circle that pulsates on gentle compression.

Step 3: Align the artery with the centerline guide on the display by moving the probe. This ensures that the artery is directly beneath the center of the probe.

Step 4: Inject lidocaine above the radial artery.

Step 5: Insert the needle into the skin directly underneath the center marking of the probe at about a 45-degree angle. Keep or move the probe close to the needle after skin puncture.

Step 6: Use short jabs (short in-and-out movements of the needle) to track the approximate course of the needle. Adjust the probe position or angulation if the tip of the needle is not seen. Adjust the needle angle or puncture location if needed to have the needle move toward the artery. Eventually, you should see the needle compress and puncture the artery wall.

Step 7: The ultrasound can be used to follow the guidewire up the arm to confirm appropriate intravascular placement.

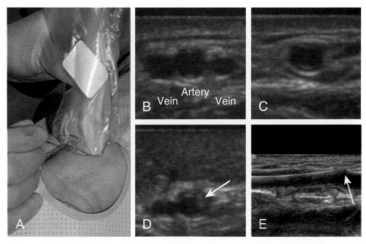

Figure 2.16 Technique of ultrasound-guided radial access. (A) Ultrasound transducer, sterilily wrapped and placed over the radial artery for needle puncture guidance. (B) Visualization of radial artery and veins. (C) Compression causes closure of radial veins and reveals pulsatility of artery. (D) Visualization of the needle tip (*arrow*) compressing and puncturing the artery. (E) Confirmation of wire position (*arrow*) in the radial artery in longitudinal plane.

Box 2.2   Medical Regimen for Radial Catheterization

Before the procedure: Topical anesthetic cream over the radial artery (optional)

1. Sedation: 0.5–1.0 mg versed and 50 mcg fentanyl
2. Typically given together, but one or the other may be used in the elderly or in patients with respiratory compromise.
3. Local anesthetic: 1% lidocaine
4. Use no more than 0.5–1 mL of lidocaine
5. After the sheath is inserted (before catheter insertion) give intra-arterial spasmolytic
6. Nitroglycerin 100–200 mcg for most patients
7. Verapamil 2.5 mg diluted into 10 mL of blood or saline
8. Intravenous unfractionated heparin 40 U/kg bolus up to a maximum of 5000 U
9. After the procedure and before sheath removal: Verapamil, 1–2.5 mg (optional) intra arterial (IA).

Medications for Radial Catheterization

Radial artery spasm is a concern for TRI, particularly for female or small patients and when using 6F or larger sheaths. Common antispasmodic medications include verapamil (2.5 5 mg IA) and nitroglycerin (100–200 mcg IA). Anxiety and high sympathetic tone are also significant contributors to vasospasm, making the use of adequate local anesthesia, sedation, and analgesia important factors for a smooth procedure.

Heparin is mandatory to reduce the risk of radial artery occlusion, but should be given intravenously after the sheath is inserted to reduce pain in the hand. Use heparin 2000–5000 U for diagnostic procedures to maintain postprocedure radial artery patency. A higher dose of heparin (70–100 U/kg) is used to prevent clotting during the PCI procedure.

Box 2.2 provides a sample regimen of drugs and doses used in our lab.

Radial Guide Catheters

In general, there are two types of radial guide catheters: (1) dedicated left and right coronary catheters and (2) universal catheters, intended to cannulate both the left and right coronaries with a single catheter. For multivessel procedures involving right and left coronaries, universal guide catheters, such as the Kimny and Tiger, may obviate the need for exchanges but may require more manipulation to intubate the coronaries. The drawback to universal guide shapes is that they may not provide sufficient guide support for procedures in both coronaries. Examples of guiding catheters are shown in Fig. 2.17.

A useful tip for guide catheter intubation from the wrist is to leave the 0.035-inch wire in the guide, feeding the back end out through the Tuohy-Borst connector and carefully flushing out air. The wire can then safely add torque control, and contrast can be injected to ensure good positioning in the coronary before the wire is withdrawn completely. If the catheter folds up in the aorta while trying to engage the left coronary ostium, the tip should be turned toward the left cusp in the aorta and the wire advanced to assist getting the proper position in the left cusp. Significant tortuosity in the subclavian or innominate artery can interfere with normal transmission of torque and catheter advancement, whereas having the patient breathe deeply can straighten subclavian tortuosity sufficiently to maneuver the catheter.

Although each catheterization lab has its own preferences for guide catheter choice, good options for left coronary cannulation include the EBU, XB, Ikari, and Judkins left catheters. If using a Judkins left (JL) guide, certain adjustments in catheter size should be made because of the different orientation of the catheter in the aorta. When approaching via the right radial artery, engagement of the left coronary typically requires a 0.5-cm smaller curve catheter than that used for transfemoral catheterization. Thus TRI from the right radial artery is typically accomplished using a JL 3.5. In contrast, the standard JL 4 can be used from the left radial artery. For very high anterior left main origins, an Amplatz guide catheter may be needed.

Preferred options for right coronary artery cannulation will vary based on operator experience. Amplatz right and left, multipurpose, and Ikari and Judkins right (JR) catheters can all be used. TRI using a JR guide from the right radial artery requires a 1-cm larger curve than that used from the leg, typically a JR 5 catheter, whereas TRI via the left radial artery can be achieved with the same size curve as from the leg, often the standard JR 4. The Amplatz left (AL) 0.75 guide shape often provides excellent support and control for more challenging PCI of the right coronary artery requiring secure backup from the right radial approach. As with transfemoral interventions, a second wire can also be used to provide extra support, especially for ostial lesions. The use of a guide catheter extension, like the GuideLiner or Guidezilla, is especially useful for marginal seating but caution is needed when it is deep seated. Withdrawal of balloons can cause countertraction on the GuideLiner, forcing it inward and potentially causing a dissection.

The most common cause of failed transradial catheterization is unsuccessful arterial access. Note that the first radial attempt has the highest chance of success. An injured artery may spasm, making subsequent attempts more difficult. Operators should thus proceed slowly and carefully, especially when first learning to obtain radial artery access. Key to reducing local vasospasm is general conscious sedation and adequate but limited local anesthesia. Ultrasound-guided access has high success rates for first-pass entry and increases the likelihood of a successful and quicker procedure.

Key Points for Radial Access

1. The ideal puncture site is greater than 2 cm proximal to the radial styloid, the bony prominence of the distal radius (Fig. 2.18).
2. Mid forearm punctures are more difficult to compress and can result in hematoma formation but may be necessary if the distal vessel is too small or obstructed.

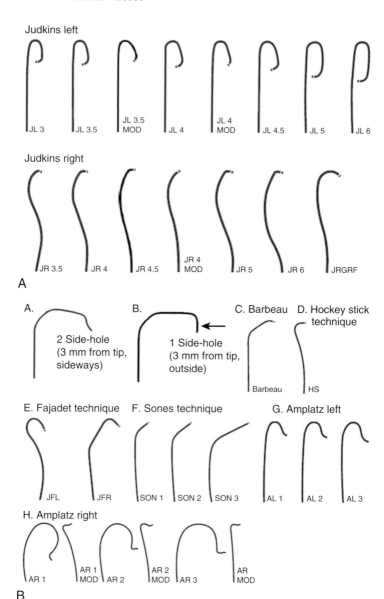

Figure 2.17 (A) Catheter configurations designed for radial artery access coronary angiography. *Top*: Judkins left catheter for left coronary access. Note: Use 0.5 cm smaller than normal if right radial access (Cordis Corp., Bridgewater, NJ). *Bottom*: Judkins right catheter for right coronary and vein graft access. Note: Can use 1 cm larger than normal if right radial access (Cordis Corp., Bridgewater, NJ). (B) Specific transradial catheter for both left and right coronaries (Terumo Medical Corp., Somerset, NJ). Optitorque catheter in Jacky (*right*) and Tiger (*left*) shapes. (C) Barbeau catheter. Specific transradial catheter for both left and right coronaries (Cordis Corp., Bridgewater, NJ). (D) Hockey stick for both right and left coronaries (Cordis Corp., Bridgewater, NJ). (E) Fajadet curve. Specific transradial catheter for left and right coronaries (Cordis Corp., Bridgewater, NJ). (F) Sones or multipurpose catheters for both right and left coronary and vein graft access (Cordis Corp., Bridgewater, NJ). (G) Amplatz left catheter for left and right coronary and vein graft access (Cordis Corp., Bridgewater, NJ). (H) Amplatz right catheter for right coronary (Cordis Corp., Bridgewater, NJ).

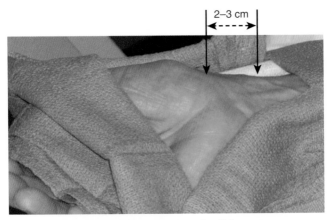

Figure 2.18 Optimal location of radial puncture.

3. The double-wall technique is very effective with the two-component needle (Fig. 2.19). Be sure to advance beyond the back wall before removing the needle.

4. There should be no resistance to wire advancement. If resistance is encountered, fluoroscopy should be used to immediately visualize the wire. Fig. 2.20 shows the steps for radial sheath insertion.

5. Use only the included metal guidewires with bare metal needles because hydrophilic wires can be shredded if they are pulled back against the bevel.

6. A small skin incision facilitates sheath introduction.

7. Hydrophilic-coated sheaths can reduce radial artery spasm and pain upon sheath withdrawal.

8. A large Tegaderm with a slit cut into it can be placed over the sheath to secure the system without the need for sutures and to provide ready access for catheters and guidewires.

9. A radial arterial loop does not necessarily preclude a transradial approach because passage of a 0.014-inch hydrophilic coronary wire can sometimes straighten out tortuous loops, allowing for smooth advancement of catheters.

10. If 7F or larger guide catheters are needed, consider using the slender guides or sheathless guide insertions. Most coronary interventions are possible through 6F guide catheters, including 1.5-mm Rotablator burrs and bifurcation stenting techniques using rapid exchange systems.

Radial Artery Hemostasis and Postprocedure Care

Radial hemostasis is achieved by application of a number of commercial radial artery compression devices. The inflatable Terumo TR Band is popular for its ease of use and the ability to directly visualize the puncture site. Regardless of the device chosen, there are a number of important steps to promote radial artery patency after hemostasis.

Given the superficial position and easy compressibility of the radial artery, checking an activated clotting time is not necessary prior to sheath removal. Another dose of antispasmotic agent may minimize radial artery spasm and patient discomfort. After applying the compression band, the sheath should be removed slowly and smoothly while slowly tightening the band. Tightening the band too aggressively before the sheath is completely removed increases patient discomfort and may strip any clot in the sheath into the artery.

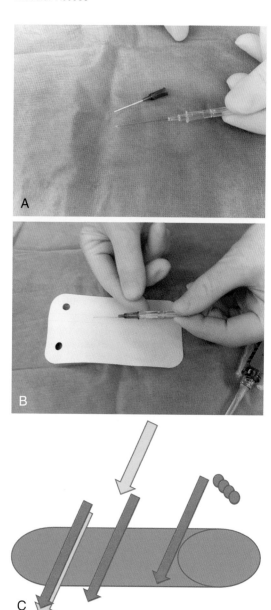

Figure 2.19 (A,B) Radial two-component needle. (C) "Through-and-through" technique for radial puncture. *(Reprinted from Nguyen TN et al., Practical Handbook of Advanced Interventional Cardiology, 3e. Malden, MA: Blackwell; 2008.)*

Figure 2.20 Radial artery access and sheath introduction. Once draped, the radial pulse is palpated. The point of puncture should be 1–2 cm cranial to the bony prominence of the distal radius. Administer a small amount of lidocaine into the skin. Use the micropuncture needle at 30- to 45-degree angulation; slowly advance until blood pulsates out of needle. It will not be a strong pulsation due to the small bore of the needle. Fix needle position and carefully introduce 0.018-inch guidewire with twirling motion. There should be little or no resistance to wire introduction. Remove needle. Make small incision over wire in preparation to introduce sheath. Advance sheath over wire into artery (A). If sheath moves easily, advance to hub. If resistance is felt with sheath halfway in artery, remove wire, and administer vasodilator cocktail. Reinsert wire and continue to advance sheath. Secure sheath with clear plastic dressing or suture (B,C). After sheath is positioned and flushed (D), the arm can now be moved to patient's side for catheter introduction.

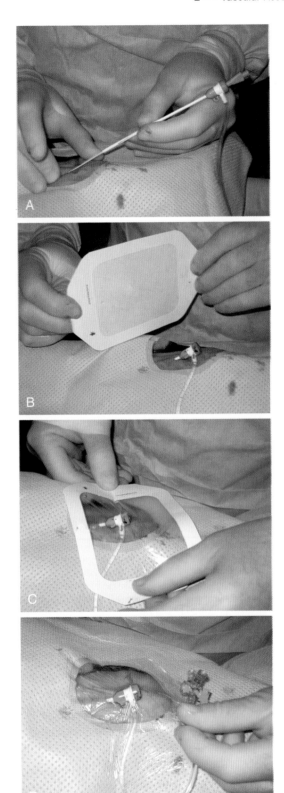

When using a TR Band, the sheath should be pulled out several centimeters (Fig. 2.21) so that the TR Band does not cover the valve portion of the sheath. After applying the TR Band, inflate with 15–17 mL air and pull the sheath out at the same time. Next, the TR Band is slowly deflated until bleeding occurs, at which point 1–2 mL of air should be reinserted into the band. This technique, known as "patent hemostasis," reduces the incidence of radial artery occlusion. In the recovery area, the TR Band is left undisturbed for 1–2 hours (for diagnostic procedures) or 2–4 hours (for interventional procedures) after achievement of hemostasis. Once the band is deflated and removed, a sterile dressing is applied. After discharge, activity restrictions include not using the affected wrist for 24 hours. Patients are instructed to elevate the arm and hold pressure in the event of small hematoma formation and to report large hematomas or significant forearm or hand pain.

Radial Spasm

Radial spasm causes resistance against catheter movement and severe arm pain to the patient. It arises frequently and can preclude completion of a procedure. Risk factors for radial artery spasm include female gender, younger age, small radial artery diameter, large sheaths, diabetes, anxiety, unsuccessful access at first attempt, and prolonged catheter manipulation. Use of sedation, analgesia, and spasmolytic agents is important for both prevention and treatment of spasm. The use of smaller sheaths (including slender systems) or guide catheters can prevent and relieve spasm.

Overcoming severe spasm during sheath removal requires gentle but steady withdrawal of the sheath to minimize patient discomfort. Excessive force should never be applied because this may result in avulsion or rupture of the radial artery. Antispasmodics, sedation, nerve blocks, and anesthesia may be used in escalating fashion for spasm that prevents easy sheath removal.

Radial Complications

Arm Hematoma

Most hematomas develop following transradial sheath removal, but a hematoma can develop during the procedure. Patients complaining of pain or paresthesia (numbness) warrant a close evaluation. During the procedure, checking under the drapes for enlarging hematoma formation is recommended.

A developing forearm hematoma can be managed with compression with a careful arm-wrapping technique. Elastic tape, compression (Ace wrap) bandage, or a manual blood pressure cuff can provide compression to the forearm. Recheck your hemostasis device and reposition if needed. After a few minutes, remove the tape and recheck the forearm; if it is not softer, re-wrap with higher tension and check for hemostasis.

The most serious complication of forearm bleeding and hematoma is a compartment syndrome with resultant hand ischemia. This extremely rare but dangerous problem requires surgical fasciotomy when it occurs. A less dangerous but debilitating complication is chronic regional pain syndrome, or reflex sympathetic dystrophy. This complication, thought to be related to prolonged access site compression, is also very rare and requires only conservative management. Fig. 2.22 provides a guide to radial artery hematoma complications and the management of these problems.

Radial Artery Occlusion

Aside from bleeding, which is typically minor, the most frequent complication of TRI is radial artery occlusion, which affects 3–5% of patients. This is typically asymptomatic, and 50% of such occlusions undergo

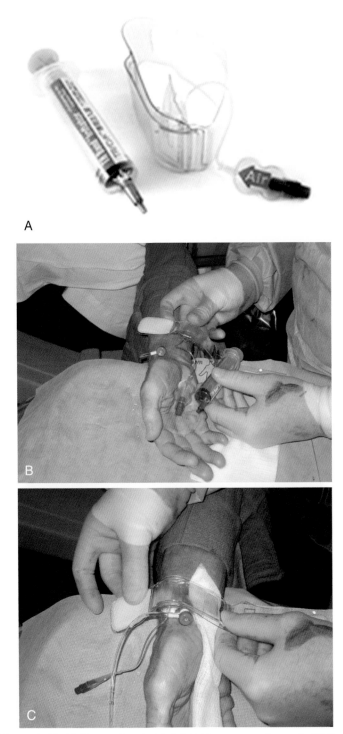

Figure 2.21 (A) Terumo band with inflatable compression pad. (B) Band applied around wrist with green dot over puncture. (C) A thin gauze wick is placed beneath band to absorb blood when pressure is released to assess proper compression pressure in pad.   *Continued*

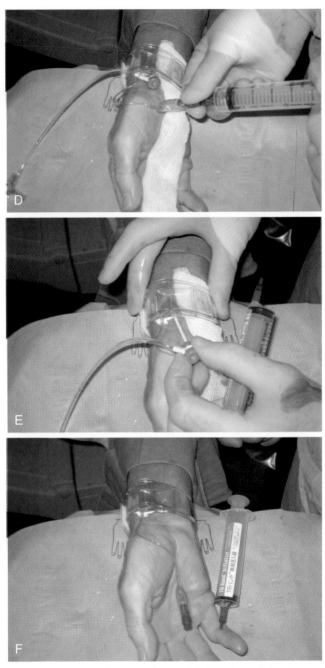

Figure 2.21, cont'd (D) Compression pad inflated. (E) Sheath removed. (F) Final result.

spontaneous recanalization at 30 days. Risk factors for radial artery occlusion include duration of catheterization time, longer sheaths, high sheath-to-artery diameter ratio, insufficient anticoagulation, and prolonged compression time. Systemic heparin is often given after radial access or after positioning of the catheter in the aortic root to help minimize radial occlusion post procedure. Patent hemostasis, confirmed with oximetry or a reverse Allen's test, is the most effective technique to avoid radial artery occlusion. Treatment of asymptomatic radial artery occlusion is typically unnecessary, although studies have described

EASY HEMATOMA CLASSIFICATION
AFTER TRANSRADIAL/ULNAR PCI

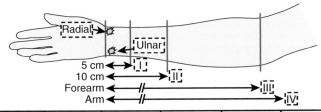

Grade	I	II	III	IV	V
Incidence	≤5%	<3%	<2%	≤0.1%	<0.01%
Definition	Local hematoma, superficial	Hematoma with moderate muscular infiltration	Forearm hematoma and muscular inflitration, below the elbow	Hematoma and muscular infiltration extending above the elbow	Ischemic threat (compartment syndrome)
Treatment	Analgesia Additional bracelet Local ice	Analgesia Additional bracelet Local ice	Analgesia Additional bracelet Local ice Inflated BP cuff	Analgesia Additional bracelet Local ice Inflated BP cuff	Consider surgery
Notes		Inform physician	Inform physician	Inform physician	STAT call to physician
Remarks	- Control blood pressure (BP) (importance of pain management) - Consider interruption of any anticoagulation and/or antiplatelet infusion - Follow forearm and arm diameters to evaluate requirement for additional bracelet and/or BP cuff inflation - Additional bracelet(s) can be placed alongside artery anatomy - Ice cubes in a plastic bag or washcloth are placed on the hematoma - Finger O_2 saturation can be monitored during inflated blood pressure cuff - To inflate blood pressure cuff, select a pressure of 20 mm Hg < systolic pressure and deflate every 15 minutes - After bracelet removal, use "Velpeau bandage" around forearm/arm for a few hours to maintan mild positive pressure				

Bertrand et al. Circulation 2006;114(24):2646-53   ©Hôpital Laval 2002   213-08

Figure 2.22 Diagram of forearm hematoma classification and its management. *(From Bertrand OF et al. Circulation 2006;114(24):2646–2653.)*

using ulnar occlusion and catheter-directed techniques to encourage recanalization.

Rare Complications

Pseudoaneurysm is an uncommon complication that can be diagnosed by ultrasound and treated with compression or thrombin injection. Radial artery dissections and perforations are also rare events that will both seal internally with guide catheter placement. The use of hydrophilic sheaths has been infrequently associated with the formation of sterile abscesses or granulomas. These typically develop 2–3 weeks postprocedure and rarely require drainage.

Percutaneous Brachial Artery Access

In general, percutaneous brachial artery puncture should be abandoned. The rate of bleeding complications is highest in the brachial artery, followed by femoral and radial arteries. The brachial approach may be advantageous in some lower extremity or renal procedures when equipment of sufficient length is unavailable.

Additional Arterial and Venous Access for High-Risk Interventions

For patients at high risk of complications who may require urgent placement of a temporary pacemaker, intra-aortic balloon pump (IABP), or percutaneous ventricular support device, an additional arterial or venous access is helpful. As a standby procedure, a small 4–5F sheath introducer can be placed in the opposite femoral artery or vein at the beginning of the procedure, permitting immediate vascular access if urgent hemodynamic or pacing support is required. Before IABP or other large device insertion, abdominal and iliac angiography should be performed to identify any significant peripheral vascular disease.

Arterial Access Management for Large-Bore Devices

The increase in percutaneous management of structural heart disease has brought increased vascular complications due to larger size (bore) catheters. Currently, the smallest delivery sheath available for TAVR is a 14F sheath. The first step in successful management of the vascular access is proper location of the arteriotomy. Ultrasound-guided access is strongly recommended to avoid the bifurcation and to ensure anterior wall puncture. Some centers will obtain contralateral access using landmarks from angiography. Initial access is often obtained with a smaller 6F sheath followed by "preclosure" preparation with a suture-mediated closure device. Currently, the Perclose ProGlide and ProStar XL devices are the only ones utilized. In both systems, the needles are deployed and the sutures set aside for closure following the procedure. Upsizing of the sheath can commence after the preclosure has been performed. At the conclusion of the procedure, completion of the vascular closure with the predelivered sutures can be performed.

Crossover Technique for Transfemoral Access and Closure (Fig. 2.23)

An additional helpful technique to control bleeding is crossover balloon hemostasis. This method uses a peripheral balloon to occlude the iliac artery after introduction from the contralateral side. It is inflated while closure is being performed. Once completed, hemostasis is confirmed with an angiogram from the contralateral catheter. For complications including incomplete closure or vessel rupture, the peripheral balloon is used for stabilization of the arteriotomy prior to placement of a covered stent.

Technique:

1. Contralateral angiography (e.g., left femoral artery access is performed with a 5F angiographic catheter positioned over the iliac bifurcation) is used to identify the desired location in the target artery (e.g., right common femoral artery). The iliac crossover is generally straightforward, using an internal mammary artery or Omniflush catheter and a standard 0.035-inch hydrophilic wire.

2. Closure of arterial access sites used for large-bore catheters uses percutaneous vascular suture devices like the Prostar XL (Abbott Vascular, Santa Clara, CA) or ProGlide (Abbott Vascular) which are placed at the beginning of access. At the conclusion of the procedure, the large-bore sheath is withdrawn over a 0.035-inch wire to the pelvic brim.

3. To reduce bleeding and have better control of the access site, a crossover balloon is advanced over the iliac bifurcation and inflated. Low-pressure balloon occlusion with a modestly oversized balloon provides proximal hemostasis, thus permitting rapid and easy

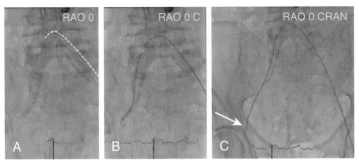

Figure 2.23 Crossover angiographic technique. Basic crossover wire technique. (A) The dotted line outlines the path of a left internal mammary 5F diagnostic catheter used to engage the iliac bifurcation. (B) A standard 0.035-inch J-wire has been passed across the bifurcation. (C) The left mammary catheter has been tracked over the wire to just above the contralateral femoral head, as noted by the white arrow. *(From Perlowski AA, Levisay JP, Salinger MH, Feldman TE. Access and closure for TAVR. Cardiac Interventions Today. September/ October 2014.)*

deployment of the closure sutures. The retrograde 0.035-inch wire is removed, provided adequate hemostasis has been achieved.

Overcoming Difficult Vascular Access Problems

Excessive Vessel Tortuosity

The most frequently encountered difficulty in advancing guide catheters is tortuosity of the iliac or subclavian vessels, a condition often found in elderly patients. A steerable 0.038-inch flexible guidewire (e.g., Wholey, Benson) is excellent for negotiating tortuous vessels. Its flexible, atraumatic, gently curved tip is steerable, thus increasing safety. In cases of extreme tortuosity, a JR diagnostic catheter may be used to help direct the guidewire tip and control the advancement of the guidewire. Angiograms will delineate the arterial course and any other obstructive lesions. Once the guidewire is beyond the tortuous or narrowed segments, further catheter exchanges should use a long exchange-length guidewire. A longer (>30 cm) or braided vascular sheath can be positioned and is often effective in straightening tortuous segments.

Commonly selected equipment for tortuous vessels includes:

1. Wholey 0.035-inch steerable guidewires (crossing)
2. Angled hydrophilic wire (crossing)
3. Angled hydrophilic glide catheter
4. Long 300-cm regular exchange guidewires
5. Long 300-cm extra-stiff exchange guidewires
6. Long arterial sheaths of 23 to 90 cm

Peripheral Vascular Disease

PVD complicates access as well as guide catheter manipulation. Weak femoral pulses often indicate atherosclerotic obstruction at the level of the femoral, common iliac, or aortoiliac bifurcation. Inability to advance the guidewire to the central aortic position requires angiography to determine further maneuvers needed to negotiate the femoral approach. In such patients, abdominal aortography and peripheral angiography are necessary to evaluate the extent of obstructive disease with focal iliac stenosis. Should a coronary intervention be required, some operators advocate iliac stent placement before proceeding with PCI. PVD may require the use of the radial approach. In patients with PVD of the lower extremities, coexistent subclavian atherosclerosis may also complicate arm access.

Access Through Inguinal Scarring, Previous Vascular Closure Device, or Synthetic Vascular Graft

Inguinal scarring may be present in patients having multiple prior interventional procedures, aortofemoral bypass surgery, femoral bypass cannula access, IABP repair, or radiation therapy. In some of these patients, a synthetic arterial conduit graft may be present but is often calcified. If possible, select an alternative access site. Otherwise, access of a severely fibrotic or scarred groin or through a femoral bypass graft may require successive dilations with 5, 6, 7, and 8F dilators before inserting a vascular sheath one size smaller than the largest dilator. Perclose and Starclose closure devices have difficulty penetrating calcified or fibrotic arteries and should be used with caution only if the tract is well dilated. Entrapment of a StarClose clip during placement in a scarred groin has been reported.

Most vascular closure device manufacturers indicate that reaccess through a site with a recently placed closure device can be performed without a problem if the device has no internal artery fixation component. Caution should be used when reaccessing all sites but especially those closed with Angio-Seal, although there are no reports of Angio-Seal anchor dislodgement during reaccess. Access of sites closed with such devices after 2–4 weeks is thought to be safe. However the contralateral femoral artery should be considered in most cases for patient comfort.

Hemostasis After Femoral PCI

Complications related to vascular access management are the most significant cause of morbidity and prolonged hospitalization. Timely and safe removal of the arterial sheath with minimal patient discomfort is the goal of a successful intervention. Improved outcomes have been associated with using smaller sheaths, discontinuation of post-PCI heparin infusions, and early removal of the sheath. Although results are improving, resources (both staff and equipment) necessary for appropriate sheath care and hemostasis are critically important to good outcomes.

Immediate Sheath Removal

The femoral arterial and venous sheaths are not routinely left in place after PCI. The presence of a vascular sheath in a heavily anticoagulated patient predisposes to hemorrhage and retroperitoneal hematoma. Most laboratories remove sheaths within a few hours after the procedure or immediately remove the sheath in the laboratory after hemostasis with a vascular closure device.

Femoral PCI Sheath Removal

Sheath removal after PCI may occur in the lab, holding area, or at patient's bedside. Manual sheath removal proceeds as described for diagnostic procedures. Several points should be kept in mind for manual sheath removal:

1. Adjust bed height or use a footstool to exert maximal pressure downward for puncture site compression with minimal fatigue.
2. Ensure good intravenous access.
3. Give local anesthetic (10–20 mL of 1% lidocaine) to the skin around the sheath and intravenous analgesics before sheath removal.
4. Have atropine and pain medication available.

5. Before removing the sheath, check that the heparin is stopped, the activated clotting time (ACT) is less than 150 seconds, vital signs are stable, no chest pain is present, and there are no plans for recatheterization.

6. If both arterial and venous sheaths were used, remove the arterial sheath first, preserving good venous access in case the peripheral IV stops working. Avoid prolonged pressure on the femoral vein. Prolonged venous occlusion, especially with pressure devices, may cause venous thrombosis. Check the leg and foot for cyanosis.

7. The duration of pressure holding, usually 15–20 minutes, depends on the sheath size, ACT, and ease of bleeding control.

8. When longer pressure application is needed after removal of a large sheath, IABP catheter, or cardiopulmonary support cannula, the FemoStop (St. Jude Medical, St. Paul, MN) or similar compression device is one of the preferred methods of mechanical arterial compression (Fig. 2.24). Compression devices provide a constant stable pressure, relative patient comfort, and easy adjustment of the degree of pressure applied. Compression devices are not intended for unsupervised use. The duration of pressure application should be kept to a minimum to decrease complications such as skin necrosis, nerve compression, or venous thrombosis.

Femoral Compression Systems

The FemoStop system (St. Jude Medical, St. Paul, MN; Fig. 2.24) is an air-filled, clear plastic compression bubble that molds to the skin contours. It is held in place by straps passing around the hips. The amount of pressure applied is controlled with an insufflator connected to a sphygmomanometer gauge. The clear plastic dome permits visualization of the puncture site. The FemoStop is mostly used for patients in whom prolonged compression is anticipated or if bleeding persists despite prolonged manual compression. The duration of FemoStop compression and time to removal of the device varies depending on the patient and staff protocols. In some hospitals, the time from application to removal may be less than 30 minutes. In other patients in whom hemostasis is required, the device may be left at a lower pressure for longer. Mechanical C-clamp systems are rarely used. Femoral compression systems should not be used in patients with lower extremity bypass grafts (fem-pop) at the access site due to the risk of graft thrombosis.

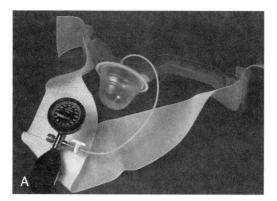

Figure 2.24 Use of the FemoStop. (A) Before proceeding, examine puncture site carefully; note and mark edges of any hematoma; record current blood pressure. *Continued*

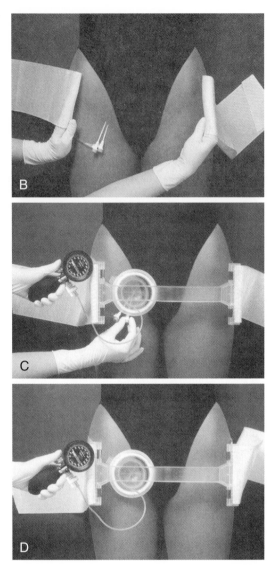

Figure 2.24, cont'd (B) Position belt. The belt should be aligned with the puncture site equally across both hips. Center the dome and adjust belt. (C) The dome should be centered over the arterial puncture site above and slightly toward the midline of the skin incision. The sheath valve should be below the rim of the pressure dome. Attach belt to ensure a snug fit. The center arch bar should be perpendicular to the body. (D) Connect dome pressure pump. Right side, for the arterial sheath, pressurize dome to 60–80 mm Hg and remove sheath and increase pressure in dome to 10–20 mm above systolic arterial pressure. Maintain full compression for 3 minutes. Reduce pressure in dome by 10–20 mm Hg every few minutes until 0 mm Hg. Check arterial pulse. Observe for bleeding. After hemostasis is obtained, remove FemoStop and dress wound. *(From Kern MJ.* The Cardiac Catheterization Handbook, *4e. Philadelphia: Mosby, 2003:67–69.)*

Vascular Closure Devices and In-Lab Hemostasis

Immediate hemostasis can be achieved in the catheterization suite using one of several vascular closure devices. Before selecting the device, femoral angiography from an oblique projection will indicate the suitability of the device insertion. Note that the ipsilateral oblique view (e.g., the right anterior oblique [RAO] for right femoral artery) best displays the bifurcation of the profunda and superficial femoral branches.

Vascular closure devices (VCDs) were developed both to obtain quick, safe hemostasis and to improve patient comfort by decreasing the time patients lie flat after the procedure. The safety of VCDs has been demonstrated in diagnostic catheterization and interventions. Most catheterization laboratories report high success rates for various closure devices used directly after PCI in fully anticoagulated patients receiving antithrombins, heparin, or glycoprotein receptor blockers. Four commonly used VCDs are shown in Table 2.1.

For repeat procedures, restick in the same vessel should be directed 1–2 cm above or below the site of the previous device placement site.

Key Points in Postprocedure Sheath Care and Hemostasis

1. "Do it right the first time." The best results stem from a meticulous arterial puncture, correct sheath placement, and careful removal and hemostasis.
2. For transport to the holding area, if the sheath is left in place, placing an appropriately sized obturator in the sheath may prevent sheath kinking (and bleeding) before sheath removal.
3. Use a clear transparent dressing over the puncture site for easy visualization of bleeding. Do not use a wad of gauze under the dressing because the combination of blood and gauze is an excellent culture media for bacteria.
4. Inspect and palpate the puncture site and distal pulses at each postprocedure check.
5. A downward trend in blood pressure and upward trend in heart rate are early warning signs of bleeding, especially occult bleeding such as a retroperitoneal hematoma (RPH). Hypotension after PCI should be assumed to be due to bleeding until the operator has identified an alternate cause (e.g., vagal reaction, ischemia, tamponade, overmedicated). If in doubt about whether there is an RPH and the patient is stable, CT scan may be helpful.

Complications of Arterial Access

Hemorrhage

The most common complication from femoral cardiac catheterization is hemorrhage and local hematoma formation, increasing in frequency with the increasing size of the sheath, the amount of anticoagulation, and the degree of obesity of the patient.

Other common complications (in order of decreasing frequency) include RPH, pseudoaneurysm, AVF formation, arterial thrombosis secondary to intimal dissection, stroke, sepsis with or without abscess formation, and cholesterol or air embolization. The frequency of these complications is increased in high-risk procedures; critically ill elderly patients with extensive atheromatous disease; patients receiving anticoagulation, antiplatelet, and fibrinolytic therapies; and patients receiving concomitant interventional procedures. Compared to the femoral approach, the brachial (but not radial) approach carries a slightly higher risk of vascular complications.

Infections and Other Rare Events

Infections are more frequent in patients undergoing repeat ipsilateral (same site) femoral punctures or prolonged femoral sheath maintenance

Table 2.1

Vascular Closure Devices

Device	On the Market	Mechanism	Advantages	Disadvantages	Sheath Sizes	Ipsilateral Access <90 Days
AngioSeal (St. Jude Medical, St. Paul, MN)	1997 to present	Collagen and suture mediated	Secure closure, long track record	Intra-arterial component, possible thromboembolic complications, infection related to suture serving as a wick	6 and 8F	1 cm higher
Perclose (Abbott Vascular, Redwood City, CA)	1997 to present	Suture mediated	Secure closure	Intra-arterial component, steep learning curve, device failure may require surgical repair	5–8F	No restrictions
StarClose (Abbott Vascular, Redwood City, CA)	2005 to present	Nitinol clip	No intra-arterial component	Adequate skin tract needed to prevent device failure	5–6F	Not fully established
Mynx (Access Closure, Mountain View, CA)	2007 to present	PEG hydrogel plug	No intra-arterial component, potential use in PVD	Possible intra-arterial injection of sealant, Failure rate	5–7F	No restrictions

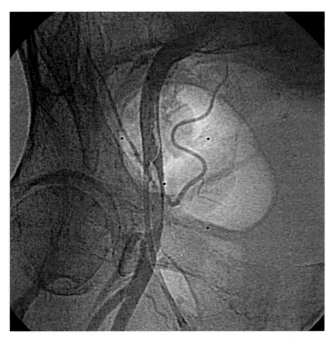

Figure 2.25 A femoral artery dissection induced by access difficulties.

(within 1–5 days). Cholesterol embolism, manifesting with abdominal pain or headache (from mesenteric or central nervous system ischemia), skin mottling ("blue toes"), renal insufficiency, or lung hemorrhage, may be a clinical finding in up to 30% of high-risk patients.

Retroperitoneal Hematomas and Pseudoaneurysms

An RPH should be suspected in patients with hypotension, tachycardia, pallor, a rapidly falling hematocrit postcatheterization, lower abdominal or back pain, or neurologic changes in the leg with the puncture. An RPH may also manifest with back pain and symptoms similar to a vagal reaction, with bradycardia and hypotension not responsive to medications. This complication is associated with *high femoral arterial puncture* and full anticoagulation. Consider a return to the cath lab to identify and control femoral bleeding. Access the contralateral artery for angiography of the suspected site and possible treatment in patients with a high clinical risk of RPH.

Pseudoaneurysm is a complication associated with *low femoral arterial puncture* (usually below the head of the femur). In the past, to avoid further neurovascular complication or rupture, the vascular surgeon routinely repaired all femoral pseudoaneurysms. With ultrasound imaging techniques, these false channels can be easily identified, and nonsurgical closure can be selected. Manual compression of the expansile growing mass, guided by Doppler ultrasound with or without thrombin or collagen injection, is an acceptable therapy for femoral pseudoaneurysm.

Fig. 2.25 shows a femoral artery dissection induced by access difficulties. Fig. 2.26 shows a femoral arteriovenous fistula. Note simultaneous contrast filling of both artery and vein. These complications are not applicable to radial artery PCI.

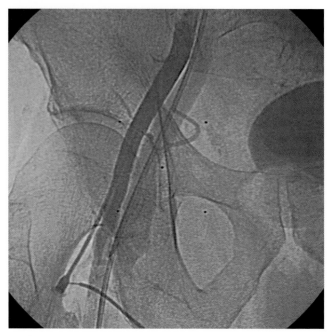

Figure 2.26 A femoral arteriovenous fistula. Note simultaneous contrast filling of both artery and vein. These complications are not applicable to radial artery PCI.

Suggested Readings

Achenbach S, et al. Transradial versus transfemoral approach for coronary angiography and intervention in patients above 75 years of age. *Catheter Cardiovasc Interv*. 2008;72:628-635.

Applegate RJ, et al. Restick following initial Angioseal use. *Catheter Cardiovasc Interv*. 2003;58(2):181-184.

Barbeau GR, et al. Evaluation of the ulnopalmar arterial arches with pulse oximetry and plethysmography: comparison with the Allen's test in 1010 patients. *Am Heart J*. 2004;147:489-493.

Burzotta F, et al. Transradial approach for coronary angiography and interventions in patients with coronary bypass grafts: tips and tricks. *Catheter Cardiovasc Interv*. 2008;72:263-272.

Chambers CE, et al. Defining the length of stay following percutaneous coronary intervention: an expert consensus document from the Society for Cardiovascular Angiography and Interventions. *Catheter Cardiovasc Interv*. 2009;73:847-858.

Chodor P, et al. RADIal versus femoral approach for percutaneous coronary interventions in patients with acute myocardial infarction (RADIAMI): a prospective, randomized, single-center clinical trial. *Cardiol J*. 2009;16:332-340.

Cura FA, Kapadia SR, Carey D, et al. Complications of femoral artery closure devices. *Cathet Cardiovasc Interv*. 2001;52:3.

Dangas G, Mehran R, Kokolis S, et al. Vascular complications after percutaneous interventions following hemostasis with manual compression versus arteriotomy closure devices. *J Am Coll Cardiol*. 2001;38:638-641.

Dauerman HL, Applegate RJ, Cohen DJ. Vascular closure devices: the second decade. *J Am Coll Cardiol*. 2007;50:1617-1626.

Doyle BJ, et al. Bleeding, blood transfusion, and increased mortality after percutaneous coronary intervention: implications for contemporary practice. *J Am Coll Cardiol*. 2009;53:2019-2027.

Jabara R, Gadesam R, Pendyala L, et al. Ambulatory discharge after transradial coronary intervention: preliminary U.S. single-center experience (Same-Day Transradial Intervention and Discharge Evaluation, the STRIDE Study). *Am Heart J*. 2008;156:1141-1146.

Kiemeneij F, et al. Hydrophilic coating aids radial sheath withdrawal and reduces patient discomfort following transradial coronary intervention: a randomized double-blind comparison of coated and uncoated sheaths. *Catheter Cardiovasc Interv*. 2003;59:161-164.

Kiemeneij F, et al. Evaluation of a spasmolytic cocktail to prevent radial artery spasm during coronary procedures. *Catheter Cardiovasc Interv*. 2003;58:281-284.

Naidu SS, Aronow HD, Box LC, et al. SCAI Expert Consensus Statement: 2016 Best Practices in the Cardiac Catheterization Laboratory. (Endorsed by the Cardiological Society of India, and Sociedad Latino Americana de Cardiologia Intervencionista; Affirmation of Value by the Canadian Association of Interventional Cardiology–Association Canadienne de Cardiologie d'intervention). *Catheter Cardiovasc Interv*. 2016.

Pancholy SB. Comparison of the effect of intra-arterial versus intravenous heparin on radial artery occlusion after transradial catheterization. *Am J Cardiol*. 2009;104:1083-1085.

Pancholy SB, et al. Prevention of radial artery occlusion—patent hemostasis evaluation trial (PROPHET study): a randomized comparison of traditional versus patency documented hemostasis after transradial catheterization. *Catheter Cardiovasc Interv*. 2008;72:335-340.

Patel MR, Jneid H, Derdeyn CP, et al.; on behalf of the American Heart Association Diagnostic and Interventional Cardiac Catheterization Committee of the Council on Clinical Cardiology, Council on Cardiovascular Radiology and Intervention, and Council on Peripheral Vascular Disease. Arteriotomy closure devices for cardiovascular procedures. A scientific statement from the American Heart Association. *Circulation*. 2010.

Patel T, Shah S, Ranjan A. *Patel's atlas of transradial intervention: the basics*. Seattle, WA: Sea Script Company; 2007.

Pristipino C, et al. Major improvement of percutaneous cardiovascular procedure outcomes with radial artery catheterization: results from the PREVAIL study. *Heart*. 2009;95:476-482.

Rao SV, et al. The transradial approach to percutaneous coronary intervention: historical perspective, current concepts, and future directions. *J Am Coll Cardiol*. 2010;55:2187-2195.

Rathore S, et al. Impact of length and hydrophilic coating of the introducer sheath on radial artery spasm during transradial coronary intervention: a randomized study. *JACC Cardiovasc Interv*. 2010;3:475-483.

Resnic FS, Blake GJ, Ohno-Machado L, et al. Vascular closure devices and the risk of vascular complications after percutaneous coronary intervention in patients receiving glycoprotein IIb–IIIa inhibitors. *Am J Cardiol*. 2001;88:493-496.

Sanborn TA, Ebrahimi R, Manoukian SV, et al. Impact of femoral vascular closure devices and antithrombotic therapy on access site bleeding in acute coronary syndromes: the Acute Catheterization and Urgent Intervention Triage Strategy (ACUITY) Trial. *Circ Cardiovasc Interv*. 2010;3:57-62.

Waksman R, King SB, Douglas JS, et al. Predictors of groin complications after balloon and new-device coronary intervention. *Am J Cardiol*. 1995;75:886-889.

Ziakas A. Safety of same-day discharge radial percutaneous coronary intervention: a retrospective study. *Am Heart J*. 2003;146:699-704.

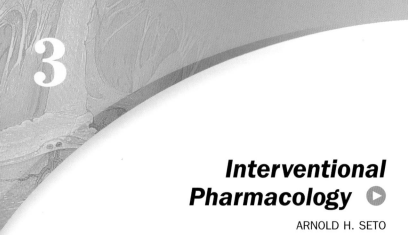

3

Interventional Pharmacology ▶

ARNOLD H. SETO

Successful coronary, structural, and peripheral interventions rely not only on mechanical tools such as balloons, wires, and stents, but also on adjunctive pharmacologic agents. Familiarity with commonly used anticoagulant and antiplatelet medications is required for the safe use of interventional equipment, while other agents such as vasodilators and vasopressors may be necessary in selected patients. Recent advances have introduced a number of agents with similar functions, and understanding the nuances of each can help tailor the pharmacology to each patient's bleeding and thrombotic risk.

Antithrombotic and antiplatelet agents for percutaneous coronary intervention (PCI) are summarized in Box 3.1, and recommendations from the American College of Cardiologists (ACC)/American Heart Association (AHA) are summarized in Table 3.1.

Anticoagulants

Unfractionated Heparin

Unfractionated heparin (UFH) is a mixture of polysaccharide molecules, one-third of which contain the key pentasaccharide sequence that binds to antithrombin. UFH accelerates the activity of antithrombin III (AT III), a molecule that breaks down the procoagulant factor IIa (thrombin) and factor Xa by forming a complex with AT III and thrombin. Fig. 3.1 diagrams the coagulation cascade and role of antithrombins.

Clinical Use

Due to variability in various heparin preparations and protein binding, monitoring of anticoagulant effect is necessary, with a goal of an activated partial thromboplastin time (aPTT) of 50–75 seconds, or 1.5–2.5 the upper limit of normal. The aPTT is not used in the catheterization laboratory because it saturates at the doses of heparin used for PCI. Instead, for PCI anticoagulation is measured using the whole blood activated clotting time (ACT), with a goal of 250–350 seconds or 200–250 seconds if using a GP IIb/IIIa inhibitor. The optimal ACT is instrument- and laboratory-dependent, with data suggesting higher rates of bleeding at higher ACT levels. Typical bolus IV UFH doses in the catheterization laboratory are 70–100 U/kg, or 50–60 U/kg with GP IIb/IIIa inhibitors. Repeated ACT measurements should be made with prolonged procedures, approximately every 20–30 minutes. Despite a theoretical risk of reactivation of coagulation with UFH discontinuation, continued heparinization following a successful PCI procedure has been associated with an increased risk of bleeding without ischemic benefits and is not recommended.

The half-life of UFH is 1.5 hours, allowing for greater control of the anticoagulant effect. Discontinuation of a UFH IV drip can normalize

Box 3.1 Antithrombotic and Antiplatelet Agents for Percutaneous Coronary Interventions

Antithrombotic Therapy

- Heparin (unfractionated)
- Low-molecular-weight heparin (enoxaparin [Lovenox], dalteparin [Fragmin], tinzaparin [Innohep])
- Direct thrombin inhibitor—Polypeptide inhibitor (bivalirudin [Angiomax])
  —Low-molecular-weight inhibitor (argatroban [Acova])

Antiplatelet Therapy

- Cyclooxygenase inhibitors (aspirin)
- Adenosine diphosphate (ADP) receptor inhibitors (clopidogrel [Plavix], prasugrel [Effient], ticlopidine [Ticlid])
- Phosphodiesterase inhibitors (cilostazol [Pletal])
- Glycoprotein IIb/IIIa receptor inhibitors (abciximab [ReoPro], eptifibatide [Integrilin], tirofiban [Aggrastat])
- Adenosine reuptake inhibitors (dipyridamole [Persantine])
- Cyclo-pentyl-triazolo-pyrimidines (CPTPs) (ticagrelor [Brilinta])
- Platelet activating receptor (PAR-1) antagonist (vorapaxar [Zontivity])

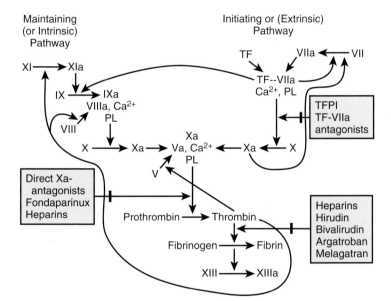

Figure 3.1 Diagrams of the coagulation cascade and role of antithrombins. *(Adapted from Wiley-Liss, Inc., a subsidiary of John Wiley & Sons, Inc. from Conde ID, Kleiman NS. Arterial thrombosis for the interventional cardiologist: from adhesion molecules and coagulation factors to clinical therapeutics.* Catheter Cardiovasc Interv. *2003;60:236–246; and Garg R, Uretsky BF, Lev EL. Anti-platelet and anti-thrombotic approaches in patients undergoing percutaneous coronary intervention.* Catheter Cardiovasc Interv. *2007;70:388–406.)*

the clotting cascade in a few hours. If there is a need to discontinue the anticoagulant effect of UFH emergently, protamine sulfate can be given, which forms an ion pair with UFH to neutralize it. Protamine dosage for UFH reversal is 1–1.5 mg IV per 100 units of remaining active UFH, based on the time course of UFH administration (max 50 mg/dose at 5 mg/min). Although most of the protamine sulfate used today is recombinant, caution should be used in patients with fish allergies because some proportion may still be derived from fish sperm. Typical protamine allergic reactions can include hypotension and bronchoconstriction due to histamine release. A slow IV infusion, while closely monitoring the patient, may mitigate the severity of the reaction. Care

Table 3.1

2013–2014 ACC/AHA Recommendations for Pharmacologic Management of Patients Undergoing Percutaneous Coronary Interventions for Acute Coronary Syndromes			
Drug	**Unstable Angina/ NSTEMI**	**STEMI**	**Comments**
Aspirin	I (LOE A)	I (LOE B)	162–325 mcg loading, 81 mg maintenance
Clopidogrel	I (LOE B)	I (LOE B)	Loading dose of 600 mg recommended as early as possible
Prasugrel	I (LOE B)	I (LOE B)	Contraindicated in patients with prior stroke or TIA. Not recommended prior to PCI.
Ticagrelor	I (LOE B)	I (LOE B)	IIa recommendation to use in preference to clopidogrel in PCI pts
Unfractionated heparin	I (LOE B)	I (LOE C)	
Low-molecular-weight heparin	I (LOE A)	I (LOE A) only for post-lytic pt	Not recommended for primary PCI
Bivalirudin	I (LOE B)	I (LOE B)	Especially for patients at high risk of bleeding
Fondaparinux	I (LOE B)	III (LOE B) for use as sole anticoagulant	Requires an additional antithrombin during PCI. Preferred for conservative strategy.
Glycoprotein IIb/IIIa inhibitors	IIb (LOE B)	IIa (LOE A-B) IIb for intracoronary or prehospital use	IIa in selected patients without preloading clopidogrel, or with significant thrombus burden; IIb otherwise

ACC, American College of Cardiology; *AHA,* American Heart Association; *NSTEMI,* non-ST-segment elevation myocardial infarction; *PCI,* percutaneous coronary intervention; *STEMI,* ST-segment elevation myocardial infarction.
　　From O'Gara et al. 2013 ACCF/AHA guideline for the management of ST-elevation myocardial infarction: executive summary: a report of the American College of Cardiology Foundation/American Heart Association Task Force on Practice Guidelines. *J Am Coll Cardiol.* 2013;61(4):485–510; and Amsterdam et al. 2014 AHA/ACC Guideline for the Management of Patients with Non-ST-Elevation Acute Coronary Syndromes: a report of the American College of Cardiology/American Heart Association Task Force on Practice Guidelines. *J Am Coll Cardiol.* 2014;64(24):e139–e228.

should also be observed in diabetic patients taking protamine-containing insulin preparations (e.g., NPH insulin) because they are at increased risk for severe protamine reactions, including anaphylaxis.

Heparin Mode of Action

1. Heparin is a mixture of glycosaminoglycans (mucopolysaccharides) that combine with a plasma protein called antithrombin III (AT III) to make the AT III a highly effective inhibitor of thrombin and several other clotting factors.
2. Heparin requires the presence of AT III to be effective.
3. Unfractionated heparin is a heterogeneous polysaccharide that binds to antithrombin to inhibit thrombin and factor Xa.

Side Effects

Heparin-Induced Thrombocytopenia. Heparin-induced thrombocytopenia (HIT) can cause an immune-mediated thrombocytopenia that can lead to thrombosis, stroke, loss of limb, or other ischemic events (e.g., heparin-induced thrombocytopenia with thrombosis [HITT]). If heparin is given after the procedure, monitor platelet count daily. If platelets fall below 100,000 or by more than 50%, discontinue heparin and consider the possible etiologies of thrombocytopenia.

There are two types of HIT (Table 3.2). Type I HIT (HIT-1) is due to direct (non–immune-mediated) platelet activation, with mild thrombocytopenia and a benign clinical course. Type II HIT (HIT-2) is due to immune-mediated platelet activation, with moderate or severe thrombocytopenia and serious thromboembolic complications. Platelet transfusions should not be used to treat HIT due to increased risk of thrombotic complications. Anticoagulation to prevent thrombosis is the main treatment of HIT-2 patients; typical drugs are the direct-acting thrombin antagonists lepirudin and argatroban.

Minor Bleeding (Puncture Site, Gums). Discontinue heparin. Monitor vital signs, aPTT, hemoglobin, hematocrit, platelet count, ACT.

Major Bleeding (Retroperitoneal, Gastrointestinal). For major bleeding complications or for reversal of anticoagulation, heparin infusion should be discontinued. Protamine sulfate (1% solution) is administered at a dose of 1 mg/100 U heparin or approximately 25 mg slow IV injection over 10 minutes. Vital signs, aPTT, hemoglobin, hematocrit, platelet count, and ACT should be monitored, with administration of blood transfusions as needed. The bleeding site should be assessed for the need for therapeutic interventions. Subcutaneous heparin administered in large doses may require repeat doses of protamine after 1 hour.

Monitor for allergic reactions to protamine and have resuscitation equipment available. Morphine or meperidine may be helpful for chills.

Low-Molecular-Weight Heparin

Low-molecular-weight heparins (LMWH: enoxaparin, tinzaparin, dalteparin) are fractionated heparins with molecular weights between 3000 and

Table 3.2

Heparin-Induced Thrombocytopenia		
	Type I Heparin-Induced Thrombocytopenia	**Type II Heparin-Induced Thrombocytopenia**
Incidence	10%	Rare (0.2%)
Mechanism	Direct platelet aggregating effect of heparin	Autoantibody (IgG) directed against platelet factor IV–heparin complex
Onset	Early (within 2 days)	Later (4–10 days)
Platelet count	50,000–150,000/mm^3	<50,000/mm^3
Duration	Transient; often improves even if heparin is continued	Requires discontinuation of all heparin; gradual recovery in platelet count in most patients
Clinical	Benign	Recalcitrant venous and arterial course thromboses and thromboembolism; may be fatal
Heparin	Unfractionated or low-molecular-weight heparin may be continued	Argatroban for longer treatment. Bivalirudin for PCI or short term treatment Danaparoid and lipirudin not available in the United States.

7000 daltons (UFH is 3000–30,000 daltons). Like UFH, LMWH binds to antithrombin and causes inhibition of factor Xa and thrombin. Due to improved subcutaneous absorption, LMWH can be administered either SQ or IV.

LMWHs have features distinct from UFH, including:

1. More predictable anticoagulation effect
2. Lack of inhibition by platelet factor 4
3. Lack of need for monitoring
4. Lower risk of HIT
5. SQ or IV bolus administration

Table 3.3 compares features of LMWHs with UFH.

Absorption and Clearance

Peak plasma anti-Xa levels are achieved 3–4 hours after SQ dosing and are detectable for up to 12 hours. LMWH is eliminated via the kidneys, and caution should be used for patients with creatinine clearance of less than 30 mL/min. LMWH can be given intravenously or subcutaneously but not intramuscularly. It has a half-life of 2–4 hours, longer than UFH.

Monitoring

The ACT assay does not reliably measure LMWH effect. LMWH activity is measured using blood anti-Xa levels. Routine monitoring is not indicated in most cases and is not readily available in many catheterization laboratories. LMWHs have very predictable antithrombotic effects; monitoring and dose adjustment is necessary only in obese patients (body mass index [BMI] >40) or patients with renal insufficiency.

Clinical Use

Enoxaparin is the best studied of the LMWH for acute coronary syndrome (ACS). The therapeutic dose is 1 mg/kg SQ every 12 hours or 0.75–1 mg/kg IV for elective PCI where no other anticoagulant has been given. To optimize anti-Xa activity for PCI, an additional IV booster dose of 0.3 mg/kg is given if PCI is performed 8–12 hours after the prior SQ dose, particularly if fewer than three previous SQ doses have been received by the patient. Switching from one anticoagulant strategy to another (i.e., LMWH to UFH) is associated with increased bleeding risk and is discouraged. Protamine may partially reverse some activity of LMWH.

Table 3.4 describes suggested doses for PCI.

Initial studies comparing LMWH to UFH in ACS have demonstrated a reduction of myocardial infarction (MI; 10.1% vs. 11%) without increases in bleeding. However, many of these trials were performed without an invasive approach. The more definitive SYNERGY trial of 9978 patients undergoing PCI for non–ST-segment elevation (NSTE) ACS demonstrated equivalent efficacy between enoxaparin and UFH (14% vs. 14.5%, $p =$ NS) with more thrombolysis in MI (TIMI) major bleeding events (9.1% vs. 7.6%, $p = 0.008$), possibly due to switching between UFH and LMWH.

Overall, LMWH is considered equivalent to UFH for ACS and PCI. Its advantages include a lack of monitoring, ease of administration, and lower risk of HIT. The lack of monitoring can be a double-edged sword because the inability to assess the adequacy of anticoagulation at the time of PCI may be perceived as a risk.

Fondaparinux

The heparinoid fondaparinux is a synthetic pentasaccharide that is derived from the binding regions of UFH and LMWH. It inhibits factor Xa with antithrombin at high potency, with a SQ dose of 2.5 mg/day. It is renally excreted with a half-life of 17 hours. Compared with LMWH, the use of fondaparinux demonstrated noninferiority for ischemic complications in the OASIS-5 trial but decreased major bleeding from

Table 3.3

Comparison of Low-Molecular-Weight and Unfractionated Heparin

Characteristic	Unfractionated Heparin	Low-Molecular-Weight Heparin
Composition	Heterogeneous mix of polysaccharides; molecular weight 3000–30,000	Homogeneous glycosaminoglycans; molecular weight 4000–6000
Mechanisms	Activates antithrombin III*; equivalent activity against factor Xa and thrombin; releases TFPI from endothelium; unable to inactivate clot-bound thrombin or FDP; inactivates fluid phase thrombin	Less activation of antithrombin III; greater activity against factor Xa than thrombin; releases TFPI for endothelium; unable to inactivate clot-bound thrombin or FDP; weaker inactivation of fluid-phase thrombin
Pharmacokinetics	Variable binding to plasma proteins, endothelial cells, and macrophages leads to unpredictable anticoagulant effects (less available to interact with antithrombin III); short half-life	Minimal binding to plasma proteins, endothelial cells, and macrophages leads to predictable anticoagulation; longer half-life
Laboratory monitoring	Unpredictable anticoagulant effects; use aPTT or ACT	Unable to use aPTT or ACT except in renal failure to body weight <50 kg or >80 kg; use anti-factor-Xa levels
Clinical uses	Venous thrombosis; unstable angina, acute myocardial infarction, ischemic stroke, PCI	Venous thrombosis in surgery and trauma patients, unstable angina, ischemic stroke. No advantage during PCI
Reversal	Protamine neutralizes antithrombin activity	Protamine neutralizes antithrombin activity but only partially reverses anti-factor-Xa activity
History of HIT-2	Should not be used in patients with a history of HIT-2	Should not be used in patients with a history of HIT-2
Cost	Inexpensive	10–20 times more expensive than unfractionated heparin

ACT, activated clotting time; aPTT, activated partial thromboplastin time; FDP, fibrin degradation product; HIT, heparin-induced thrombocytopenia; PCI, percutaneous coronary intervention; TFPI, tissue factor pathway inhibitor.
*Antithrombin III is now commonly referred to as antithrombin.
  Modified from Safian R, Grines C, Freed M. *The New Manual of Interventional Cardiology*. Birmingham, MI: Physicians' Press, 1999.

4.1% to 2.2% (HR 0.52, $p < 0.001$). Major bleeding was associated with mortality, which was reduced with fondaparinux (2.9% vs. 3.5%, $p = 0.02$). Unexpected episodes of catheter thrombosis were noted with fondaparinux (0.9% vs. 0.4%) but can be avoided with a standard bolus of UFH at the time of PCI.

Fondaparinux carries a Class I recommendation for anticoagulation for ACS but with a lower level of evidence than UFH, LMWH, and

Table 3.4

Suggested Dosing of Enoxaparin Prior to Percutaneous Coronary Intervention	
Preprocedure Enoxaparin	**IV Bolus Enoxaparin Dose at Time of PCI**
No prior enoxaparin	0.75 mg/kg IV
Prophylactic doses of enoxaparin only	0.5 mg/kg IV
One–two 1 mg/kg SQ doses, last <8 hr prior	0.3 mg/kg IV
One–two SQ doses, last 8–12 hr prior	0.3–0.5 mg/kg IV
Adequate (>3) SQ doses, last <8 hr prior	No additional enoxaparin
Adequate (>3) SQ doses, last 8–12 hr prior	0.3 mg/kg IV
Any doses, >12 hr	Can use alternative antithrombin

Table 3.5

Direct Thrombin Inhibitors
Polypeptide Inhibitors
Hirudin (lepirudin,[*,†] desirudin)
Bivalirudin
Low-Molecular-Weight Inhibitors
Argatroban[†]
Dabigatran
Ximelagatran[*]

*Not commercially available.
†Approved for use in patients with HIT.

bivalirudin. Despite a mortality benefit in the OASIS-5 trial, fondaparinux has not been widely accepted by practicing interventionalists due to the small risk of catheter thrombosis. However, it is the preferred agent for patients when a conservative, noninvasive approach is selected.

Direct Thrombin Inhibitors

Direct thrombin inhibitors are polypeptide or low-molecular-weight inhibitors of thrombin that do not require antithrombin for anticoagulant effect (Table 3.5). Low-molecular-weight inhibitors such as argatroban inactivate circulating thrombin at the active binding site but do not inactivate clot-bound thrombin. Intravenous infusion of argatroban is approved for treatment of HIT, with limited case reports of its use in PCI. Oral dabigatran is a direct thrombin inhibitor approved for use in atrial fibrillation and venous thromboembolism.

Bivalirudin is a 20-amino acid polypeptide with a chemical structure similar to hirudin that is frequently used in PCI. It binds bivalently (at both the active site and exosite-1) and reversibly to both circulating and clot-bound thrombin. The amino terminal region of bivalirudin is cleaved by thrombin from the active site, which weakens the bond between the remaining segment of bivalirudin and exosite-1, causing prompt recovery of thrombin function after drug discontinuation (half-life of 25 minutes). This specific pharmacology potentially leads to reductions in bleeding complications and increased efficacy against thrombus.

Pharmacokinetics

Bivalirudin is given as an IV bolus of 0.75 mg/kg, with an infusion of 1.75 mg/kg per hour. It has a rapid onset of action of 5 minutes. It does

Table 3.6

Comparison of Unfractionated Heparin and Bivalirudin

	Unfractionated Heparin	Bivalirudin
Effect on clot-bound thrombin	None	Inactivation
Effect on thrombin	High-affinity interaction; inhibits thrombin and factor Xa	High-affinity interaction
Effect on factor Xa bound to platelets	None	Inactivation
Binding to endothelium and plasma proteins	High; results in less heparin availability to activate antithrombin	None
Risk of heparin-induced thrombocytopenia	High	None
Anticoagulant effects	Highly variable	Predictable
Laboratory monitoring	Essential	May be unnecessary with bivalirudin

not bind to plasma proteins or endothelium and thus generates a predictable anticoagulant effect that can be measured with the aPTT and ACT. Bivalirudin is excreted by the kidney and has a half-life of 25 minutes in patients with normal renal function. This short half-life may allow for prompt sheath removal after discontinuation of a bivalirudin infusion. The infusion should be dose-adjusted in renal insufficiency, although PCI procedures may be so brief that dose adjustment may be unnecessary unless the infusion is continued post-PCI.

Clinical Use

Compared with UFH with glycoprotein inhibitors, bivalirudin demonstrates equal efficacy with a reduced risk of bleeding in patients with unstable angina/non–ST-segment elevation MI (UA/NSTEMI) (REPLACE-2 and ACUITY trials) and in ST-segment elevation MI (STEMI) (HORIZONS-AMI). These trials mandated preprocedural clopidogrel administration; however, the bivalirudin infusion may be extended at full dose for up to 4 hours following the procedure if antiplatelet agents are delayed. Failure to extend the infusion in a patient may explain the increased risk of acute stent thrombosis seen with bivalirudin because the drug's short duration of action may not sufficiently protect against thrombosis while dual antiplatelet medications take effect. The reduction in major bleeding with bivalirudin may be attenuated with other bleeding reduction strategies, especially transradial access.

Table 3.6 compares UFH with direct thrombin inhibitors.

Warfarin

Warfarin is a coumarin derivative that acts by inhibiting the gamma-carboxylation of glutamic acid residues in the clotting proteins II (prothrombin), VII, IX, and X. It is indicated for patients with atrial fibrillation, prosthetic heart valves, cardiomyopathies, and venous thromboembolism. Limited evidence suggests a benefit in prevention of stroke after large anterior MI. Prior to the development of thienopyridines, warfarin was utilized for PCI but provided minimal benefit in stent thrombosis at the cost of significant periprocedural bleeding, and it has little role in the current era. Nevertheless it is frequently encountered due to the comorbidities of the coronary artery disease population.

Oral absorption is rapid and nearly complete. Warfarin is cleared from the blood and taken up by the liver over several hours. Daily warfarin takes 4–7 days to produce a therapeutic international normalized ratio (INR). Large loading doses do not markedly shorten the time to achieve a full therapeutic effect. After any dose change or any new diet or drug interaction, 4–5 days of the therapy is required to reach a new antithrombotic steady state.

Warfarin is typically held for 5 days prior to procedures to allow for a recovery of coagulation function, particularly when anticoagulation for PCI is anticipated. For femoral procedures, a preprocedure INR of less than 1.8 is desirable due to an increased risk of bleeding, whereas transradial procedures can often be safely performed regardless of the INR. The practice of "bridging" anticoagulation with LMWH or UFH prior to most surgical procedures has been found to be largely nonbeneficial and associated with higher bleeding rates. Bridging anticoagulation should thus be reserved for patients with mechanical heart valves or active venous thromboembolism. With careful management of the vascular access site, interventional procedures also can be performed with uninterrupted, full anticoagulation from warfarin on board.

Oral Anti-Xa Inhibitors

The newer oral anti-Xa inhibitors are an evolving class of medications that may prove to have a role in ACS. Rivaroxaban, the first of these to be released, has recently been demonstrated to have a benefit in ACS patients following stabilization and revascularization (ATLAS ACS 2-TIMI 51) and in the presence of aspirin and clopidogrel. Prolonged treatment with an oral dose of 2.5 or 5 mg/day reduced the risk of cardiovascular death, MI, or stroke from 10.7% to 8.9% (HR 0.84, $p = 0.008$) but increased the risk of major bleeding from 0.6% to 2.1% ($p < 0.001$). Further studies may justify a role of these agents in the future, including potentially as anticoagulation for PCI, but presently these agents are best held prior to planned procedures because they likely increase the risk of bleeding from other anticoagulants for PCI.

Antiplatelet Agents

Antiplatelet drugs decrease platelet aggregation and inhibit thrombus formation to prevent both acute and chronic stent thrombotic occlusion. These drugs are highly effective in the arterial circulation, where anticoagulants have reduced effect. Coupled with antithrombin drugs (e.g., heparin or bivalirudin), the antiplatelet drugs are the mainstay of PCI pharmacology. Antiplatelet agents are required for stenting and are very useful for primary and secondary prevention of thrombotic cerebrovascular or cardiovascular disease.

There are multiple classes of antiplatelet drugs, each with different mechanisms of action. Several drugs are often given together for synergistic inhibition of platelet activity while weighing the risk of bleeding against benefit of preventing thrombosis. The classes of antiplatelet drugs are:

- Cyclooxygenase inhibitors (aspirin)
- Adenosine diphosphate (ADP) receptor inhibitors (clopidogrel [Plavix], prasugrel [Effient], ticlopidine [Ticlid])
- Phosphodiesterase inhibitors (cilostazol [Pletal])
- Glycoprotein IIb/IIIa receptor inhibitors (abciximab [ReoPro], eptifibatide [Integrilin], tirofiban [Aggrastat])
- Adenosine reuptake inhibitors (dipyridamole [Persantine])
- Cyclo-pentyl-triazolo-pyrimidines (CPTPs; ticagrelor)
- Thrombin receptor (PAR-1) antagonist (vorapaxar)

Aspirin

Aspirin acetylate irreversibly binds and inactivates platelet cyclooxygenase, inhibiting production of thromboxane A2 (TXA2), which is a potent inducer of platelet aggregation and vasoconstriction via the production of cyclic adenosine monophosphate (cAMP). Platelet resistance to

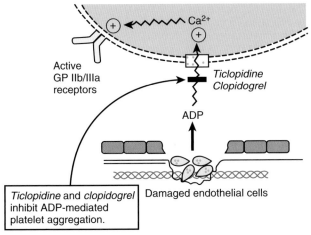

Figure 3.2 Thienopyridines block ADP receptors. *ADP,* adenosine diphosphate.

aspirin is rare. Doses range between 81 and 325 mg/day PO. After oral ingestion, rapid absorption occurs, with peak plasma levels in 20 minutes. It is rapidly cleared, but its effects last for the lifetime of the platelet. The template bleeding time can be used to gauge aspirin's effect on platelet function, but this is rarely necessary.

Indications

- Stable angina
- Unstable angina
- Acute MI
- Coronary angioplasty
- Primary and secondary prevention of MI
- Carotid or primary cerebrovascular disease (stroke prevention)
- Peripheral vascular disease
- Atrial fibrillation (not as effective as warfarin; use when warfarin is contraindicated)
- Prosthetic heart valves (adjunctive therapy with warfarin).

Aspirin should be used with caution in those with aspirin allergies (asthma), active peptic ulcer disease, or predisposition to bleeding.

Clopidogrel

Together with aspirin, the most commonly used antiplatelet agent is clopidogrel, a thienopyridine. This drug class affects the adenosine diphosphate (ADP)-dependent activation of platelet aggregation and adhesion through the IIb/IIIa receptors (Fig. 3.2). The platelet IIb/IIIa receptor is a glycoprotein responsible for platelet linkage to fibrinogen and von Willebrand factor. These links result in platelet–platelet attachment (fibrinogen) and platelet–vessel wall adhesion (von Willebrand factor), respectively. Clopidogrel is rapidly absorbed, with peak plasma level in 2 hours; it has a plasma half-life of 6–8 hours and achieves steady-state drug levels in 14–21 days.

An unidentified hepatic metabolite of clopidogrel interferes with platelet membrane function by inhibiting ADP-induced platelet–fibrinogen binding and platelet–to-platelet interactions. Platelets exposed to the active metabolite are inhibited for their lifetime, about 7–10 days. Patients with variants of the CYP2C19 allele are poor metabolizers of clopidogrel and exhibit resistance to its effect.

The dose of clopidogrel is a 300–600 mg PO load prior to or at the time of PCI, then 75 mg/day PO for 6–12 months. Because of the rare potential of neutropenia or thrombotic thrombocytopenic purpura (TTP) with the previous thienopyridine ticlopidine, routine complete blood counts are recommended with this drug. However, no instances of TTP were seen in more than 32,000 clopidogrel phase III trial patients, and TTP is estimated to occur in only 4 cases per million, making routine monitoring optional.

Indications

- Prevention of stent thrombosis as part of a dual antiplatelet regimen
- Prevention of MI and stroke in patients who cannot take aspirin or fail aspirin therapy
- Treatment of acute MI with or without PCI
- Stroke prevention in patients with risk factors or previous stroke

Prasugrel

Prasugrel is a thienopyridine prodrug whose metabolite irreversibly inhibits the ADP receptor. Similar to clopidogrel, it requires a two-step metabolism; however one step is mediated by serum esterases. Prasugrel as a result exhibits a high degree of platelet inhibition regardless of CYP inhibitors or variants. Its onset of action is rapid at 30 minutes. Its duration of effect is longer than clopidogrel at 5–10 days and thus should be discontinued 7 days prior to major surgery.

The TRITON-TIMI 38 trial randomized 13,608 patients with ACS to either prasugrel (60-mg loading dose and 10-mg maintenance dose) or clopidogrel (300-mg loading dose and 75 mg/day). Among patients undergoing PCI, prasugrel was administered only after diagnostic angiography. The primary efficacy end point of cardiovascular death, MI, or stroke occurred in 9.9% of patients on prasugrel versus 12.1% of patients taking clopidogrel (HR 0.81, $p <0.001$), mainly driven by recurrent MI. However, the rate of major bleeding was increased with prasugrel from 1.8% to 2.4% (HR 1.32, $p = 0.03$), including fatal bleeding and coronary artery bypass graft (CABG)-related bleeding. Patients with a history of stroke or transient ischemic attack (TIA), patients older than 75 years of age, and patients with low body weight had a higher risk of bleeding and no net benefit with prasugrel over clopidogrel.

Ticagrelor

Ticagrelor is a newer ADP-receptor antagonist called a *cyclopentyltri-azolopyrimidine*. It binds reversibly to the P2Y12 receptor and has a half-life of 12 hours. Ticagrelor requires no metabolism for activity, exhibits a rapid onset of action, and produces high levels of platelet inhibition. Based on its shorter half-life and reversible inhibition, ticagrelor may be held for as little as 1–3 days prior to CABG. It must be administered twice daily, however. There is also up to a 15% rate of dyspnea and an increase in heart block with ticagrelor, which may be complicating factors after MI.

The PLATO trial randomized 18,624 patients with ACS to clopidogrel (300 mg/75 mg) or ticagrelor (180-mg loading dose with 90 mg b.i.d. maintenance). Patients receiving PCI were given an additional 300 mg load of clopidogrel, or 90 mg ticagrelor if PCI occurred more than 24 hours after the initial loading dose. Major adverse cardiovascular events were reduced from 11.7% in the clopidogrel group to 9.8% in the ticagrelor group (HR 0.84, $p <0.001$). This benefit to ticagrelor appeared to result without any difference in the rates of major bleeding from clopidogrel (11.2% vs. 11.6%, $p = 0.43$). Finally ticagrelor was found to have an overall mortality benefit compared with clopidogrel (4.7% vs. 9.7%, $p <0.01$), which was driven by reductions in cardiovascular death.

Cilostazol

Cilostazol is a phosphodiesterase-3 inhibitor with modest antiplatelet activity due to increases in cAMP within platelets. Cilostazol provides vasodilatation, improves endothelial function, and may reduce restenosis after PCI. It has a clinical role in the treatment of claudication from peripheral arterial disease. Based on small trials, cilostazol may reduce the risk of stent thrombosis or major adverse cardiac events (MACE) in conjunction with other antiplatelet agents after PCI, especially in Asian populations with clopidogrel resistance. It is relatively contraindicated in patients with heart failure.

Dipyramidole

Dipyramidole is an adenosine reuptake and phosphodiesterase inhibitor with modest antiplatelet activity. It is used clinically for stroke prevention as an adjunct to aspirin and historically as a hyperemic agent for nuclear stress testing. It has little clinical use in contemporary interventional cardiology. However, the presence of dipyramidole can prolong and accentuate the effect of IV adenosine given for hemodynamic assessments in the cardiac cath lab. This combination should be avoided when possible.

Vorapaxar

Vorapaxar is a thrombin receptor (PAR-1) antagonist that inhibits thrombin-activated platelet aggregation, a mechanism distinct from other antiplatelet agents. This newer agent was initially tested in conjunction with aspirin and clopidogrel in the TRACER trial of 12,944 patients with ACS. Vorapaxar was associated with no significant reduction in MACE, but with an increase in major bleeding especially intracranial hemorrhage. Vorapaxar was subsequently tested for secondary prevention in the TRA 2°P–TIMI 50 study of 26,449 patients with a history of MI, peripheral artery disease, or stroke. After 30 months, compared with standard therapy of aspirin and selective clopidogrel, vorapaxar reduced the risk of MACE (9.3% vs. 10.5%, p <0.001) but increased the risk of moderate or severe bleeding. Patients with prior stroke were at particularly increased risk of intracranial hemorrhage with vorapaxar. Vorapaxar thus has potentially a secondary prevention role in patients at low bleeding risk but no role in acute interventions.

Glycoprotein IIb/IIIa Receptor Blockers

The most potent antiplatelet agents are the glycoprotein IIb/IIIa receptor blockers (abciximab [ReoPro], eptifibatide [Integrilin], tirofiban [Aggrastat]), which are administered intravenously. These agents exhibit high levels (>90%) of platelet inhibition because they act on the final step in platelet aggregation, the binding of the platelet to fibrinogen. These agents reduce ischemic complications (~9% relative risk reduction) but also increase risks of bleeding.

GPIIb/IIIa inhibitors have primarily demonstrated a benefit in patients treated with an invasive approach; patients managed conservatively with a dual antiplatelet regimen of aspirin and clopidogrel may not benefit. The benefits of GPIIb/IIIa inhibition are highest in those patients with elevated TIMI-risk scores (>4), especially those with positive troponin assays. It is reasonable to delay the administration of GPIIb/IIIa agents until the time of PCI because the benefit of "upstream" treatment is nearly balanced by an increased risk of bleeding.

Although the ischemic benefits of GPIIb/IIIa inhibitors were primarily demonstrated in the pre-clopidogrel era, they have been shown to persist in more contemporary studies. Their role in the era of potent oral P2Y12 inhibition with prasugrel and ticagrelor remains unclear. However, in patients with STEMI or NSTEMI not pretreated with P2Y12 inhibitors, the onset of action of all oral P2Y12 inhibitors is delayed by 2–6 hours, thus putting the patient at risk of stent thrombosis following PCI. As a result, an intravenous antiplatelet agent may "bridge" the patient to the onset of activity of clopidogrel, prasugrel, or ticagrelor.

Table 3.7 summarizes the use of glycoprotein receptor blockers for PCI.

Cangrelor. Cangrelor is a recently approved intravenous P2Y12 antagonist with a rapid onset of action (2–3 minutes) and recovery of platelet function after discontinuation. In the CHAMPION-PHOENIX trial, compared with patients treated with oral clopidogrel at the time of or immediately after PCI, cangrelor-treated patients had a lower risk of recurrent MI or stent thrombosis at the cost of an increase in minor but not major bleeding. As a result, in patients who were not adequately pretreated with clopidogrel prior to PCI, cangrelor may provide sufficient platelet inhibition to conduct PCI safely.

The efficacy of cangrelor compared with oral ticagrelor or prasugrel at the time of PCI is unclear but may persist, given the known delays in absorption and activity of all oral P2Y12 inhibitors. Cangrelor binds competitively with the P2Y12 receptor and prevents the binding of prasugrel or clopidogrel. Oral loading doses of these agents should be administered only after cangrelor is discontinued, making cangrelor less useful for bridging to the onset of absorption and action of these agents compared with the glycoprotein inhibitors. The effect of ticagrelor is unchanged by the presence of cangrelor.

Platelet Function Testing

Significant proportions of patients have clopidogrel or aspirin resistance on in vitro platelet function testing. A large number of platelet function assays are available as commercial point-of-care testing systems (Table 3.8). The use of different point-of-care assays provides slightly different information on platelet function.

Although there is considerable literature on the subject of platelet function testing and resistance, evidence linking post-treatment platelet reactivity to long-term ischemic events is weak. It remains unclear how platelet function results should change management because the recent GRAVITAS study demonstrated that a protocol of routinely doubling the dose of clopidogrel in patients with clopidogrel resistance as defined by the VerifyNow assay was not associated with improved outcomes. The other P2Y12 inhibitors, prasugrel and ticagrelor, show significantly lower rates of resistance and should be used when clopidogrel resistance is detected or suspected.

At this time, it is not justified to routinely test for platelet resistance in the clinical setting.

Platelet function testing may be helpful in a patient with recent subacute stent thrombosis, although such patients should likely be changed to a potent antiplatelet agent in most cases. Patients with a recently implanted stent who require surgery may benefit from platelet function testing. If platelet function is near normal, one can proceed with surgery as needed. If platelet function is greatly impaired, then the timing of surgery must be balanced against the timing of clopidogrel withdrawal.

Vasodilators

Adenosine

Adenosine is an endogenous nucleoside with various actions throughout the body. The A_{2a} receptor causes vasodilatation and hyperemia (increased flow) in the coronary circulation, whereas the A_1 receptor causes bradycardia. The A_{2b} receptor causes bronchoconstriction. Adenosine is rapidly inactivated by adenosine deaminases in red blood cells and endothelium, resulting in a short duration of action.

Table 3.7

Platelet Glycoprotein IIb/IIIa Antagonists for Percutaneous Coronary Intervention

	Abciximab	Eptifibatide	Tirofiban
Dose for PCI	0.25 mg/kg IV bolus plus 0.125 µg/kg/min (maximum 10 µg/min) IV infusion for 12 hr. Low-dose heparin and early sheath removal to minimize bleeding. For patients with unstable angina planning to undergo PCI within 24 hr, bolus plus infusion of abciximab (PCI dose) can be started up to 24 hr prior to PCI and continued at the same rate until 1 hr after the procedure.	*Acute coronary syndromes (PURSUIT dose):* 180 µg/kg IV bolus plus 2.0 µg/kg/min IV infusion. If arrive in cath lab >4 hr after initiating therapy, no additional bolus is required. *Percutaneous intervention (ESPRIT dose):* 2 × 180 µg/kg/min IV bolus 10 min apart, plus 2.0 µg/kg/min IV infusion for 18–24 hr.	25 mcg/kg IV bolus (over 5 min) followed by an infusion of 0.15 mcg/kg/min for 18 hr (high dose bolus). Patients with creatinine clearances <60 mL/min should receive the same bolus but half the usual infusion rate.
Heparin (unfractionated)	Maintain ACT at 200–250 sec to minimize bleeding. Initial IV heparin dose based on ACT: ACT (sec) Heparin (bolus) <150 70 µ/kg, 150–199 50 µ/kg, >200 no additional. Discontinue heparin immediately after PCI.	100 µ/kg bolus, titrate to ACT 300–350 sec. May also consider lower doses, as recommended for abciximab. In ESPIRIT, the recommended initial heparin dose was 60 µ/kg to achieve a target ACT of 200–300 sec.	100 u/kg bolus, titrate to ACT 300–350 sec. May also consider lower doses, as recommended for abciximab.
Aspirin	325 mg started at least 1 day prior to PCI and continued indefinitely; four chewable baby aspirin (325 mg total) for urgent intervention. For stents, add clopidogrel 300 mg oral load, then 75 mg PO daily for 2–4 weeks.	See abciximab.	See abciximab.

ACT, activated clotting time; *PCI,* percutaneous coronary intervention, *PO,* per os (by mouth).
Modified from Safian R, Grines C, Freed M. *The New Manual of Interventional Cardiology.* Birmingham, MI: Physicians' Press, 1999.

Table 3.8

Point-of-Care Platelet Function Assays

Platelet Function Assay	Mechanism	Method	Comments
VerifyNow Assay (Accumetrics, San Diego, CA)	Agonist-induced activated platelets bind to fibrinogen-coated polystyrene beads.	Whole blood added in mixing chamber with different receptor-coated beads causing agglutination; reflected light transmitted through the chamber is reduced. Assays for P2Y12, ADP, and IIb/IIIa are available.	Advantages: Automated cartridge-based bedside device, rapid assay for aspirin.
Plateletworks System (Helena Laboratories, Beaumont, TX)	Single platelet disappearance, expressed as platelet count after exposure to ADP.	Minimal sample preparation testing for platelet aggregation.	Sample preparation more time consuming.
PFA-100 Analyzer (Dade Behring, Marburg, Germany)	Adhesion and aggregation in whole blood under high shear conditions, exposed to collagen-epinephrine and/or collagen-ADP.	Whole blood put in citrated tubes, inserted through capillary collagen-coated membrane infused with ADP or epinephrine. Platelet formation and plugging is measured.	Advantage: Measures variety of platelet disorders. Disadvantage: Testing cartridge insensitive to clopidogrel. Device is used for research studies only.
Cone and Platelet Analyzer (DiaMed, Cressier sur Morat, Switzerland)	Measures interaction with platelets and shear forces.	Citrated whole blood is incubated with ADP. Tests the physiologic milieu of high shear stress. Microaggregate formation tested after exposure to clopidogrel.	Tests platelets more precisely than ex vivo. Limitations: No published studies demonstrating low-surface coverage associated with clopidogrel response.
Impedance Aggregometer (Chrono-Log, Havertown, PA)	Electrical impedance between two electrodes immersed in whole blood.	500 μL whole blood diluted and inserted into cuvette, which is incubated. Agonist added and resistance impedance computed.	A good correlation with optical aggregometry. Sample preparation 2 minutes, results available in 10 minutes. Limitation: No prospective studies.

ADP, adenosine diphosphate.

From Kern M. Do we need platelet function testing in PCI intervention? *Cath Lab Digest*. June 2009. Available at http://cathlabdigest.com/articles/Do-We-Need-Platelet-Function-Testing-Percutaneous-Coronary-Intervention.

Exogenous adenosine is the most frequently used agent for hemodynamic measurements requiring hyperemia due to its low cost, short half-life, and relatively few persistent side effects. It is injected via the intravenous (typically 140 mcg/kg per minute) or intracoronary route (40–200 mcg). Intracoronary adenosine (60–100 mg) may be helpful in resolving cases of slow or no reflow following PCI, and smaller doses may prevent no reflow. Adenosine is administered in larger doses (6–12 mg IV) for suppression of atrioventricular node conduction, which is a diagnostic and therapeutic maneuver in the treatment of supraventricular tachycardia. Adenosine should be used with caution in patients at risk for bronchospasm and is contraindicated in patients on dipyramidole. Caffeine at high doses may inhibit the response to adenosine, but the effect is modest at clinically relevant doses.

Regadenoson

Regadenoson is a selective A_{2a} receptor antagonist designed to recreate the hyperemic effects of adenosine with a lower risk of off-target effects such as bradycardia or bronchospasm. Because it has a longer half-life than adenosine at 2–3 minutes, it is administered as a single 0.4 mg/5 mL intravenous bolus for convenience. Clinical trials utilizing the agent in nuclear perfusion imaging suggested it was noninferior to adenosine. Despite its selective antagonism of the A_{2a} receptor, side effects including dyspnea and chest pain occur at similar rates compared with adenosine and occasionally require reversal with aminophylline. Regadenoson has been utilized in the cardiac catheterization laboratory as a substitute for adenosine during hemodynamic measurements; however due to its increased cost and lack of definitive benefits, it is rarely used.

Nitroglycerin

Nitroglycerin is a vasodilator with multiple uses in the cath lab. It is administered via the intra-arterial route to relieve coronary spasm and prevent spasm from intracoronary tools such as intravascular ultrasound catheters or coronary wires. Nitroglycerin relieves angina and heart failure by causing coronary dilatation and reducing preload and afterload.

Nitroglycerin can be administered via the intracoronary (IC), IV, transdermal, and sublingual route. Typical doses range from 50 to 300 mcg IC, 20–200 mcg/min IV, and 0.3 to 0.4 mg sublingual. Doses can be repeated until the desired effect is generated or hypotension develops. Tachyphylaxis can occur with chronic nitroglycerin use. Of note, nitroglycerin is not effective in vessels of less than 200 microns in diameter. Nitroglycerin therefore should not be used to treat no-reflow phenomenon unless there is superimposed epicardial vasospasm.

Nicorandil

Nicorandil is an anti-anginal medication with properties of nitrates and K+ATPase agonist. Nicorandil stimulates guanylate cyclase to increase cyclic guanosine monophosphate (cGMP) formation, which increases protein kinase G to cause increased activity of the K+ATPase, resulting in hyperpolarization and inhibition of smooth muscle constriction. It causes dilatation of the epicardial coronary arteries at low concentrations and reductions in coronary vascular resistance at high concentrations. It has been demonstrated to be safe and potentially cardioprotective during PCI. Nicorandil (2 mg IC) is administered for hyperemia for hemodynamic measurements and has fewer side effects (heart block) compared with adenosine. Nicorandil may be useful to prevent and treat no reflow. It is available around the world, but not available in the United States. Oral nicorandil is associated with adverse reactions including headaches and oral ulcers.

Papaverine

Papaverine is an opioid derivative that inhibits phosphodiesterase, resulting in elevated cAMP levels. It has actions as a direct smooth muscle vasodilator that affect both the coronary and peripheral circulation. It is approved to treat spasms of the gastrointestinal tract and is also used to treat erectile dysfunction and migraine headaches. In its injectable form, it causes consistent vasodilatation and hyperemia, making it useful for fractional flow reserve measurements. However it is associated with occasional side effects including polymorphic ventricular tachycardia and ventricular fibrillation (2%–3%), constipation, hypotension, and tachycardia.

Verapamil

Verapamil is a non-dihydropyridine calcium channel blocker used in supraventricular tachycardia. Although, compared with dihydropyridines, it has minimal vasodilatory effects, in patients with no reflow or slow flow after PCI, verapamil is effective in improving distal perfusion. The typical dose ranges from 100 mcg to 1000 mcg IC, with heart block and bradycardia as the main side effects.

Nitroprusside

Nitroprusside is a direct arterial vasodilator, acting by supplying nitric oxide to the arteriole smooth muscle. It is used for patients with hypertensive crisis as a continuous infusion. IC nitroprusside (0.6 mcg/kg IC bolus) acts as a hyperemic agent for hemodynamic measurements but is infrequently used because it causes significant hypotension. Nitroprusside may be beneficial in patients with no reflow, typically at a dose of 100 mcg IC, but this benefit was not confirmed in a larger trial.

    Nitroprusside is inactivated by light and must be stored in protective (dark) intravenous bags. It has a very short onset and duration of action of less than 3 minutes. Cyanide toxicity can occur in patients with renal insufficiency with prolonged use.

Nicardipine

Nicardipine is a dihydropyridine intravenous calcium channel blocker that causes arteriolar vasodilation with minimal inotropic or chronotropic effects. It is used in hypertensive crisis, where it can be infused at up to 15 mg/hour. It may be helpful in prevention or treatment of no reflow.

    Tables 3.9 and 3.10 list the vasodilators and doses typically used for hemodynamic measurements and treatment of no reflow.

Inotropes

Dobutamine

Dobutamine is an exogenous inotropic agent that stimulates the adrenergic beta$_1$ and beta$_2$ receptors. It increases cardiac inotropy and chronotropy, making it useful in congestive heart failure, cardiogenic shock, and bradycardia. In the cath lab, dobutamine is used infrequently to differentiate true low-flow, low-gradient aortic stenosis from pseudostenosis.

Vasoconstrictors

Dopamine

Dopamine is an endogenous amine with multiple actions. In normal subjects, dopamine stimulates the dopamine receptor at low doses

Table 3.9

Vasodilatory Agents for Hyperemia Induction

Agent	Route	Dose	Comments
Adenosine	IV	140 mcg/kg/min	Reference standard used in trials. Side effects of dyspnea, chest pain, bradycardia. Inconsistently causes sustained hyperemia.
Adenosine	IC	60–100 mcg (RCA) 100–200 mcg (LCA)	Fewer systemic side effects than IV, rapid onset of hyperemia that lasts 15–20 seconds. Rapidly repeatable. Requires guide catheter engagement that may risk dampening
Regadenoson	IC	0.4 mg	Expensive. Variable duration of hyperemia, potentially prolonged.
Nitroprusside	IC	0.6 mcg/kg	Easy to use, but causes significant hypotension.
Nicorandil	IC	2 mg	Fewer side effects than adenosine. Not available in the United States.
Papaverine	IC	10–20 mg	Rare side effect of polymorphic VT (2–3%).

Table 3.10

Agents for Treatment of No Reflow

First-line agents	Adenosine (10–100 mcg IC, for treatment, 24–48 mcg IC for prevention) Verapamil (100 mcg IC, up to 1500 mcg total) Nitroprusside (100 mcg IC, repeated boluses) Nicorandil (2 mg IC, single dose)
Second-line	Diltiazem (0.5–2.5 mg IC bolus, up to 5–10 mg) Papaverine (10 mg IC) Nicardipine (200 mcg IC, mean dose 460 mcg)
Controversial, probably ineffective	Glycoprotein Inhibitors (effective in prevention but unclear benefit in treatment) Forceful injection of saline
Ineffective	Nitroglycerin (but can resolve superimposed spasm) Stenting, bypass surgery Thrombolytics

Table 3.11

Activity of Catecholamines					
	Activity at Receptors				
Agent	**alpha$_1$**	**alpha$_2$**	**beta$_1$**	**beta$_2$**	**Dopamine**
Dobutamine	+	−	+++	+	−
Dopamine	++	+	++	+++	++++
Norepinephrine	+++	+++	+	−	−
Epinephrine	+++	++	+++	++	−
Phenylephrine	+++	+	−	−	−

(3.5 mcg/kg per minute IV), the beta receptor at intermediate doses (5–10 mcg/kg per minute), and the alpha receptor at high doses (10–20 mcg/kg per minute). The specific action of dopamine may vary with the dose and the patient's particular condition. At low doses, dopamine increases renal perfusion, although the effect is not clinically meaningful. Dopamine is readily available and useful for shock, but because of its various actions has been largely supplanted by norepinephrine.

Norepinephrine

Norepinephrine stimulates the alpha and to a lesser extent the beta adrenergic receptors. It provides a vasoconstrictive effect with some inotropic activity, making it the preferred choice in shock. It is useful for high-risk PCI procedures or in patients with hypotension.

Epinephrine

Epinephrine is an endogenous agent that stimulates the beta and alpha adrenergic receptors. It is used at high dose (1 mg) for patients with cardiac arrest or asystole. Shock or symptomatic bradycardia in the cath lab is better treated with smaller doses (50–100 mcg IV) of epinephrine because excessive adrenergic activity worsens myocardial ischemia.

Phenylephrine

Phenylephrine is a selective alpha adrenergic agonist that causes arterial vasoconstriction. Phenylephrine increases cardiac afterload without increasing inotropy, potentially reducing cardiac output. It is useful as a resuscitative agent because it provides a rapid increase in blood pressure when given as an intravenous bolus (100 mcg). It is less effective and should be avoided in cardiogenic shock because systemic vascular resistance is typically elevated.

Table 3.11 lists the relative receptor activity of the commonly used catecholamines.

4

Intravascular Lesion Assessment: Physiology and Imaging ▶

MORTON J. KERN · MICHAEL J. LIM

Introduction

The rationale for using intravascular lesion assessment tools arises from two principles: (1) that revascularization (via percutaneous coronary intervention [PCI] or coronary artery bypass graft [CABG]) is justified best by the presence of ischemia, which depends on the hemodynamic significance of a lesion; and (2) that the coronary angiogram frequently fails to establish the hemodynamic significance of coronary stenoses with accuracy, particularly for the intermediately narrowed (between 30% and 80% diameter stenosis) lesions. This limitation of angiography has been documented repeatedly by poor correlations to stress testing and is attributable to the anatomic complexity of the atherosclerotic lumen.

Coronary angiography can only produce a two-dimensional silhouette image of the three-dimensional vascular lumen. Angiographic accuracy is further limited by the inability to identify diffusely "diseased" and "normal" vessel segments. In addition, unlike intravascular ultrasound (IVUS), angiography does not provide vascular wall detail sufficient to characterize plaque size, length, and eccentricity. The eccentric lumen produces conflicting degrees of angiographic narrowing when viewed from different angulations, causing uncertainty related to lumen size and its impact on coronary blood flow (Fig. 4.1). Moreover, there are at least six morphologic features that determine resistance to flow, most of which can be measured from the angiogram or even IVUS (Fig. 4.2). Additional artifacts including contrast streaming, branch overlap, vessel foreshortening, calcifications, and ostial origins further contribute to uncertain angiographic lesion interpretation.

The uncertainty of angiographic lesion assessment is a significant clinical problem. When evidence of ischemia is lacking, before stenting all intermediate lesions indiscriminately, the functional significance of a stenosis by fractional flow reserve should be identified as the first step in PCI. After the lesion is shown to be flow limiting, the anatomic and morphologic features of the stenosis and reference vessel segment can be assessed by IVUS. More detail on structure and composition can be obtained by optical coherence tomography (OCT), and, in the future, a determination of the plaque character (e.g., lipid pool content with near infrared spectroscopy [NIRS]) may assist in appropriate stenting in regions beyond the most stenotic segment.

Thus, the three most common technologies for intravascular coronary lesion assessment tools available at this time are the (1) coronary pressure wire, (2) IVUS, and (3) OCT. The thermodilution flow measurements of the St. Jude pressure wire, the Doppler flow wire that measures flow velocity, and their use as research tools to study

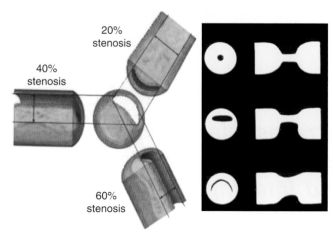

Figure 4.1 *Left*: Diagram of angiographic projections demonstrating markedly different diameter narrowings illustrating the greatest limitation of angiography for eccentric lesions. *Right*: Orthogonal projections of different orifice configurations that complicate determination of physiologic impact of narrowing.

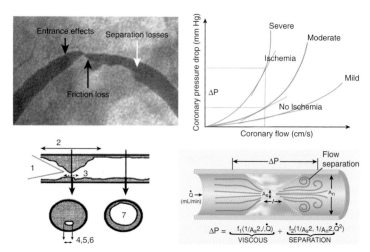

Figure 4.2 *Top left*: Frame from cineangiogram of left coronary artery (LCA) with an intermediate left anterior descending (LAD) lesion. *Bottom right*: Diagram of regions of stenosis resistance causing poststenotic pressure loss (1, entrance angle; 2, length of disease; 3, length of stenosis; 4, minimal lumen diameter; 5, minimal lumen area; 6, eccentricity of lesion; 7, area of reference vessel segment). *Top right*: Pressure gradient–coronary flow curves demonstrating effect of increasing hemodynamic severity. Straight lines indicate portion of curves where pressure and flow are linearly related, permitting the derivation of fraction flow reserve (FFR) to function.

the microcirculation, as well as new imaging modalities such as near infrared spectroscopy imaging will also be addressed briefly.

Coronary Pressure and Fractional Flow Reserve

Pijls and De Bruyne developed and validated an index for determining the physiologic impact of coronary stenoses, called the *fractional flow reserve (FFR)*. FFR is measured as the ratio of mean distal coronary pressure divided by the mean proximal aortic pressure during maximal hyperemia. The coronary pressure beyond the stenosis is measured with a 0.014-inch guidewire with a high-fidelity pressure transducer mounted 3 cm from the tip of the wire, at the junction of the radiopaque and radiolucent segments. A full discussion of the FFR method and results can be found elsewhere (see suggested reading).

Concept of Fractional Flow Reserve

FFR is defined as the ratio of maximal hyperemic flow across an epicardial coronary stenosis compared to maximal hyperemic flow in the same artery without the stenosis. FFR is expressed as the percentage of normal maximal flow through the stenotic artery. FFR can be separately computed for the myocardium (FFR_m), the epicardial coronary artery (FFR_c), and the collaterals (FFR_{collat}), based on translesional pressure measured during maximal hyperemia and, in some cases, coronary occlusion wedge pressure. Figs. 4.3 and 4.4 illustrate the

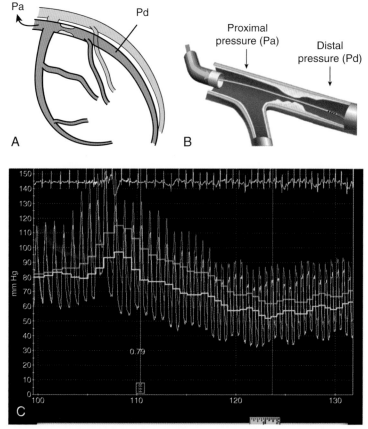

Figure 4.3 (A) Diagrams of the theory of fractional flow reserve (FFR). FFR is the ratio of maximal myocardial perfusion in the stenotic territory divided by maximal hyperemic flow in that same region in the hypothetical case the lesion was not present (the faint pink artery is the hypothetical normal artery without the stenosis.). FFR represents that fraction of hyperemic flow that persists despite the presence of the stenosis. FFR is defined as myocardial flow (Qs) across stenosis/myocardial flow (Qn) without stenosis. (B) Diagram of pressure wire inside guide catheter across a target lesion. (C) pressure signals used to calculate FFR. Mean aortic pressure (red) and distal coronary pressure (yellow) are recorded at rest and then during hyperemia induced by adenosine. The nadir of Pd/Pa pressures (green line) is used for the FFR calculation which is 0.79.

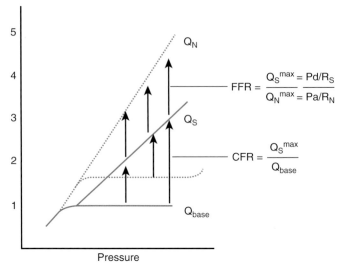

Figure 4.4 Differences between coronary flow reserve (CFR) and fractional flow reserve (FFR). Graph displays flow increase from baseline on vertical axis and pressure along horizontal axis. Baseline flow, Q_{base}, can increase to the line of maximal hyperemia (*dark angled line*) at different points corresponding to translesional pressure. If the line of hyperemia changes or the basal flow changes, the CFR changes, as represented by different arrow sizes. In contrast, FFR is the change from the measured flow across the stenotic artery, Q_s, to the normal flow, Q_N. Since the measurements are made at maximal hyperemia in the target vessel comparing it to theoretic maximal hyperemia in a normal vessel, there is little change in FFR despite changing hemodynamics, microcirculation, or contractility. *Pd*, distal pressure; *Pa*, aortic pressure; R_s, R_N, stenotic and normal vessel resistance.

Table 4.1

Calculations of Fractional Flow Reserve From Pressure Measurements Taken During Maximal Arterial Vasodilation

Myocardial fraction flow reserve (FFR_{myo}):

$$FFR_{myo} = 1 - \Delta P/Pa - Pv$$
$$= Pd - Pv/Pa - Pv$$
$$= Pd/Pa$$

Coronary fractional flow reserve (FFR_{cor}): $FFR_{cor} = 1 - \Delta P(Pa - Pw)$
Collateral fractional flow reserve (FFR_{coll}): $FFR_{coll} = FFR_{myo} - FFR_{cor}$

Note: All measurements are made during hyperemia except Pw. *Pa*, mean aortic pressure; *Pd*, distal coronary pressure; *ΔP*, mean translesional pressure gradient; *Pv*, mean right atrial pressure; *Pw*, mean coronary wedge pressure or distal coronary pressure during balloon inflation.
From Pijls NHJ, van Som AM, Kirkeeide RL, et al. Experimental basis of determining maximum coronary, myocardial, and collateral blood flow by pressure measurements for assessing functional stenosis severity before and after percutaneous transluminal coronary angioplasty. *Circulation*. 1993;87:454–67.

concept and data used to derive FFR. Table 4.1 lists the calculations for FFR, and Table 4.2 lists the thresholds for clinical applications of FFR.

FFR differs from absolute coronary flow reserve (CFR, maximal flow/basal flow) because it does not depend on basal flow levels but is computed only at maximal flow (hyperemia). FFR has several advantages over CFR:

1. It has an absolute normal value of 1.0 for every artery, every patient.

Table 4.2

Physiologic Criteria Associated With Clinical Applications

FFR and Other FFR-Like Indices

Index	Normal Value	Ischemic Threshold	Comments
FFR	1	≤0.80	See Table 4.1
cFFR	1	≈0.83	Avoids adenosine by using contrast media; may correlate with FFR better than iFR and P_d/P_a
iFR	1	≈0.90	Avoids need for hyperemia; 80% accurate when compared with FFR
Rest P_d/P_a	1	≈0.92	Avoids need for hyperemia; 80% accurate when compared with FFR

cFFR, contrast FFR; *FFR*, fractional flow reserve; *iFR*, instantaneous wave-free ratio; P_d/P_a, distal coronary pressure/proximal coronary pressure.

From Fearon W. Invasive coronary physiology for assessing intermediate lesions in advances in interventional cardiology. *Circ Cardiovasc Interv.* 2015;8;e001942.

2. It is not affected by changing hemodynamics or status of the microcirculation.

3. It is specific for epicardial coronary stenoses.

Technique of Fractional Flow Reserve

FFR can be easily measured using a 5F or 6F guide catheter and any of several available pressure wire/microcatheter systems (St. Jude Medical, Minneapolis, MN, or Volcano Therapeutics, Rancho Cordova, CA; Opsens, Quebec City, Quebec; Acist Medical Inc, Minneapolis, MN, Boston Scientific, Boston, MA). After diagnostic angiography with a guide catheter seated in the coronary ostium, the steps to measure FFR are as follows:

1. The pressure wire is connected to the system's pressure analyzer, calibrated and zeroed on the table, outside the body.

2. Anticoagulation (IV heparin usually 40 u/kg) and intracoronary nitroglycerin (100–200 mcg bolus) are administered.

3. The wire is advanced through the guide to the coronary artery. The pressure wire signal and the guide pressure are matched (i.e., equalized, also called *normalized*) before crossing the stenosis. By early convention, the guidewire transducer was positioned at the end of the guide catheter. In fact, it does not matter exactly where the wire is in relation to the guide catheter or coronary ostium except that both should be in the aortic sinus when equalizing the signals.

4. The wire is then advanced across the stenosis about 2 cm distal to the coronary lesion (about 10 artery diameters).

5. Maximal hyperemia is induced with IV adenosine (140 mcg/kg/min) or intracoronary (IC) bolus adenosine (50–100 mcg for the right coronary artery, 100–200 mcg for the left coronary artery). Alternative hyperemic agents are rarely used but include nitroprusside (50–100 mcg) or ATP (50–100 mcg). FFR is measured at the lowest Pd/Pa ratio after the onset of hyperemia, usually within 2 minutes for IV adenosine and at 15–20 seconds after IC adenosine.

6. FFR is calculated as the ratio of the mean distal pressure to mean proximal pressure during maximal hyperemia. An FFR of less than 0.80 has a strong ischemic correlation and is an indication to proceed with PCI/CABG. If a PCI is deemed necessary, it can be performed using the pressure wire as the angioplasty guidewire.

After the procedure, FFR can be remeasured to assess the adequacy of the intervention and residual disease impact in the target or other vessels.

7. Finally, at the end of the procedure (either the diagnostic assessment or after the PCI), the pressure wire should be pulled back into the guide to confirm pressure signal stability (equal pressure readings) and the lack of pressure signal drift.

Coronary Hyperemia for Fractional Flow Reserve

Maximal coronary hyperemia is required for accurate FFR. Table 4.3 lists available pharmacologic agents suitable for inducing hyperemia. The most common in use today is adenosine.

IV adenosine is weight-based, operator-independent, and the preferred method of inducing hyperemia. By providing a sustained hyperemic stimulus, IV adenosine allows for a slow pullback of the pressure wire, useful to identify the exact location of the pressure dropoff or the presence of diffuse disease. IV adenosine is often required for the assessment of aorto-ostial narrowings without the guide catheter in place to permit maximal coronary flow without obstruction. However, IV adenosine may not always produce a stable Pd/Pa ratio, and, at times, no stable period can be identified. Johnson and Seto reported various patterns of pressure changes induced by IV adenosine (Fig. 4.5). Johnson et al. have demonstrated that the lowest distal/aortic pressure ratio (Pd/Pa), called a *smart minimum,* during the adenosine infusion is the right value with the highest reproducibility. The smart minimum FFR is the lowest Pd/Pa without pressure wave artifact that occurs any time after the adenosine effect has begun, and most FFR signal monitors have incorporated software that automatically computes and displays the lowest Pd/Pa. The operator and team must continue to view the recording to ensure that FFR is the smart value and not just "a value" that might be artificial. Thus, as noted, the best and most reproducible point at which to take the FFR (Pd/Pa during hyperemia) is the minimum Pd/Pa ratio excluding any artifact.

IC adenosine is equivalent to IV infusion for determination of FFR. Although IV adenosine has been the standard for FFR for more than three decades and used successfully in generating the datasets that demonstrated superior FFR-guided outcomes in the FAME and other studies, recent examinations of hemodynamic variability during IV adenosine has prompted a return to using IC adenosine.

There are many reports of different doses of IC adenosine, ranging from 16 mcg to 700 mcg. The most recent IC dose investigation by Adjedj et al. provides a modern and definitive demonstration that the optimal doses appear to be 100 mcg for the right coronary artery (RCA) and 200 mcg for the left (LCA) (Fig. 4.6A). A greater than 10% incidence of heart block is observed with RCA IC adenosine in doses noted. These doses will eliminate any uncertainty that the operator achieved maximal hyperemia or did not give enough adenosine to get the most accurate FFR. The concentration of IC adenosine should be mixed to provide 10 or 20 mcg/mL. One liter of the adenosine/saline mix can supply the entire lab's needs for the day. A stopcock and flush syringe connected to the adenosine syringe make delivery of the drug easy (Fig. 4.6B).

A full discussion of alternative agents can be found in *The Cardiac Catheterization Handbook,* 6e (2015), Chapter 13, "Non-angiographic Lesion Assessment."

Pitfalls of Fractional Flow Reserve

As a cautionary note, catheters with sideholes should not be used to measure FFR because proximal pressure gradients may occur and

Table 4.3

Pharmacologic Agents Used to Induce Maximal Coronary Hyperemia in the Cath Lab

	Adenosine	Adenosine	Papaverine	NTP	Regadenoson
Route	IV	IC	IC	IC	IV
Dosage	140 mcg/kg/min	100–200 mcg LCA, 50–100 mcg RCA	15 mg LCA, 10 mg RCA	50–100 mcg	0.4 mg
Half-life	1–2 min	30–60 sec	2 min	1–2 min	2–4 min (up to 30 min)
Time to max hyperemia	<1–2 min	5–10 sec	20–60 sec	10–20 sec	1–4 min
Advantage	Gold standard	Short action	Short action	Short action	IV bolus
Disadvantage	↓BP, chest burning	AV Block, ↓BP	Torsades, ↓BP	↓BP	↑HR, ? redose, long action

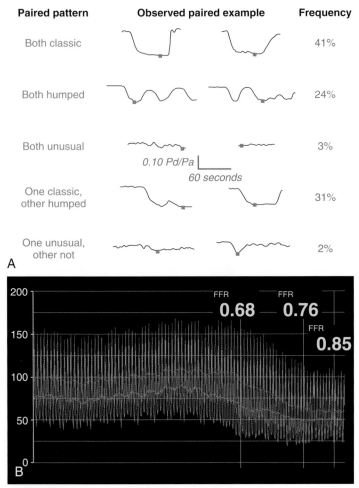

Figure 4.5 (A) Adenosine variability. Paired patterns of Pd/Pa during hyperemia. Each lesion underwent repeat study separated by 2 minutes of rest, producing five observed paired patterns of varying frequency. For each observed example, the red dot marks the smart minimum fractional flow reserve (FFR). The blue scale for Pd/Pa and time applies to the example tracings. Even with the same patient/lesion, the two paired tracings differ 31% of the time. (B) When to take the correct FFR? Typical coronary hemodynamic response to intravenous adenosine. The lowest Pd/Pa (0.68) occurs early in hyperemia, at point A. Values obtained at the earliest nadir of Pd (point B, 0.76) and during stable hyperemia (point C, 0.83–0.85) are significantly higher. Johnson et al. recommend choosing the lowest 5-beat average Pd/Pa value (the lowest point on the Pd/Pa plot line, point A) as the FFR. *(A is from Johnson N, et al. Repeatability of fractional flow reserve despite variations in systemic and coronary hemodynamics. J Am Coll Cardiol Interv. 2015;8(8):1018–27; B is from Seto AH, Tehrani DM, Bharmal MI, Kern MJ. Variations of coronary hemodynamic responses to intravenous adenosine infusion: Implications for fractional flow reserve measurements. Catheter Cardiovasc Interv. 2014;84:416–25.)*

complicate distal gradient evaluations. Larger guide catheters can partially occlude the coronary ostium as hyperemia is induced, impairing maximal flow. Removing the guide catheter from the coronary ostium after giving the hyperemic agent will avoid this pitfall.

Errors in the performance of accurate FFR involve hemodynamic artifacts and failure to induce maximal hyperemia. Tables 4.4 and 4.5 list a number of factors that can reduce the accuracy of FFR. Figs. 4.7–4.9 show artifacts that may produce false FFR readings.

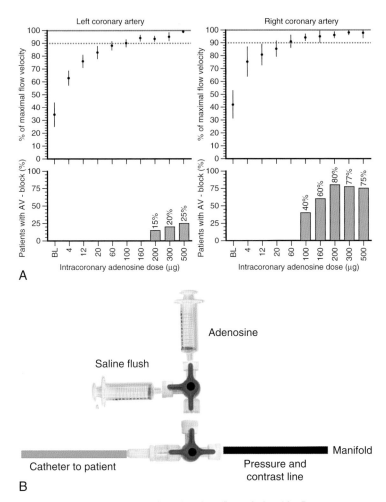

A

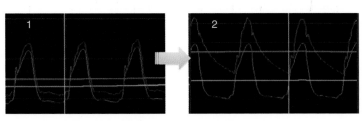

B

Figure 4.6 (A) Intracoronary adenosine dose-flow relationship. Dose–response data for the right coronary artery (RCA) (*left panel*) and the left coronary artery (LCA) (*right panel*). The data are expressed as the percent of maximum flow for each patient (Q/Q$_{max}$) at each dose of intracoronary (IC) adenosine. The error bars represent the 95% confidence intervals for each value. *Lower panels*: The bars represent the percent of patients in whom high-grade atrioventricular (AV) block occurred with that dose of adenosine. *BL,* baseline. (B) Syringe and stopcock assembly for rapid intracoronary adenosine injection. *(A is from Adjedj J, Toth GG, Johnson NP, et al. Intracoronary adenosine: dose-response relationship with hyperemia. J Am Coll Cardiol Interv. 2015;8:1422–30.)*

Figure 4.7 Example of pressure signals during damping (*left*) and after withdrawal of guide catheter (*right*).

Table 4.4

Factors Involved in Fractional Flow Reserve Accuracy

Hemodynamic Artifacts or Errors

1. *Signal drift.* This is rare and can be determined by careful observation of pressure waveform and presence of dichrotic notch. If suspicious, check with rematching of signals on pullback to aortic location.
2. *Incorrect height of pressure transducer.*
3. *Loss of pressure due to guidewire introducer.* Remove and tighten Touhey-Borst Valve.
4. *Damping of pressure by guiding catheter.* Observe aortic pressure wave. Use IV adenosine and keep catheter in aorta, not coronary ostium.
5. *Guiding catheters with side holes* produce pseudostenosis across the catheter into the coronary ostium. Use IV adenosine and keep catheter in aorta, not coronary ostium.
6. *Pressure damping with 4 or 5F catheters if not flushed with saline.* Contrast media viscosity will produce unreliable aortic pressure wave.

Failure to Induce Hyperemia

A. Adenosine, intracoronary bolus administration
   1. *Submaximum stimulus in some patients.* Very rare; if suspected, select alternative agent (e.g., nitroprusside, papaverine, ATP)
   2. *Failure to capture pressure change at peak hyperemia.* Maximum gradient is underestimated when calculated from mean signal, unless it is taken on beat-to-beat basis.
   3. *No pullback curve possible with bolus administration.*
   4. *Guiding catheter fails to seat and deliver drug.*
   5. *Guide catheter flow is obstructed.*
   6. *Incorrect dose mix or dilution.*
B. Adenosine, IV Adenosine
   1. Check infusion, pump system, and lines.
   2. Infuse through central vein.
   3. Avoid Valsalva maneuver during infusion.
   4. Decrease of blood pressure by 10–15%.
   5. *Burning or angina-like chest pain during infusion.* This is harmless and does not indicate ischemia. IV adenosine is not to be used in patients with severe obstructive lung disease (bronchospasm).
   6. *If peripheral vein is used, avoid kinking of arm/elbow.*
   7. *Avoid Valsalva maneuvers.*

Table 4.5

Confounding Technical Factors for Fractional Flow Reserve

1. Equipment factors
   Erroneous zero
   Incomplete pressure transmission (tubing/connector leaks)
   Faulty electric wire connection
   Pressure signal drift
   Hemodynamics recorder miscalibration
2. Procedural factors
   Guide catheter damping
   Incorrect placement of pressure sensor
   Inadequate hyperemia
3. Physiologic factors
   Serial lesion
   Reduced myocardial bed
   Acute myocardial infarction
4. Theoretical conditions that might influence FFR
   Severe left ventricular hypertrophy
   Exuberant collateral supply
   Adenosine insensitivity

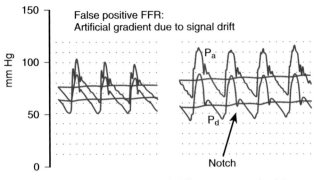

Figure 4.8 Example of pressure signal drift as a cause for false-positive fractional flow reserve (FFR). Note preservation of dichrotic notch on distal pressure indicating normal transmission of pressure.

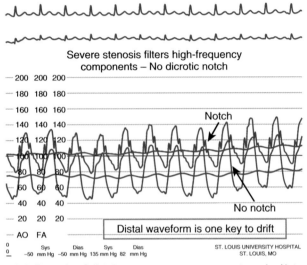

Figure 4.9 Example of distal pressure across severe stenosis. Note distal pressure wave configuration with wide pulse pressure and loss of dichrotic notch indicative of severe stenosis.

Use of Fractional Flow Reserve for Specific Angiographic Subsets

The Intermediate Coronary Lesion

FFR assists the operator in deciding to treat or not treat coronary lesions based on ischemia. Some operators are concerned that not stenting intermediate but hemodynamically insignificant lesions will result in harm to the patient later. This concern is unfounded based on the 5-year outcomes of the DEFER study. The DEFER study randomized 325 patients scheduled for PCI into three groups: a deferral group (n = 91) in whom FFR was 0.75 or greater and medical therapy was continued; patients who had an FFR of greater than 0.75, the PCI performance group (n = 90), in which the lesions were treated with stents. The third group was the reference group (n = 144) who had an FFR of less than 0.75, and stents were placed as planned. For the deferred and performed groups, the event-free survival was the same (80% and 73%, respectively; $p = 0.52$), and both were significantly better than in the reference group (63%, $p = 0.03$). The composite rate of cardiac death and acute myocardial infarction (MI) in the deferred, performed, and reference groups was 3%, 8%, and 16%, respectively ($p = 0.21$ for deferred vs. performed and $p = 0.003$ for reference vs.

both the deferred and performed groups; Fig. 4.10A). The 15-year outcomes of deferred PCI based on FFR is shown in Fig. 4.10B. The percentage of patients free from chest pain on follow-up was not different between the deferred and performed groups. The 5-year risk of cardiac death or MI in patients with a normal FFR is less than 1% per year and not decreased by stenting. Treating patients with intermediate lesions

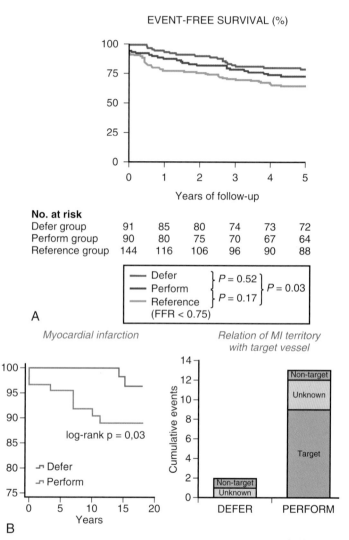

Figure 4.10 (A, top panel) The DEFER Study results. Kaplan-Meier survival curves for freedom from adverse cardiac events during 5-year follow-up for the defer group (*blue line*), treatment group (*red line*), and reference group (*yellow line*). (B, lower panel) DEFER 15-year outcomes. Kaplan-Meier of myocardial infarction (MI) (B, lower right) and relation of myocardial infarction with study vessel territory (*B*). The rate of MI was significantly lower in the DEFER group (2.2%) compared with the Perform group (10.0%), p = 0.03. This was almost exclusively due to less target vessel–related infarctions. Patients with a baseline fractional flow reserve (FFR) of 0.75 or higher had a significantly lower rate of MI compared with patients with an FFR of less than 0.75 (6.1 vs. 12.5%, p = 0.044). (*A is from Pijls NHJ, Van Schaarden-burgh P, Manoharan G, et al. Percutaneous coronary intervention of functionally non-significant stenoses: 5-year follow-up of the DEFER study. J Am Coll Cardiol. 2007;49:2105–11; B is from Zimmermann FM, et al. The deferral vs. performance of percutaneous coronary intervention of functionally non-significant coronary stenosis: 15-year follow-up of the DEFER trial. Eur Heart J. 2015 Dec 1;36(45):3182–88.)*

assisted by FFR is associated with a low event rate, comparable to event rates in patients with normal noninvasive testing. Fig. 4.11 is an example of FFR for intermediate lesion assessment. Similar outcomes for deferment of lesions with an FFR of greater than 0.80 were also reported in patients in the FAME study described next.

Multivessel Disease PCI

The FAME (FFR Versus Angiography for Multivessel Evaluation) trial by Tonino et al. compared a physiologically guided PCI approach (FFR-PCI) to a conventional angiographic guided PCI (Angio-PCI) in patients with multivessel coronary artery disease (CAD). A total of 1005 patients with multivessel CAD undergoing PCI with drug-eluting stents (DES) were enrolled. Operators identified all lesions by visual angiographic appearance (>50% diameter stenosis) to be treated in advance

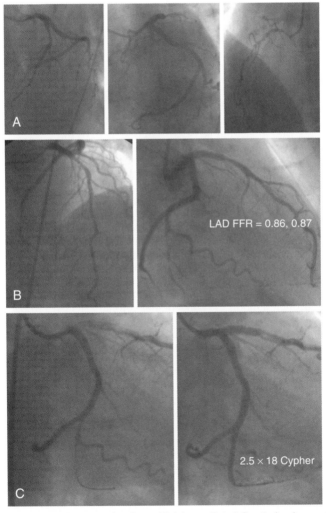

Figure 4.11 Angiograms of patient with intermediate left anterior descending (LAD) LAD and severe OM1 branch lesion. (A) *Left panel*, LAO view of LAD, middle LAO caudal view of left coronary artery (LCA), and *right panel*, occluded right coronary artery (RCA) of 2 years ago. (B) *Left panel*, RAO cranial shows intermediate LAD; *right panel*, severe OM1 branch stenoses. Fractional flow reserve (FFR) of LAD is 0.86, 0.87. (C) *Left panel*, pre-percutaneous coronary intervention (PCI) of OM1 and post PCI. Patient became pain free and did well.

of randomization to a stenting strategy. For the FFR-PCI group (n = 496), all lesions had FFR measurements and only those with an FFR of less than 0.80 were stented. For the Angio-PCI group (n = 509), all lesions identified were stented. Clinical characteristics and angiographic findings were similar in both groups, with average SYNTAX scores of 14.5 (indicating low–intermediate risk patients).

Compared to the Angio-PCI group, the FFR-PCI group used fewer stents per patient (1.9 ± 1.3 vs. 2.7 ± 1.2; $p < 0.001$) and less contrast (272 mL vs. 302 mL; $p < 0.001$), and had a lower procedure cost ($5332 vs. $6007; $p < 0.001$) and shorter hospital stay (3.4 vs. 3.7 days; $p = 0.05$). More importantly, the 2-year rates of mortality or MI were 13% in the Angio-PCI group compared with 8% in the FFR-PCI group ($p = 0.02$). Composite rates of death/nonfatal MI, or revascularization were 22% and 18%, respectively ($p = 0.08$). For lesions deferred on the basis of an FFR of greater than 0.80, the rate of MI was only 0.2% and the rate of revascularization was 3.2 % after 2 years (Fig. 4.12A).

FAME demonstrated that PCI guided by FFR in patients with multivessel CAD significantly reduces mortality and MI at 2 years when compared with standard angiography-guided PCI. A related cost-effectiveness evaluation showed that FFR-guided PCI not only improved outcomes, but did so at a significantly lower cost.

The Fractional Flow Reserve-Guided PCI Versus Medical Therapy in Stable Coronary Disease (FAME 2) trial compared optimal medical therapy to optimal medical therapy with PCI in patients who have proven ischemia by FFR. FAME 2 compared effectiveness of treating ischemic lesions (i.e., those with FFR ≤0.80) by optimal medical therapy alone (OMT) or revascularization with PCI plus OMT. A total of 1220 patients with angiographic disease in one, two, or three vessels that was suitable for PCI underwent FFR. All patients with lesions having an FFR of 0.80 or less were randomized to either PCI or medical therapy. A composite of all-cause mortality, nonfatal MI, or unplanned hospitalization leading to urgent revascularization during a 2-year follow-up was the primary end point. As in prior studies following those lesions that did not undergo PCI for an FFR of more than 0.80, in the FAME 2 trial, those lesions that had FFR values of greater than 0.80 were entered into a registry and followed. These patients had a low rate of the primary end point of death (0), MI (1.8%), or urgent revascularization (2.4%) over the follow-up 12 months, thus reproducing the findings of the pre-DES era DEFER trial (Fig. 4.12B).

Together these data are the core source of FFR-related outcomes. They strongly support the concept that coronary stenoses whose FFR is not physiologically significant (i.e. >0.80) have an exceptionally good prognosis without PCI and should be treated with optimal medical therapy alone.

Left Main Stenosis

Accurate assessment of the hemodynamic significance of left main (LM) coronary lesions is of critical importance when a patient faces possible CABG surgery. Because of the inherent limitations discussed earlier, angiography alone may not be reliable in intermediate LM stenoses, and FFR is useful for decision-making.

Numerous studies of FFR support its use in equivocal LM disease (Table 4.6). Most recently, Hamilos et al. in a large multicenter prospective trial examined FFR and 5-year outcome in 213 patients with an angiographically equivocal LM coronary artery stenosis. When FFR was greater than 0.80, patients were treated medically or another stenosis was treated by coronary angioplasty (nonsurgical group; n = 138). When FFR was less than 0.80, CABG surgery was performed (surgical group; n = 75). The 5-year survival estimates were 90% in the nonsurgical (FFR >0.80) group and 85% in the surgical (FFR <0.80) group (p = 0.48). The 5-year event-free survival estimates were 74% and 82% in the two groups, respectively (p = 0.50) (Fig. 4.13). Of note, only 23% of

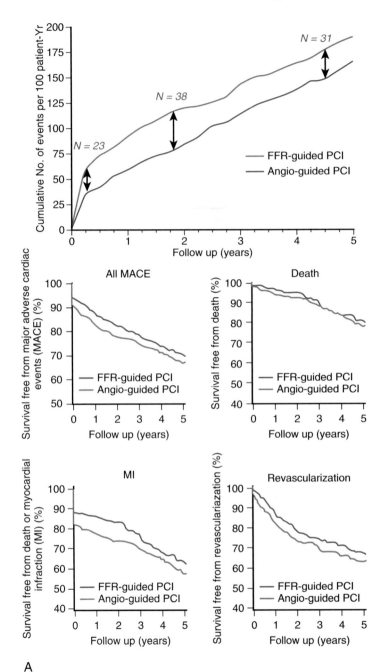

A

Figure 4.12 (A) The FAME study results. Kaplan-Meier survival curves according to study group. Results confirm the long-term safety of fractional flow reserve (FFR)-guided percutaneous coronary intervention (PCI) in patients with multivessel disease. A strategy of FFR-guided PCI resulted in a significant decrease of major adverse cardiac events for up to 2 years. From 2 years to 5 years, the risks for both groups developed similarly. This clinical outcome in the FFR-guided group was achieved with a lower number of stented arteries and less resource use. These results indicate that FFR guidance of multivessel PCI should be the standard of care in most patients. *(From Lokien X, et al. Fractional flow reserve versus angiography for guidance of PCI in patients with multivessel coronary artery disease (FAME): 5-year follow-up of a randomised controlled trial. The Lancet 2015;386;1853–1860.)*

Continued

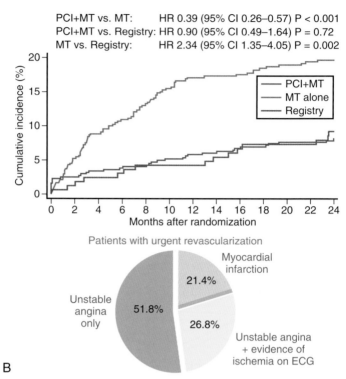

PCI+MT vs. MT: HR 0.39 (95% CI 0.26–0.57) P < 0.001
PCI+MT vs. Registry: HR 0.90 (95% CI 0.49–1.64) P = 0.72
MT vs. Registry: HR 2.34 (95% CI 1.35–4.05) P = 0.002

Figure 4.12, cont'd (B) FAME 2 study results. Kaplan-Meier curve for primary end point of death, myocardial infarction, or urgent revascularization at 12 months in the group assigned to PCI and optimal medical therapy (*blue*) versus optimal medical therapy alone (*red*) versus those who did not undergo revascularization (*green*). The pie chart shows the events prompting revascularization with about 50% unstable angina, 25% MI, and 25% UA with ECG changes. *(Modified from De Bruyne B, et al. Fractional flow reserve-guided PCI versus medical therapy in stable coronary disease. N Engl J Med 2012;367(11):991–1001.)*

patients with a diameter stenosis of greater than 50% had a hemodynamically significant LM by FFR.

The assessment of an isolated LM is straightforward. The pressure wire can be put into either the left anterior descending (LAD) artery or the circumflex artery (CFX) and FFR measured. For distal LM, FFR is measured twice, once in each branch. However, the LM FFR assessment becomes more complex when there is additional potentially significant LAD disease that may reduce flow to anterior wall thus creating a falsely elevated LM FFR.

Fearon et al. demonstrated that the LM FFR measured in the setting of downstream LAD disease was only affected when the FFR of both the LM and LAD was less than 0.45. In 25 patients, Fearon and colleagues created an intermediate narrowing in the LM with a balloon catheter after stenting the LAD, or the left circumflex (LCx), or both. FFR was measured in the LAD and LCx coronary arteries before and after creation of "downstream" stenosis by inflating an angioplasty balloon within the newly placed stent thus mimicking the LM/LAD anatomy. The true FFR (FFR_{true}) of the LM, measured in the nondiseased downstream vessel in the absence of stenosis in the other vessel, was compared with the apparent FFR (FFR_{app}) measured in the presence of stenosis. LM FFR was significantly lower than apparent FFR (FFR_{app}, 0.81 ± 0.08 vs. 0.83 ± 0.08, $p < 0.001$), although the numerical difference was small. This difference correlated with the severity of downstream disease ($r = 0.35$, $p < 0.001$). In all cases in which FFR_{app} was greater than 0.85, FFR_{true} was greater than 0.80. In most cases, downstream

Table 4.6

Fractional Flow Reserve (FFR) Studies Assessing Intermediate Left Main Stenosis

Study	FFR Threshold	N	Medical Therapy			Surgical Therapy			Follow-Up Time
			N (%)	MACE	Death	n (%)	MACE	Death	
Hamilos (2009)	0.8	213	136 (65%)	26%	9 (6.5%)	73 (35%)	17%	7 (9.6%)	35 ± 25
Courtis (2009)	0.75 surg; >0.80 med	142	82 (58%)	13%	3 (3.6%)	60 (42%)	7%	3 (5%)	14 ± 11
Lindstaedt (2006)	0.75 surg; >0.80 med	51	24 (47%)	31%	0	27 (53%)	34%	5 (19%)	29 ± 16
Suemaru (2005)	0.75	15	8 (53%)	0	0	7 (47%)	29%	0	33 ± 10
Legutko (2005)	0.75	38	20 (53%)	10%	0	18 (46%)	11%	2	24 mean
Jimenez-Navarro (2004)	0.75	27	20 (74%)	10%	0	7 (26%)	29%	2	2 ± 12
Bech (2001)	0.75	54	24 (44%)	24%	0	30 (56%)	17%	1	29 ± 15

From Lokhandwala J, Hodgson J. Assessing intermediate left main lesions with IVUS or FFR. *Cardiac Interventions Today.* October 2009.

Kaplan-Meier mortality curves showing percent survival (A) and major adverse cardiac events (MACE; B) in the 2 study groups

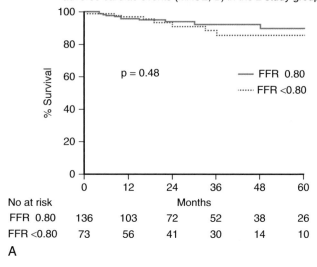

No at risk					
FFR 0.80	136	103	72	52	38	26
FFR <0.80	73	56	41	30	14	10

A

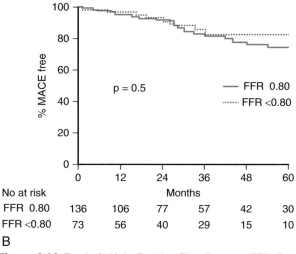

No at risk					
FFR 0.80	136	106	77	57	42	30
FFR <0.80	73	56	40	29	15	10

B

Figure 4.13 The Left Main Fraction Flow Reserve (FFR) 5-year outcome study. (A) Total survival. (B) Major adverse cardiac event-free survival by Kaplan-Meier mortality curves in the two study groups. *(From Hamilos M, et al. Long-term clinical outcome after fractional flow reserve–guided treatment in patients with angiographically equivocal left main coronary artery stenosis. Circulation. 2009;120:1505–12.)*

disease does not have a clinically significant impact on the assessment of FFR across an intermediate LMCA stenosis with the pressure wire positioned in the nondiseased vessel (Fig. 4.14G and H).

Fig. 4.14A–E shows an example of FFR in multivessel CAD. Table 4.7 lists FFR studies and outcomes over the past decade that support the concept that FFR-directed interventions and diagnostic studies have superior outcomes compared to angiography-guided studies alone.

Ostial and Side Branch Lesions

Ostial narrowings of side branches or newly produced narrowings in side branches within stents ("jailed" branches) are particularly difficult to assess by angiography because of their overlapping orientation relative to the parent branch, stent struts across the branch, and image foreshortening (Fig. 4.14). Koo et al. compared FFR to angiography in 97 "jailed" side branch lesions (vessel size >2.0 mm, percent stenosis >50% by visual estimation) after stent implantation. No lesion with less than 75% stenosis had an FFR of less than 0.75. Among 73 lesions with ≥75% stenosis or greater, only 20 lesions (27%) were functionally significant. Of 91 patients, side branch intervention was performed in 26 of 28 patients with an FFR of less than 0.75. In this subgroup, FFR increased to greater than 0.75 despite residual stenosis of 69 ± 10%. At 9 months, functional restenosis was 8% (5/65) with no difference in events compared to 110 side branches treated by angiography alone (4.6% vs. 3.7%, $p = 0.7$) (Fig. 4.15A and B). Measurement of FFR for ostial and side branch assessment thus identifies the minority of lesions that are functionally significant, reducing the need for complex, time-consuming, and potentially detrimental side-branch interventions.

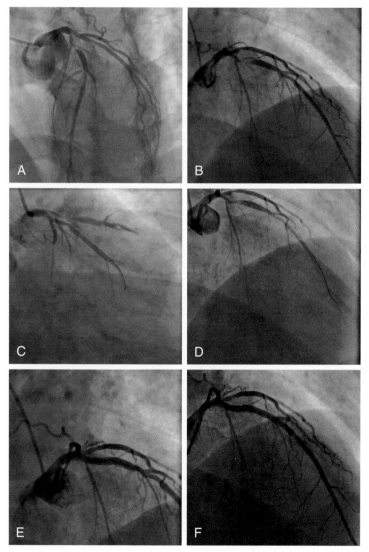

Figure 4.14 Cine frames from multivessel percutaneous coronary intervention (PCI)-guided by fractional flow reserve (FFR). (A) LAO cranial view of left coronary artery (LCA) showing severe and moderate lesions in the left anterior descending (LAD) and circumflex (CFX) arteries. (B) RAO view of LCA. (C) FFR of CFX was 0.88. (D) PCI of LAD performed. (E) After stent of proximal LAD, Mid-LAD lesion assessed by FFR at 0.68, an additional stent was placed; (F) Final result of fully deployed stents, guided by FFR. *Continued*

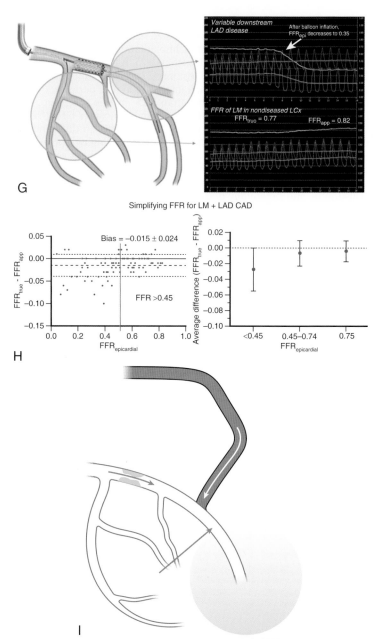

Figure 4.14, cont'd (G) *Left*: Cartoon of experimental layout to test relationship between left main (LM) and LAD lesions of increasing severity. There is a deflated ("winged") balloon in the LM coronary artery with a variably inflated balloon within the newly placed LAD coronary artery stent and pressure wires down the LAD and the left CFX coronary artery. The circles represent changing bedside when the LAD balloon is inflated. Only when the LAD lesion is very severe does the FFR apparent in the CFX rise. (H) *Left*: Bland-Altman plot demonstrating the relationship between the difference in FFR$_{true}$ and FFR$_{app}$ based on the severity of downstream disease as assessed by FFR of the left middle coronary artery (LMCA) and the downstream stenosis (FFR$_{epi}$). *Right*: Chart demonstrating the average difference between the FFR$_{true}$ and FFR$_{app}$ depending on the severity of the downstream stenosis (FFR$_{epi}$). (I) Diagram of SVG (red) to LAD. Blood flow to distal bed (blue circle) is result of 3 flows: 1, native LAD, collaterals from other native vessels (red arrow) and flow from SVG. *(G, H are from Fearon W, et al. The impact of downstream coronary stenosis on FFR assessment of intermediate left main CAD: human validation. J Am Coll Cardiol Interv. 2015;8(3):398–403.*

Table 4.7

Fractional Flow Reserve Studies on Long-Term Outcomes

FFR Outcome Studies	N =	Study Design	Question	Outcome	Journal
DEFER (2007)	325	Prospective MC RCT	Is it safe to defer FFR normal intermediate lesions?	Less MACE in FFR >0.75 when rx'd medically	JACC
FAME (2009)	750	Prospective MC RCT	Does FFR-guided PCI vs. angio-guided for MVD improve outcomes?	Less MACE, lower cost w FFR	NEJM
FAME II (2012)	1220	Prospective MC RCT	Does FFR-guided PCI + OMT vs. OMT alone improve outcomes?	Less MACE w FFR, cost effective	NEJM
FAMOUS-NSTEMI (2014)	350	Prospective MC Randomized (UK)	Does FFR-guided PCI in NSTEMI change angio decisions for revasc? Outcomes?	FFR reclass revasc decision in 22%, Less revasc w FFR	EHJ
DANAMI3-PRIMULTI (2015)	600	Prospective MC Randomized (Denmark)	Dose FFR-guided PCI in MV STEMI vs. IRA only revasc improve outcomes?	Less MACE w FFR	Lancet
Mayo (2013)	7358	Retrospective SC Registry	Does FFR-guided vs. angio-guided PCI improve outcomes in routine practice?	Less MACE w FFR	EHJ
R3F (2014)	1.075	Prospective MC Registry (France)	Does FFR change angio decisions for revasc? Outcomes?	FFR reclass revasc decision in 47%, similar outcomes	Circulation
POST-IT (2015)	918	Prospective MC Registry (Portugal)	Does FFR change angio decisions for revasc? Outcomes?	FFR reclass revasc decision in 44% (follow-up data in press)	In press
Asan registry (2013)		Prospective SC Registry	Does FFR-guided vs. angio-guided PCI improve outcomes in routine practice?	Fewer stents and less MACE w FFR	EJHJ

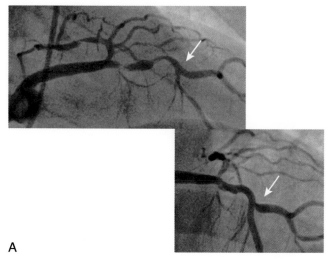

A

FFR VS. OSTIAL LESION SEVERITY

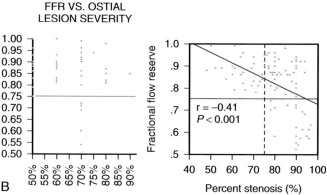

B

$r = -0.41$
$P < 0.001$

Percent stenosis (%)

Figure 4.15 (A) Angiographic frames showing jailed side branch before (*left*) and after (*right*) left anterior descending (LAD) artery stenting. (B) *Left*: Comparison of fractional flow reserve (FFR) and percent stenosis for ostial lesions. *(From Zaiee A, et al. FFR vs ostial lesion severity. Am J Cardiol. 2004;93:1404–07; and (right) Koo BK, et al. Comparison of FFR and percent stenosis for jailed side branches. J Am Coll Cardiol. 2005;46:633–37.)*

Saphenous Vein Graft Lesions

When assessing a lesion in a saphenous vein graft (SVG), recall that there are three sources of coronary blood flow to the myocardium: the epicardial artery, the bypass conduit, and collateral flow (Fig. 4.14I). The FFR is the summed responses of three competing flows (and pressure) from (1) the native vessel, (2) the CABG conduit, and (3) the collateral flow induced from long-standing native coronary occlusion. In the most uncomplicated situation of an occluded native vessel with minimal distal collateral supply, the theory of FFR will apply just as much to a lesion in a SVG as to a native right coronary artery feeding a normal myocardial bed. For more complex situations, the FFR will reflect the summed responses of the three supply sources and yield a net FFR indicating potential ischemia in that region.

Interesting is the fate of SVG conduits implanted distal to hemo-dynamically *insignificant* lesions. Surgeons and cardiologists have recognized that late patency is reduced and native CAD can be acceler-ated by placement of an unneeded graft. Although most surgical consultants typically recommend bypassing all lesions with greater than 50% diameter narrowing in patients with multivessel disease, the patency rate of SVGs on vessels with hemodynamically nonsignificant lesions has rarely been questioned. Botman et al. found that there was a 20–25% incidence of graft closure in 450 coronary artery bypass grafts when placed on non-hemodynamically significantly stenosed arteries (preoperative FFR >0.80) at 1-year follow-up (Fig. 4.16A). Toth et al. also demonstrate improved CABG patency in hemodynamically significantly stenosed arteries compared to those with angiographic-only guided surgery (Fig. 4.16B). In patients requiring CABG for multivessel revascularization, angiographic lesions of uncertain significance may benefit from FFR assessment, providing prognosis of graft patency and potentially reducing unnecessary graft placement.

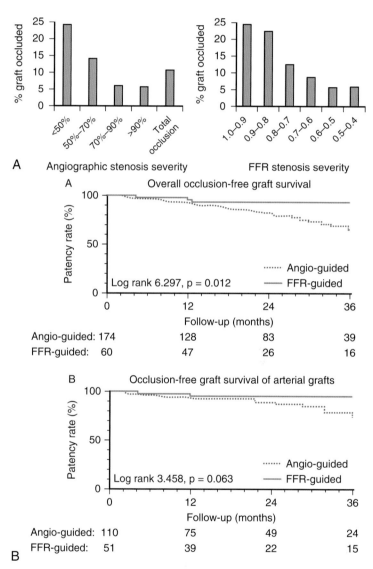

Figure 4.16 The fate of bypass grafts and fractional flow reserve (FFR) at time of surgery. (A) High FFR is associated with high occlusion rates. (B) Clinical events in the angio-guided and FFR-guided group during 36-month follow-up. *Panel A*: overall survival (log rank 2.216, *p* = 0.137). *Panel B*: Myocardial infarction (MI)-free survival (log rank 0.064, *p* = 0.780). *Panel C*: Target vessel revascularization (TVR)-free survival (log rank 0.777, *p* = 0.378). *Panel D*: Major adverse cardiac event (MACE)-free survival (log rank 0.013, *p* = 0.908). *(A is from Botman CJ, Schonberger J, Koolen S, et al. Does stenosis severity of native vessels influence bypass graft patency? A prospective fractional flow reserve-guided study. Ann Thorac Surg. 2007;83:2093–97. B is from Toth G, et al. Fractional flow reserve-guided versus angiography-guided coronary artery bypass graft surgery. Circulation. 2013;128(13):1405–11.)*

Coronary Lesions in Acute Coronary Syndrome

In acute coronary syndrome (ACS) settings and especially in acute MI (AMI), the pathophysiology of the infarcted artery and its subtended microvascular bed is both dynamic and complex. The predictive ability of FFR in ACS has several limitations: (1) the microvascular bed in the infarct zone may not have uniform, constant, or minimal resistance; (2) the severity of stenosis may evolve as thrombus and vasoconstriction abate; and (3) FFR measurements are not meaningful when normal perfusion has not been achieved. Thus FFR has limited utility in the infarct-related artery during the first 24–48 hours after ACS. However, FFR has demonstrated value in remote lesion assessment and in target lesion assessment during the recovery phase of MI.

The role of FFR in ST-elevation MI (STEMI) patients was reported in the Primulti Study. Following the PCI of the STEMI vessel, FFR was used in any noninfarct artery considered angiographically significant and treated if the FFR was less than 0.80. A total of 313 patients were in the culprit-only group and were compared to 314 patients with complete revascularization, guiding nonculprit lesion stenting by FFR. At a 2-year follow-up major adverse cardiac events (MACE) occurred in 68 (22%) patients of the culprit-only group compared to 40 (13%) in the FFR-guided STEMI revascularization group (hazard ratio 0.56, 95% CI 0.38–0.83; $p = 0.004$).

Despite the PRIMULTI study findings, there remains a question whether FFR will be reliable in the ACS setting. FFR is directly related to flow; flow is directly related to the myocardial territory or mass supplied by the stenotic vessel; for a given stenosis, the higher the flow, the lower the FFR and vice versa. Thus for the same stenosis at two points in time, the FFR could decrease if the flow measured at a later time increased due to myocardial bed changes, as might be expected with infarct healing. This problem, the visual-functional mismatch between the angiographic stenosis and the FFR, is commonly seen with severe angiographic lesions in small branches supplying a small mass having a high FFR or mild lesions in large branches supplying a large myocardial mass having a low FFR (Fig. 4.17).

Because of a changing myocardial bed during the recuperation phase after an acute infarction, FFR is not used in the STEMI culprit artery until 4.6 days after the event, when myocardial function is believed to stabilize. For the noninfarct-related artery (non-IRA) in STEMI/NSTEMI patients, the zone of myocardial injury of the culprit vessel is unknown but may extend close to the region supplied by the non-IRA. Thus a normal FFR at the time of STEMI might be lower several days later if the myocardial flow improves to the remote non-IRA zone, changing the initial treatment decision based on a high FFR. The stability

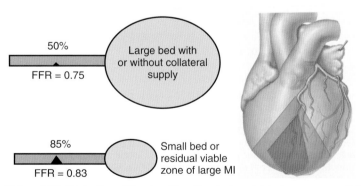

Figure 4.17 Illustration of the visual-functional mismatch between myocardial mass and fractional flow reserve (FFR). Because flow is related to myocardial bed size, a moderate lesion (*top*, 50%) serving a large territory could have low FFR (0.75) whereas a more severe appearing lesion (*bottom*, 85%) serving a small bed (such as after infarction) could have high FFR (0.83).

of FFR in the noninfarct artery in STEMI/NSTEMI patients was examined in a subset of the FAME study. A total of 101 patients undergoing PCI for both STEMI and NSTEMI had 112 nonculprit lesions assessed by FFR at the index procedure and again repeated 35 ± 4 days later. The FFR of these nonculprit stenoses was 0.77 ± 0.13 during the index procedure and was an identical 0.77 ± 0.13 at the time of follow-up. In those with unstable angina or NSTEMI, there was no evidence for a changing FFR over 3 months of follow-up.

Preliminary data from the COMPARE-ACUTE multicenter trial 8 reported on results in 408 patients with multivessel disease and STEMI undergoing primary PCI. A total of 613 FFR measurements were made in nonculprit lesions. FFR measured in a nonculprit lesion was negative in 57% (>0.80) and positive in 43%, highlighting the fact that nonculprit lesions identified during STEMI may be innocent bystanders and may not need to be treated.

Given the results of the FFR for non-IRA and the PRIMULTI study, wherein long-term outcomes remain durable and a function of the FFR, as in the 5-year FAME data presented at the ESC 2015, the use of FFR for decisions about treating non-IRA may emerge as a dominant strategy for the revascularization of multivessel disease in the STEMI patient.

Serial (Multiple) Lesions in a Single Vessel

When more than one discrete stenosis is present in the same vessel, the hyperemic flow and pressure through the first lesion will be attenuated by the second and vice versa (Fig. 4.18A and B). One stenosis will

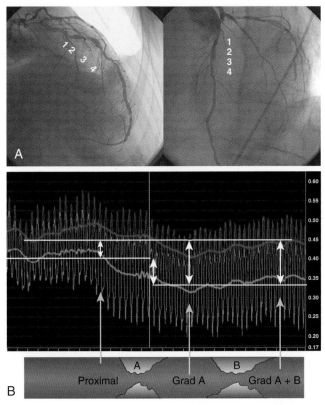

Figure 4.18 (A) Example of serial lesion fractional flow reserve (FFR). Individual lesion FFR cannot be determined without a coronary occlusion wedge pressure. In practice, treatment of largest translesional gradient is performed, then reassessment of remaining lesion will determine treatment approach. (B) Serial lesion assessment. Diagram of pressures and pressure gradients across lesions in series. *Pa,* aortic pressure; *Pm,* mid pressure between lesions; *Pd,* distal pressure. *ΔP1 and ΔP2,* pressure gradients produced by each lesion.

Continued

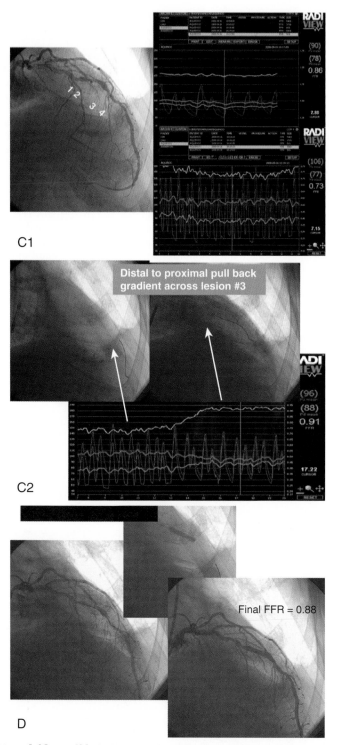

Figure 4.18, cont'd (C) Example of serial lesion assessment. Panels show RAO and LAO cine frames of lesions with numbers. (C1) shows resting pressure across all lesions (*top*) and FFR across all lesions (*bottom*). FFR = 0.73. (C2) Distal to proximal pressure wire pullback shows that step-up of pressure gradient was present only across lesion 3. (D) Angiographic frames of percutaneous coronary intervention (PCI) for lesion 3. Final FFR was 0.88.

mask the true effect of its serial counterpart. When the distance between two lesions is greater than 6 times the vessel diameter, the stenoses generally behave independently and the overall pressure gradient is the sum of the individual pressure losses at any given flow rate.

The interaction between two stenoses is such that the FFR of each individual lesion cannot be calculated by the simple equation for isolated stenoses applied to each separately, but can be predicted by more complete equations taking into account Pa, Pm, Pd, and coronary occlusion pressure, Pw. The requirement for the coronary occlusion pressure makes this approach unsuitable for most diagnostic purposes.

In clinical practice, the use of a pressure pullback recording is particularly well suited to identify the specific regions of a vessel with large pressure gradients that may benefit from treatment. The one stenosis with the largest gradient can be treated first and the FFR remeasured for the remaining stenoses to determine the need for further treatment (Fig. 4.18B–D).

Diffuse Coronary Disease

Using FFR during continuous pressure wire pullback from a distal to a proximal location, the impact of diffuse atherosclerosis can be documented. Diffuse atherosclerosis, rather than a focal narrowing, is characterized by a continuous and gradual pressure recovery during pullback, without any abrupt increase in pressure related to a focal region. The pressure pullback recording at maximum hyperemia will provide the necessary information to decide if and where stent implantation may be useful (Fig. 4.19). The location of a focal pressure drop superimposed on diffuse disease can be identified as an appropriate location for treatment.

Assessing Collateral Flow by Poststenotic Pressure

The pressure-derived fractional collateral flow is defined as the mean coronary wedge pressure (distal coronary pressure during balloon occlusion) divided by the mean aortic pressure (if the central venous pressure is abnormal, then it should be subtracted from both the wedge and aortic pressures). In general, a pressure-derived fractional collateral flow of 0.25 or more suggests sufficient collaterals to prevent ischemia during PCI. Furthermore, these patients have a significantly lower adverse event rate during follow-up compared to those with insufficient collaterals at the time of PCI (pressure-derived collateral flow <0.25). Pressure-derived collateral flow has also been studied in patients with AMI and has been shown to be the major determinant of left ventricular recovery after primary PCI. Unfortunately this technique for assessing collaterals is limited by the requirement for coronary artery occlusion.

Resting Pd/Pa and Instantaneous Wave-Free Pressure Ratio, iFR, Coronary Stenosis Significance

Utilization of an adenosine-independent pressure-derived index of coronary stenosis severity may facilitate an easier assessment of stenosis severity. FFR requires that coronary resistance is stable and minimal, usually achieved by the administration of adenosine. Sen et al. determined that the period of diastole, in which equilibration or balance between pressure waves from the aorta and distal microcirculatory reflection was a "wave-free period," has low and fixed resistance. This period of low resistance may be sufficiently low to be equal to the FFR measurement (Fig. 4.19B and C). The ratio of Pd/Pa during the wave-free period was called the *instantaneous wave-free pressure ratio* (iFR). In the ADVISE study, 157 stenoses were assessed with pressure and flow distal to the stenosis, with 118 stenoses assessed as a second segment of the research using pressure alone. The intracoronary resistance at rest during the wave-free period was similar in variability and magnitude to that during FFR, and the iFR correlated closely with FFR ($r = 0.90$). However there were limitations to this analysis despite having high sensitivity, specificity, and negative and positive predictive values for iFR versus FFR. In particular, there is concern that the iFR at rest was different from the iFR during hyperemia, suggesting that the wave-free period does not have as low a resistance as would a hyperemic period.

Subsequently, Petraco et al. demonstrated that at iFR cutpoints of greater than 0.93 or less than 0.86, there was a strong correlation with normal and abnormal FFR values (using 0.80 as an FFR cutpoint). Thus

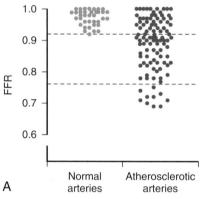

Diffuse disease as measured by FFR may result in ischemia despite no significant focal narrowing

A

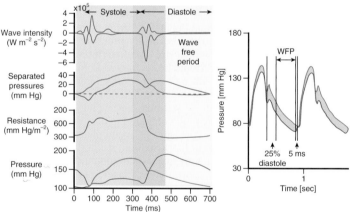

Resting (i.e. no adenosine) instantaneous pressure during wave free period = iFR

Davies JE et al. Circulation 2006;113:1767–1778

Davies JE et al. JACC 2012;59:1392–402

B

Figure 4.19 Fractional flow reserve (FFR) in diffuse coronary artery disease (CAD). (A) Graphs of individual values of FFR in normal arteries and in atherosclerotic coronary arteries without focal stenosis on arteriogram. The upper dotted line indicates the lowest value of FFR in normal coronary arteries. The lower dotted line indicates the 0.75 threshold level. (*From De Bruyne B, et al. Circulation. 2001;104:2401–2406*). (B) *Left*: The instantaneous wave-free ratio (iFR). Wave-intensity analysis demonstrates the proximal and microcirculatory (distal) originating waves generated during the cardiac cycle. A wave-free period can be seen in diastole when no new waves are generated (*shaded*). This corresponds to a time period in which there is minimal microcirculatory (distal)–originating pressure, minimal and constant resistance, and a nearly constant rate of change in flow velocity. (Separated pressure above diastole is the residual pulsatile separated pressure component after subtraction of the diastolic pressure.)

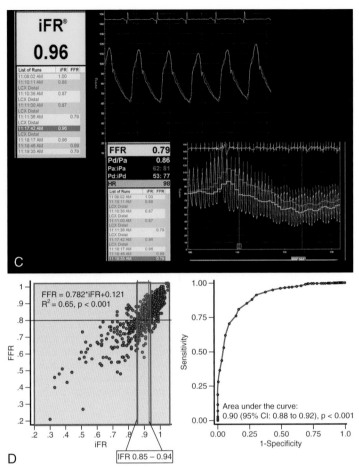

Figure 4.19, cont'd (C) Pressure tracings of iFR (*top left*) and FFR (*bottom*). (D) ADVISE study. Pd/Pa and FFR relationship. Scatterplot of the Pd/Pa and FFR relationship. Receiver-operating characteristic curves of iFR and Pd/Pa compared with FFR ≤0.80. *CI,* confidence interval; *Pd/Pa,* baseline distal coronary pressure to aortic pressure. *(A is from De Bruyne B, et al. Circulation. 2001;104:2401–06; B is from Sen S, et al. Development and validation of a new adenosine-independent index of stenosis severity from coronary wave–intensity analysis results of the ADVISE (ADenosine Vasodilator Independent Stenosis Evaluation) Study. Am Coll Cardiol. 2012;59:1234; D is from Escaned J, et al. Diagnostic accuracy of baseline distal-to-aortic pressure ratio to assess coronary stenosis severity: a post-hoc analysis of the ADVISE II Study. J Am Coll Cardiol Interv. 2015;8(6):834–836.)*

potentially 57% of the patients with intermediate stenosis could be assessed without the need for hyperemic stimulus (Fig. 4.19D).

The RESOLVE study compared the diagnostic accuracy of iFR and resting pressure ratio (Pd/Pa) to FFR in a core laboratory. The IFR, Pd/Pa, and FFR were measured in 1768 patients from 15 clinical sites. Core lab technicians were used to analyze the data. Thresholds corresponding to 90% accuracy in predicting ischemic versus nonischemic FFR were then identified. In 1974 lesions, the optimal iFR to predict an FFR of less than 0.8 was 0.90 with accuracy of 80%. For the resting Pd/Pa ratio, the cutpoint was 0.92, with an overall accuracy of 80% with no significant differences between iFR and Pd/Pa. Both measures have 90% accuracy to predict positive or negative FFR in 65% and 48% of lesions, respectively. These data suggest that the overall accuracy of iFR with FFR was about 80%, which can be improved to 90% in a subset of lesions. Clinical outcome studies are in progress to determine whether the use of iFR or some variation thereof might obviate the need for hyperemia in selected patients.

Coronary Doppler Blood Flow Technique

IC Doppler flow velocity measurements are most useful for research investigations into the status of the microcirculation with normal epicardial conduits. The Doppler flow wire can provide an objective, physiologic measurement of coronary blood flow and can measure flow velocity responses to pharmacologic or mechanical interventions. It is also useful in the study of collateral blood flow responses.

The Doppler angioplasty guidewire (Volcano Therapeutics, Del Mar, CA) is a flexible, steerable guidewire 175 cm long and 0.014 inch in diameter with a piezoelectric ultrasound transducer integrated into the tip. The forward-directed ultrasound beam diverges in a 27-degree arc from the long axis (measured to the −6 dB round-trip points of the ultrasound beam pattern). A pulse repetition frequency of more than 40 kHz, pulse duration of +0.83 msec, and sampling delay of 6.5 msec are standard for clinical usage. The system is coupled to a real-time spectrum analyzer, a videocassette recorder, and a video page printer. The quadrature/Doppler audio signals are processed by the spectrum analyzer using online fast Fourier transformation to provide a scrolling grayscale spectral display. The frequency response of the system calculates approximately 90 spectra per second. Simultaneous electrocardiographic and arterial pressure is also input to the video display. The fundamentals and artifacts of flow velocity measurements have been described in detail elsewhere (see Suggested Readings).

Coronary Flow Velocity Signal Analysis

The velocity of red blood cells flowing past the ultrasound emitter/receiver on the end of a guidewire can be determined from the frequency shift, defined as the difference between the transmitted and returning frequency, where:

$$V = (F_1 - F_0) \times (C/2F_0) \times Cos\emptyset$$

where V = velocity of blood flow, F_0 = transmitting (transducer) frequency, F_1 = returning frequency, C = constant for the speed of sound in blood, and $\emptyset$ = angle of incidence. Volumetric flow is the product of the vessel area (cm^2) and the flow velocity (cm/sec), yielding a value in cm^3/sec.

The parameters of IC flow velocity, including maximal peak velocity (MPV) and mean or average peak velocity (APV) diastolic and systolic velocities, are displayed and recorded (Fig. 4.20).

Coronary flow velocity reserve (CFR or CFVR) is the ratio of the hyperemia average peak velocity (APV) to resting APV. CFR measures the summed response of both the epicardial artery and the microcirculation. For this reason, a patient without epicardial disease but with abnormal microcirculatory function can have an abnormal CFVR, thus limiting the utility of CFVR for assessment of intermediate epicardial stenoses in patients with microvascular disease.

Technique of Coronary Doppler Measurements

The technique of Doppler wire flow velocity signal acquisition is identical to that of the FFR pressure wire. Prior to introducing the sensor wire, heparin and IC nitroglycerin (200 mcg) are given. Nitroglycerin blocks changes in epicardial lumen dimension during the

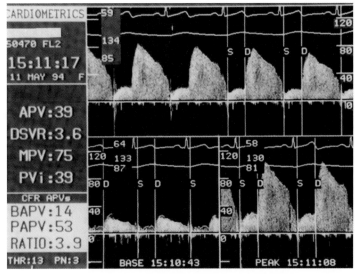

Figure 4.20 Panel of flow velocity signals for measurement of coronary vasodilatory flow reserve. Flow panel was divided into upper and lower parts. The upper panel is a continuous display in real time of the flow spectra. The normal phasic pattern is seen shortly after hyperemia. The electrocardiogram (ECG) and aortic pressure is displayed on top of the flow signals. The numbers in the upper left corner box are the heart rate, systolic pressure, and diastolic pressure. The lower panel is divided into left and right for storage of baseline and hyperemic signals, respectively. The codes at the left are the values for the flow parameters of the top panel (*far right*). *APV*, average peak velocity; *DSVR*, diastolic-systolic velocity ratio; *MPV*, maximal peak velocity; *PVI*, peak velocity interval; *Ratio*, coronary flow reserve; *BAPV/PAPV*, base and hyperemic APV, respectively.

measurements, which may alter the flow velocity down the vessel. Using standard angioplasty equipment, the wire is introduced through the guide catheter to the coronary artery. The tip of the wire should be positioned in a mid-vessel segment (about 3 mm in diameter). Attempts should be made to position the wire in the middle of a major vessel and, by gentle torquing, maximize the velocity signal. The wire should not be moved between the resting velocity measurement and the hyperemic velocity measurement. Coronary hyperemia is induced exactly as done for determining FFR (see earlier discussion).

Although earlier studies report a coronary vasodilatory reserve ratio of 3.5–5 in normal patients, lower values are more commonly observed in patients with chest pain and angiographically normal arteries (normal 2.7 ± 0.6). Changes in cardiovascular hemodynamics (heart rate, contractility, blood pressure) can impact the CFVR (but not FFR), a limitation when performing follow-up or serial CFVR measurements.

Methodological Considerations

Doppler coronary velocity only measures relative changes in velocity. To measure absolute blood flow, APV × CSA is calculated. The following assumptions must be made:

1. The cross-sectional area of the vessel being studied remains fixed during hyperemia.
2. The velocity profile across the vessel is not distorted by arterial disease.
3. The angle between the crystal and sample volume remains constant and less than 30 degrees from the horizontal flow stream.

Assessing Collateral Flow by IC Doppler

In order to quantify the presence and degree of collaterals, a Doppler collateral flow index (CFI) has been described. CFI is defined as the amount of flow via collaterals to a vascular region, divided by the amount of flow to the same region via the normally patent vessel. It is determined by summing the integral of systolic and diastolic flow velocities during balloon occlusion. In the case of temporally shifted bidirectional flow velocity signals, the antegrade and retrograde velocity integrals are added. The total velocity integral during balloon occlusion is then divided by the velocity integral after successful PCI, in order to calculate the CFI. A Doppler CFI of greater than 0.30 has been shown to accurately predict collateral circulation adequate enough to prevent myocardial ischemia during PCI. Moreover the Doppler CFI is a more sensitive determinant of collateral flow than is angiographically visible collateral circulation. In another study, patients undergoing PCI who had a Doppler CFI of greater than 0.25 had a fourfold decrease in the MACE rate at approximately 2 years compared to those with a CFI of less than 0.25. The obvious limitation of this technique is that it requires performance of PCI (Fig. 4.21).

Assessing the Microcirculation by Thermodilution Blood Flow Measurements

For the St. Jude pressure wire system, proprietary software has been developed that allows simultaneous measurement of FFR, CFR, and the index of microcirculatory resistance (IMR) using the pressure wire. CFR and IMR are measured using a novel coronary thermodilution technique, whereby the pressure transducer serves as a distal thermistor and the shaft of the pressure wire as a proximal thermistor. In this manner, the resting mean transit time of room temperature saline injected down the coronary artery can be measured with the pressure wire and compared to the hyperemic mean transit time. The ratio of resting to hyperemic mean transit times serves as an estimate of CFR. FFR using the standard technique can be measured simultaneously (Fig. 4.21B). Coronary thermodilution CFR was initially validated in an in vitro model and an in vivo animal model. Subsequently it has been shown to correlate with CFVR measured with a Doppler wire in humans. A similar wire system that measures pressure-derived FFR and Doppler-derived CFVR is also available.

The ratio of distal coronary pressure to the inverse of the mean transit time during maximal hyperemia defines the IMR. IMR is superior to CFR because it is not affected by resting hemodynamics, making it more reproducible even after hemodynamic perturbations. It is also specific for the microvasculature, whereas CFR is affected by epicardial stenosis. IMR, when measured immediately after primary PCI for STEMI, predicts the amount of myocardial damage as well as left ventricular recovery better than other indices, such as CFR, ST segment resolution, or thrombolysis in myocardial infarction (TIMI) myocardial perfusion grade. IMR can also be useful for identifying microvascular dysfunction in patients with chest pain and no epicardial artery disease.

Safety of Intracoronary Sensor-Wire Measurements

Qian et al. examined the safety of intracoronary Doppler wire measurements in 906 patients. Fifteen patients (1.7%) had severe transient bradycardia after intracoronary adenosine, 14 in the right coronary artery and one in the left coronary artery. Nine patients (1%) had coronary spasm during passage of the Doppler guidewire (five in the right coronary and four in the LAD). Two patients (0.2%) had ventricular fibrillation during the procedure. Hypotension with bradycardia and ventricular asystole occurred in one patient. Transplant recipients had more of these complications than either diagnostic or interventional procedures.

Collateral flow reversal during
balloon occlusion

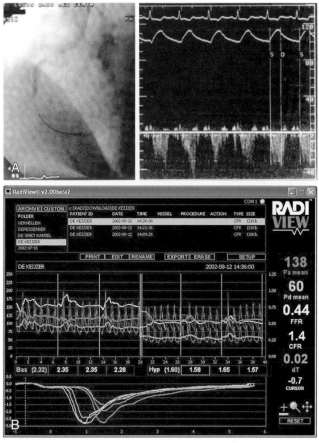

Figure 4.21 (A) Flow velocity signal reversal characteristic of epicardial collateral flow. (B) Example of simultaneous pressure and temperature tracings. The top tracings represent central aortic pressure (Pa) and distal coronary pressure (Pd), and fractional flow reserve (FFR) (Pd/Pa). The lower tracings are temperature tracings recorded by the proximal (shaft) and distal sensors. The half-time of injection was derived from the proximal thermodilution curve. Coronary flow velocity is calculated from the distal thermodilution. Tmn at hyperemia, CFR = V/Tmn at hyperemia, V/Tmn at rest CFR = Tmn at rest. *(Courtesy of Radi Medical, Uppsala, Sweden.)*

All complications could be managed medically. These data support the safety of using sensor wire measurements.

Intravascular Imaging With Ultrasound and Optical Coherence Tomography

IVUS provides anatomic information, including plaque characteristics, lesion length, and lumen dimensions. It is complementary to both angiography and physiology, allowing a thorough investigation of the disease within the vessel wall. By determining plaque characteristics, IVUS also is useful in selection of interventional equipment and procedures, such as atherectomy for plaque debulking.

OCT is similar to IVUS but uses infrared light to create images from reflected wavelength interference; it produces 10× resolution of ultrasound images. The OCT technique is discussed later. American Heart Association/American College of Cardiologists and Society of Cardiovascular Angiography and Interventions (AHA/ACC/SCAI) recommendations for coronary IVUS are shown in Table 4.8.

Two types of IVUS systems exist, both utilizing 20–40 MHz silicon piezoelectric crystals:

(1) A mechanical system that relies on a rotating internal cable and (2) a solid-state system externally mounted on a catheter and controlled electronically (Fig. 4.22). With the mechanical systems, the imaging core rotates via a flexible drive shaft to sweep the transducer

Table 4.8

Recommendations for Coronary Intravascular Ultrasound (IVUS) and Optical Coherence Tomography (OCT)

Intravascular Ultrasound

DEFINITELY BENEFICIAL:

IVUS is an accurate method for determining optimal stent deployment (complete stent expansion and apposition and lack of edge dissection or other complications after implantation) and the size of the vessel undergoing stent implantation.

PROBABLY BENEFICIAL:

IVUS can be used to appraise the significance of left main coronary artery (LMCA) stenosis and, employing a cutoff minimum lumen area (MLA) of greater than 6 mm^2, assess whether revascularization is warranted. IVUS can be useful for the assessment of plaque morphology.

NO PROVEN VALUE/SHOULD BE DISCOURAGED:

IVUS measurements for determination of non-LMCA lesion severity should not be relied upon in the absence of additional functional evidence for recommending revascularization.

Optical Coherence Tomography (OCT)

PROBABLY BENEFICIAL:

Determination of optimal stent deployment (sizing, apposition, and lack of edge dissection), with improved resolution compared with IVUS.

POSSIBLY BENEFICIAL:

OCT can be useful for the assessment of plaque morphology.

NO PROVEN VALUE/SHOULD BE DISCOURAGED:

OCT should not be performed to determine stenosis functional significance.

From Lofti A, Jeremias A, Fearon WF, et al. Expert consensus statement on the use of fractional flow reserve, intravascular ultrasound, and optical coherence tomography: a consensus statement of the Society of Cardiovascular Angiography and Interventions. *Cath Cardiovasc Interv.* 2014;83:509–18.

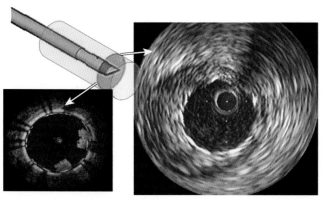

Figure 4.22 Intravenous ultrasound (IVUS) catheter has either rotating imaging core or multiple microtransducers at tip to generate IVUS image (*right side*). Optical coherence tomographic imaging uses a rotating core of the imaging fibers to generate image (*left*).

Table 4.9

Common Clinical Applications for Intravascular Ultrasound (IVUS), Optical Coherence Tomography (OCT), and Near Infrared Spectroscopy (NIRS)			
Guide PCI strategy	**IVUS**	**OCT**	**NIRS**
Establish reference vessel size	+	+	+
Determine lesion length/extent of disease	+	+	+
Examine post PCI angiographic anomalies	+	+	−
Ambiguous angiography			
Ostial left main	+	−	−
Unusual lesion morphology	+	+	+
ACS plaque vulnerability?	+	+	+
In-stent restenosis-mechanisms			
Stent underexpansion	++	+	−
Neointimal hyperplasia	+	++	−

+, useful; −, not useful.

continuously through a 360-degree arc in the vessel. The rotation rate is 1800 rpm, generating 30 images per second. The solid-state catheter (Volcano Therapeutics, Rancho Cordova, CA) has 64 ultrasound transducers arranged circumferentially around the catheter tip and sequentially activated to produce a 360-degree image. Both IVUS catheters range in size from 3.2F to 3.5F and have a tapered tip and shaft. They are designed to fit through a 6F guide catheter. The IVUS catheter connects to a console, which displays and records the images digitally. Images from both systems are displayed in a tomographic, real-time video format. Currently IVUS has a resolution of approximately 100–150 microns.

Common clinical applications for IVUS (Table 4.9) include:

1. Assessment of lesion calcium
2. Vessel and lesion dimensions
3. Confirmation of atherosclerotic plaque
4. Adequacy of stent deployment

Technique of Intravascular Imaging Catheter Use

The technique of IVUS/OCT is identical to that of PCI balloon or stent catheter placement. After administration of heparin and positioning of an angioplasty guidewire in the distal coronary vessel, IC nitroglycerin is given to dilate the vessel and avoid vasospasm. The IVUS/OCT catheter is then advanced along the guidewire, until the transducer is beyond the region of interest. The imaging core or the IVUS catheter can then be pulled with an automated pullback device. An accurate pullback run is necessary to determine lesion length and volumetric analyses.

The mechanical system requires an initial flush of saline to remove air microbubbles from the plastic sheath housing the rotating imaging core. Nonuniform rotational distortion (NURD) can occur with the mechanical system due to uneven drag on the catheter driveshaft leading to changes in the rotational speed. This artifact most commonly occurs in tortuous vessels and manifests as a smearing of one side of the image. A ring-down artifact, seen with the solid-state system, results in white circles surrounding the ultrasound catheter and precluding near-field imaging and is due to acoustic oscillations in the transducer resulting in high-amplitude signals. Adjustments can now be made on the newer solid-state systems to minimize this problem.

Setup

Integration of IVUS into the laboratory is critical for optimal use of the technology (Fig. 4.23). To minimize problems, it is important for several

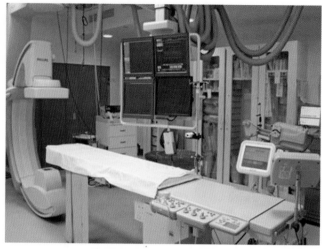

Figure 4.23 Cath lab with integrated intravenous ultrasound (IUVS) and fractional flow reserve (FFR) monitors.

members of the support staff to take specialized training and assume responsibility for the equipment. Commercially available IVUS systems are fully integrated into the angiographic imaging system and do not require transport of a separate console into the laboratory. The following preparations make the most efficient use of IVUS:

1. Specialized support staff familiar with operation of the equipment and image interpretation

2. Use of an automated pullback device, which standardizes the procedure to prevent too rapid scanning and eliminate much of the physician operator effect on image quality

3. A system of maintenance for IVUS-related records, videotapes, and CD-ROMs

4. An image review station that is separate from the IVUS machine itself; direct transfer of the DICOM images to an image-archival network allows review at many stations

Image Features

Regardless of the imaging system used, the basic image features described here are from the center outward. A normal IVUS image is shown in Fig. 4.24.

1. *Dead zone.* The black circular ring in the middle of the image is caused by the space occupied by the catheter.

2. *Catheter artifact.* A "halo" artifact around the catheter usually encroaches onto lumen areas and therefore may affect analysis. It may also encroach onto the signals transmitted from the vessel wall. These artifacts are related to either the imaging sheath or a property of ultrasonic imaging termed "ringdown" (disorganized near-field echo signals).

3. *Lumen.* The dark, echolucent area surrounding the catheter artifact signal is the lumen. With some higher frequency scanners or under conditions of slow blood velocity, a fine speckle pattern may be seen in the lumen (Fig. 4.25).

4. *Inner layer.* In a normal artery, the intima is often too thin to be seen reliably. The thin inner echogenic layer surrounding the lumen usually represents the internal elastic lamina. In a diseased coronary artery, the atheromatous intima is seen as a thick echogenic layer surrounding the lumen. In vessels with mild to

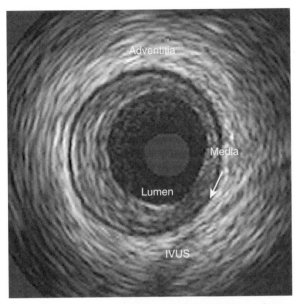

Figure 4.24 Normal intravascular ultrasound (IVUS) image demonstrating the three normal layers of the coronary artery—the adventitia is the outermost, separated by a dark echolucent line from the media. The lumen and media border defines the intima. This artery has an eccentric plaque from 11 o'clock to 4 o'clock.

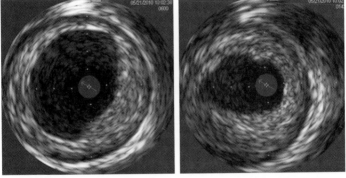

Figure 4.25 Eccentric plaque by intravascular ultrasound (IVUS) in large ectatic vessel.

moderate atherosclerosis, a thin echodense layer at the intima–media interface can be seen, correlating histologically to the internal elastic lamina. This may be obscured in severely diseased atherosclerotic arteries.

5. *Middle hypoechoic layer.* The media, packed with smooth muscle cells and a few elastin fibers, appears as a relatively echolucent area. The external elastic lamina may sometimes be seen as an echodense layer at the media–adventitia interface.

6. *Outer echogenic layer.* The adventitia is seen as an echodense layer surrounding the hypoechoic media. The adventitia shows increased echodensity due to both the inhomogeneous histologic structures and the high elastin and collagen content. This structure has the most intense echoes in normal arteries. Echoes that are more intense than the adventitia are therefore abnormal. In this region, perivascular structures may also be observed (i.e., veins and pericardium).

Dimensional Measurements

One of the major advantages of IVUS is its ability to provide precise measurements (Figs. 4.26–4.28). Several studies have analyzed the accuracy of ultrasound images for measuring lumen size and wall thickness. Correlations with histologic measurements have been uniformly high, although measurements of the dimensions of the layers and overall wall thickness have been reported to be less accurate than lumen area determinations. The lumen–intima and media–adventitia interfaces are generally accurate using ultrasound scanning; both interfaces show a relatively large increase in acoustic impedance as the beam passes through the layers. The intima–media interface may also provide a significant change in impedance, particularly in the presence of prominent internal elastic lamina. At this interface, however, there is a "trailing-edge" effect that can result in the spreading or blooming of the intimal image. The net result is that the transition is

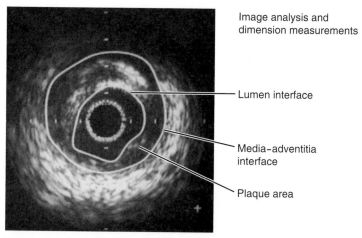

Image analysis and dimension measurements

— Lumen interface

— Media–adventitia interface

— Plaque area

Figure 4.26 Intravascular ultrasound (IVUS) images showing how ultrasound-derived measurements are obtained from planimetry of the lumen and media–adventitia interfaces. Halo is term given for lucency around the central black space of the IVUS catheter. *(Courtesy of John McB. Hodgson, MD.)*

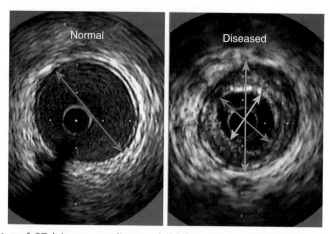

Figure 4.27 Intravenous ultrasound (IVUS) measurements for dimensions in *(left)* normal and *(right)* diseased coronary artery. Inter-dot distance = 1 mm. Vessel diameter computed from leading edge to leading edge adventia *(red arrow)*. Lumen diameter on right has two dimensions of an eccentric plaque *(yellow and red arrows)*. Vessel dimension here is from green arrow.

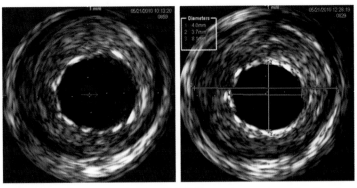

Figure 4.28 Intravenous ultrasound (IVUS) measurements made after stent implantation.

obscured, the intima appears thicker than by histologic determination, and the media appears correspondingly thinner. However wall thickness using the combined intima and media corresponds closely to the histological dimensions.

All ultrasound measurements are performed on *end-diastolic images* unless specified otherwise. Artery lumen dimensions are quantified from images of proximal, distal, or reference vessel segments and within the target lesion(s) or stent. The following measurements are routinely obtained.

1. *Lumen and vessel diameters.* Minimal, maximal, and mean diameters may be obtained.

2. *Percentage diameter or area stenosis* is the lumen diameter or area within the lesion segment divided by the lumen diameter or area within the reference segment. This is similar to the measures made by angiography.

3. *Total vessel area.* The vessel cross-sectional area is the area confined within the external elastic lamina or the media–adventitia interface.

4. *Lumen area* is the integrated area central to the leading-edge echo. The area is confined within the lumen–intima interface. If the catheter is tangential, the lumen area is slightly overestimated.

5. *Wall area* (intima and media) equals total area minus lumen area. In abnormal vessels, this is the plaque area (also called *plaque plus media area*).

6. *Percentage plaque area* (also called *plaque burden or percentage cross-sectional narrowing* [%CSN]) equals total vessel area minus lumen area divided by total vessel area:

Percentage plaque area = (total area − lumen area/total area) × 100

7. *Indices of eccentricity.* A lesion eccentricity index (L_{ECC}) is calculated by lumen dimensions:

$$L_{ECC} = \text{maximum diameter/minimum diameter}$$

Plaque distribution is classified into three categories:

1. *Concentric plaque.* Maximum plaque thickness (leading-edge plus sonolucent zone) of less than 1.3 times minimum plaque thickness

2. *Moderately eccentric plaque.* Maximum plaque thickness (leading edge plus sonolucent zone) 1.3–1.7 times minimum plaque thickness

3. *Severely eccentric plaque.* Maximum plaque thickness (leading edge plus sonolucent zone) greater than 1.7 times minimum plaque thickness

Intravascular Ultrasound Plaque Morphology

In general, plaque may be classified as "soft" or "hard" based on whether the echodensity is less than or similar to the adventitia.

Soft plaque. More than 80% of the plaque area in an integrated pullback throughout the lesion is composed of thickened intimal echoes with homogeneous echo density less than that seen in adventitia (Fig. 4.29).

Fibrous plaque. More than 80% of plaque in an integrated pullback throughout the lesion is composed of thick and dense echoes involving the intimal leading edge, with homogeneous echo density greater than or equal to that seen for adventitia.

Calcified plaque. Bright echoes within a plaque demonstrate acoustic shadowing and occupy more than 90% of the vessel wall circumference in at least one cross-sectional image of the lesion. The extent of calcification, defined as the presence of any hyperechogenic structure that shadows underlying ultrasound anatomy, is reported as the degree of circumference in which shadowing is present. Calcium is also classified as deep or superficial (Fig. 4.30). Detection of calcium using IVUS can guide appropriate device selection, such as the need for high-speed rotational atherectomy.

Mixed plaque. Bright echoes with acoustic shadowing encompass less than 90% of the vessel wall circumference, or a mixture of soft and fibrous plaque is seen with each component occupying less than 80% of the plaque area in an integrated pullback through the lesion (Fig. 4.31).

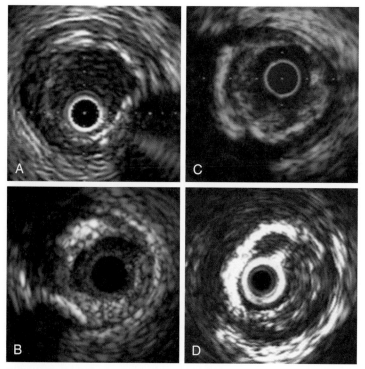

Figure 4.29 Intravenous ultrasound (IVUS) images for various types of coronary arterial diseases. (A) Mixed plaque type. (B) Mild atherosclerosis. (C) Soft atheromata. (D) Calcified atheromata. *(Courtesy of John McB. Hodgson, MD.)*

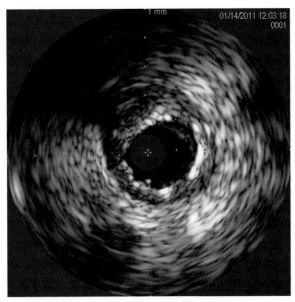

Figure 4.30 Calcium is quantified by measuring the "arc" it encompasses. Calcium is classified by its location within the plaque. Superficial calcium is closer to the lumen than to the adventitia. Deep calcium is closer to the adventitia than to the lumen.

Subintimal thickening. Subintimal thickening involving reference vessel segments is defined as a concentric prominent leading-edge echo and a widened subintimal echolucent zone with a combined thickness of more than 500 microns.

Additional Plaque Features

Plaque location. Plaque may be described as concentric or eccentric, with or without ulceration. In describing a nonconcentric plaque, its location is noted in relation to a clock (i.e., "Plaque is present, extending from the 8 o'clock position to the 11 o'clock position, with calcium deposits seen at 9 o'clock").

Intimal flap or dissection. This is seen as a linear structure with or without a free edge. True and false channels can also be visualized. The characteristic motion of an intimal flap may be seen within the lumen. Radiographic contrast injection can assist in defining the lumen and indicating whether there is communication of the lumen with an echo-free area below a flap. In some systems, blood flow can be colorized and may assist in defining dissections (Fig. 4.32).

Thrombus. Fresh thrombus is a low to moderately echogenic or granular mass that occupies part of the lumen and adjoins the adjacent wall; often it is mobile and has an irregular border. Edge definition is possible with contrast injection.

Aneurysm. Aneurysmal areas are expanded, thin-walled structures adjoining the lumen. They can be mistaken for branches, which have a similar appearance.

Side branches. Side branches appear as "buds" with a loss of the intimal border. The location of the lesion in relation to branch vessels and, in particular, in relation to the coronary ostium, can be well visualized with IVUS, which can aid decisions regarding stent placement.

"Vulnerable plaque" or atherosclerotic lesions at high risk for rupture. IVUS studies suggest that lesion eccentricity and the presence of echolucent zones within the plaque (representing large necrotic lipid pools) are major determinants of plaque vulnerability and increased propensity for rupture (Fig. 4.33). The limited resolution of IVUS makes it unable to directly detect the thin (<65 microns) fibrous caps, hence the presence of a necrotic core in contact with the lumen (no IVUS

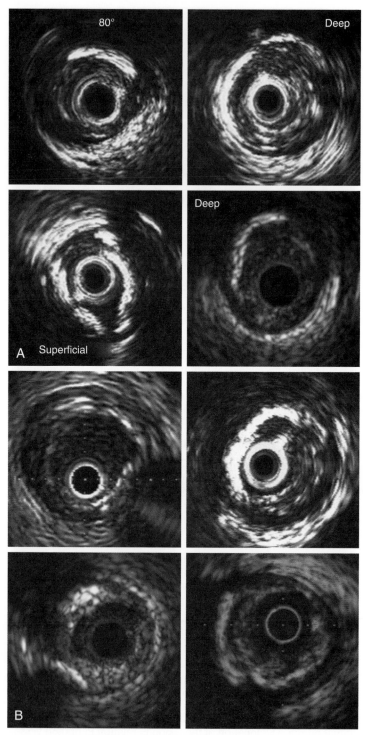

Figure 4.31 Mixed plaque types.

evidence of a fibrous cap) has been used to identify vulnerable plaques. Unstable lesions may demonstrate ulceration or thin mobile dissection flaps by IVUS. In addition, the presence of "positive remodeling" or compensatory enlargement of the vessel to accommodate plaque and maintain lumen has also been found more commonly in unstable than in stable coronary lesions.

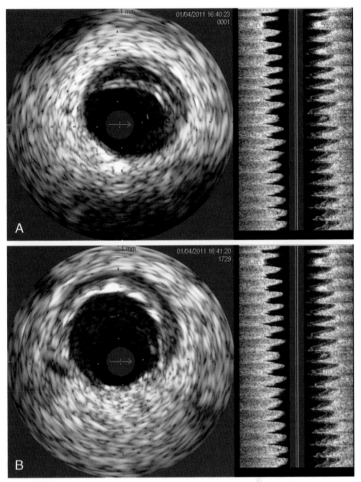

Figure 4.32 (A) Intravenous ultrasound (IVUS) demonstration of intimal flap or dissection. (B) IVUS showing stent in place.

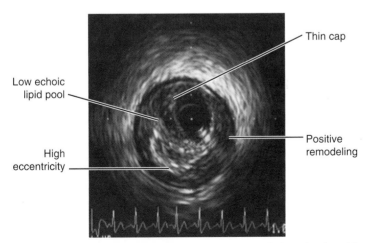

Figure 4.33 Intravenous ultrasound (IVUS) characteristics of vulnerable plaque.

Assessing Coronary Lesions Before PCI: Anatomy Is Not Always Equal to Physiology

IVUS parameters for predicting the clinical (hemodynamic) significance of intermediate coronary lesions have been compared to FFR. IVUS was compared to thallium stress imaging in one study of 70 patients. A minimum lumen area (MLA) of less than 4.0 mm^2 had a sensitivity of 88% and specificity of 90% for predicting ischemia on the noninvasive nuclear test. Furthermore in a large retrospective study of patients with intermediate lesions in whom PCI was deferred Abizad et al. found that an IVUS MLA of greater than 4 mm^2 predicted freedom from adverse events.

When comparing IVUS to FFR Takagi et al. demonstrated in 51 lesions that an IVUS MLA of less than 3.0 mm^2 had a sensitivity of 83% and a specificity of 92% for predicting an FFR of <0.75. An area stenosis of greater than 0.6 had a sensitivity of 92% and specificity of 88% for predicting an FFR of less than 0.75. Kang et al. showed more recently in 236 lesions that an FFR of less than 0.80 was associated with IVUS MLA, plaque burden, lesion length of 3.1 mm with MLA of less than 3.0 mm^2, and LAD vessel location. In their study, the best IVUS cutoff value to predict an FFR of less than 0.80 was an MLA of as little as less than 2.4 mm^2. Among 117 lesions with an MLA of greater than 2.4 mm^2, 96% had an FFR of greater than 0.80. Fig. 4.34 compares IVUS to FFR.

IVUS and LM Stenosis

Interrogating intermediate LM coronary lesions is another area where IVUS is commonly employed. Unfortunately there is no universal

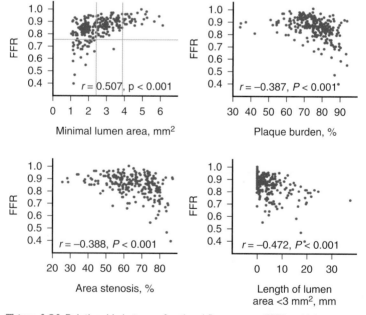

Figure 4.34 Relationship between fractional flow reserve (FFR) and Intravenous ultrasound (IVUS) parameters. FFR significantly correlated with MLA ($r = 0.507$, $p < 0.001$), PB ($r = -0.387$, $p < 0.001$), area stenosis ($r = -0.388$, $p < 0.001$), and length with a lumen area <3.0 mm^2 ($r = -0.472$, $p < 0.001$). *(From Kang SJ, Lee JY, Ahn JM, et al. Validation of intravascular ultrasound-derived parameters with fractional flow reserve for assessment of coronary stenosis severity. Circ Cardiovasc Interv. 2011;4:65–71.)*

agreement on IVUS criteria for a significant LM coronary lesion. However, a lesion with an IVUS MLA of less than 6.0 mm^2 and/or a percentage area stenosis of greater than 60% has been generally considered a significant stenosis. One study showed an increased 1-year event rate in patients with LM diameter of less than 3.0 mm, especially in patients with diabetes. The most recent comparison of IVUS-derived parameters to FFR for assessing intermediate LM lesions found that an MLA area of 5.9 mm^2 correlated best with an FFR of less than 0.75.

In summary, the IVUS parameters for predicting ischemia have variable cutoff values when compared to FFR. Because of the complexity of any individual stenosis, including size of the reference vessel segment not accounted for in IVUS studies, lesion assessment for functional significance is best determined by FFR.

Assessing Percutaneous Coronary Interventions by Intravenous Ultrasound

IVUS has been studied extensively in the setting of assessing and optimizing PCI. It is a valuable tool for ensuring optimal stent expansion and strut apposition after stenting. IVUS allows a more thorough evaluation of arterial dissections, particularly involving the stent edges. After stenting, use of IVUS universally leads to improved stent expansion and larger final lumen dimensions, which, in many studies, has translated into lower restenosis rates and better long-term outcomes. Both absolute and relative criteria have been put forth for gauging an optimal stent result. Complete stent apposition to the vessel wall, a minimum stent area of greater than 90% of the average reference area or 100% of the smallest reference area, and symmetric stent expansion with the minimum/maximum lumen diameter of greater than 0.7 are commonly cited relative criteria. An absolute minimum stent area that is greater than 7 mm^2 is a useful absolute criterion.

There are data to suggest that an IVUS-guided PCI results in a lower target vessel revascularization rate during follow-up. This has been attributed to the improved stent expansion achieved with IVUS guidance compared to angiography alone. One randomized study documented cost savings over 2 years of follow-up. With the advent of DES, in which maximal expansion may not be as critical (although still important), IVUS guidance may appear less valuable. However, ensuring complete lesion coverage by accurate length measures, selection of the appropriate diameter stent, evaluating for calcium that may impair expansion or delivery, documenting appropriate apposition, and ensuring the absence of peri-stent dissection or hematoma remain important features associated with better clinical results.

Assessing Complications

Following coronary interventions, vessel stretching, plaque redistribution or shifting, plaque removal, plaque fissuring, and dissections can be clearly outlined by IVUS. IVUS studies have shown that dissections are dependent on differential plaque types, usually occurring at the edge of calcified segments.

Diagnosis of Allograft Vasculopathy

IVUS has been an excellent means of diagnosing and quantifying cardiac transplant vasculopathy. Routine annual angiographic studies often reveal "normal" vessels in the transplant patient, whereas IVUS studies of the same cohort reveal diffuse intimal hyperplasia. Serial assessments of the progression of intimal proliferation in cardiac transplant patients with angiography and IVUS have documented accelerated vasculopathy, occurring most actively within the first year following transplant.

Progression and Regression of Coronary Atherosclerosis

Because of the limitations of angiography in defining wall structure and pathology, IVUS has been useful in assessing the extent and progression or regression of atherosclerosis in trials of primary or secondary intervention for CAD. Several studies to assess atheroma progression after randomization to a lipid-lowering regimen or "regular care" have been completed and documented slowing of lesion progression and enhanced echogenicity, possibly indicating reduced lipid content. The REVERSAL trial showed that intensive statin therapy could cause plaque regression using IVUS parameters.

Optical Coherence Tomography

Intracoronary OCT is a catheter-based optical imaging modality in many ways similar to IVUS, but it provides higher resolution (about 7 microns axial and 30 microns transverse resolution) cross-sectional images of the coronary wall. OCT uses an interferometric technique, typically with near-infrared light. By analyzing the coherence of the light reflections, the OCT imaging catheter permits tissue characterization with a 10–20-microns level of resolution.

The OCT catheter has a fiberoptic imaging core that replaces the ultrasound imaging core. The catheter is introduced into the artery over a guidewire exactly like the IVUS catheter. A relatively recent modification of the signal acquisition method, called *frequency-domain imaging*, improves signal-to-noise ratio, permitting faster image acquisition. Images are acquired during rapid automated pullback after an injection of saline or contrast to displace blood and clear the viewing field. Compared with conventional imaging modalities, OCT has a superior resolution to evaluate certain features of the vulnerable plaque, such as plaque rupture, intracoronary thrombus, thin-capped fibroatheroma, and macrophages within the fibrous caps. Furthermore OCT can visualize stent malapposition and tissue protrusion after stenting and neointimal hyperplasia at late follow-up. One drawback of OCT in comparison to IVUS is its shallow depth of penetration (1–2 mm), limiting assessment of plaque composition. Figs. 4.35–4.39 show examples of OCT in coronary artery interventions.

The exact role of OCT in imaging coronary vessels remains to be determined. It may replace IVUS for certain applications, such as assessing stent deployment, but IVUS may remain the standard for

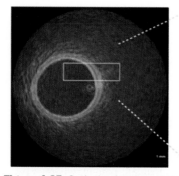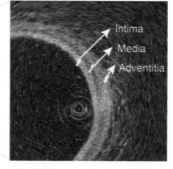

Figure 4.35 Optical coherence tomography (OCT) is a light-based imaging modality utilizing recently developed laser and fiber optic technologies to create real-time, high-resolution tomographic images most notably in medical applications. The fascinating point of OCT is its excellent resolution: enough to distinguish the edge among intima, media, and adventitia. Images show features of a normal coronary artery in man.

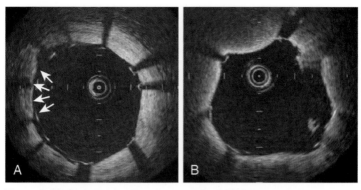

Figure 4.36 Optical coherence tomography (OCT) images of (A) stent strut incomplete apposition and (B) full apposition with some tissue prolapse at 1 o'clock.

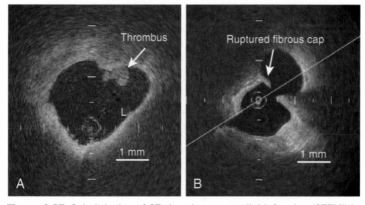

Figure 4.37 Culprit lesion of ST-elevation myocardial infarction (STEMI) by optical coherence tomography (OCT). *(Courtesy of Dr. Shigeo Takarada.)*

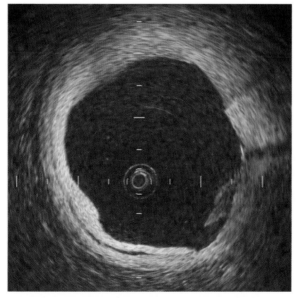

Figure 4.38 Optical coherence tomography (OCT) image of coronary dissection with flap at 4 o'clock. *(Courtesy of Dr. Shigeo Takarada.)*

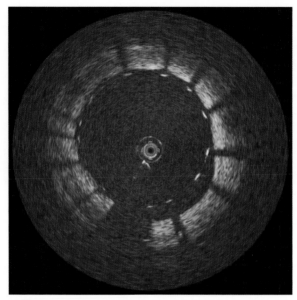

Figure 4.39 Optical coherence tomography (OCT) image of incomplete stent apposition (3 to 6 o'clock). *(Courtesy of Dr. Shigeo Takarada.)*

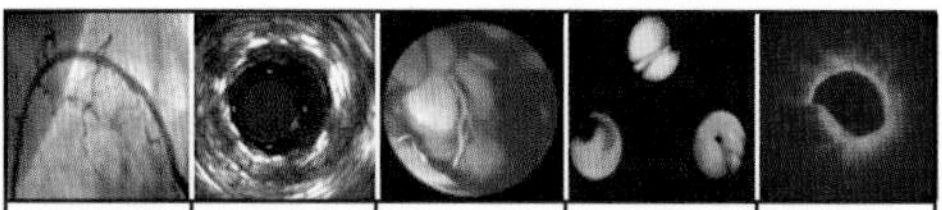

	CAG	IVUS	CT, MRI	Angioscopy	OCT
Resolution (μm)	100–200	80–120	80–300	<200	10–15
Probe size (μm)	N/A	700	1000	800	140
Contact	No	Yes	No	No	No
Ionizing radiation	Yes	No	No	No	No
Other	Flow only	N/A	N/A	Surface only	Plaque character

Figure 4.40 Comparison of coronary imaging devices in the cath lab. *CT,* computed tomography; *IVUS,* intravascular ultrasound; *MRI,* magnetic resonance imaging; *OCT,* optical coherence tomography.

assessing plaque composition. Combination coregistered OCT/IVUS catheters are in development. Fig. 4.40 compares coronary imaging modalities that can be used in the cath lab today.

Compositional Intravascular Imaging: Near Infrared Spectroscopy Coronary Imaging System

Invasive imaging of the coronary artery with IVUS provides a detailed anatomic quantitative description with some information relating to tissue composition (calcification, fibrosis, lipid or soft plaque).

Combining an IVUS catheter system with optical fiber transmission of near infrared (NIR) wavelength light, the NIR spectroscopy (NIRS)/IVUS catheter can be used to detect cholesterol content in a vessel localized by IVUS. The presence of a large lipid pool is intimately associated with vulnerable coronary plaques.

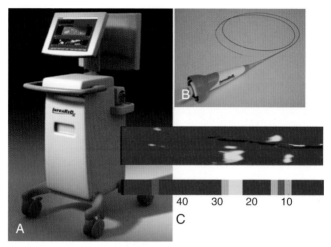

Figure 4.41 InfraReDx LipiScan System. (A) Console. (B) 3.2F catheter (monorail, 0.014-inch compatible; no priming required; automated pullback; no occlusion blood flow). (C) Validated lipid core plaque (LCP) detection algorithm.

The NIRS LipiScan catheter uses the basic principle of spectroscopy, a technique used by chemists to identify molecules based on their distinct spectroscopic signature. Using this principle, an intravascular imaging catheter was equipped with a laser, emitting a specific wavelength of light specific for linoleic acid, the major chemical constituent of cholesterol within plaques. The fiberoptic core transmits near infrared light and is used in a manner analogous to an IVUS catheter. An automatic pullback device pulls the infrared catheter within the artery from distal to proximal during the scanning for cholesterol. As the spectrum of light goes through the blood and into the vessel wall, its reflection is collected and analyzed. Because the vessel wall absorbs some of the spectra, the spectroscopic signature is a function of the light sent out and the light returned (the difference is the absorbed light). Cholesterol signal is designated as yellow, nonlipid as red or black. No signal is white.

The LipiScan Console (Fig. 4.41) performs several functions. In brief, it provides (1) the near-infrared light source for spectroscopy, (2) a data processing system that analyzes the signals returned from the pullback interface, (3) a user interface to the system, (4) a means of data storage, and (5) communication to the pullback interface that drives the automated scanning of the LipiScan Coronary Imaging Catheter core. The major components of the console are a laser and laser delivery system, computer system and software, and power module.

This technique provides a "chemographic" map of cholesterol deposits within the artery, displayed as if the artery had been laid open and spread out from distal to proximal. The "chemogram" is based on an algorithm that quantitates the likelihood of a lipid-core plaque in any particular 2 mm block of vessel. The chemogram is color-coded, with bright yellow indicating a greater than 90% likelihood of a lipid-core plaque and red indicating no evidence of a lipid-core plaque. The chemogram approach was validated against diseased human coronary artery ring segments in vitro. The U.S. Food and Drug Administration (FDA) approved the LipiScan catheter for the detection of lipid core plaques. The risks and limitations of the LipiScan catheter are similar to the IVUS catheter; it is currently available in a combined device (Fig. 4.42).

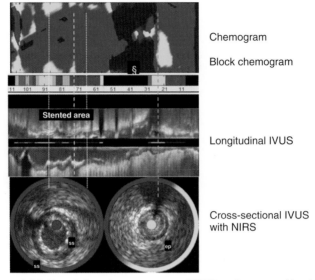

Chemogram

Block chemogram

Longitudinal IVUS

Cross-sectional IVUS with NIRS

Figure 4.42 Near infrared spectroscopy (NIRS) catheter combined with intravenous ultrasound (IVUS). *(Courtesy of Dr. Patrick Serruys, Rotterdam.)*

Suggested Readings

Abizaid A, Mintz G, Mehran R, et al. Long-term follow-up after percutaneous transluminal coronary angioplasty was not performed based on intravascular ultrasound findings: importance of lumen dimensions. *Circulation*. 1999;100:256-261.

Adjedj J, Toth GG, Johnson NP, et al. Intracoronary adenosine. dose-response relationship with hyperemia. *J Am Coll Cardiol Interv*. 2015;8:1422-1430.

Botman CJ, Schonberger J, Koolen S, et al. Does stenosis severity of native vessels influence bypass graft patency? A prospective fractional flow reserve-guided study. *Ann Thorac Surg*. 2007;83:2093-2097.

Christou MA, Siontis GC, Katritsis DG, et al. Meta-analysis of fractional flow reserve versus quantitative coronary angiography and noninvasive imaging for evaluation of myocardial ischemia. *Am J Cardiol*. 2007;99(4):450-456.

De Bruyne B, Pijls NH, Heyndrickx GR, et al. Pressure-derived fractional flow reserve to assess serial epicardial stenoses: theoretical basis and animal validation. *Circulation*. 2000;101:1840-1847.

De Bruyne B, et al. Fractional flow reserve in patients with prior myocardial infarction. *Circulation*. 2001;104(2):157-162.

DeBruyne B, Bartunek J, Sys SU, et al. Simultaneous coronary pressure and flow velocity measurements in humans: feasibility, reproducibility and hemodynamic dependence of coronary flow velocity reserve, hyperemic flow versus pressure slope index and fractional flow reserve. *Circulation*. 1996;94:1842-1849.

Engstrøm T. The third DANish study of optimal Acute treatment of patients with ST-segment elevation Myocardial Infarction: PRImary PCI in MULTIvessel disease. Presented at: American College of Cardiology/i2 Scientific Session; March 16, 2015; San Diego, CA.

Fearon W. Invasive coronary physiology for assessing intermediate lesions in advances in interventional cardiology. *Circ Cardiovasc Interv*. 2015;8:e001942.

Fearon WF, Shah M, Ng M, et al. Predictive value of the index of microcirculatory resistance in patients with ST-segment elevation myocardial infarction. *J Am Coll Cardiol*. 2008;51:560-565.

Fearon WF, Yong AS, Lenders G, et al. The impact of downstream coronary stenosis on fractional flow reserve assessment of intermediate left main coronary artery disease: human validation. *J Am Coll Cardiol Intv*. 2015;8(3):398-403.

Fischer JJ, Wang XQ, Samady H, et al. Outcome of patients with acute coronary syndromes and moderate lesions undergoing deferral of revascularization based on fractional flow reserve assessment. *Catheter Cardiovasc Interv*. 2006;68:544-548.

Gardner CM, Tan H, Hull EL, et al. Detection of lipid core coronary plaques in autopsy specimens with a novel catheter-based near-infrared spectroscopy system. *JACC Cardiovasc Imaging*. 2008;1(5):638-648.

Hamilos M, Muller O, Cuisset T, et al. Long-term clinical outcome after fractional flow reserve–guided treatment in patients with angiographically equivocal left main coronary artery stenosis. *Circulation*. 2009;120:1505-1512.

Johnson NP, Johnson DT, Kirkeeide RL, et al. Repeatability of fractional flow reserve (FFR) despite variations in systemic and coronary hemodynamics. *J Am Coll Cardiol Intv*. 2015;8(8):1018-1027.

Kang SJ, Lee JY, Ahn JM, et al. Validation of intravascular ultrasound-derived parameters with fractional flow reserve for assessment of coronary stenosis severity. *Circ Cardiovasc Interv.* 2011;4:65-71.

Kern MJ, Samady H. Current concepts of integrated coronary physiology in the cath lab. *J Am Coll Cardiol.* 2010;55:173-185.

Koo BK, Kang HJ, Youn TJ, et al. Physiologic assessment of jailed side branch lesions using fractional flow reserve. *J Am Coll Cardiol.* 2005;46(4):633-637.

Koo BK, Park KW, Kang HJ, et al. Physiological evaluation of the provisional side-branch intervention strategy for bifurcation lesions using fractional flow reserve. *Eur Heart J.* 2008;29(6):726-732.

Koo BK, Waseda K, Kang HJ, et al. Anatomic and functional evaluation of bifurcation lesions undergoing percutaneous coronary intervention. *Circ Cardiovasc Interv.* 2010;3:113-119.

Lofti A, Jeremias A, Fearon WF, et al. Expert consensus statement on the use of fractional flow reserve, intravascular ultrasound, and optical coherence tomography: a consensus statement of the society of cardiovascular angiography and interventions. *Catheter Cardiovasc Interv.* 2014;83:509-518.

Magni V, Chieffo A, Colombo A. Evaluation of intermediate coronary stenosis with intravascular ultrasound and fractional flow reserve: its use and abuse. *Catheter Cardiovasc Interv.* 2009;73:441-448.

McClish JC, Ragosta M, Powers ER, et al. Recent myocardial infarction does not limit the utility of fractional flow reserve for the physiologic assessment of lesion severity. *Am J Cardiol.* 2004;93(9):1102-1106.

McGeoch RJ, Oldroyd KG. Pharmacological options for inducing maximal hyperaemia during studies of coronary physiology. *Catheter Cardiovasc Interv.* 2008;71:198-204.

Meuwissen M, Chamuleau SAJ, Siebes M, et al. The prognostic value of combined intra-coronary pressure and blood flow velocity measurements after deferral of percutaneous coronary intervention. *Catheter Cardiovasc Interv.* 2008;71:291-297.

Nam C-W, Yoon H-J, Cho Y-K, et al. Outcomes of percutaneous coronary intervention in intermediate coronary artery disease: fractional flow reserve–guided versus intravascular ultrasound–guided. *J Am Coll Cardiol Intv.* 2010;3:812-817.

Ng MK, Yeung AC, Fearon WF. Invasive assessment of the coronary microcirculation: superior reproducibility and less hemodynamic dependence of index of microcirculatory resistance as compared to coronary flow reserve. *Circulation.* 2006;113:2054-2061.

Nishioka T, Amanullah AM, Luo H, et al. Clinical validation of intravascular ultrasound imaging for assessment of coronary stenosis severity: comparison with stress myocardial perfusion imaging. *J Am Coll Cardiol.* 1999;33:1870-1878.

Ntalianis A, Sels JW, Davidavicius G, et al. Fractional flow reserve for the assessment of nonculprit coronary artery stenoses in patients with acute myocardial infarction. *JACC Cardiovasc Interv.* 2010;3(12):1274-1281.

Piek JJ, van Liebergen RA, Koch KT, et al. Clinical, angiographic and hemodynamic predictors of recruitable collateral flow assessed during balloon angioplasty coronary occlusion. *J Am Coll Cardiol.* 1997;29:275-282.

Pijls NH, Bech GJ, el Gamal MI, et al. Quantification of recruitable coronary collateral blood flow in conscious humans and its potential to predict future ischemic events. *J Am Coll Cardiol.* 1995;25:1522-1528.

Pijls NH, De Bruyne B, Bech GJ, et al. Coronary pressure measurement to assess the hemodynamic significance of serial stenoses within one coronary artery: validation in humans. *Circulation.* 2000;102:2371-2377.

Pijls NH, De Bruyne B, Peels K, et al. Measurement of fractional flow reserve to assess the functional severity of coronary-artery stenoses. *N Engl J Med.* 1996;334:1703-1708.

Pijls NH, De Bruyne B, Smith L, et al. Coronary thermodilution to assess flow reserve: validation in humans. *Circulation.* 2002;105:2482-2486.

Pijls NH, Klauss V, Siebert U, et al. Fractional flow reserve (FFR) post-stent registry investigators. coronary pressure measurement after stenting predicts adverse events at follow-up: a multicenter registry. *Circulation.* 2002;105:2950-2954.

Pijls NHJ, Fearon WF, Tonino PAL, et al. Fractional flow reserve versus angiography for guiding percutaneous coronary intervention in patients with multivessel coronary artery disease: 2-year follow-up of the FAME (Fractional Flow Reserve Versus Angiography for Multivessel Evaluation) study. *J Am Coll Cardiol.* 2010;56:177-184.

Pijls NHJ, Kern MJ, Yock PG, et al. Practice and potential pitfalls of coronary pressure measurement. *Catheter Cardiovasc Interv.* 2000;49:1-16.

Pijls NHJ, Van Gelder B, Van der Voort P, et al. Fractional flow reserve: a useful index to evaluate the influence of an epicardial coronary stenosis on myocardial blood flow. *Circulation.* 1995;92:318-319.

Pijls NHJ, Van Schaardenburgh P, Manoharan G, et al. Percutaneous coronary intervention of functionally non-significant stenoses: 5-year follow-up of the DEFER study. *J Am Coll Cardiol.* 2007;49:2105-2111.

Potvin JM, Rodés-Cabau J, Bertrand OF, et al. Usefulness of fractional flow reserve measurements to defer revascularization in patients with stable or unstable angina pectoris, non-ST-elevation and ST-elevation acute myocardial infarction, or atypical chest pain. *Am J Cardiol.* 2006;98:289-297.

Samady H, Lepper W, Powers ER, et al. Fractional flow reserve of infarct-related arteries identifies reversible defects on noninvasive myocardial perfusion imaging early after myocardial infarction. *J Am Coll Cardiol.* 2006;47:2187-2193.

Samady H, McDaniel M, Veledar E, et al. Baseline fractional flow reserve and stent diameter predict optimal post-stent fractional flow reserve and major adverse cardiac events after bare-metal stent deployment. *J Am Coll Cardiol Intv.* 2009;2:357-363.

Samady H, et al. Fractional flow reserve of infarct-related arteries identifies reversible defects on noninvasive myocardial perfusion imaging early after myocardial infarction. *J Am Coll Cardiol.* 2006;47(11):2187-2193.

Seiler C, Fleisch M, Billinger M, et al. Simultaneous intracoronary velocity- and pressure-derived assessment of adenosine-induced collateral hemodynamics in patients with one- to two-vessel coronary artery disease. *J Am Coll Cardiol.* 1999;34:1985-1994.

Sels JW, Tonino PA, Siebert U, et al. Fractional flow reserve in unstable angina and non-ST-segment elevation myocardial infarction experience from the FAME (Fractional flow reserve versus Angiography for Multivessel Evaluation) study. *JACC Cardiovasc Intv.* 2011;4(11):1183-1189.

Seto AH, Tehrani DM, Bharmal MI, et al. Variations of coronary hemodynamic responses to intravenous adenosine infusion: implications for fractional flow reserve measurements. *Catheter Cardiovasc Interv.* 2014;84:416-425.

Smits P, et al. Fractional flow reserve guided primary multivessel percutaneous coronary intervention to improve guideline indexed actual standard of care for treatment of ST-elevation myocardial infarction in patients with multivessel coronary disease. https://clinicaltrials.gov/ct2/show/NCT01399736.

Takagi A, Tsurumi Y, Ishii Y, et al. Clinical potential of intravascular ultrasound for physiological assessment of coronary stenosis: relationship between quantitative ultrasound tomography and pressure-derived fractional flow reserve. *Circulation.* 1999;100:2505.

Tarkin JM, Nijjer S, Sen S, et al. Hemodynamic response to intravenous adenosine and its effect on fractional flow reserve assessment: results of the Adenosine for the Functional Evaluation of Coronary Stenosis Severity (AFFECTS) study. *Circ Cardiovasc Intv.* 2013;6(6):654-661.

Tonino PAL, De Bruyne B, Pijls NHJ, et al. Fractional flow reserve versus angiography for guiding percutaneous coronary intervention. *N Engl J Med.* 2009;360:213-224.

Tonino PAL, Fearon WF, De Bruyne B, et al. Angiographic versus functional severity of coronary artery stenoses in the FAME study, fractional flow reserve versus angiography in multivessel evaluation. *J Am Coll Cardiol.* 2010;55:2816-2821.

Topol EJ, Nissen SE. Our preoccupation with coronary luminology. The dissociation between clinical and angiographic findings in ischemic heart disease. *Circulation.* 1995;92:2333-2342.

Wald DS, Morris JK, Wald NJ, et al. Randomized trial of preventive angioplasty in myocardial infarction. *N Engl J Med.* 2013;369(12):1115-1123.

Waxman S, Dixon SR, L'Allier P, et al. In vivo validation of a catheter-based near-infrared spectroscopy system for detection of lipid core coronary plaques: initial results of the SPECTACL study. *JACC Cardiovasc Imaging.* 2009;2(7):858-868.

Werner GS, Ferrari M, Betge S, et al. Collateral function in chronic total coronary occlusions is related to regional myocardial function and duration of occlusion. *Circulation.* 2001;104:2784-2790.

Zimmermann FM, Ferrara A, Johnson NP, et al. Deferral vs. performance of percutaneous coronary intervention of functionally non-significant coronary stenosis: 15-year follow-up of the DEFER trial. *Eur Heart J.* 2015;36(45):3182-3188.

5

Adjunctive Devices for Non-Balloon Coronary Interventional Techniques and Devices: Rotational Atherectomy, Thrombectomy, Cutting Balloons, and Embolic Protection ▶

KEVAL K. PATEL · RAHIL RAFEEDHEEN · TAREK HELMY

Introduction

Over the past several decades, percutaneous coronary procedures have evolved significantly to allow for interventions on advanced, calcified, and complex lesions. However prior to this era of stenting and complex interventions, animal models revealed that the neointimal response of a vessel after percutaneous transluminal coronary angioplasty (PTCA) is directly proportional to the injury of the vessel during the procedure. The hypothesis speculating that directly modifying the plaque without injury to the vessel wall would decrease restenosis led to an advent of technologies such as rotational atherectomy (PTRA, introduced in 1988), helium laser angioplasty (ELCA, introduced in 1990), cutting balloon (CBA, introduced in 1991), and orbital atherectomy (OA, introduced in 2008). Although the long-term results of these devices in several studies did not fulfill the promise of lowering the rates of target vessel revascularization with PTCA, in the current era there is a niche for these devices to debulk heavily calcified vessels in order to facilitate delivery of stents and improve procedural results.

Rotational Atherectomy

Mechanism of Action

The principal mechanism for rotational atherectomy (RA) is differential cutting in which the diamond-tipped burr drills through rigid atherosclerotic plaque and calcium but spares the underlying elastic arterial structure. The resultant particulate matter is generally less than 10 μm in diameter, which passes through the microcirculation and is picked up by the reticuloendothelial system.

Indications and Contraindications

Although studies have shown that routine use of RA may not render a clinical benefit, there are several clinical scenarios in which RA can improve angiographic results. Most commonly it is used to prepare vessels with severe fibrocalcific disease where otherwise balloons or stents could not be passed. Additionally, attempts to pass stents through such lesions may render them susceptible to inappropriate positioning, stent dislodgement, or erosion of the polymer–drug coating and inadequate drug delivery to the vessel wall.

Another scenario is with vessels that have highly calcified nonyielding lesions that may require high-pressure balloon expansion due to increased vessel stiffness. This can increase the probability of balloon rupture as well as vessel dissection or perforation. Delivering a stent in an incompletely dilated vessel can increase the risk of restenosis long term and stent thrombosis acutely or subacutely. RA can be used to modify plaque in such situations to improve angiographic results.

RA has also been proposed to debulk bifurcation lesions with heavy disease burden to reduce plaque shift or the "snow-plowing" effect. However, caution is advised in these scenarios due to risk of dissection or perforation. Angulation of more than 60 degrees is a relative contraindication for RA, and bends of more than 90 degrees have a strong contraindication. Other contraindications are summarized in Table 5.1. A lesion that is more than 25 mm in length has a relative contraindication for RA. However if RA is being considered for these patients, a smaller burr size should be used. A reduced ejection fraction (<30%) was previously a contraindication to RA, but the advent of mechanical support devices such as the Impella catheter has allowed physicians to consider RA for a select few of these patients.

Device

The Rotablator system (Boston Scientific, Natick, MA) consists of a nickel-coated brass burr (Fig. 5.1A and B) that is coated with 2000–3000 microscopic diamond crystals that are 20 μm in size (with only 5 μm protruding from the nickel coating on its leading face). The burr is available in 1.25 to 2.50 mm sizes (0.25-mm increments) and is attached to a long, flexible drive shaft that is covered in a 4.3F Teflon sheath. The drive shaft can be inserted through various coronary guide catheters based on size (Table 5.2) over a RotaWire, which is 0.009 inch in diameter and 330 cm in length. The drive shaft is connected to an advancing console (Fig. 5.2) that houses a turbine driven by compressed

Table 5.1

Indications and Contraindications to Rotational Atherectomy		
Indicated	**High-Risk**	**Contraindicated**
Single-vessel atherosclerotic coronary artery disease with a calcified plaque that *can* be passed with a guidewire	Severe, diffuse multivessel coronary artery disease	Occlusions where a guidewire cannot be passed
	Unprotected left main PCI	Saphenous vein graft PCI
	Patients with compromised LV function (LVEF <30%)	Angiographic evidence of significant dissection Type C or greater at the treatment site
	De novo lesion >25 mm in length	
Low-risk, multivessel coronary artery disease	Severely angulated (>45 degrees) lesions	
	Last remaining conduit with compromised LV function	
De novo lesion <25 mm in length	Angiographic evidence of thrombus	

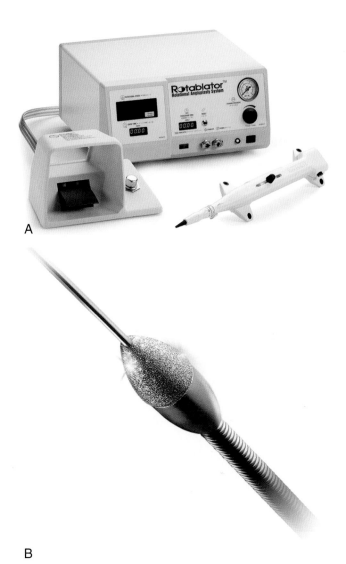

A

B

Figure 5.1 (A) Rotablator Rotational Atherectomy System. (B) Diagram of the rotational atherectomy burr. *(Courtesy of Boston Scientific Corp., Marlborough, MA.)*

Table 5.2

Recommended Guide Catheter Sizes for Use With the Coronary Rotablator		
Rotablator Burr Size (mm)	**Recommended Guide Catheter Internal Diameter (inch)**	**Guide Size (French)***
1.25	0.053	6–8
1.50	0.063	6–8
1.75	0.073	6–8
2.00	0.083	7–9
2.15	0.089	7–9
2.25	0.093	7–9
2.50	0.102	9–10

*For a given size of catheter, the inside diameter varies from manufacturer to manufacturer. French sizes assume thin-wall (high-volume flow) catheters with side holes.

Rotalink™ system components

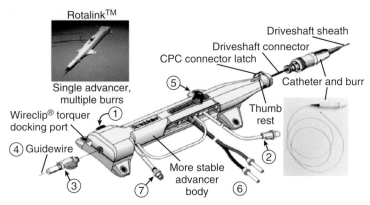

Figure 5.2 Rotablator advancer unit with removable catheter and burr attachment: 1, brake defeat knob; 2, air pressure close; 3, wire clip; 4, rotablator wire; 5, burr position control knob; 6, fiberoptic tachometer; 7, pressurized saline infusion port with lubricant. The guidewire comes with a 0.017-inch (maximum) spring tip (0.43 mm diameter), facilitating negotiation of the wire through the vasculature. *(Courtesy of Boston Scientific Corporation, Boston, MA.)*

Table 5.3

Recommended Rotablator Advancer Turbine Speed			
Burr Size (mm)	Burr Size (French)	Design Rotational Speed Range (rpm)*	Optimum Rotational Speed Range (rpm; No Tissue Contact)
1.25	3.75	150,000–190,000	180,000
1.50	4.50	150,000–190,000	180,000
1.75	5.25	150,000–190,000	180,000
2.00	6.00	150,000–190,000	180,000
2.15	6.45	140,000–180,000	160,000
2.25	6.75	140,000–180,000	160,000
2.50	7.50	140,000–180,000	160,000

Rotablator Catheter Sheath Outer Diameter		
Size (mm)	Size (French)	Size (inch)
1.35	4.0	0.058

*Preset speed outside of the body at the higher rotational speed—for example, for a 1.25 mm Rotablator advancer, set speed outside body at 190,000 rpm.

nitrogen gas and that can rotate at speeds ranging from 140,000 to 190,000 rpm (Table 5.3). An emulsifier solution (Rotaglide) made of egg yolk, EDTA, and olive oil is infused along with saline via a pressurized system through the driveshaft to reduce friction and improve heat dissipation.

Technical Tips

Once the choice to use RA is made based on the indications and contraindications discussed earlier, the next step is to determine the burr size. For vessels where one can determine the size of the artery, a burr-to-artery ratio of less than 0.8 is appropriate because even though a larger ratio (>0.85) can aggressively debulk the lesion, it can increase the propensity for complications such as dissection and perforations. For subtotal occlusions where the arterial size is difficult to ascertain, it is prudent to start with a small burr size (1.25 or 1.5 mm) to create a pilot channel and then upsize to a ratio of less than 0.8. Additionally, a smaller burr-to-artery ratio should also be used for vessels with lesions that are longer than 25 mm or if the vessel has mild tortuosity.

The next step is preparing the patient for RA. The patients usually already have aspirin on board; some operators use verapamil pre-emptively to prevent spasm. Heparin or bivalirudin can be given next to fully anticoagulate the patients. Traditionally, operators have chosen heparin due to reversibility in case of vessel perforation but studies have shown safety with bivalirudin as well. RA is associated with speed-dependent platelet activation, and glycoprotein (GP) IIb/IIIA receptor antagonists can be used to counter this. In patients undergoing intervention for lesions in the right coronary artery or a dominant circumflex artery, placement of a temporary pacing wire is recommended.

A guide catheter with a gentle curve should be sized depending on the burr size (Table 5.2). It is important to make sure that the guide catheter is coaxial to the vessel to prevent dissection of the vessel and retraction of the wire during RA. The RotaFloppy wire should be used for lesions that are more proximal and easily crossable to prevent guidewire bias in which a burr would differentially debride more on the lesser curvature of the vessel, which is straightened out by a stiffer wire. The extra-support RotaWire can be used for difficult-to-cross, heavily calcified lesions or distal lesions. If a lesion cannot be crossed by the RotaWire, a 0.014-inch guidewire can be used to cross the lesion and then be exchanged for the RotaWire using a low-profile balloon or a tracking catheter.

Once the RA manifold is assembled, the burr speed is adjusted outside the body (160,000–180,000 rpm for burrs ≤2.0 mm, 140,000–160,000 rpm for burrs >2.0 mm). Either saline or the Rotaflush solution (mix 4 mg of nitroglycerin and 5 mg of verapamil in 500 mL of saline to decrease spasm) is used to flush the system. The Rotaglide solution is added to reduce friction. Before inserting the burr into the Y-adapter, one must also check for free movement of the burr with the advancer and test that the braking system holds the wire in place during rotation.

After this, the burr is inserted via a Y-adapter and advanced over the wire through the guide catheter into the vessel to about 1–2 cm proximal to the lesion. The operator should hold the back end of the wire and apply gentle traction on the guidewire and catheter to limit acquired tension and thereby prevent the burr from leaping forward during the initial pass. This acquired tension is alleviated further by transiently activating the system proximal to the lesion. The system is then activated and the burr is brought into contact with the lesion in a "pecking" fashion in which 1–3 seconds of contact with the plaque is followed by pulling back the burr from the plaque surface for 3–5 seconds. This decreases the risk of sudden deceleration of the burr and allows the debris to clear from the distal circulation. It is important to prevent deceleration over 5000 rpm because such decelerations can lead to plaque heating, torsional dissection of the vessel, and formation of larger particles that can lead to slow reflow or no reflow. Another important consideration during RA is that the operator should hold gentle forward pressure on the guide catheter and the wire to maintain wire position in the distal vessel. The total time taken for each pass should not exceed 30 seconds. Fig. 5.3 and Videos 5.1A–G demonstrate the use of RA in a severe left main stenosis. The slow pecking technique is important to prevent device entrapment beyond the target lesion, which is a rare but serious complication requiring expertise to extract the device or emergent surgery if other measures fail.

The most important factor in successfully using RA is to reduce complications such as dissection, perforation, and preventing no reflow or slow reflow (reduction in blood flow by 1 thrombolysis in myocardial infarction [TIMI] grade) despite having a patent vessel and stent thrombosis after RA. Technical tips to prevent these adverse effects

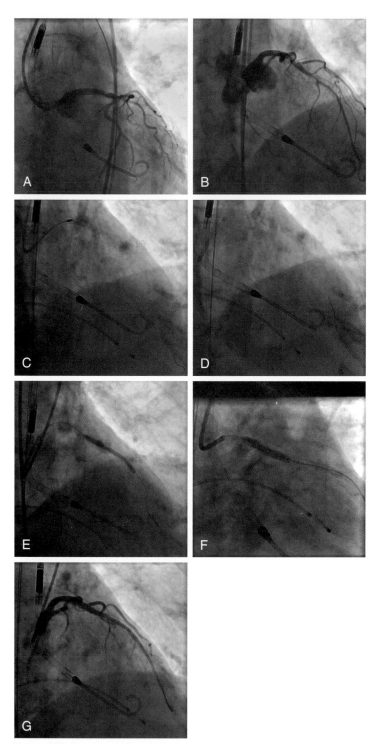

Figure 5.3 Case example using rotational atherectomy in the treatment of fibrocalcific left main and LAD disease. (A,B) Baseline angiography demonstrating calcified plaque of the LM and LAD in caudal and cranial projections. (C) RA using a 1.5-mm burr. (D) Post- RA Angiography. (E) Stent deployment into the LAD. (F) Stenting of the LM into the LAD. (G) Angiography of the LM and LAD post stenting. LM, left main; LAD, left anterior descending; PTCA, percutaneous transluminal coronary angioplasty; RA, rotational atherectomy.

> **Box 5.1** Technical Notes and Tips on Performing Rotational Atherectomy
>
> - A nitrogen compressed-gas cylinder with pressure regulator capable of delivering a minimum 140 L/min at 90–100 psi is required.
> - The compressed-gas cylinder valve must be open to supply compressed gas to the console. The regulator should be adjusted so that the pressure does not exceed 100 psi.
> - Angulated lesions and branch ostial lesions have a higher incidence of dissection and/or perforation: downsize initial burrs and stepwise increase burr size to achieve the final result.
> - Rotational atherectomy (RA) can be performed on chronic total occlusions only if the guidewire is confirmed to be in true lumen distally.
> - Perforations are uncommon. Covered stents should be available in all cardiac catheterization laboratories performing RA.

are listed in Box 5.1. When performed by an experienced operator with the appropriate precaution, RA proves to be an excellent method to debulk and modify plaque in preparation for stenting. This lesion preparation is especially important in cases for which bioabsorbable stents are planned for use.

Clinical Outcomes

The mechanistic hypothesis of RA allowing for differential plaque modification with lower vessel injury as compared to traditional PTCA was studied in three clinical trials (ERBAC, COBRA, and DART) where RA was compared to PTCA for definitive therapy. All three trials yielded either unfavorable or neutral results. RA was then studied as an adjunct therapy for aggressive debulking prior to PTCA. Unfortunately, STRATAS showed no reduction in restenosis rates and CARAT showed no reduction in major adverse cardiac events (MACE). Similarly, for in-stent restenosis ARTIST showed that PTCA was superior to RA in reducing MACE, and, as such, use of RA carries a class III indication for in-stent restenosis. With the advent of stenting there were two clinical trials (SPORT and EDRES) looking at RA as an adjunct to bare metal stenting (BMS) versus traditional PTCA and BMS. EDRES showed a trend toward decreased restenosis rates ($p = 0.05$) and SPORT showed a minimal reduction in target lesion revascularization (TLR) that was not statistically significant. However, in patients with chronic total occlusion (CTO) there was a significant reduction in restenosis rates when RA was used as an adjunct to BMS.

Drug-eluting stents (DES) ushered in a new era in PCI with reduction in restenosis rates due to neointimal hyperplasia, which would potentially ameliorate the failures seen in previous clinical trials due to high restenosis rates. The ROTAXUS study was a large multicenter randomized controlled trial (RCT) comparing RA with DES as opposed to DES alone in treatment of complex coronary lesions. There was a high crossover rate between the two groups leading to greater procedural success rates when RA was used as an adjunct to DES. But the cost of this initial success was greater rates of lumen loss at 9 months. This was likely due to greater vessel injury in RA leading to more neointimal hyperplasia. Thus RA should only be used in highly calcified complex lesions that may not be crossable or dilatable. The use of RA with second-generation stents with smaller stent struts and newer medications or bioabsorbable scaffolding may have lower restenosis rates, but these have not been studied extensively.

Orbital Atherectomy

The Diamondback 360-degree OA system (Cardiovascular Systems, St. Paul, MN) uses a diamond-coated crown (available in sizes 1.25 to

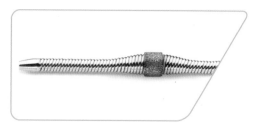

Figure 5.4 A diamond-coated crown for orbital atherectomy system. *(Cardiovascular Systems, St. Paul, MN).*

2.00 mm at 0.25 mm increments) (Fig. 5.4) that orbits eccentrically over a coil made of three spiral wires. The elliptical motion of the crown is different from the burr used for RA such that the diameter and the depth of the OA depend on the velocity of crown rotation (80,000–200,000 rpm). Theoretically this elliptical motion of the crown makes deeper cuts and can ablate plaque in both antegrade and retrograde fashion and, at the same time, allows for greater blood flow and heat dissipation during atherectomy. The additional advantages of OA over RA are that the risk of entrapment of the device on the plaque is theoretically lower and the sanding motion results in smaller particulate matter.

The procedural technique for OA is similar to that of PTRA except that, when selecting lesions, the operator should ensure the presence of calcium on both sides of the arterial wall using fluoroscopy or a 270-degree arc of calcium within the plaque via intravenous ultrasound (IVUS). A ViperWire (0.012-inch) can be used to cross the lesion instead of the RotaWire, and care should be taken not to advance the crown within 5 mm of the distal end of the ViperWire. The ViperSlide (composed of soybean oil, egg yolk phospholipids, glycerin, and water) solution is used for flush in place of the RotaFlush, and, unlike the RA system where the adequacy of flushing is determined by the operator, the OA system requires continuous flow of flush and automatically disables if the flow is interrupted. Finally, the preferred motion for the OA crown is slow continuous advancement as opposed to the pecking motion preferred for RA. The potential complications of OA are similar to those of RA and were discussed earlier.

The ORBIT I study was a pilot study of 50 patients looking at OA prior to DES placement; it showed that 94% of patients had procedural success. MACE was reported to be 4% in hospital, 6% at 30 days, and 8% at 6 months, with a TLR rate of 2%. A follow-up analysis showed a MACE rate of 18.2% and a TLR rate of 3%. ORBIT II was a follow-up multicenter trial done in the United States in which 443 patients underwent OA prior to DES placement; it had a procedural success rate of 88.2%, with a MACE rate of 16.4% and TLR rate of 5.9% at 1 year. Overall these rates of clinical events are comparable to those of RA and DES, and OA thus provides another option for plaque modification in patients with severely calcified atherosclerotic disease.

Laser Angioplasty

The ELCA system emits UV laser light (300 nm wavelength) that ablates plaque using vaporization (photothermal effect), direct breakdown of chemicals (photochemical dissociation), and ejection of the debris from tissue (photoacoustic effect). The process is associated with formation of a vapor bubble that can be mitigated by infusing saline at a rate of 2–3 mL/sec via the guide catheter during the ablation. Another complication is dissection or perforation of the vessel, which can be reduced by limiting the size of the laser catheter to less than two-thirds the size of the reference vessel. The clinical experience in RCTs comparing ELCA to other modalities have failed to show benefit. However, in some trials, ELCA was successful in recanalizing CTO or subtotal occlusions that were not crossable with conventional guidewires. ELCA should thus be considered for such lesions; additionally, ELCA also has approval for saphenous vein graft (SVG) lesions and ostial lesions that are not amenable to RA and OA.

Cutting Balloon Angioplasty

Mechanism of Action

CBA involves three to four 0.1–0.4-mm-thick atherotomes (long stainless steel blades) mounted on a noncompliant balloon designed to make microincisions on plaque during inflation. CBA requires lower inflation pressures as compared to PTCA and thus theoretically renders the advantage of lower barotrauma and thereby reduces neointimal proliferation. The atherotomes make controlled incisions that do not exceed the entire radius of the plaque and thereby reduce the incidence of plaque fracture. Since the incisions are limited within the plaque, theoretically there is a lower chance of vessel dissection.

Indications and Contraindications

Routine use of CBA for standard lesions is not supported by current guidelines, and CBA is particularly disadvantageous for vessels that are very tortuous or are less than 2 mm in size; lesions that are greater than 20 mm long; heavily calcified lesions; and CTOs. CBA does have a specific role for bifurcation lesions, ostial lesions, and in-stent restenosis (ISR). For bifurcation lesions, the challenges for routine PTCA are plaque shift and high restenosis rates. The lower inflation pressure and microincisions of CBA reduce plaque shift and neointimal proliferation, resulting in lower restenosis rates than does PTCA. There is a lower incidence of balloon slippage (watermelon seeding) with CBA as compared to PTCA, thereby reducing trauma to the healthy vessel beyond the target lesion; this gives CBA an advantage in the treatment of ostial lesions and ISR. Current guidelines give CBA a class IIb indication for use in ISR.

Equipment

The Flextome Cutting Balloon (Boston Scientific, Natick, MA) is available in monorail and over-the-wire configurations and has a flex point at every 5 mm on the atherotomes to allow for greater flexibility. The Cutting Balloon Ultra-2 is an older monorail device that has 30% less deliverability. The flextome device is available in lengths of 6, 10, and 15 mm and sizes of 2.0 to 4.0 mm. There are three atherotomes mounted on sizes 2.0 to 3.25 mm and four atherotomes on 3.5- to 4.0-mm devices. The atherotomes are concealed within the folds of the balloon to allow safe delivery to the lesion; balloon inflation allows the atherotomes to rise to the surface to make microscopic incisions into plaque (Fig. 5.5).

Technique and Technical Tips

The atherotomes make cutting balloons less flexible than conventional balloons and hence more difficult to deliver. One can predilate the lesion with a conventional 1.5- or 2-mm balloon to allow the cutting balloon to pass. Inflation should be performed slowly to allow for appropriate deployment of the atherotomes in a perpendicular fashion to the atheroma in the vessel wall. Another technique is to partially inflate the cutting balloon as it enters the lesion and then advance the balloon through the lesion as it deflates. For difficulty in crossing lesions, operators can consider using a (buddy) 0.014-inch wire in addition to the guidewire to support the guide catheter while advancing the cutting

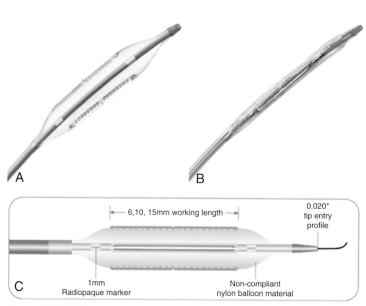

Figure 5.5 (A) Flextome cutting balloon in its inflated state. Microtomes can be seen extending outward from the balloon. (B, C) The cutting balloon (*above*) in the deflated state and (*below*) in the inflated state. The microtomes can be seen extending outward from the balloon. *(Courtesy of Boston Scientific Corp., Marlborough, MA.)*

balloon through a lesion within a stent or in a tortuous segment. In addition, for tortuous vessels, there is a potential for guidewire bias. This can be reduced using a Wiggle wire (Abbott Vascular, Abbott Park, IL).

The potential complications of CBA are atherotome fracture or retention, vessel perforation, and inappropriate folding of the device on deflation (device "winging") making it difficult to retrieve. These can be mitigated by ensuring that the ratio of balloon to vessel size is 1 : 1, not exceeding the recommended inflation pressures for given balloon and desired vessel size, and slowly inflating the balloon during angioplasty, followed by slow deflation of the balloon before pulling negative prior to retrieval. Multiple slow inflations maintained over 60–90 seconds allow for smooth, flat incisions and provide good angiographic results.

Clinical Results

The initial results from single-center trials comparing CBA to PTCA in de novo lesions showed promise; however, in large, multicentered trials such as the Cutting Balloon Global Randomized Trial (GRT) and REDUCE, the results were equivalent for an end point of binary restenosis at 6-month follow-up (GRT: CBA 31.4% vs. PTCA 30.4%, $p = 0.75$; REDUCE: CBA 32.7% vs. PTCA 25.5%, $p = 0.75$). There was also no reduction in MACE (CBA 13.6% vs. PTCA 15.1%) in GRT, and the rates of coronary perforation were higher with CBA (0.8% vs. PTCA 0%).

The role of CBA prior to stenting with BMS was studied in REDUCE 3, which showed lower restenosis rates with CBA (11.8% vs. PTCA 19.6%, $p < 0.05$). However, there was no difference in MACE (CBA 11.5% vs. PTCA 16.8%, $p = 0.082$), and the role of CBA prior to DES placement has not been studied.

Several trials have looked at the role of CBA in the setting of ISR. In the Restenosis Cutting Balloon Evaluation Trial (RESCUT), 428 patients with ISR were randomized to CBA versus PTCA with no reduction in restenosis rates at 7 months (CBA 29.8% vs. PTCA 31.4%, $p = 0.82$). Similarly, the REDUCE 2 trial did not show any reduction in restenosis rates with CBA as compared to PTCA in ISR. RESCUT did show a lower rate of balloon slippage, earning CBA a class IIb indication for angioplasty in ISR.

Scoring Balloon Angioplasty

The AngioSculpt Scoring Balloon (AngioScore, Freemont, CA) has a ninitol spiral element with three spiral struts that wrap around a semicompliant balloon. This provides a more flexible alternative to the CBA catheter, which has three or four linear struts on a noncompliant balloon. The increased flexibility provides better crossing capability compared to CBA, but the data for clinical use are limited. One non-randomized study showed greater stent expansion when compared to direct stenting or conventional PTCA prior to stenting. Currently there are no randomized trials to evaluate the use of scoring balloon angio-plasty in coronary intervention.

Thrombectomy

Primary PCI has been shown to improve clinical outcomes when compared with conservative medical therapy using fibrinolytic or thrombolytic agents; it has become the treatment of choice, and is the standard of care, for patients with acute ST-elevation myocardial infarction (STEMI).

One of the main concerns during primary PCI, or in lesions with large thrombus burden, is embolization of thrombotic or plaque debris and vasoactive substances into the distal coronary circulation resulting in no reflow or slow reflow phenomena. The frequency of this complica-tion has been reported to be between 15% and 20% during primary PCI. Despite distal embolization, the reduction of distal coronary flow is usually transient; however, adverse outcomes have been associated even with transient minimal reductions in coronary microvascular flow during PCI. This was the main premise that raised the concept of thrombectomy using manual or mechanical catheters. The goal was to develop a technique to aspirate intracoronary debris during PCI to reduce the incidence of distal embolization. Initial studies did not demonstrate any benefit of mechanical thrombectomy during primary PCI in patients with STEMI. However, some studies were able to dem-onstrate a reduction of distal coronary embolization as measured by either myocardial blush or TIMI flow grades on postprocedure coronary angiograms and improved clinical outcomes in patients treated with mechanical thrombectomy.

Background

Angiographically, thrombus is visualized in 75.90% of patients with non-STEMI acute coronary syndrome (ACS) and almost 100% of patients with STEMI. Fig. 5.6 shows angiographic thrombus.

Thrombectomy should be considered when thrombus is present in a culprit artery of sufficient diameter such that it can allow safe passage of the thrombectomy catheters. Fiberoptic angioscopy is the gold standard for detection of intracoronary thrombus; however, most cardiac catheterization laboratories do not possess this technique. As a result, IVUS or optical coherence tomography (OCT) is an alternate method for detection of intracoronary thrombus. On coronary angiog-raphy, thrombus is recognized as a filling defect in the lumen of the coronary artery with or without persistent contrast staining. IVUS and OCT reveal the presence of thrombus as a low echogenic mass with a globular or layered appearance protruding from the attached vessel wall. It is challenging to definitively differentiate thrombus from soft plaque on IVUS imaging, and OCT is a better modality for thrombus imaging and diagnosis.

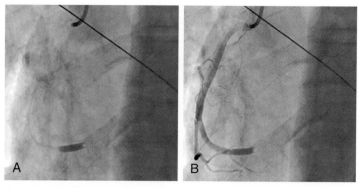

Figure 5.6 Angiographic appearance of intracoronary thrombus. (A) Contrast staining noted in distal right coronary artery (RCA) suggestive of intracoronary thrombus. (B) Complete occlusion of flow distal to the intracoronary thrombus.

Aspiration of the intracoronary thrombus can be performed manually using any one of the several available manual aspiration catheters or a high-pressure rheolytic thrombectomy system (AngioJet, Boston Scientific, Maple Grove, MN). Of these, the AngioJet catheter uses high-pressure water jets that are directed backward into the catheter to create a strong negative suction (Venturi current) at the space of the catheter tip (Fig. 5.7). This not only evacuates the thrombus effectively but also macerates the thrombus into very small particles.

Mechanical Thrombectomy

Technical Tips

Mechanical aspiration thrombectomy devices are dual-lumen catheters that are passed across the culprit lesion over a standard 0.014-inch guidewire. Of the two lumens, the smaller lumen consists of the guidewire using a rapid exchange monorail system. The larger lumen connects the distal opening to the proximal port and serves as the aspiration lumen, using a large (30–50 mL) lockable aspiration syringe that is attached to the proximal port. Currently, the most frequently used aspiration thrombectomy catheters are the Export XT Aspiration Catheter (Medtronic, Inc., Minneapolis, MN, Fig. 5.8), the Pronto V3 Extraction Catheter (Vascular Solutions, Inc., Minneapolis, MN), and the Extract Catheter (Volcano Therapeutics, Rancho Mirage, CA). All these catheters are available in both 6F and 7F sizes. These catheters also vary in the degree of rigidity or support to cross difficult lesions. The Pronto LP has a stiletto, stiffening the catheter and allowing more pushability and crossability.

Mechanical aspiration should be performed in an antegrade fashion (i.e., from proximal to distal) while crossing the lesion, and this should be continued while the aspiration catheter is being withdrawn into the guide catheter. This can be repeated multiple times as long as there is continuous collection of the thrombus into the lockable syringe. Continuous aspiration ensures that there is no premature release of the distal thrombus into the proximal part of the coronary artery, other coronary branches, or into the aortic root. Operators should exercise caution because large thrombus particles may be attached to the tip of the aspiration catheter even if there is no flow into the syringe. At the end of aspiration, sufficient back-bleeding should be performed to ensure that both the guide catheter and the connector are clear of the entire thrombus burden.

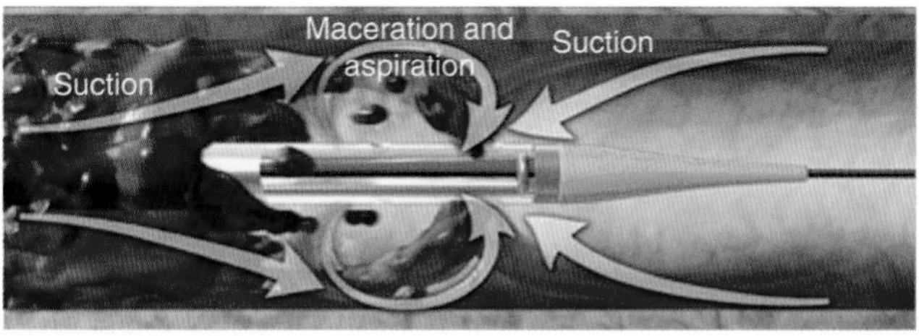

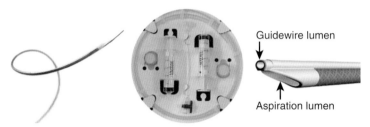

Figure 5.7 AngioJet Rheolytic Thrombectomy System cross-stream technology.

Figure 5.8 The Medtronic Export XT Aspiration Catheter. *(Courtesy of Medtronic, Inc., Minneapolis, MN.)*

Clinical Outcomes Data

There are mixed results with the use of aspiration thrombectomy during PCI. The Thrombus Aspiration During Percutaneous Coronary Intervention in Acute Myocardial Infarction Study (TAPAS) is the largest randomized trial revealing the benefits of using aspiration thrombectomy during primary PCI. There was reduction in mortality in those who received aspiration thrombectomy along with primary PCI. Benefits were also noted in the Multidevice Thrombectomy in Acute ST-Segment ELevation Acute Myocardial Infarction (MUSTELA) trial revealing reduced microvascular obstruction at 3 months as well as increased incidence of postprocedural ST elevation resolution on electrocardiogram. However, benefits were not noted in the Intracoronary Abciximab and Aspiration Thrombectomy in Patients with Large Anterior Myocardial Infarction (INFUSE AMI) trial. The Thrombus Aspiration During ST-Segment Elevation Myocardial Infarction (TASTE) trial performed in Scandinavia revealed no mortality benefit at 30 days if routine aspiration thrombectomy was performed during primary PCI, and the lack of benefit persisted at 1-year follow-up.

Fluoroscopy or procedural time is an important aspect; in the TAPAS trial, fluoroscopy times were reported to be similar when thrombectomy was performed during PCI when compared to PCI alone. However, this was not the case in the other studies, in which fluoroscopy times were higher if thrombectomy was performed. Quality of thrombectomy technique is also important, with concern for air or thrombus embolism into the distal coronary bed or risk of stroke if not performed appropriately. Figs. 5.9 and 5.10 illustrate use of thrombectomy for STEMI.

Rheolytic Thrombectomy

The AngioJet Rheolytic Thrombectomy system (AngioJet, Boston Scientific, Maple Grove, MN) works by removing the thrombus or plaque debris by utilizing high-velocity, high-pressure water jets situated around the catheter tip and directed into the aspiration catheter. This allows transport of the thrombus toward the inflow windows. This method has the ability to fragment thrombus using the saline jets. This technique

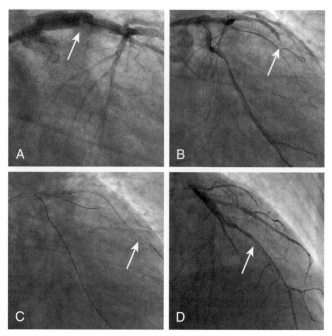

Figure 5.9 Case example using mechanical thrombectomy. (A) Heavy thrombus burden in the left main coronary artery (*arrow*). (B) Embolization of thrombus to the mid left anterior descending (LAD) artery occluding distal flow (*arrow*). (C) Aspiration thrombectomy (*arrow*). (D) Restoration of flow to the distal LAD.

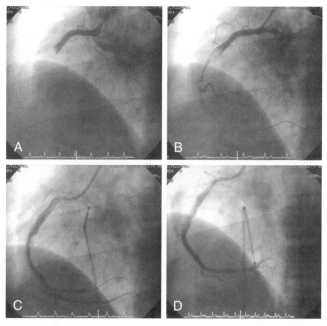

Figure 5.10 Example of AngioJet thrombectomy in a 37-year-old man 8 hours after the onset of chest pain for acute inferior wall myocardial infarction. (A) Right coronary artery with thrombus in proximal portion. (B) Angioplasty guidewire traversing lesion with large amount of clot in the proximal portion of the artery. (C) Right coronary artery after 4F AngioJet. A temporary pacemaker was also inserted. (D) The thrombus was almost completely extracted from the vessel. The final angiogram demonstrates residual distal embolic occlusions but good patency, with TIMI grade 3 flow.

creates a strong suction of approximately 600 mm Hg at the space near the catheter tip, leading to a Venturi effect. The cross-stream allows a small amount of saline to wash into the coronary artery prior to maceration and extraction, leading to augmented removal of the intracoronary thrombus. The Rheolytic Thrombectomy system can be used in the setting of ACS, stent thrombosis, and coronary artery and vein graft thrombosis, as well as for thrombosis of peripheral vessels or grafts for efficient removal of thrombus from the vessel.

The Device

The AngioJet Thrombectomy system utilizes three components: the driver, the pump set, and replaceable catheters. The driver essentially works as a pump set that generates high pressures of up to 10,000 pounds per square inch and also monitors aspiration and system flow during the procedure, which helps to maximize patient safety. The pump set drives the saline into the aspiration catheter and ensures that there is a balance between the fluid leaving the catheter and the fluid entering the catheter, thus maintaining a constant pressure within the target vessel. The AngioJet catheters are 135–140 cm long and taper from the distal 5 cm to the tip. They are available in 4F, 5F, and 6F sizes. The AngioJet Spiroflex, SpiroflexVG, and XMI catheters can be used in both the native coronary arteries as well as in SVGs.

Technical Tips

The AngioJet catheter needs to be prepped and primed while submerged in saline prior to use. The prepared catheter is then advanced to reach the proximal end of the target thrombus, after which the system is activated and the catheter is slowly advanced across the thrombotic lesion at a rate of 0.5 mm/sec and then retracted at the same rate back toward the starting point at the proximal end of the lesion. This process can be repeated multiple times as long as angiographic improvement of coronary flow is noted.

There is concern for hemolytic anemia with prolonged use of the rheolytic thrombectomy system; therefore total device time use should be limited to 10 minutes. Hemolysis induces the release of adenosine, which can precipitate bradyarrhythmias. Placement of a temporary pacing wire is recommended, especially when performing thrombectomy in the right coronary artery of a dominant left circumflex coronary artery in the event that significant bradyarrhythmia occurs.

This technique provides an advantage over manual aspiration thrombectomy because a large thrombus burden may be removed more effectively. However its use is limited by the added procedure time required for prepping and priming the device and placement of temporary pacing wires, which can lead to delays in revascularization of the target vessel especially in the setting of ACS.

Although initial studies showed improvement in myocardial perfusion and reduction in infarct size using this technique, there was no difference in clinical outcomes at 6 months (Albiero et al. 2004). In later studies, there was no difference noted in the reduction of infarct size; the main study evaluating this technique was the AngioJet Rheolytic Thrombectomy in Patients Undergoing Primary Angioplasty for Acute Myocardial Infarction (AIMI) trial, which was a large randomized trial comparing primary PCI alone to primary PCI with rheolytic thrombectomy (Mauri et al. 2002). One of the limitations of this study was randomization after the diagnostic coronary angiogram was performed, which may have led to selection bias because patients with higher thrombus burden were potentially selected for thrombectomy. The other limitation was the finding that patients who underwent PCI alone were found to have TIMI 3 grade flow in the culprit artery prior to PCI, which is known to be associated with smaller infarct area. Another important concept is the retrograde thrombectomy technique (i.e., distal to proximal thrombectomy), wherein the device is placed at the distal end of the thrombus prior to initiation of thrombectomy. This may promote distal embolization during placement of the thrombectomy catheter.

There is a greater appeal to using manual aspiration catheters as compared to the mechanical rheolytic technique. In addition to being comparatively inexpensive, the manual aspiration catheters are easier to use. Apart from flushing the aspiration catheter, there is no other preparation required. This ensures there is no significant delay in revascularization of the coronary artery, although there may be technical challenges in advancing the catheter, especially in smaller and tortuous vessels. In addition, use of the smaller 6F catheters limits the rate of thrombus extraction due to a smaller lumen diameter. The 7F catheters may allow faster rates of extraction (up to 3 times faster compared to 6F catheters); however, catheter delivery using a 7F catheter is more challenging and may restrict its use to only the larger epicardial arteries and may carry a higher risk of vessel injury including dissection and perforation.

Embolic Protection Devices

SVGs develop atherosclerotic luminal disease much more commonly than do arterial grafts. In fact, within 10 years, approximately half of these vein grafts develop complete or significant occlusion. In the majority of these cases, PCI is preferred over redo CABG surgery due to the inherent risks associated with repeat surgical revascularization. PCI of the SVGs are associated with multiple technical challenges, the most concerning being the high risk of no reflow phenomenon due to embolization of thrombotic debris into the distal vessel. Epicardial vasodilators such as nitroglycerin are of little value in restoring distal flow, but microvascular vasodilators such as adenosine or nicardipine may have a beneficial role in treating the no reflow phenomenon. This has led to the development of embolic protection devices to prevent or minimize distal embolization and in turn improve both procedural as well as clinical outcomes.

Embolic protection devices are developed to decrease embolization of thrombotic or friable plaque material into the distal vessel during PCI. Although the data do not support the use of embolic protection devices during primary PCI in STEMI patients, these devices have been shown to improve outcomes in patients undergoing PCI on SVGs.

Several embolic protection systems have been developed over the years. There are two primary mechanisms to trap the embolic debris. The balloon occlusion technique requires placement of the device either proximal or distal to the lesion where the device traps the emboli, which are subsequently aspirated. These devices are no longer commercially available. The alternative method is to deploy a filter device distal to the lesion in order to ensure that debris that gets embolized is captured and does not occlude the microcirculation, so distal flow in the vessel is maintained.

Balloon Occlusion Technique

The most commonly used device utilizing the balloon occlusion system is the Proxis Embolic Protection System (St. Jude Medical Inc., St. Paul, MN, Fig. 5.11). This consists of a 3.5F infusion catheter that contains the device and is advanced using a 7F guide catheter over a standard guidewire. The device is placed proximal to the lesion, after which the balloon is inflated to occlude distal antegrade blood flow. A stagnant column of blood is created that is aspirated immediately after the PCI is performed. This allows removal of all debris before antegrade distal flow is restored in the target vessel upon balloon deflation.

The main benefit of using the Proxis system is the protection against distal embolization before the lesion is crossed with a guidewire

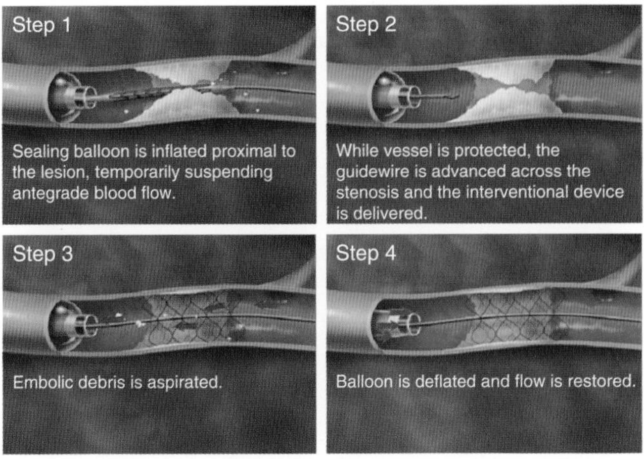

Figure 5.11 The Proxis Embolic Protection System. *(Courtesy of St. Jude Medical Inc., St. Paul, MN.)*

by occluding the vessel. However, the Proxis device should only be used in vessels ranging between 3.0 and 5.0 mm in diameter. These should not be used in vessels with a larger diameter because complete occlusion of the vessel may not be achieved using this system, thus resulting in partial antegrade flow into the distal vessel with subsequent embolization of thrombotic debris.

The Proxis system can be used during PCI of all SVGs as long as there is an adequate "landing zone" to deploy the system proximally. The advantage of the Proxis system over the distal filter device is the ability to utilize this system in cases where there is lack of an adequate "landing zone" distal to the lesion where the filter device would need to be deployed. In contrast, use of balloon occlusion devices leads to occlusion of distal blood flow, leading to temporary myocardial ischemia, which is not seen in distal filter devices.

The Proximal Protection During Saphenous Vein Graft Intervention Using the Proxis Embolic Protection System (PROXIMAL) trial compared the Proxis system to distal embolic protection devices and evaluated their efficacy in preventing clinical events during PCI of SVGs. The trial showed that there was no difference in MACE in both arms. As such, it was deemed a noninferior technique for preventing distal embolization during PCI.

The GuardWire Temporary Occlusion and Aspiration System (Medtronic, Inc., Minneapolis, MN) is another balloon occlusion technique wherein the balloon occludes the vessel several centimeters distal to the lesion. This ensures that all thrombotic debris released during PCI is trapped in the stagnant column of blood distal to the lesion, which can be aspirated prior to deflating the balloon. The use of this system is limited due to the fact that it needs an adequate "landing zone" distal to the lesion, and it also causes temporary myocardial ischemia.

The Saphenous Vein Graft Angioplasty Free of Emboli Randomized (SAFER) trial compared the GuardWire system to conventional PCI of SVGs without the use of distal embolic protection devices. The trial revealed that, at 30 days, there was significant reduction in MACE, which was the primary end point. The relative risk reduction of MACE was 42% ($p = 0.004$).

Distal Filter Device Technique

The Filterwire EZ Embolic Protection System (Boston Scientific Corporation, Natick, MA, Fig. 5.12) is the most commonly utilized device for this technique. This device consists of a symmetric 110-micron pore

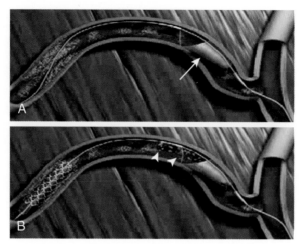

Figure 5.12 The Boston Scientific Filterwire EZ Embolic Protection System. (A) The filter (*arrow*) is deployed distal to the lesion. (B) Embolic material (*arrowheads*) is captured during intervention. *(Courtesy of Boston Scientific Corp., Natick, MA.)*

basket filter fixed to a guidewire. When this filter is released, it expands up to 5.5 mm. This technique requires crossing the lesion and placing the Filterwire EZ System distal to the lesion prior to deploying the filter. After completing the PCI, the filter is collapsed into a retrieval catheter thus trapping the thrombotic debris and preventing distal embolization.

The main benefit of utilizing the filter device technique over the balloon occlusion devices is maintenance of continuous antegrade blood flow while trapping larger debris during the procedure and avoiding myocardial ischemia. In theory, the drawback of these filter devices is the inability to trap smaller particles or vasoactive substances due to limitations in filter pore sizes, resulting in incomplete protection of the microvascular circulation. However the evidence from clinical studies comparing filter devices to balloon occlusion devices suggests that there is similar debris size distribution as well as outcomes with either technique. In practice, the major limitation is the need for an adequate "landing zone" approximately 25–30 mm distal to the edge of the lesion to deploy the device.

The SpiderFX Embolic Protection Device (ev3, Inc., Plymouth, MN, Fig. 5.13) is another device that utilizes the distal filter technique and can be used during PCI of SVGs. This device is heparin-coated and comes in a range of sizes from 3.0 mm to 7.0 mm. This device has an advantage over the Filterwire EZ Embolic Protection System in that it does not have a fixed guidewire and allows use of any standard 0.014-inch interventional guidewire. The filter is delivered distal to the lesion using a 3.2F catheter by means of a rapid exchange system (SpideRX); at the end of the procedure, it is retrieved using a separate 4.2F or 4.6F SpideRX retrieval catheter.

The Filterwire EX Randomized Evaluation (FIRE) trial evaluated the efficacy of the Filterwire EX embolic protection device to the GuardWire balloon occlusion system during PCI of SVGs. The primary end point, which was a composite of death, MI, and TVR at 30 days, was noted to be similar in both groups (9.9% of patients treated with the Filterwire EX device vs. 11.6% of patients treated with the GuardWire system).

The Saphenous Vein Graft Protection in a Distal Embolic Protection Randomized (SPIDER) trial compared the SpiderFX embolic protection device to a control group treated with either the Filterwire EZ embolic protection system or a GuardWire system during PCI of SVGs. The

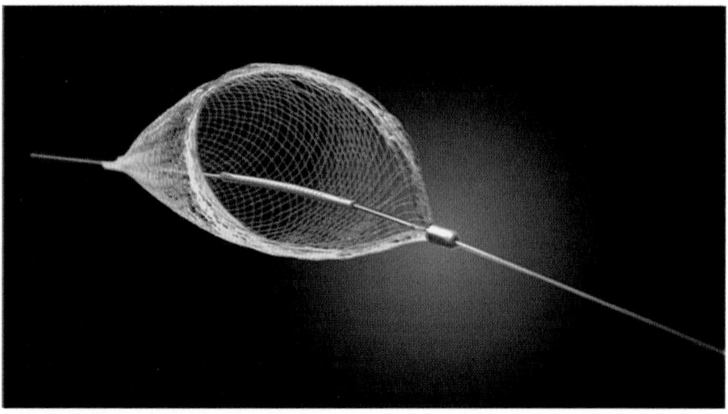

Figure 5.13 The SpiderFX Embolic Protection Device. *(Courtesy of ev3, Inc., Plymouth, MN.)*

SpiderFX device was found to be noninferior, with MACE occurring in 9.1% of the patients versus 8.4% in the control group at 30 days.

Suggested Readings

Abdel-Wahab M, Richardt G, Joachim Büttner H, et al. High-speed rotational atherectomy before paclitaxel-eluting stent implantation in complex calcified coronary lesions: the randomized ROTAXUS (Rotational Atherectomy Prior to Taxus Stent Treatment for Complex Native Coronary Artery Disease) trial. *JACC Cardiovasc Interv.* 2013;6:10-19.

Ahn SS, Auth D, Marcus DR, et al. Removal of focal atheromatous lesions by angioscopically guided high-speed rotary atherectomy. Preliminary experimental observations. *J Vasc Surg.* 1988;7:292-300.

Albiero R, Silber S, Di Mario C, et al. Cutting balloon versus conventional balloon angioplasty for the treatment of in-stent restenosis: results of the restenosis cutting balloon evaluation trial (RES-CUT). *J Am Coll Cardiol.* 2004;43:943-949.

Bittl JA, Chew DP, Topol EJ, et al. Meta-analysis of randomized trials of percutaneous transluminal coronary angioplasty versus atherectomy, cutting balloon atherotomy, or laser angioplasty. *J Am Coll Cardiol.* 2004;43:936-942.

Buchbinder M, Fortuna R, Sharma S, et al. Debulking prior to stenting improves acute outcomes: early results from the SPORT trial. *J Am Coll Cardiol.* 2000;35:8A.

Chambers JW, Feldman RL, Himmelstein SI, et al. Pivotal trial to evaluate the safety and efficacy of the orbital atherectomy system in treating de novo, severely calcified coronary lesions (ORBIT II). *JACC Cardiovasc Interv.* 2014;7:510-518.

Cho GY, Lee CW, Hong MK, et al. Side-branch occlusion after rotational atherectomy of in-stent restenosis: incidence, predictors, and clinical significance. *Catheter Cardiovasc Interv.* 2000;50:406-410.

Dauerman HL, Higgins PJ, Sparano AM, et al. Mechanical debulking versus balloon angioplasty for the treatment of true bifurcation lesions. *J Am Coll Cardiol.* 1998;32:1845-1852.

Delhaye C, Wakabayashi K, Maluenda G, et al. Safety and efficacy of bivalirudin for percutaneous coronary intervention with rotational atherectomy. *J Interv Cardiol.* 2010;23:223-229.

de Ribamar Costa J Jr, Mintz GS, Carlier SG, et al. Nonrandomized comparison of coronary stenting under intravascular ultrasound guidance of direct stenting without predilation versus conventional predilation with a semi-compliant balloon versus predilation with a new scoring balloon. *Am J Cardiol.* 2007;100:812-817.

Dill T, Dietz U, Hamm CW, et al. A randomized comparison of balloon angioplasty versus rotational atherectomy in complex coronary lesions (COBRA study). *Eur Heart J.* 2000;21:1759-1766.

Ergene O, Seyithanoglu BY, Tastan A, et al. Comparison of angiographic and clinical outcome after cutting balloon and conventional balloon angioplasty in vessels smaller than 3 mm in diameter: a randomized trial. *J Invasive Cardiol.* 1998;10:70-75.

Hamburger JN, Gijsbers GH, Ozaki Y, et al. Recanalization of chronic total coronary occlusions using a laser guide wire: a pilot study. *J Am Coll Cardiol.* 1997;30:649-656.

Hamburger JN, Serruys PW, Scabra-Gomes R, et al. Recanalization of total coronary occlusions using a laser guidewire (the European total surveillance study). *Am J Cardiol.* 1997;80:1419-1423.

Hansen DD, Auth DC, Hall M, et al. Rotational endarterectomy in normal canine coronary arteries: preliminary report. *J Am Coll Cardiol.* 1988;11:1073-1077.

Hansen DD, Auth DC, Vracko R, et al. Rotational atherectomy in atherosclerotic rabbit iliac arteries. *Am Heart J.* 1988;115:160-165.

Ito H, Piel S, Das P, et al. Long-term outcomes of plaque debulking with rotational atherectomy in side-branch ostial lesions to treat bifurcation coronary disease. *J Invasive Cardiol.* 2009;21:598-601.

Kini A, Reich D, Marmur JD, et al. Reduction in periprocedural enzyme elevation by abciximab after rotational atherectomy of type B2 lesions: results of the Rota Reopro randomized trial. *Am Heart J.* 2001;142:965-969.

Koch KC, vom Dahl J, Kleinhans E, et al. Influence of a platelet GPiib/iiia receptor antagonist on myocardial hypoperfusion during rotational atherectomy as assessed by myocardial Tc-99m sestamibi scintigraphy. *J Am Coll Cardiol.* 1999;33:998-1004.

Levine GN, Bates ER, Blankenship JC, et al. 2011 ACCF/AHA/SCAI guideline for percutaneous coronary intervention. A report of the American College of Cardiology Foundation/ American Heart Association Task Force on Practice Guidelines and the Society for Cardiovascular Angiography and Interventions. *J Am Coll Cardiol.* 2011;58:e44-e122.

Mauri L, Bonan R, Weiner BH, et al. Cutting balloon angioplasty for the prevention of restenosis: results of the cutting balloon global randomized trial. *Am J Cardiol.* 2002;90:1079-1083.

Mauri L, Reisman M, Buchbinder M, et al. Comparison of rotational atherectomy with conventional balloon angioplasty in the prevention of restenosis of small coronary arteries: results of the dilatation vs ablation revascularization trial targeting restenosis (DART). *Am Heart J.* 2003;145:847-854.

Nageh T, Kulkarni NM, Thomas MR. High-speed rotational atherectomy in the treatment of bifurcation-type coronary lesions. *Cardiology.* 2001;95:198-205.

Oesterle SN, Bittl JA, Leon MB, et al. Laser wire for crossing chronic total occlusions: "Learning phase" results from the U.S. Total trial. Total occlusion trial with angioplasty by using a laser wire. *Catheter Cardiovasc Diagn.* 1998;44:235-243.

Ozaki Y, Yamaguchi T, Suzuki T, et al. Impact of cutting balloon angioplasty (CBA) prior to bare metal stenting on restenosis. *Circ J.* 2007;71:1-8.

Parikh K, Chandra P, Choksi N, et al. Safety and feasibility of orbital atherectomy for the treatment of calcified coronary lesions: the ORBIT I trial. *Catheter Cardiovasc Interv.* 2013;81:1134-1139.

Reifart N, Vandormael M, Krajcar M, et al. Randomized comparison of angioplasty of complex coronary lesions at a single center. Excimer laser, rotational atherectomy, and balloon angioplasty comparison (ERBAC) study. *Circulation.* 1997;96:91-98.

Safian RD, Feldman T, Muller DW, et al. Coronary angioplasty and rotablator atherectomy trial (CARAT): immediate and late results of a prospective multicenter randomized trial. *Catheter Cardiovasc Interv.* 2001;53:213-220.

Schwartz RS, Huber KC, Murphy JC, et al. Restenosis and the proportional neointimal response to coronary artery injury: results in a porcine model. *J Am Coll Cardiol.* 1992;18:267-274.

Takebayashi H, Haruta S, Kohno H, et al. Immediate and 3-month follow-up outcome after cutting balloon angioplasty for bifurcation lesions. *J Interv Cardiol.* 2004;17:1-7.

Tian W, Lhermusier T, Minha S, et al. Rational use of rotational atherectomy in calcified lesions in the drug-eluting stent era: review of the evidence and current practice. *Cardiovasc Revasc Med.* 2015;16:78-83.

Whitlow PL, Bass TA, Kipperman RM, et al. Results of the study to determine rotablator and transluminal angioplasty strategy (STRATAS). *Am J Cardiol.* 2001;87:699-705.

Stents, Restenosis, and Stent Thrombosis ▶

CHENG-HAN CHEN · AJAY J. KIRTANE

Introduction

Stents are cylindrical mesh scaffolds designed to maintain durable vessel patency after revascularization of diseased coronary arteries. Initially developed three decades ago to combat the limitations (namely, vessel recoil as well as excessive neointimal hyperplasia) of balloon angioplasty, stents have evolved from simple stainless steel wire coils to complex systems consisting of various metallic, polymeric, and pharmacologic components. A broad base of clinical trial data collected over the past few decades has established stenting as the most common revascularization modality for patients suffering from ischemic coronary artery disease. Despite improvements in vessel patency with each generational iteration of stent technology, stent thrombosis and restenosis continue to be causes of both short- and long-term revascularization failure. This chapter describes the basics of stent design and technology and reviews the biological responses that lead to stenting failure in the form of restenosis and thrombosis.

Stents

Design Characteristics

The ideal stent should be made of a nonthrombogenic material that is sufficiently flexible and low-profile to facilitate delivery in its unexpanded state through guiding catheters and tortuous vessels yet have an expanded configuration providing sufficient radial strength with minimal recoil. It should also provide uniform scaffolding to the treated vessel but also conform to vessel bends. Radiopacity should be sufficient to adequately visualize on fluoroscopy, but not overly so as to obscure important vessel features. During expansion, there should be minimal trauma to the underlying tissue, which can stimulate an injury response causing neointimal proliferation potentially resulting in restenosis. There should be minimal risk of stent fracture. In the case of drug-eluting stents (DES), the bioactive agent should be delivered to the surrounding tissue at a tissue dose and uptake rate that can effectively limit neointimal hyperplasia without excess toxicity. Multiple design characteristics of stent platforms have been identified and engineered to better optimize these parameters.

Stents can be classified based on their underlying structural composition (e.g., metallic vs. nonmetallic polymeric), configuration (e.g., slotted tube vs. coiled wire and open vs. closed cell), chemical stability and presence of a coating (either biostable or bioabsorbable), presence of a bioactive pharmacologic agent (such as a sirolimus analogue or paclitaxel), and method of implantation (either balloon-expandable or self-expanding).

Composition

Until recently, all commercial stent systems were based on an underlying scaffold structure composed of inert metal. Initial generations of metallic stents primarily utilized 316L stainless steel, a medical grade steel selected for its strength, corrosion resistance, and biocompatibility. More recent stent designs have employed cobalt chromium and platinum chromium alloys that are able to provide sufficient radial strength and visibility while enabling lower profile thin stent struts (~75 µm compared to 100–150 µm for most stainless steel–based designs). While these materials have formed the basis for balloon-expandable stent systems, the super-elastic material nitinol allows for self-expanding stents. Composed of an alloy of nickel and titanium, nitinol is able to be set into a particular expanded shape by annealing at high temperature. After cooling, the stent is squeezed down and constrained on a delivery system, able to return to the original shape when released into a blood vessel.

An area of intense interest is the development of bioresorbable scaffolds that are able to provide essential mechanical support during the initial healing process of an expanded coronary artery (over 3–6 months) yet resorb after this period when it is no longer needed. In an idealized form, such a device would result in possible restoration in physiologic coronary vasomotion as well as offering the potential benefit in reducing late events due to the persistence of a metallic prosthesis within the coronary artery (e.g., restenosis and/or thrombosis). In addition, the absence of permanent material would eliminate the potential for persistent side branch obstruction by stent struts, obstruction to potential future surgical graft anastomoses, and stent fracture–related restenosis. The materials with properties best suited for this purpose are generally polymeric in nature, although certain metallic alloys such as magnesium-zinc have been studied for their ability to corrode (degrade into its constitutive ions) in aqueous biological environments. The bioresorbable polymer at the most advanced stage of investigation for stent applications is poly-L-lactic acid (PLLA), notably used as the backbone of the Absorb Bioresorbable Vascular Scaffold (BVS, Abbott Vascular, Santa Clara, CA). Other polymers that have been studied include tyrosine-polycarbonate and poly-salicylic acid/adipic acid, but these platforms have not reached the level of development of polyester-based PLLA scaffolds.

Configuration

Although originally conceived as a wire coil, the vast majority of stent configurations are based on either a slotted tube design or on modular construction (Fig. 6.1). The former involves laser cutting of a metallic tube into specific patterns that influence the flexibility of the stent while maintaining maximal radial strength and minimizing elastic recoil after expansion. Modular stents, in contrast, are created by welding multiple repeating short units to each other. The most common form of this construction involves corrugating either round or elliptorectangular subunits, followed by welding of the subunits to each other at specific points in order to regulate flexibility and structural strength.

Stent designs can be further classified by the size and shapes of the resultant cells, broadly divided into either open-cell or closed-cell configurations. Open-cell designs generally incorporate openings of various sizes and shapes along the length of the stent and can provide improved flexibility and deliverability with minor loss in radial strength. However, these designs may potentially provide lower coverage on the outer curve of angulated segments. Closed-cell designs typically involve a repeating element throughout the stent area, providing uniform wall coverage with decreased tendency for plaque prolapse. Limitations of this design include potentially reduced flexibility and deliverability and an increased tendency to straighten vessel bends when compared

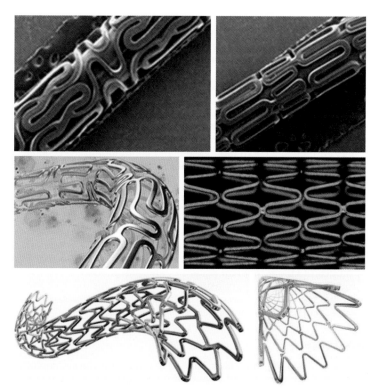

Figure 6.1 Cell designs of drug-eluting stents: Cypher (*top left*), Taxus (*top right*), Xience (*middle left*), Synergy (*bottom left*), and BioFreedom (*bottom right*) are all of slotted tube design. The Endeavor stent (*middle right*) is modular in design.

to open-cell designs. Differences in stent designs are thought to significantly influence both early and late vessel responses: stents that are more conformable and less rigid produce less injury, thrombosis, and neointimal hyperplasia.

Stent strut thickness is also thought to be a factor in vessel biological response. The thinner struts found in more recent stent designs are associated in ex vivo and clinical studies with reduced thrombogenicity, less neointimal hyperplasia, and lower rates of thrombosis and restenosis. However, these thin-strutted stents may potentially provide somewhat lower mechanical strength, resulting in a slightly greater tendency for recoil, longitudinal deformation, and compression.

A special category of stent classification involves stents designed specifically for bifurcations. Developed to address the limitations of a single-stent technique (with provisional side branch stenting) and the multitude of two-stent techniques, these devices are either still under clinical investigation or available only outside the United States. This category ranges from stents that are designed primarily for the main branch but maintain access to facilitate side branch stenting (e.g., Multi-Link Frontier by Abbott Vascular, Santa Clara, CA), stents that treat the side branch first and require a second stent for the main branch (e.g., Tryton by Tryton Medical, Durham, NC), to fully bifurcated stents (e.g., Medtronic Bifurcation Stent System by Medtronic, Minneapolis, MN). Further research is required to better define the patient population and lesion subsets that would benefit most from this technology.

Indications

Stents were originally developed to prevent abrupt vessel closure due to dissection and/or recoil after balloon angioplasty, thus obviating the need for emergent repeat intervention or coronary artery bypass surgery. While initially tested after failed balloon angioplasty ("bail-out" stenting), routine planned stenting has now become the standard of care due to multiple studies (starting with STRESS and BENESTENT-1) demonstrating superior acute results and greater event-free survival compared to balloon angioplasty. In these studies, although stents were associated with a greater amount of neointimal hyperplasia compared with balloon angioplasty, the acute gain in vessel size provided by the scaffolding stent increased more than the late loss in luminal diameter, resulting in improved results over balloon angioplasty alone. Further data (both randomized and nonrandomized) generated over the ensuing decades have demonstrated the advantage of stenting over traditional balloon angioplasty across a broad range of patient and lesion subsets and have relegated balloon dilation to lesions that are too small for stenting (typically <2.0 mm), lesions to which stents cannot be delivered (either due to vessel tortuosity or calcification), or in patients who cannot tolerate the traditional course of dual-antiplatelet therapy (DAPT). While mostly avoiding the potential for acute vessel closure, stents are, however, still susceptible to a variety of modes of failure that can result in either thrombosis or restenosis through neointimal hyperplasia and/or stent expansion. To address these limitations, various coatings were developed to improve on bare metal stent (BMS) platforms.

Coatings

A variety of coatings have been studied to reduce the thrombogenicity and restenotic potential of stents. One category of coating involves modifying the stent to be more biocompatible by presenting a more inert surface to the surrounding tissue. This category includes coatings composed of gold, as well as elemental carbon-based silicon carbide and diamond-like films. Polymer coatings have also been widely employed, ranging from formulations designed to be bio-inert (e.g., fluorinated copolymer in the Xience V DES (Abbott Vascular, Santa Clara, CA), Polyzene-F, and the proprietary Biolinx polymer in the Resolute DES (Medtronic, Santa Rosa, CA) to polymers meant to mimic the cell membrane (e.g., phosphorylcholine). Another category of stent coating involves tethering a bioactive molecule to elicit a specific biological response. These coatings include the early heparin-coated stents (covalently heparin-bonded Palmaz-Schatz and Bx Velocity stents) as well as CD34 antibody-coated stents designed to capture endothelial progenitor cells and facilitate re-endothelialization after stent deployment.

Covered Stents

A third more specialized type of stent "coating" category comprises covered stents, in which an elastic membrane (composed of polytetrafluoroethylene in the Graftmaster stent (Abbott Vascular, Santa Clara, CA) or polyethylene terephthalate in the MGuard stent (InspireMD, Israel) is stretched over an underlying metallic stent substrate. Originally designed to exclude and contain atheroemboli from the vessel lumen, randomized clinical trials found no benefit compared with control BMSs for this purpose. However, these stents are clearly of value in treating life-threatening perforations, as well as in treating aneurysms, pseudoaneurysms, and clinically significant fistulae.

By far the most successful coating category involves utilizing polymers as carrier vehicles for controlled release of pharmacologically active agents to surrounding tissue after stent implantation, most commonly for the purpose of inhibiting neointimal hyperplasia due to vessel injury. The following section describes the various iterations of this DES technology that have been developed over the past decade and a half.

Drug-Eluting Stents

Restenosis after traditional balloon angioplasty generally occurs through some combination of dissection, elastic recoil, negative vessel remodeling, and neointimal hyperplasia (Fig. 6.2). BMSs serve as a scaffold to prevent acute closure and limit elastic recoil and negative remodeling but are still subject to luminal renarrowing due to neointimal formation after vessel injury. DES maintain the mechanical advantages of the underlying metal scaffold but also deliver a pharmacologic agent to interrupt the natural cellular response to injury that results in the activation, proliferation, and migration of vascular smooth muscle cells that cause in-stent restenosis. A variety of antiproliferative drugs have been studied, but the clinically relevant agents fall into two categories: paclitaxel and sirolimus analogues. To control the drug release from the stent system, a polymeric coating and delivery vehicle is typically

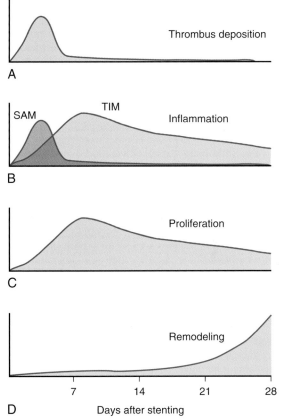

Figure 6.2 The four phases of vascular repair after stent-induced arterial injury in terms of time after stenting. (A) Platelet-rich thrombus accumulates at areas of deep strut injury and peaks at 3–4 days after stent deployment, accounting for most early lumen loss. (B) Coincident with thrombus deposition, inflammatory cells are recruited to the injury site, both at and between stent struts. At 3–7 days after stenting, the surface-adherent monocytes (SAMs) migrate into the neointima as tissue-infiltrating monocytes (TIMs) and remain in place. (C) Proliferation of smooth muscle cells and monocyte macrophages within the neointima peaks at 7 days after implantation and continues above baseline levels for weeks thereafter. (D) Collagen deposition in the adventitia and throughout the tunica media and neointima leads to arterial shrinkage or remodeling, causing compression of the artery on stent struts from the outside in. *(Modified from Garasic J, Edelman E, Rogers C. Stent design and the biologic response. In Beyar R, Keren G, Leon M, Serruys PW, eds.* Frontiers in Interventional Cardiology. *London: Martin Dunitz, 1997:95–100.)*

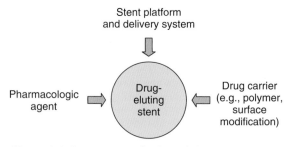

Figure 6.3 Components of a drug-eluting stent system.

employed. These three components—BMS platform/delivery system, active pharmacologic agent, and polymeric drug carrier—form the traditional basis for the DES systems in use today (Fig. 6.3).

Initial DES systems relied on commercially available BMS designs in order to facilitate device development and regulatory approval. These stents were universally 316L stainless steel in construction and employed polymers that were not necessarily ideal as platforms for drug-release coatings. Subsequent DES designs have employed newer metallic scaffold materials, such as cobalt chromium and platinum chromium, that allow for improved performance and device delivery. Stent geometrical design has been modified for its role as the underlying scaffold for drug delivery to the surrounding tissue. Homogeneous drug distribution was improved by adjusting the interstrut distances and considering the relative impact of closed- versus open-cell configurations. These newer designs resulted in better stent conformability to the vessel wall, thus increasing the stent-to-vessel contact necessary for optimal drug delivery to the underlying vessel. Other modifications in newer DES designs have included changes to the delivery polymer itself, with designs to make it more biocompatible or even bioresorbable over time. Additionally, changes to the coating distribution to limit total drug dose (e.g., abluminal-only coatings) and even polymer-free DES systems that rely on stent surface modification (e.g., drug release wells) to carry and deliver drug have been developed. Perhaps the most radical DES design iteration forgoes a metallic stent substrate altogether in favor of a bioabsorbable polymer that provides initial mechanical support after vessel expansion but resorbs after the drug is released and it is no longer needed.

Pharmacology

A wide range of pharmacologic agents have been tested clinically for their ability to limit restenosis after stent deployment. These compounds are typically antiproliferatives that target and inhibit the vascular smooth muscle cells that result in neointimal tissue formation. In addition to their important biological attributes, including mechanism of action, potency, and therapeutic window, many chemical attributes of these compounds (e.g., lipophilicity) also play a role in their suitability for use in DES systems. The two most clinically important classes of agents are paclitaxel and the rapamycin (also known as sirolimus) family of analogues including zotarolimus, everolimus, biolimus, novolimus, myolimus, and amphilimus.

Isolated from the Pacific Yew tree (*Taxus brevifolius*), paclitaxel is a highly lipophilic diterpenoid compound initially utilized as a chemotherapeutic drug. Its principal action is to stabilize intracellular microtubules and prevent their depolymerization. Because microtubules are essential to the mitotic spindle and mitosis, paclitaxel inhibits mitotic progression and cell proliferation particularly in the G0–G1 and G2–M phases of the cell cycle (Fig. 6.4). At low doses (such as those used in DES applications), paclitaxel arrests the G0–G1 and G1–S phases resulting in cytostasis without cell death. Paclitaxel is, however, limited

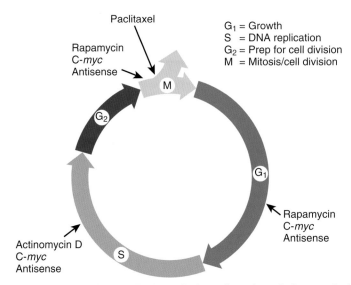

Figure 6.4 Sites of action in the cell phase for selected pharmacologic stent coating to inhibit restenosis.

by a relatively narrow therapeutic window because higher doses can cause cytotoxicity in the form of focal medial necrosis. Other effects of paclitaxel include dose-dependent impaired signal transduction, decreased cytokine and growth factor release and activity, antiangiogenic effects, and reduced smooth muscle cell migration.

Rapamycin (also known as sirolimus) is a macrolide first isolated from *Streptomyces hygroscopicus* in 1972 from samples of the bacterium found on Easter Island (also known as Rapa Nui). Although initially developed as an antifungal agent, it was soon discovered to have significant immunosuppressive and antineoplastic properties through an inhibitory effect on mammalian target of rapamycin (mTOR). Rapamycin first forms a complex with the cytosolic protein FK-binding protein 12 (FKBP12), after which the sirolimus–FKBP12 complex then binds to and inhibits the cell cycle–specific kinase mTOR Complex 1 (mTORC1). Because mTORC1 regulates transcription, translation, and cell cycle progression, inhibition of mTORC1 prevents progression in the cell cycle, particularly in the late G1 to S phase, resulting in cytostasis. Sirolimus was used as the antiproliferative agent in the first commercially available DES: the Cypher stent. Multiple analogues of rapamycin have been developed. Zotarolimus is a semisynthetic derivative (first developed in 1997) of rapamycin in which a lipophilic tetrazole ring is substituted for the native hydrophilic hydroxyl group at position 42. Due to this change, zotarolimus is highly lipophilic, increasing tissue retention time as well as its cell membrane permeability. Zotarolimus is the agent used in the Medtronic Endeavor and Resolute DES. Similarly, everolimus is a hydroxyethyl ether semisynthetic analogue of sirolimus, in which a 2-hydroxyethyl group substitutes for the native hydroxyl group at position 40. It is the active agent in the Abbott Xience and Boston Scientific Promus and Synergy families of DES. Biolimus A9 (also known as *umirolimus*) is another semisynthetic sirolimus analogue, with the hydroxyl group at position 40 substituted for an ethoxyl ethyl group. This results in much greater lipophilicity than sirolimus, enhancing tissue uptake and cellular penetration. Biolimus A9 is used in the Biosensors BioMatrix and Terumo Noburi DES, as well as the Biosensors BioFreedom polymer-free DES.

Of note, two other sirolimus analogues that have been studied for DES applications—tacrolimus and pimecrolimus—have a different mechanism of action. These agents block the calcineurin receptor and inhibit smooth muslce cell activity through binding FKBP506. Unlike the aforementioned mTOR inhibitors, neither tacrolimus nor pimecrolimus has been demonstrated to be beneficial for decreasing restenosis.

Polymers for Drug Delivery

Polymers are long-chain macromolecules composed of many repeating subunits. In DES applications, polymers are typically employed as drug carrier vehicles for the controlled release of a pharmacologic agent to the surrounding tissue after stent deployment. Depending on the chemical structure and subunits that are designed into a specific synthetic polymer, a wide range of properties and processing parameters can be adjusted and tuned for a desired performance characteristic. The primary attributes of a polymer include its chemical composition and its molecular weight distribution. These in turn define the secondary characteristics of a polymer that affect its role as a drug carrier, such as crystallinity, charge, relative hydrophobicity, potential biodegradability, porosity, solvent solubility, miscibility, and compatibility with specific drugs. All these characteristics will ultimately influence the drug release profile of a drug from a polymer. As a component of an implanted device, polymers ideally must also be biocompatible (nontoxic and noninflammatory), durable, sterilizable, and easily processed.

Many synthetic polymers have been developed and investigated as controlled-release carriers in DES. The vast majority are biostable (durable), although newer systems have employed biodegradable polymers that can undergo hydrolytic degradation. Drug release from a durable polymer occurs primarily through diffusion of the drug out of the polymer coating, with small components of drug release from swelling of the coating. With biodegradable polymer coatings, drug is also released from direct dissolution after degradation of the polymer chains. Drug elution kinetics depend not only on the polymer characteristics just described, but also on drug–polymer interactions. These include drug binding with the polymer, drug loading ratio, and the partition coefficient of the drug in polymer.

Although polymer carriers enable controlled release of drug, their presence can potentially result in undesirable biological responses. The polymer coating of some first-generation DES have been implicated in hypersensitivity and eosinophilic inflammatory reactions leading to delayed re-endothelialization that were not previously seen with BMS. This may have contributed to findings of an increased risk of late stent thrombosis compared to BMS. In addition, it is thought that continued inflammation resulting from the presence of polymer may result in late stent malapposition, aneurysm formation, and restenosis. For these reasons, there has been great interest in biodegradable polymer drug-carrier coatings and even polymer-free DES (Fig. 6.5).

First-Generation Drug-Eluting Stents

The first-generation DES devices include the Cypher sirolimus-eluting stent and the Taxus paclitaxel-eluting stent, the first two devices approved for clinical use. They were both based on existing BMS platforms coupled with available nonbiodegradable polymers that were not specifically designed for biocompatibility or drug release. In contrast, second-generation devices comprise the vast majority of DES currently used and combine more deliverable and thinner strut stents with polymers designed for biocompatibility and release of a specific pharmacologic agent. Newer generation DES platforms have moved toward biodegradable and polymer-free drug-release coatings and even biodegradable polymer scaffolds.

Multiple industry- and investigator-initiated studies corroborated highly favorable initial results, and, as a result of the approval and availability of the first DES platforms (Cypher and Taxus), DES became the predominant intracoronary device used for percutaneous coronary intervention.

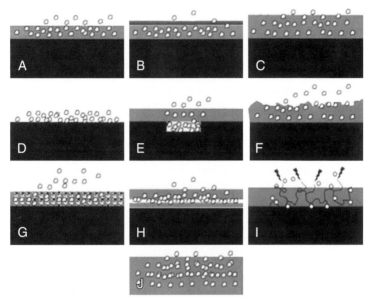

Figure 6.5 Schematic representation of different modalities of drug-eluting stent platforms. (A) Drug–polymer blend, release by diffusion. (B) Drug diffusion through additional polymer coating. (C) Drug release by swelling of coating. (D) Non–polymer-based drug release. (E) Drug loaded in stent reservoir. (F) Drug release by coating erosion. (G) Drug loaded in nanoporous coating reservoirs. (H) Drug loaded between coatings (coating sandwich). (I) Polymer-drug conjugate cleaved by hydrolysis or enzymic action. (J) Bioerodible polymeric stent. Black represents the stent strut; gray represents the coating. *(From Price MJ (ed):* Coronary Stenting, *1st ed. Philadelphia, Elsevier Saunders, 2014, p. 20, Fig. 2.12.)*

Second-Generation Drug-Eluting Stents

Second-generation DES platforms are distinguished by the use of more deliverable thinner strut stents (typically composed of either cobalt chromium or platinum chromium alloys) mated with coatings specifically developed for drug release and biocompatibility. In particular, design changes were made to alleviate some of the abnormal biological responses associated with the first-generation systems (such as delayed endothelialization and increased inflammation) that could potentially lead to complications such as late malapposition, stent thrombosis, and restenosis. The most studied durable polymer second-generation DES are the zotarolimus-eluting Endeavor and Resolute DES and the everolimus-eluting Xience and Promus families.

The zotarolimus-eluting Endeavor stent consists of a phosphoryl-choline (PC)/zotarolimus coating applied to the MP35N cobalt chromium Driver modular BMS (strut thickness 91 μm). Phosphorylcholine is a hydrophilic polymer based on the major lipid head group component of cell membranes and is designed to increase biocompatibility through biomimicry. A PC base coat forms the first layer of the Endeavor coating, on top of which sits the polymer–drug matrix. To slow drug elution, a drug-free PC overcoat covers the matrix. Drug elution is relatively rapid from this system, with 90% of zotarolimus released within 7 days and 100% within 30 days. Approval of Endeavor by the U.S. Food and Drug Administration (FDA) was based on the ENDEAVOR series of clinical trials. Although this series of trials demonstrated that the Endeavor DES was superior to a BMS comparator and clinically noninferior to other first-generation DES platforms, the angiographic late loss of this stent (~0.6 mm) was greater than in other DES platforms, likely related to the lack of a sustained elution of zotarolimus. Notably this early clinical disadvantage of the stent was offset by improvements in clinical safety end points at long-term follow-up. These findings support the hypothesis that there is a finite and optimal period for drug elution, beyond which an emphasis should be placed upon biocompatibility.

As with the Endeavor DES system, the Resolute DES is a zotarolimus-eluting stent based on an iterated cobalt-alloy BMS platform. Whereas Endeavor was based on the Driver BMS, in which multiple sinusoidal rings are welded together, the Resolute system utilizes the single-wire Integrity and Onyx chromium BMS. Instead of the PC polymer, a proprietary BioLinx tripolymer consisting of both hydrophobic and hydrophilic components is used in the Resolute to better modulate the elution of zotarolimus (60% elution in 30 days, 100% by 180 days). The large ($N = 2292$) RESOLUTE All-Comers trial compared Resolute with the Xience V everolimus-eluting stent in patients with a wide range of clinical and anatomical variability and found that Resolute was non-inferior in regards to the primary endpoint of target lesion failure (composite of death, cardiac death, myocardial infarction [MI], and target lesion revascularization) at 1 year (8.2% vs. 8.3%, p for noninferiority < 0.001). Longer term follow-up from this trial as well as others had demonstrated nearly indistinguishable results from other second-generation DES platforms.

The Xience V everolimus-eluting stent family is based on a durable biocompatible fluorinated copolymer (consisting of vinylidene fluoride and hexafluoropropylene) matrix releasing everolimus (polymer to everolimus at a 83% to 17% ratio) applied to a low-profile (81 μm) flexible L605 cobalt chromium alloy stent. The polymer is elastomeric and experiences minimal deformation with expansion. In addition, fluoropolymers have been shown to be resistant to platelet and thrombus deposition. Xience V, the original member of the family, is based on the MultiLink Vision metal stent platform, whereas the updated Xience PRIME stent moved to the more deliverable MultiLink 8 platform. Improvements in the stent delivery system catheter led to the Xience Xpedition and Xience Alpine systems, although the DES itself remains unchanged from the Xience PRIME. Approximately 80% of the drug is released after 30 days, and 100% is released after 120 days.

The SPIRIT series of trials evaluated the safety and efficacy of the Xience system. FDA approval in 2008 was based on the pivotal SPIRIT IV trial in which 3687 patients were randomized to Xience versus Taxus Express. This trial demonstrated a reduction in the primary end point of target vessel failure (composite of cardiac death, MI, and/or target vessel revascularization) with the Xience system (4.2% vs. 6.8%, $p = 0.001$).

The Promus family (consisting of Promus Element and Promus Premier) of everolimus-eluting stents utilizes the identical coating formulation (fluorinated copolymer releasing everolimus) as the Xience family. However, the stent platform is based on the Omega platinum chromium stent. Because platinum chromium is denser than 316L stainless steel or cobalt chromium, thinner struts can be employed without compromising stent radial strength. This enables a more flexible and deliverable system that still maintains adequate radiopacity. Although the stent remains unchanged, the Promus Premier improved upon the delivery system of the original Promus Element and additionally reinforced the proximal portions of the stent in order to address initial concerns regarding longitudinal compression of the stent platform. The PLATINUM trial ($N = 1530$) established Promus as noninferior to Xience V in regards to the primary endpoint of target vessel failure and led to commercial device approval.

Next-Generation Technologies

Although polymer matrices have been an essential component of DES stent platforms in modulating drug release, the persistence of a permanent polymer coating long after the drug supply has been exhausted (or needed) may contribute to chronic inflammation. This in turn could play a role in late and very late stent thrombosis as well as in late restenosis. Newer (i.e., "second-generation") DES designs have addressed this through improving the biocompatibility of the polymer layer. Another approach has been to eliminate the permanent polymer layer altogether, either through the use of biodegradable polymer carriers or with novel polymer-free DES designs.

The Synergy everolimus-eluting stent system is based on the same platinum chromium BMS platform and pharmaceutical agent as the current generation Promus system. However, the polymer coating is composed of abluminal-only biodegradable poly(D,L-lactide-co-glycolide) (PDLGA) in a 85:15 lactide:glycolide ratio instead of permanent fluorinated copolymer. Both the PDLGA polymer and the everolimus are fully absorbed after 3–4 months, thus eliminating long-term polymer exposure. Approval in the United States in 2015 was based on the pivotal EVOLVE II study ($N = 1684$), which found that the Synergy stent was noninferior to the Promus Element Plus in regards to the primary end point of target lesion failure at 12 months. More recent data suggest that this stent platform may have a very low rate of late and very late stent thrombosis, and ongoing studies are being conducted to further investigate whether these results are sustained over longer term follow-up. Furthermore, due to the disappearance of both drug and polymer from this platform, studies are ongoing to investigate the safety of shorter term dual antiplatelet therapy after Synergy stent implantation.

Bioresorbable Drug-Eluting Stents

The vast majority of stent systems in use today are based on permanent metallic stents. While the concept of a completely bioresorbable stent was investigated long before the DES era, it was only recently that stent designs combining a bioresorbable scaffold with an antiproliferative pharmacologic agent entered widespread clinical study. Since the mechanical benefit of a stent scaffold on acute results, vessel recoil, and negative remodeling is thought to be only necessary for the first 3–6 months after implantation, bioresorbable stents offer potential advantages in restoring the treated artery to its state of natural vasomotion and function. Additionally, the resorption of a stent could relieve side branch obstruction and could facilitate future revascularization (either percutaneous or surgical) in patients who require further interventions. Finally, the absence of a permanent implant could mitigate the effects of late inflammation and neoatherosclerosis that occur following permanent metallic stents, which may form the basis for such complications as late stent thrombosis and restenosis.

The first completely bioresorbable DES to be approved for clinical use (currently outside the United States) is the Absorb Bioresorbable Vascular Scaffold (BVS) (Fig. 6.6). Its underlying structure is composed of PLLA is coupled with an everolimus-eluting bioresorbable coating composed of poly-D,L-lactic acid (PDLLA) that releases the agent at a similar profile to the Xience V family of DES (80% after 30 days). Small platinum markers at the scaffold edges provide fluoroscopic landmarking because the remainder of the scaffold is radiolucent. The native strut thickness (including the drug layer) of 156 μm (which may be greater following implantation when the polymer takes on water) is comparable to earlier generation stainless steel stent platforms but is notably larger than the current generation of cobalt chromium and platinum chromium stents, reflecting the challenge of constructing scaffolds with polymeric materials that inherently have less mechanical strength than metallic alloys.

The initial iteration of the Absorb BVS (Cohort A design) was studied in the ABSORB FIM trial, in which 30 patients received the BVS scaffold in simple, de novo coronary lesions. Acute recoil and radial strength were found to be similar to contemporary metallic stents. However, late loss was noted to be 0.44 mm, largely due to late recoil

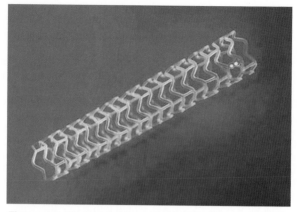

Figure 6.6 Bioabsorbable scaffold (BVS, Abbott Vascular).

with a smaller component of neointimal hyperplasia. As a result, a redesigned scaffold (Cohort B design) incorporated changes in the scaffold processing parameters in order to decrease the rate of hydrolysis and resorption, thereby lengthening the duration of structural support and resulting in improved outcome, as observed using multiple imaging modalities within the ABSORB Cohort B trial ($N = 101$). In this trial, scaffold enlargement was seen on intravascular ultrasound (IVUS) and optical coherence tomography (OCT) (likely due to remodeling), countered by increases in plaque area, resulting in late loss comparable to metallic DES.

The ABSORB II trial randomized 501 patients in a 2:1 ratio to receive either Absorb BVS ($N = 335$) or Xience ($N = 166$) and found similar rates of all death, all MI, and revascularization at 2 years (11.6% for BVS vs. 12.8% for Xience V, $P = 0.70$). The co-primary end points of vasomotion and minimum lumen diameter will be analyzed at 3 years. One-year results from the pivotal ABSORB III trial comparing Absorb BVS ($N = 1322$) to Xience ($N = 686$) found no significant difference between the groups (7.8% for BVS vs. 6.1% for Xience, $P = 0.007$ for noninferiority) in regards to the primary end point of target lesion failure (cardiac death, target vessel MI, or ischemia-driven target lesion revascularization). The FDA approved this stent in 2016. Data from both trials, however, have suggested that while the ABSORB BVS is statistically noninferior to its comparator stent, the Xience V stent, there are numerically greater rates of stent thrombosis. Within ABSORB III, for example, the overall rate of stent thrombosis was 1.5% for ABSORB versus 0.7% for Xience V at 1 year ($p = 0.13$). Further analyses have indicated that the greatest differences between the two stents occurred among patients with smaller vessels (e.g., vessels <2.25 mm in reference vessel diameter), in whom the larger struts of the ABSORB stent may have resulted in worsened outcomes. As a result, assiduous attention to vessel sizing as well as adequate pre- and postdilation is recommended when using this device.

Numerous other bioresorbable vascular scaffolds are currently in development, ranging from other polymeric designs to magnesium-based platforms. The potential for an abrogation of even the small number of late events that occur with the best-in-class current-generation DES platforms has spurred continued innovation within the DES landscape. Ultimately the clinical outcomes trials with these and future devices will be the arbiter of whether these systems can deliver on their promise.

Stent Restenosis

Despite tremendous advances in the technology used for PCI over the past 40 years, restenosis continues to affect a small but significant number of patients. Initial percutaneous balloon angioplasty resulted in restenosis rates of almost 50%—a combination of acute vessel closure, elastic recoil, negative remodeling, and mild amounts of neointimal hyperplasia. BMSs reduced the rate of restenosis compared to balloon angioplasty by reducing the incidence of acute recoil and acute vessel closure, and, further, by stimulating positive remodeling of the stented vessel. However the more aggressive neointimal hyperplasia after BMS implantation still resulted in restenosis rates that ranged from 20% to 40% despite efforts to maximize luminal area by increasing stent gain. This concept of "bigger is better" (or stent optimization) has remained a mainstay of coronary stenting techniques. The advent of DES led to dramatically lower rates of restenosis (of <10%) through pharmacologic suppression of smooth muscle cell proliferation, and future treatment advances may improve on this further with novel antiproliferative agents and improved stent platform designs. Nonetheless, achieving optimal stent expansion acutely has still resulted in improved outcomes, even within the DES era.

Definitions

Restenosis is most commonly defined as luminal renarrowing of greater than 50% (*binary angiographic restenosis*), either within the stent (*in-stent restenosis*) or within the stent and including 5 mm proximal or distal to the stent margin (*in-segment restenosis*) on follow-up angiography (typically 6 or 9 months later). While binary restenosis is the standard used in most clinical trials, it should be noted that restenosis is a continuous variable, with percentage stenosis after PCI that can range anywhere within a normal Gaussian distribution (Fig. 6.7). Restenosis can also

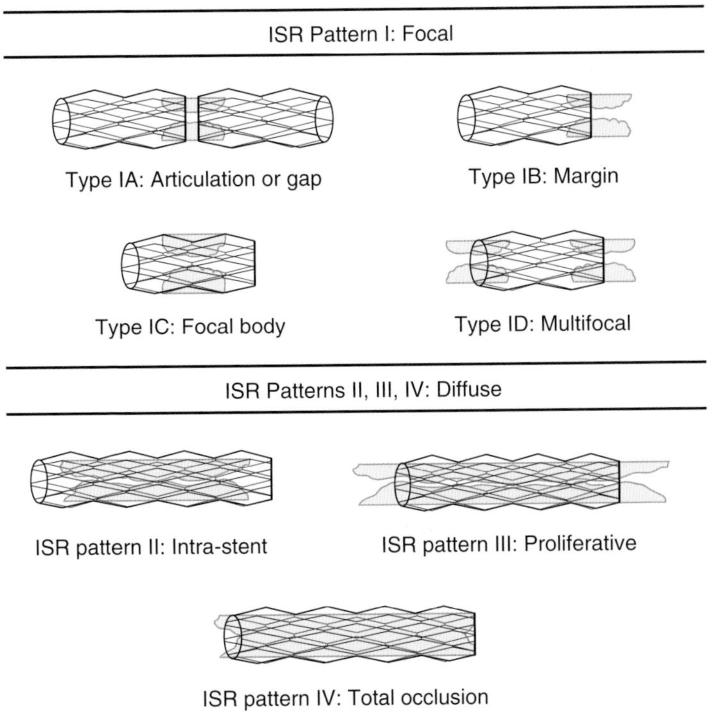

ISR Pattern I: Focal

Type IA: Articulation or gap

Type IB: Margin

Type IC: Focal body

Type ID: Multifocal

ISR Patterns II, III, IV: Diffuse

ISR pattern II: Intra-stent

ISR pattern III: Proliferative

ISR pattern IV: Total occlusion

Figure 6.7 Mehran classification schematic for four typical patterns of in-stent restenosis (ISR). Pattern I (focal) contains four types (A–D). Patterns II through IV (diffuse) are defined according to geographic position of ISR in relation to the previously expanded stent. *(From Mehran R, Dangas G, Abizaid AS, et al. Angiographic patterns of in-stent restenosis: classification and implications for long-term outcome. Circulation. 1999;100:1872–1878.)*

be measured in terms of *late loss*, the difference in millimeters between the minimal luminal diameter (MLD) of the segment after PCI and the MLD on follow-up angiography. The *late loss index* describes the late loss divided by the *acute gain* (difference between the post- and pre-procedural MLD of the treated segment) (Fig. 6.8). *Clinical restenosis* (as proposed by the Academic Research Consortium) occurs with (1) a luminal renarrowing of greater than 50% of the MLD associated with either symptoms of ischemia or abnormal results of invasive diagnostic testing such as FFR (<0.80) or IVUS (<6 mm for left main or <4 mm for non-left main) or (2) luminal renarrowing of greater than 70% even in the absence of ischemic signs or symptoms. Clinical restenosis typically leads to repeat target lesion revascularization (TLR), either through PCI or coronary artery bypass surgery.

Pathophysiology

Restenosis occurs as a direct consequence of traumatic local expansion and injury to a treated vessel. Acute elastic recoil and negative vessel remodeling, while initially common in the era of balloon angioplasty, have been practically eliminated with stenting. Instead, restenosis is now mostly a result of neointimal hyperplasia, a complex biological response to stenting involving the activation, proliferation, and migration of smooth muscle cells into the endovascular lumen as well as increased production and deposition of extracellular matrix (Fig. 6.9).

The vascular response to stenting stems from the initial insult to the endothelial cell layer and internal elastic lamina, which stimulates the release of thrombogenic and vasoactive cytokines from injured cells and tissue. Within the first few days after injury, this results in apoptosis of the smooth muscle cells in the vascular media, macrophage activation, increased leukocyte accumulation, increased platelet

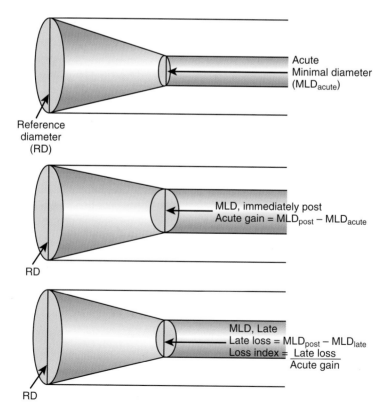

Figure 6.8 Calculations of acute gain, late loss, and loss index.

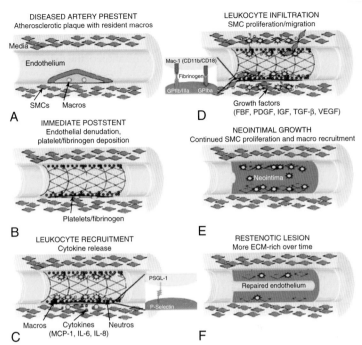

Figure 6.9 Mechanism of restenosis after stent placement. (A) Mature atherosclerotic plaque before intervention. (B) Immediate result of stent placement with endothelial denudation and platelet/fibrinogen deposition. (C, D) Leukocyte recruitment, infiltration, and smooth muscle cell proliferation and migration in the days after injury. (E) Neointimal thickening in the weeks after injury, with continued smooth muscle cell proliferation and monocyte recruitment. (F) Long-term (weeks to months) change from a predominantly cellular to a less cellular and more extracellular matrix–rich plaque. *ECM,* extracellular matrix; *FBF,* fibroblast growth factor; *GP,* glycoprotein; *IGF,* insulin-like growth factor; *IL,* interleukin; *MCP-1,* monocyte chemoattractant protein-1; *PDGF,* platelet-derived growth factor; *PSGL-1,* P-selectin glycoprotein ligand-1; *SMC,* smooth muscle cell; *TGF,* transforming growth factor; *VEGF,* vascular endothelial growth factor. *(From Welt FGP, Rogers C. Arterioscler Thromb Vasc Biol. 2002;22:1769–1776.)*

aggregation, and thrombus formation. Vascular smooth muscle cells then undergo phenotypic modification and activation due to a host of growth factors (including fibroblast growth factor [FBF], platelet-derived growth factor [PDGF], insulin-like growth factor [IGF], transforming growth factor [TGF]-β, vascular endothelial growth factor [VEGF]) from this inflammatory response. Over the next few months, neointimal tissue accumulates as a result of smooth muscle cell proliferation and migration along with increased extracellular matrix production, leading eventually to obstruction of the vessel lumen and restenosis.

Time Course

Very early restenosis (restenosis occurring <24 hours after PCI in the absence of stent thrombosis) can occur as a result of acute elastic recoil or plaque prolapse through stent struts. It is quite rare to observe this phenomenon, which was far more often seen following balloon angioplasty without stenting. Early restenosis (occurring <3 months after PCI) is not common but is associated with more aggressive subsequent restenosis. In general, the incidence of restenosis after stenting then rises gradually, peaking approximately 5 months after PCI with BMS and between 8 and 13 months with DES (depending on the specific DES system). This discrepancy is thought to be related to the effect of the antiproliferative drug eluted by the DES on slowing the natural injury response to stenting, with perhaps a contribution from a hypersensitivity reaction to the polymer coating (especially of the first-generation DES). Late restenosis due to neointimal hyperplasia is fairly uncommon because continued organization of the extracellular matrix typically results in a small increase in luminal area. However, late restenosis has occurred years after both BMS and DES, with more recent studies implicating neoatherosclerosis (new development of lipid-laden plaque with potential for plaque rupture) as a possible cause of restenosis years after stenting. In cases of Neoatherosclerosis leading to late restenosis, the clinical presentation can often mimic de novo acute coronary syndromes, and the angiographic findings within the stent can be indistinguishable from late stent thrombosis.

Risk Factors

There are multiple biological, device, and procedural factors that can contribute to restenosis after stent implantation. Genetic mutations in the genes encoding mTOR may result in resistance to rapamycin and its analogues, while mutations in the genes involved in paclitaxel metabolism may affect biological response to paclitaxel. Some studies have found an association between nickel (found in stainless steel and to a lesser extent cobalt-chromium and platinum-chromium) allergy and restenosis. The polymers used in the first-generation DES have been implicated in hypersensitivity reactions potentially resulting in restenosis, particularly eosinophilic reactions to paclitaxel-eluting stents and granulomatous reactions to sirolimus-eluting stents.

Procedural and device factors associated with restenosis include stent underexpansion, edge dissections, geographic miss, stent fracture, stent gap, and nonuniform drug distribution in DES. Stent expansion can be best evaluated by IVUS or OCT, with an MLA of greater than 90% of the reference lumen area indicative of excellent expansion. Of note, stent malapposition (in which space is seen between the stent struts and the vessel wall on IVUS or OCT) in conjunction with stent underexpansion is potentially associated with stent thrombosis rather than restenosis. Failure to cover areas that have been subjected to balloon barotrauma (at the margins of the deployed stent), including gaps between stents, has been shown to be associated with increased restenosis. In the case of DES, gaps in coverage can result in decreased level of drug elution at the gap site, potentially increasing the risk of restenosis. Stent fracture, defined as the complete or partial separation of stent struts after PCI, is thought to occur in 1–8% of cases. This results in decreased drug availability and lower radial strength at the site of fracture, predisposing the site to restenosis.

Certain patient and lesion subtypes are also known to be associated with an increased risk of restenosis. Diabetes mellitus (especially if insulin-dependent) has been shown to increase the risk of restenosis between 30% and 50% after BMS implantation, although the risk is smaller after DES. Patients with end-stage renal disease have restenosis rates reported as high as 50%. Cardiac allograft vasculopathy after orthotopic heart transplantation is a rapidly progressive form of atherosclerosis sometimes treated by stent implantation, but studies have found greater rates of restenosis and worse clinical outcomes compared to PCI of native coronary arteries. Lesion characteristics associated with increased risk of restenosis include a small reference vessel diameter and a long lesion length. Other lesion subtypes at higher risk of restenosis are ostial lesions, calcified lesions, true bifurcation lesions requiring stents in the main and side branches, chronic total occlusions, and saphenous vein graft lesions.

Management

Management of in-stent restenosis is predicated on an understanding of the underlying etiology of the specific restenotic lesion. Intravascular imaging with IVUS or OCT provides valuable anatomic information by depicting the layers of the coronary vessel, the vessel lumen, and the stent itself. This may provide information as to whether the restenosis resulted from underexpansion of the stent for the vessel size, excessive neointimal hyperplasia, geographic miss, strut fracture, a combination of these mechanisms, or another cause. Based on the etiology, various treatment options can then be weighed to reduce the potential for recurrent restenosis.

The pattern of restenosis can either be focal or diffuse, with several subtypes seen within each category depending on the location of the restenosis in relation to the stent body and margins. If the restenosis is secondary to an underexpanded area of stent limited to a focal area, treatment with balloon angioplasty alone may be sufficient. However, if there is diffuse in-stent restenosis due to excessive neointimal hyperplasia, other treatment modalities including restenting are frequently necessary.

During the BMS era, various treatments for in-stent restenosis including restenting with BMS, cutting balloon, excimer laser angioplasty, and directional or rotational atherectomy were studied and found to be no better than balloon angioplasty alone. Multiple studies did show that vascular brachytherapy with either beta or gamma radiation was effective in reducing recurrent restenosis at the 1-year time point (compared to balloon angioplasty) but resulted in high rates of late stent thrombosis and restenosis likely due to delayed healing and re-endothelialization.

The advent of DES led to a significant change in the management of in-stent BMS restenosis. Trials conducted with first-generation DES platforms demonstrated the superiority of these devices over vascular brachytherapy. In the randomized ISAR-DESIRE trial, treatment with either sirolimus-eluting stents (SES) or paclitaxel-eluting stents (PES) was found to significantly decrease BMS restenosis at 6-month follow-up (14.3% for SES, 21.7% for PES, vs. 44.6% for balloon angioplasty alone). Based on the results of this and other trials, DES is now the standard of care for the treatment of BMS restenosis. However, the optimal treatment for DES restenosis is somewhat less well defined. Contemporary treatment involves restenting with a second DES, typically with a sirolimus-analogue-eluting second-generation system. Depending on the underlying mechanism of restenosis, other treatment options may include conventional, cutting, or scoring balloon angioplasty; vascular brachytherapy; or bypass surgery. An emerging alternative treatment strategy involves the use of drug-eluting balloons (not currently approved for coronary use in the United States). Initial trials utilizing a paclitaxel-eluting balloon demonstrated a decrease in late loss, angiographic restenosis, and 12-month major adverse cardiac events when compared to uncoated balloons. The larger ($N = 402$) ISAR-DESIRE 3 trial found a paclitaxel-eluting balloon to be superior to standard balloon angioplasty in terms of diameter stenosis at 6- to 8-month follow-up angiography, and noninferior to the Taxus Liberte paclitaxel-eluting stent when treating DES restenosis. Further studies are necessary to characterize and understand the mechanism of restenosis after DES implantation (especially of the second-generation and newer systems) and to develop optimal treatment strategies tailored to these mechanisms.

Stent Thrombosis

Stent thrombosis, although rare (occurring in <1% patients within the first year), is one of the most serious complications following stent placement. More than 80% of patients who experience stent thrombosis present with acute MI, and 30-day mortality rates in patients with stent thrombosis range from 10% to 25%. As a result, prevention and treatment of this complication are of utmost importance.

Definitions

The most widely used definition involving the classification and timing of stent thrombosis was developed by the Academic Research Consortium (Table 6.1). *Definite* stent thrombosis is confirmed by angiographic or autopsy evidence of thrombus in the setting of an acute coronary syndrome, and *probable* stent thrombosis is defined as unexplained death within 30 days after stent implantation or acute MI involving the target vessel territory without angiographic confirmation. *Acute* thrombosis occurs within 24 hours (excluding *intraprocedural* events within the catheterization laboratory), *subacute* between 1 day and 30 days, *early* within 30 days (counting both *acute* and *subacute* events), *late* between 30 days and 1 year, and *very late* after 1 year. The thrombotic occlusion is classified as *primary* if it is directly related to the stent implantation and *secondary* if it occurs at the stent site after a subsequent intervention to the target lesion.

It is noteworthy that the initial studies describing the poor outcomes following stent thrombosis were conducted almost entirely following the examination of subacute stent thrombosis events. More recent data assessing the outcomes of very late stent thrombosis (occurring beyond 1 year) have shown that the mortality of these later events is approximately half of that following an early event, perhaps due to a different pathophysiology (e.g., neoatherosclerotic plaque rupture).

Risk Factors

Stent thrombosis can occur as a result of many reasons, including various patient-related factors, procedural factors, and postprocedural factors (Box 6.1). Patients who present with thrombotic acute coronary syndromes, smokers, and patients with diabetes and/or chronic kidney disease as well as severely depressed left ventricular function are all more prone to stent thrombosis. High residual platelet reactivity after treatment, which can be seen in patients with genetic mutations in the enzyme responsible for converting clopidogrel to its active metabolite, has been associated with stent thrombosis. Lesion factors that increase risk of thrombosis include diffuse disease with long stented segments, small vessels, bifurcation disease, and significant inflow or outflow lesions proximal or distal to the stent.

Procedural factors associated with stent thrombosis include inadequate stent expansion and/or apposition, the stent type used (i.e., BMS or DES), excessive stent overlap, and the presence of edge

Table 6.1

Academic Research Consortium Definitions of Stent Thrombosis	
Classification	
Definite	An acute coronary syndrome with angiographic or autopsy evidence of thrombus or occlusion within or adjacent to a stent
Probable	Unexplained death within 30 days after stent implantation or acute myocardial infarction involving the target-vessel territory without angiographic confirmation.
Possible	Any unexplained death beyond 30 days after the procedure
Timing	
Acute	Within 24 hours (excludes intraprocedural events)
Subacute	1–30 days
Early	Within 30 days
Late	30 days to 1 year
Very late	After 1 year

Box 6.1 Potential Mechanisms of Stent Thrombosis

Patient-related factors relating to increased thrombogenicity:
- Smoking
- Diabetes
- Chronic kidney disease
- Acute coronary syndrome presentation
- Thrombocytosis
- High post-treatment platelet reactivity
- Premature discontinuation or cessation of dual antiplatelet therapy
- Surgical procedures (unrelated to the PCI)

Lesion-based factors relating to rheology/thrombogenicity within stents:
- Diffuse coronary artery disease with long stented segments
- Small vessel disease
- Bifurcation disease
- Thrombus-containing lesions
- Significant inflow or outflow lesions proximal or distal to the stented segment

Stent-related factors:
- Poor stent expansion
- Edge dissections limiting inflow or outflow
- Delayed or absent endothelialization of stent struts
- Hypersensitivity/inflammatory and/or thrombotic reactions to drug-eluting stent polymers
- Strut fractures
- Late malapposition/aneurysm formation
- Development of neoatherosclerosis within stents with new plaque rupture

From Kirtane AJ, Stone GW, *Circulation.* 2011;124(11):1283-7.

dissections limiting inflow or outflow. The thicker struts of earlier generation BMS and DES systems have been associated with increased risk of stent thrombosis, and this may have implications in the thrombosis risk of first-generation bioabsorbable scaffolds. In addition, the polymers used in certain first-generation DES systems may be inherently thrombogenic and/or prone to mechanical deformation after implantation, serving as a nidus for thombus formation. Strut fracture has also been linked to increased thrombosis risk.

Postprocedural risk factors for stent thrombosis include early discontinuation of dual-antiplatelet therapy (although the ideal length of treatment varies by the specific stent system), the delayed re-endothelialization of stent struts seen in DES systems as a result of the antiproliferative agent, and the development of neoatherosclerosis within the stent leading to plaque rupture.

Specific strategies aimed at reducing the occurrence of stent thrombosis are shown in Box 6.2.

Treatment

The treatment of stent thrombosis, especially when presenting as acute MI, is almost always emergent PCI. Options for restoring perfusion include thrombectomy (either aspiration or mechanical) and/or balloon angioplasty, with the administration of more potent pharmacologic agents such as glycoprotein IIb/IIIa inhibitors at the discretion of the operator. Adjunctive imaging with modalities such as IVUS or OCT can be very helpful in discerning the underlying etiology of the thrombosis (e.g., stent underexpansion/malapposition or residual dissection) and is recommended prior to further balloon manipulation of the stented site. Additional stents are typically avoided unless a mechanical reason for the thrombosis (such as edge dissection) is seen. Evaluation for nonmechanical causes of thrombosis such as hypercoagulable state, thrombocytosis, or aspirin/clopidogrel resistance should be considered. Finally, escalation of maintenance antiplatelet therapy (e.g., from

---

Box 6.2 Strategies to Minimize the Occurrence of Stent Thrombosis

Patient selection:
- Screening for likely adherence to prescribed medical regimens (including ability to afford dual antiplatelet therapy)
- Careful screening for bleeding risk (or ability to tolerate dual antiplatelet therapy)
- Confirmation of no upcoming surgical procedures in the recent future (6 weeks for BMS, 6–12 months for DES)

Stent selection and deployment:
- Consider use of stents with proven lower stent thrombosis rates
- Appropriate vessel sizing
- High-pressure stent deployment and postdilation
- Ensuring absence of edge dissections
- Ensuring adequate inflow and outflow
- Avoiding the use of two stents in bifurcation lesions (if possible)

Peri- and postprocedure care:
- Use of more potent oral antiplatelet regimens (e.g., prasugrel, ticagrelor) in appropriately indicated clinical scenarios such as acute coronary syndromes in patients with acceptable bleeding risk
- Patient education and clinical follow-up emphasizing the importance of adherence to prescribed dual antiplatelet therapy
- Continuation of dual antiplatelet therapy without interruption whenever possible if a dental, endoscopic, or surgical procedure is necessary (which is feasible for most surgeries other than neurovascular)

From Kirtane AJ, Stone GW, *Circulation*. 2011;124(11):1283-7.

---

clopidogrel to more potent oral antiplatelet therapies such as prasugrel or ticagrelor) is standard.

Suggested Reading

Cook S, Lenawee P, Togni M, et al. Incomplete stent apposition and very late stent thrombosis after drug-eluting stent implantation. *Circulation*. 2007;115:2426-2434.

Dangas G, Claessen BE, Caixeta A, et al. In-stent restenosis in the drug-eluting stent era. *J Am Coll Cardiol*. 2010;56:1897-1907.

Ellis SG, Kereiakes DJ, Metzger C, et al. Everolimus-eluting bioresorbable scaffolds for coronary artery disease. *N Engl J Med*. 2015;373:1905-1915.

Gupta A, Mancini D, Kirtane AJ, et al. Value of drug-eluting stents in cardiac transplant recipients. *Am J Cardiol*. 2009;103(5):659-662.

Fischman DL, Leon MB, Balm DS, et al. A randomized comparison of coronary-stent placement and balloon angioplasty in the treatment of coronary artery disease. Stent Restenosis Study Investigators. *N Engl J Med*. 1994;331:496-501.

Garasic JM, Edelman ER, Squire JC, et al. Stent and artery geometry determine intimal thickening independent of arterial injury. *Circulation*. 2000;101:812-818.

Holmes DR Jr, Kereiakes D, Garg S, et al. Stent thrombosis. *J Am Coll Cardiol*. 2010;56:1357-1365.

Kandzari D, Leon M, Popma J, et al. Comparison of zotarolimus-eluting and sirolimus-eluting stents in patients with native coronary artery disease: a randomized controlled trial. *JACC Cardiovasc Interv*. 2006;48(12):2440-2447.

Kereiakes DJ, Meredith IT, Windecker S, et al. Efficacy and safety of a novel bioabsorbable polymer-coated, everolimus-eluting coronary stent: the EVOLVE II Randomized Trial. *Circ Cardiovasc Interv*. 2015;8:e002372.

Kirtane AJ, Gupta A, Iyengar S, et al. Safety and efficacy of drug-eluting and bare metal stents: comprehensive meta-analysis of randomized trials and observational studies. *Circulation*. 2009;119:3198-3206.

Kirtane AJ, Stone GW. How to minimize stent thrombosis. *Circulation*. 2011;124:1283-1287.

Kolandaivelu K, Swaminathan R, Gibson WJ, et al. Stent thrombogenicity early in high-risk interventional settings is driven by stent design and deployment and protected by polymer-drug coatings. *Circulation*. 2011;123:1400-1409.

Lee MS, Kobashigawa J, Tobis J. Comparison of percutaneous coronary intervention with bare-metal and drug-eluting stents for cardiac allograft vasculopathy. *JACC Cardiovasc Interv*. 2008;1:710-715.

Leon MB, Nikolsky E, Cutlip DE, et al. Improved late clinical safety with zotarolimus-eluting stents compared with paclitaxel eluting stents in patients with de novo coronary lesions: 3-year follow-up from the ENDEAVOR IV (Randomized Comparison of Zotarolimus- and Paclitaxel-Eluting Stents in Patients With Coronary Artery Disease) trial. *JACC Cardiovasc Interv*. 2010;3:1043-1050.

Leon MB, Teirstein PS, Moses JW, et al. Localized intracoronary gamma-radiation therapy to inhibit the recurrence of restenosis after stenting. *N Engl J Med.* 2001;344:250-256.

Morice MC, Serruys PW, Sousa JE, et al. A randomized comparison of a sirolimus-eluting stent with a standard stent for coronary revascularization. *N Engl J Med.* 2002;346: 1773-1780.

Mehran R, Dangas G, Abizaid AS, et al. Angiographic patterns of in-stent restenosis: classification and implications for long-term outcome. *Circulation.* 1999;100:1872-1878.

Moses JW, Leon MB, Popma JJ, et al. Sirolimus-eluting stents versus standard stents in patients with stenosis in a native coronary artery. *N Engl J Med.* 2003;349:1315-1323.

Price MJ, ed. *Coronary Stenting.* 1st ed. Philadelphia: Elsevier Saunders; 2014.

Serruys PW, de Jaegere P, Kiemeneij F, et al. A comparison of balloon-expandable-stent implantation with balloon angioplasty in patients with coronary artery disease. Benestent Study Group. *N Engl J Med.* 1994;331:489-495.

Serruys PW, Silber S, Garg S, et al. Comparison of zotarolimus-eluting and everolimus-eluting coronary stents. *N Engl J Med.* 2010;363:136-146.

Silber S, Windecker S, Vranckx P, et al. Unrestricted randomised use of two new generation drug-eluting coronary stents: 2-year patient-related versus stent-related outcomes from the RESOLUTE All Comers trial. *Lancet.* 2011;377:1241-1247.

Stone GW, Ellis SG, Cox DA. A polymer-based, paclitaxel-eluting stent in patients with coronary artery disease. *N Engl J Med.* 2004;350:221-231.

Stone GW, Miei M, Newman W, et al. Comparison of an everolimus-eluting stent and a paclitaxel-eluting stent in patients with coronary artery disease: a randomized trial. *JAMA.* 2008;299:1903-1913.

Stone GW, Teirstein PS, Meredith IT, et al. A prospective, randomized evaluation of a novel everolimus-eluting coronary stent: the PLATINUM (a Prospective, Randomized, Multicenter Trial to Assess an Everolimus-Eluting Coronary Stent System [PROMUS Element] for the Treatment of Up to Two de Novo Coronary Artery Lesions) trial. *J Am Coll Cardiol.* 2011;57:1700-1708.

Topol E, ed. *Textbook of Interventional Cardiology.* 6th ed. Philadelphia: Elsevier Saunders; 2012.

Urban P, Meredith IT, Abizaid A, et al. Polymer-free drug-coated coronary stents in patients at high bleeding risk. *N Engl J Med.* 2015;373:2038-2047.

Welt FG, Rogers C. Inflammation and restenosis in the stent era. *Arterioscler Thromb Vasc Biol.* 2002;22:1769-1776.

Windecker S, Serruys PW, Wandel S, et al. Biolimus-eluting stent with biodegradable polymer versus sirolimus-eluting stent with durable polymer for coronary revascularisation (LEADERS): a randomised non-inferiority trial. *Lancet.* 2008;372:1163-1173.

7

Treatment of Coronary Bifurcations

EMMANOUIL S. BRILAKIS ·
YVES LOUVARD · PHILIPPE GENEREUX ·
SUBHASH BANERJEE

Definition and Classification

The European Bifurcation Club (EBC) has defined bifurcation lesions as lesions occurring at, or adjacent to, a significant division of a major epicardial coronary artery. What is "significant" remains subjective and is determined by the treating physician as branches that, if compromised during percutaneous coronary intervention (PCI), can cause symptoms or periprocedural myocardial infarction.

There are multiple classifications of bifurcation lesions, but one of the simplest and most commonly used currently is the Medina classification (Fig. 7.1) that records any narrowing of 50% or more in each of the three arterial segments of the bifurcation in the following order: proximal main vessel (MV), distal main vessel, and proximal side branch (SB). The presence of significant stenosis is marked as "1" and the absence as "0." A limitation of the Medina classification is that it does not account for angulation that can affect the technical difficulty of the procedure.

Basics of Bifurcation Lesion PCI

The PCI of bifurcation lesions can result in both acute (such as SB occlusion and periprocedural myocardial infarction) and long-term (such as restenosis and/or stent thrombosis) complications. Several strategies for bifurcation PCI have been developed and are summarized in the Main, Across, Distal, Side (MADS) classification based on the manner in which the first stent has been implanted (Fig. 7.2).

Using large (such as 7F or 8F) guide catheters may facilitate bifurcation PCI because these allow more treatment options, especially for two-stent strategies or if a complication occurs. However, 6F guides (with or without radial access) are adequate for most bifurcations and are used by most operators. Wiring both the MV and SB should be

Disclosures

Dr. Brilakis is a consultant and speaker receiving honoraria from Abbott Vascular, Asahi, Cardinal Health, Elsevier, GE Healthcare, and St. Jude Medical; has research support from InfraRedx and Boston Scientific; and his spouse is an employee of Medtronic. Dr. Louvard receives honoraria for workshop participation from Terumo, Abbott, and Medtronic. Dr. Genereux receives speaker fees from Abbott Vascular and CSI and is a consultant for CSI. Dr. Banerjee receives research grants from Gilead and the Medicines Company, is a consultant and receives speaker honoraria from Covidien and Medtronic; has ownership in MDCARE Global through his spouse; and has intellectual property in HygeiaTel.

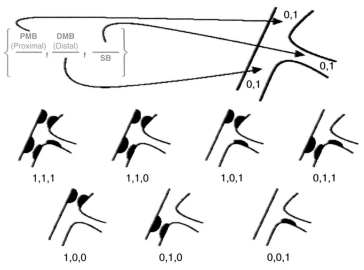

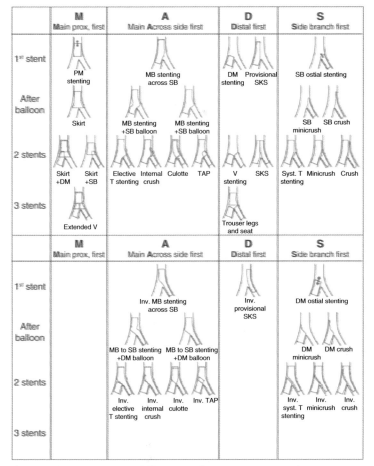

Figure 7.1 The Medina classification of bifurcation lesions. The first number describes the proximal main vessel, the second number the distal main vessel, and the third number the side branch. Each segment is described as "1" if the segment has a diameter stenosis of ≥50% by visual estimation; otherwise, it is described as "0."

Figure 7.2 The MADS classification of bifurcation lesion stenting. (*Reprinted from Lassen JF, Holm NR, Stankovic G, et al. Percutaneous coronary intervention for coronary bifurcation disease: consensus from the first 10 years of the European Bifurcation Club meetings. EuroIntervention 2014;10:545–560, with permission from Europa Digital & Publishing.*)

done for all bifurcations with important SBs, ideally with different wire types. The most challenging branch to wire should be wired first, and the wires should be kept in the same position on the table as on the working projection to prevent twisting. Drug-eluting stents (DES) significantly reduce the risk for in-stent restenosis and are preferred for bifurcation lesions. The minimum number of stents should be used, and imaging should be strongly considered to optimize stent expansion and stent strut apposition. Several dedicated bifurcation systems have been developed, but none has been approved for use in the United States and are used infrequently in Europe.

A practical approach for selecting a treatment strategy for bifurcation lesion PCI follows.

Algorithmic Approach to Bifurcation PCI

Determine Whether a Side Branch Needs to Be Preserved

Small side branches supplying a small amount of myocardium that are unlikely to cause symptoms if they be become occluded or highly stenotic do not require any specific treatment (see Fig. 7.3). Hence, such lesions are approached with main vessel stenting without attempts to maintain the side branch patency.

Determine the Likelihood of Side Branch Occlusion During Bifurcation PCI

The likelihood of SB occlusion is estimated based on vessel size, angulation, and proximal disease. A study of 1601 consecutive bifurcation PCIs demonstrated SB occlusion in 7.37%. SB occlusion was associated with the following six parameters:

1. Plaque distribution at the same side as the SB
2. Lower MV thrombolysis in myocardial infarction (TIMI) flow grade before stenting

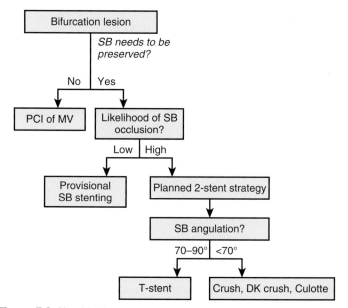

Figure 7.3 Algorithmic approach to bifurcation percutaneous coronary intervention.

3. Higher preprocedure diameter stenosis of the bifurcation core

4. Higher bifurcation angle

5. Higher diameter ratio between MV/SB

6. Higher diameter stenosis of SB before MV stenting

Important SBs at high risk for compromise are best treated with an upfront two-stent strategy.

Significant Side Branch at Low Risk for Occlusion

The preferred strategy for such lesions is *provisional SB stenting*: both branches are wired and the MV is stented first, followed by stenting of the SB only if the SB develops a severe stenosis or its flow is compromised (Figs. 7.4 and 7.5). Predilation of the MV is usually performed to ensure subsequent expansion of the stent, whereas predilation of the SB is not needed for most cases unless there is significant ostial SB disease or reduced flow after wiring. DES are preferred, sized to the diameter of the distal vessel, but allowing expansion to the reference diameter of the proximal MV. According to the Finet's formula, the diameter of the proximal main vessel is equal to (distal main vessel diameter + SB diameter) $\times$ 0.678. Hence, the chosen stent has to accommodate two diameters: the one of the distal main vessel (no oversizing to avoid carina shift and compromise of the SB) and the one of the proximal segment (to prevent stent underexpansion and malapposition). Expansion of the proximal MV portion of the stent is achieved using the Proximal Optimization Technique (POT) (Fig. 7.4A–C) (i.e., inflation with a short balloon adequately sized for the proximal MV (based on Finet's formula). POT facilitates rewiring of the SB (if needed), thus minimizing the risk of outside wire crossing and facilitating equipment advancement through the proximal portion of the MV stent.

Several studies have shown improved outcomes with provisional SB stenting as compared with a routine two-stent strategy. These studies nonetheless have been criticized for including non-true bifurcation lesions, stenting small SBs, and not performing a two-step final kiss. In general, two-stent techniques are easier to perform when the SB is stented first, but a provisional SB technique may obviate the need for SB stenting in the majority of treated bifurcations.

Routine SB ballooning after main vessel stenting is generally *not* recommended except when the SB ostium is compromised by significant diameter stenosis, dissection, and/or reduced flow. Kissing balloon can cause SB dissection requiring SB stenting and should be done with noncompliant short balloons to push back the carina in its flow divider position. Fractional flow reserve of jailed SBs can be useful because many lesions that appear severe by angiography may not be hemodynamically significant (FFR was <0.75 in only 27% of 73 jailed SBs with ≥75% angiographic stenosis) and may not require stenting. However, advancing the pressure wire through the jailed SB can be challenging.

Rewiring a jailed SB can be challenging (although POT can significantly facilitate rewiring) and should be performed through a distal stent strut because wiring through a proximal stent strut can result in suboptimal SB ostium coverage and metal overhang into the main vessel. As discussed earlier, the POT technique should be performed prior to rewiring attempts if there is a mismatch between the proximal and distal main vessel diameter. Rewiring through a jailed side branch may be facilitated by (Fig. 7.6):

- Having a jailed wire in the side branch that marks the SB origin and changes the access angle
- Use of polymer-jacketed guidewires
- Use of a microcatheter, especially angled microcatheter such as the Supercross and the Venture (Vascular Solutions, Minneapolis, MN) (Fig. 7.5D) or through a dual-lumen microcatheter,

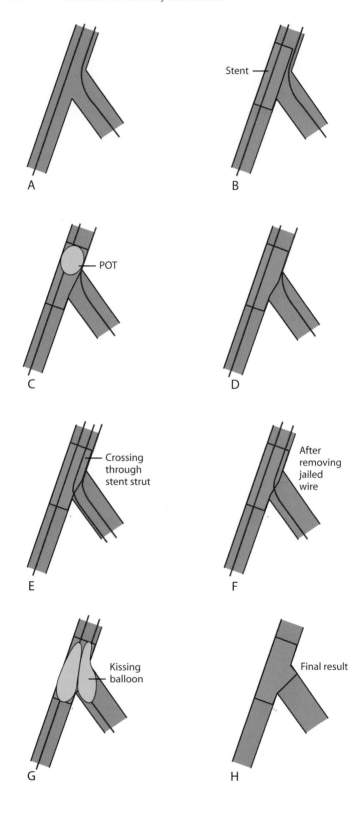

Figure 7.4 Illustration of provisional side branch stenting. (1) The MV and SB are both wired (panel A). (2) Consider predilation of the SB (if it has significant disease: most times predilation is not needed because it may cause dissection that can lead to implantation of an SB stent). (3) The MV is stented with a stent sized for the distal MV reference diameter (see panel B). (4) Consider using the proximal optimization technique (POT) (panel C) if the proximal MV reference diameter is significantly larger than the distal MV reference diameter or if rewiring of the SB appears to be necessary. (5) Rewire the SB (using the jailed guidewire as a marker of the vessel course; panel D) if the SB becomes compromised after MV stenting. Rewiring should be performed through a distal stent strut (panel E). (6) After rewiring, the jailed guidewire is removed (panel F), followed by kissing balloon inflation (panel G) that optimizes SB ostium coverage with a stent. (7) A SB stent may or may not be required, depending on the result of balloon inflation.

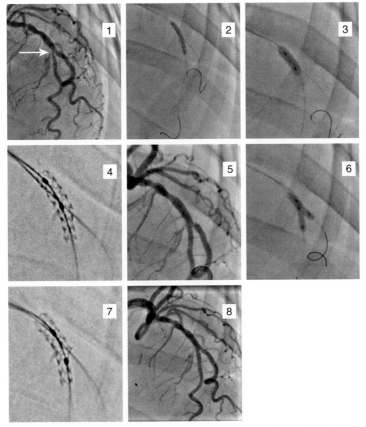

Figure 7.5 Illustrative case of bifurcation stenting using the provisional side branch stenting technique. A bifurcation of the left anterior descending artery and the diagonal branch (panel 1) was treated with crossover stenting after wiring both branches (panel 2). After proximal optimization technique (panel 3), the side branch (diagonal) was rewired (panel 4) and given a proximal side branch lesion (panel 5), kissing balloon inflation was performed (panel 6) with an excellent final result (panel 7 and 8). *(Courtesy of Dr. Yves Louvard.)*

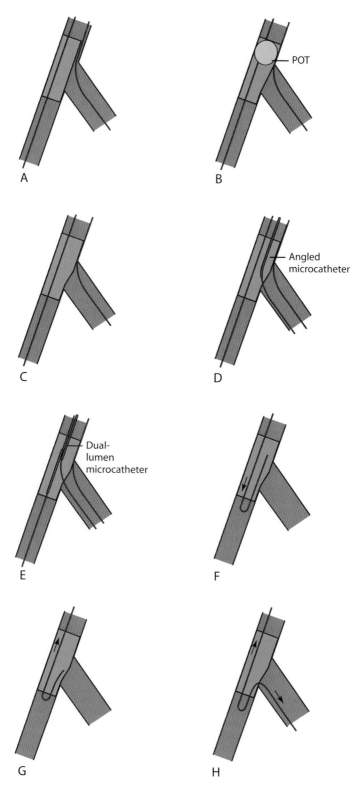

Figure 7.6 How to rewire a jailed side branch. (1) Before rewiring, the proximal optimization technique (POT) is performed if the proximal main vessel is larger than the distal main vessel to optimize proximal stent strut apposition and prevent substent guidewire advancement (panels A–C). (2) An angled microcatheter (panel D), a dual-lumen microcatheter (panel E), or a knuckled guidewire (panels F–H) can be used to prevent inadvertent substent guidewire entry. Alternatively, the SB could be rewired by withdrawing the main vessel guidewire.

such as the Twin-Pass (Vascular Solutions) (Figs. 7.6E and 7.16) that can prevent crossing through proximal stent struts
- Use of a hairpin wire or reversed guidewire technique (Fig. 7.6F–H)

If the SB cannot be rewired after stenting and flow is compromised, a small balloon can be advanced over the jailed guidewire to restore flow into the SB prior to continued rewiring attempts.

After SB rewiring, balloon advancement through the stent struts can be challenging and can be facilitated by:
- Use of a small balloon (1.20–1.50 mm)
- Use of the Threader (Boston Scientific, Natick, MA) or the Glider (Trireme Medical, Pleasanton, CA) balloon, or a microcatheter

If everything else fails, rewiring with another wire through another strut can be attempted.

If SB stenting is needed in provisional SB technique after MV stenting, the following techniques can be used depending on SB angulation (Fig. 7.7):
- Nearly 90 degrees: Use T- stenting; an SB stent is deployed without protrusion in the MV stent (Fig. 7.8).

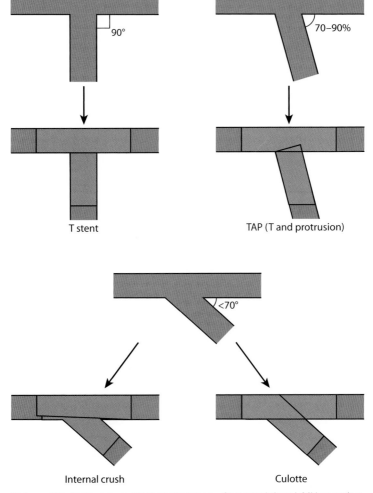

Figure 7.7 Bailout two-stent techniques after provisional MV stenting. Technique selection depends on SB angulation.

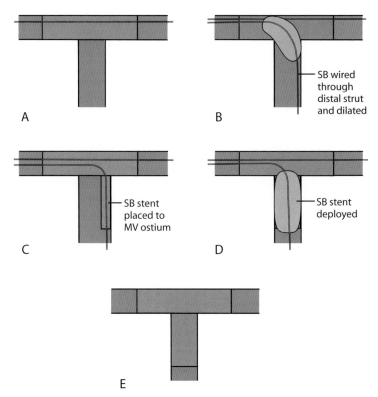

Figure 7.8 Bailout T-stent technique after MV stenting. (1) In the T-stent technique, after stenting the main vessel and performing the proximal optimization technique (POT) (panel A), the SB is rewired through a distal stent strut (panel B). (2) A stent is placed in the SB up to the MV ostium (panel C). (3) The SB stent is deployed (panel D). (4) In the end, both MV and SB are stented (panel E).

- 70–90 degrees: Use the T and protrusion (TAP) technique (Fig. 7.9); the SB stent is deployed with minimal protrusion while an uninflated balloon is kept in the MV, followed by slight withdrawal of the SB balloon and kissing balloon inflation (without rewiring the SB).

- Less than 70 degrees: Use an internal mini crush or a culotte. In an internal mini crush (Fig. 7.10), the SB is deployed with more protrusion in the MV stent, followed by rewiring of the SB stent, high-pressure balloon inflation, and final kiss balloon inflation. In a culotte (Fig. 7.11), the SB stent is deployed into the MV stent, followed by rewiring of the MV stent, high-pressure balloon inflation into the MV, and final kissing balloon inflation. The culotte technique may be preferred when the MV diameter is similar to the SB diameter, but both techniques require rewiring and final kissing balloon inflation.

Significant Side Branch at High Risk for Occlusion

Such bifurcation lesions are best treated with an upfront two-stent strategy (MV and SB). Lesion preparation (with balloon angioplasty and/or cutting balloon inflation or atherectomy) is important for both MV and SB prior to stenting to facilitate stent delivery and expansion. The most commonly used two-stent strategies are the T-stent and TAP

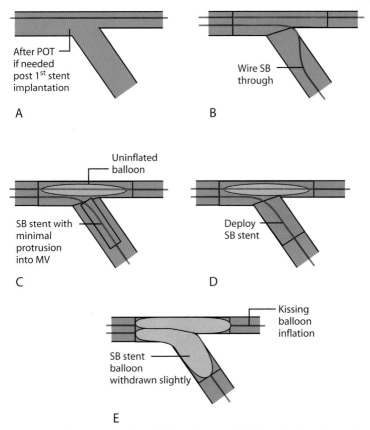

Figure 7.9 T and protrusion (TAP) technique. (1) After stenting the main vessel and performing the proximal optimization technique (POT) (panel A), the SB is rewired through a distal stent strut (panel B). (2) A stent is placed in the SB with minimal protrusion in the MV with an uninflated balloon placed in the MV (panel C). (3) The SB stent is deployed (panel D). (4) The SB stent balloon is slightly withdrawn into the MV, and kissing balloon inflation is performed (panel E).

technique (for 70- to 90-degree angulation) and the crush or culotte (for <70-degree angulation):

- Nearly 70–90 degrees: Use T-stenting; a SB stent is deployed without protrusion in the MV stent (Fig. 7.12).
- Less than 70 degrees: Use a crush, double-kiss (DK) crush, or culotte. Crush is preferred when the SB is of smaller size, whereas either crush or culotte are good options when both branches are of nearly equal size.
- Crush is performed as illustrated in Fig. 7.13. The optimal location for SB recrossing is controversial: distal recrossing carries the risk of abluminal rewiring leaving part of the SB uncovered by stent. The EBC recommends recrossing in a middle to distal position. Mini-crush (that involves limited protrusion of the SB stent in the MV) is preferred to minimize the area of the three-stent layer in the MV. Also a two-step kissing technique (high-pressure inflation of the SB stent after crushing and rewiring, followed by kissing balloon inflation) is preferred over standard kissing balloon to minimize the residual stenosis of the SB ostium.
- DK crush (Figs. 7.14 and 7.15) is currently the preferred crush bifurcation technique and involves kissing balloon inflation
Text continued on p. 216

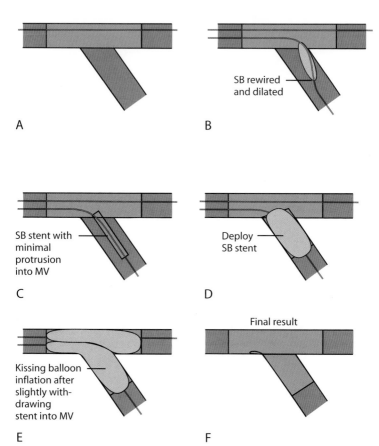

A

B
SB rewired
and dilated

C
SB stent with
minimal
protrusion
into MV

D
Deploy
SB stent

E
Kissing balloon
inflation after
slightly with-
drawing
stent into MV

F
Final result

Figure 7.10 Internal crush technique after MV stenting. (1) After stenting the main vessel and performing the proximal optimization technique (POT) (panel A), the SB is rewired through a distal stent strut and dilated (panel B). (2) A stent is placed in the SB extending into the MV (panel C). (3) The SB stent is deployed (panel D). (4) After withdrawing the SB stent into the MV, kissing balloon inflation is performed (panel E). (5) Final result is achieved (panel F).

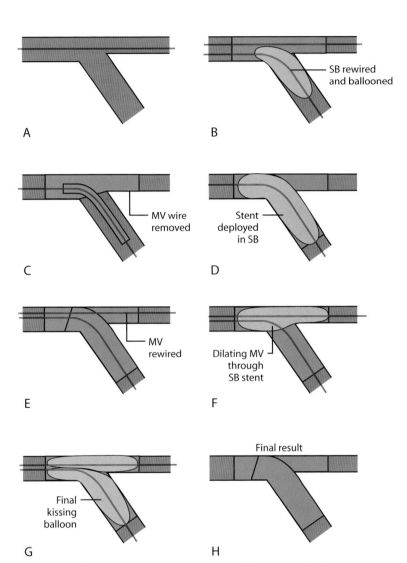

Figure 7.11 Bailout culotte technique after MV stenting. (1) After stenting, the main vessel and performing the proximal optimization technique (POT) (panel A), the SB is rewired through a distal stent strut (panel B). (2) A stent is placed in the SB extending into the MV, and the MV wire is removed (panel C). (3) The SB stent is deployed (panel D). (4) The MV is rewired through the SB stent (panel E). (5) The MV is dilated through the SB stent (panel F). (6) Final kissing balloon inflation is performed (panel G). (7) Final result is achieved (panel H).

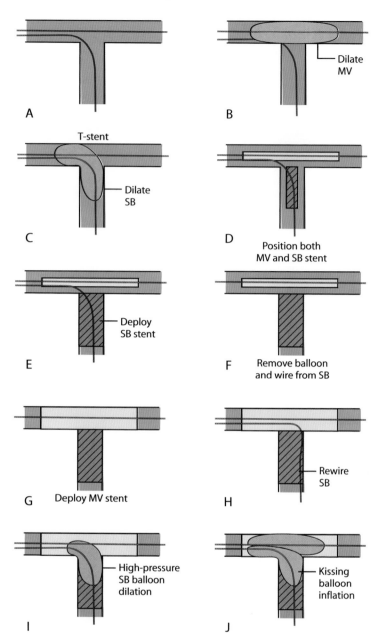

Figure 7.12 T-stenting technique. (1) Both the MV and SB are wired (panel A). (2) Both the MV and the SB are predilated (panels B and C). (3) The MV and SB stents are positioned with the SB stent positioned at the SB ostium (panel D). (4) The SB stent is deployed (panel E). (5) The balloon and wire are removed from the SB (panel F). (6) The MV stent is deployed (panel G), and proximal optimization is performed if the size of the proximal MV is larger than the distal MV. (7) The SB is rewired through a distal stent strut (panel H). (8) High-pressure SB dilation is performed (panel I). (9) Kissing balloon inflation is performed (panel J).

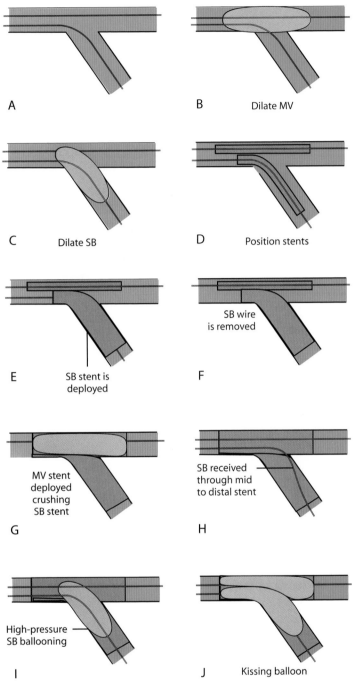

Figure 7.13 Crush technique. (1) Both the MV and SB are wired (panel A). (2) Both the MV and SB are dilated (panel B and C). (3) Both MV and SB are positioned with the SB stent protruding into the MV (for about one-third of its length in the classic crush or adjacent to the proximal end of the SB in the mini-crush technique) (panel D). (4) The SB stent is deployed (panel E). (5) The SB guidewire is removed (panel F). (6) The MV stent is deployed, crushing the portion of the SB stent lying in the MV (panel G), and proximal optimization is performed if the size of the proximal MV is larger than the distal MV. (7) The SB stent is rewired (panel H). (8) High-pressure SB balloon inflation is performed (panel I). (9) Final kissing balloon inflation is performed (panel J).

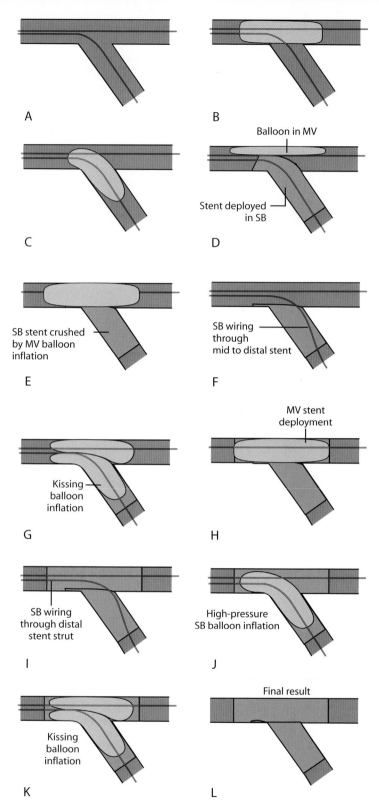

Figure 7.14 The double kiss crush (DK Crush) technique. (1) Both the MV and SB are wired (panel A). (2) Both the MV and SB are dilated (panel B and C). (3) Both MV and SB are positioned with the SB stent protruding into the MV (about 1–2 mm) (panel D). (4) After removing the SB guidewire, the MV balloon is inflated, crushing the SB stent (panel E). (5) The SB is rewired through a proximal stent strut (panel F). (6) Kissing balloon inflation is performed (first kiss) (panel G). (7) After removal of the SB guidewire, the MV stent is deployed (panel H). (8) The SB is rewired through a distal strut (panel I). (9) High-pressure SB balloon inflation is performed (panel J). (10) Kissing balloon inflation is performed (second kiss) (panel K). (11) After use of the proximal optimization technique (POT) technique, the final result is achieved (panel L).

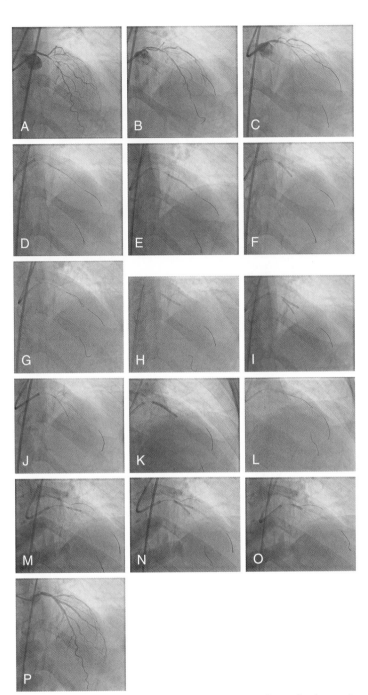

Figure 7.15 Illustration of the DK-crush technique. (1) Left anterior descending (LAD) artery and first diagonal bifurcation lesion (panel A). Both the main branch (LAD) and side branch (diagonal) are wired and predilated (panel B and C). A stent is placed in the SB (diagonal) protruding about 3 mm in the LAD and a balloon is advanced in the MB adjacent to the SB stent (panel D). The SB stent is deployed (panel E). The stent balloon is removed, followed by crushing of the SB stent by inflating the MV balloon (panel F). The SB is rewired, followed by removal of the trapped guidewire (panel G). Two-step kiss is performed by first inflating a noncompliant SB balloon to 20 atm (panel H), followed by kissing balloon inflation at 12 atm (panel I). The MV stent is advanced (panel J) and deployed (panel K). The SB rewired through the MV struts using a TwinPass catheter (panel L) to minimize the risk of wiring under the MV stent struts. Following removal of the trapped SB guidewire, two-step kiss is performed again with high-pressure balloon inflation in the SB (Panel M) followed by kissing balloon inflation at 12 atm (panel N). Proximal optimization is performed (panel O) with a larger (3.0 × 8 mm) short balloon, with an excellent final angiographic result (panel P).

Continued

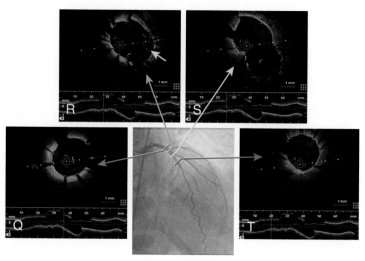

Figure 7.15, cont'd Optical coherence tomography at the end of the procedure demonstrated good stent expansion and stent strut apposition proximal (panel Q) and distal (panel T) to the bifurcation, with excellent scaffolding of the SB ostium (panel S) and a triple layer of stent proximal to the bifurcation (*arrow*, panel R).

twice: after crushing the first stent with a balloon before deploying the second stent, and after deploying the second stent following rewiring of the SB. DK crush can facilitate access to the side vessel, which is a limitation of the standard crush technique.

- Culotte is performed as illustrated in Fig. 7.16. Culotte is preferred when the MV and SB have similar diameters; however, the DK-Crush III trial demonstrated higher rates of restenosis and target vessel revascularization in unprotected left main bifurcation lesions treated with the culotte versus DK crush technique.

There are several other two-stent techniques, such as the simultaneous kissing stent (SKS) technique, in which two stents are positioned in both the MV and SB with their proximal portions being parallel to each other and deployed. Although SKS allows continuous wire access to both MV and SB, it is not currently recommended because it creates a long, new metal carina and, recrossing may be challenging to achieve.

Intravascular Imaging for Bifurcation Stenting

Intravascular imaging (intravascular ultrasounds [IVUS] and optical coherence tomography [OCT]) is highly recommended for bifurcation PCI, both before stenting (to assess lesion composition and the need for pretreatment and to select the optimal stent sizes) and after stenting (to confirm adequate stent expansion, stent-strut apposition, and lack of stent distortion). Minimum stent areas that should be achieved at various locations during left main stenting are shown in Fig. 7.17. Particular attention should be paid to the circumflex ostium that is the most common site of in-stent restenosis during left main stenting.

Imaging of a jailed side branch should be avoided to prevent stent deformation, but imaging of both branches is recommended for two-stent bifurcation PCI techniques.

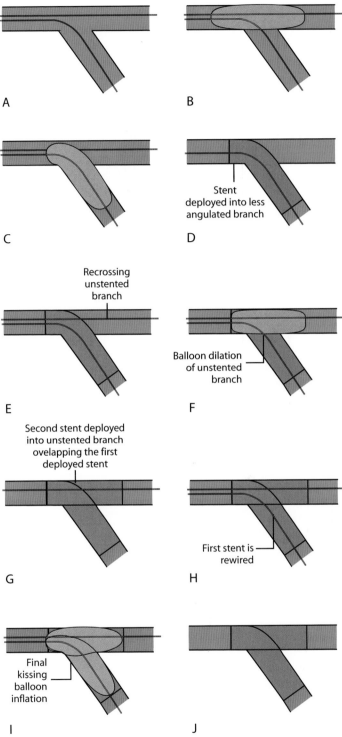

Figure 7.16 The culotte technique. (1) Both the MV and SB are wired (panel A). (2) Both the MV and SB are dilated (panels B and C). (3) After removing the wire from the straighter branch, a stent is deployed into the more angulated branch (panel D). (4) The stent is recrossed with a guidewire into the straighter branch (panel E). (5) The unstented straighter branch is dilated with a balloon (panel F). (6) After removing the guidewire from the already stented branch, a second stent is deployed into the unstented branch overlapping the initially deployed stent (panel G). (7) The first stent is rewired (panel H). (8) Final kissing balloon inflation is performed (panel I). (9) Final result is achieved (Panel J).

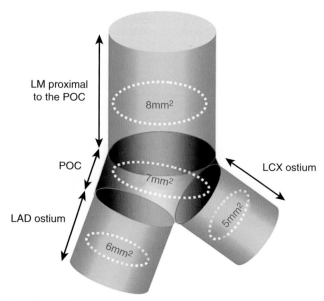

Figure 7.17 Minimum stent areas during left main stenting to minimize the risk for restenosis. LM, left main; POC, point of confluence; LAD, left anterior descending; LCX, left circumflex.

Antiplatelet Therapy After Bifurcation Stenting

Patients undergoing bifurcation stenting may be at increased risk for stent thrombosis. As a result, more intensive (e.g., aspirin + ticagrelor or aspirin + prasugrel) or prolonged (>12 months) dual antiplatelet therapy may be considered after bifurcation stenting, especially for two-stent bifurcation PCI techniques.

SUMMARY

Several treatment techniques are available for treating bifurcation lesions. A provisional SB stenting strategy is preferred for lesions with insignificant SB or SB at low risk for occlusion. For bifurcations requiring an upfront two-stent strategy, the T-stent technique is preferred when the bifurcation angle is 70 degrees or greater and a DK crush or culotte technique when the bifurcation angle is less than 70 degrees. The proximal optimization technique (for all bifurcations) and the two-step kiss technique (for two-stent bifurcation stenting) can help optimize bifurcation stenting results.

Suggested Reading

Chen SL, Xu B, Han YL, et al. Comparison of double kissing crush versus Culotte stenting for unprotected distal left main bifurcation lesions: results from a multicenter, randomized, prospective DKCRUSH-III study. *J Am Coll Cardiol.* 2013;61:1482-1488.

Colombo A, Bramucci E, Sacca S, et al. Randomized study of the crush technique versus provisional side-branch stenting in true coronary bifurcations: the CACTUS (Coronary Bifurcations: Application of the Crushing Technique Using Sirolimus-Eluting Stents) study. *Circulation.* 2009;119:71-78.

Dou K, Zhang D, Xu B, et al. An angiographic tool for risk prediction of side branch occlusion in coronary bifurcation intervention: the RESOLVE score system (Risk prEdiction of Side branch OccLusion in coronary bifurcation interVEntion). *JACC Cardiovasc Interv.* 2015;8:39-46.

Ferenc M, Gick M, Kienzle RP, et al. Randomized trial on routine vs. provisional T-stenting in the treatment of de novo coronary bifurcation lesions. *Eur Heart J.* 2008;29:2859-2867.

Iakovou I, Schmidt T, Bonizzoni E, et al. Incidence, predictors, and outcome of thrombosis after successful implantation of drug-eluting stents. *JAMA*. 2005;293:2126-2130.

Kang SJ, Ahn JM, Song H, et al. Comprehensive intravascular ultrasound assessment of stent area and its impact on restenosis and adverse cardiac events in 403 patients with unprotected left main disease. *Circ Cardiovasc Interv*. 2011;4:562-569.

Koo BK, Kang HJ, Youn TJ, et al. Physiologic assessment of jailed side branch lesions using fractional flow reserve. *J Am Coll Cardiol*. 2005;46:633-637.

Lassen JF, Holm NR, Stankovic G, et al. Percutaneous coronary intervention for coronary bifurcation disease: consensus from the first 10 years of the European Bifurcation Club meetings. *EuroIntervention*. 2014;10:545-560.

Louvard Y, Thomas M, Dzavik V, et al. Classification of coronary artery bifurcation lesions and treatments: time for a consensus! *Catheter Cardiovasc Interv*. 2008;71:175-183.

Medina A, Suarez de Lezo J, Pan M. A new classification of coronary bifurcation lesions]. *Rev Esp Cardiol*. 2006;59:183.

Ormiston JA, Webster MW, Webber B, et al. The "crush" technique for coronary artery bifurcation stenting: insights from micro-computed tomographic imaging of bench deployments. *JACC Cardiovasc Interv*. 2008;1:351-357.

Steigen TK, Maeng M, Wiseth R, et al. Randomized study on simple versus complex stenting of coronary artery bifurcation lesions: the Nordic bifurcation study. *Circulation*. 2006;114:1955-1961.

Watanabe S, Saito N, Bao B, et al. Microcatheter-facilitated reverse wire technique for side branch wiring in bifurcated vessels: an in vitro evaluation. *EuroIntervention*. 2013;9:870-877.

Zhang JJ, Chen SL. Classic crush and DK crush stenting techniques. *EuroIntervention*. 2015;11(suppl V):V102-V105.

8

Percutaneous Coronary Interventions of Chronic Total Occlusions ▶

BARRY F. URETSKY · EMMANOUIL BRILAKIS ·
MAURO CARLINO · STEPHANE RINFRET

Introduction

Percutaneous coronary intervention (PCI) of a chronic total occlusion (CTO), defined as a total occlusion (with thrombolysis in myocardial infarction [TIMI] grade 0 flow) of greater than 3 months' duration, is one of the most technically challenging coronary subsets. "Getting there from here" is a phrase that refers not only to methods of recanalizing the CTO but to the interventionalist's learning the advanced techniques not used in non-CTO lesions in order to maximize success rates and minimize complications. If the interventionist becomes facile with the methods described in this chapter, then the expected success rate at the time of this writing is in the 85%–90% range. This chapter introduces the subject; the interested reader is referred to texts devoted to this subject, such as those cited in the bibliography.

Some lesions have minimal antegrade flow. These lesions, often called *CTOs* or *functional CTOs*, are not truly totally occluded and, by virtue of the small antegrade channel, have a higher probability of being recanalized antegrade.

Indications for CTO PCI should be patient-dictated rather than operator-dependent. That is, indications for PCI should be identical to non-CTO PCI; namely, to improve patient outcomes. Technical challenges for the interventionist should not be a reason to refer for bypass surgery or medical therapy; rather, the interventionist should refer to a colleague with requisite skills.

Pre-Intervention Essentials

Planning the Procedure

Careful planning ("a game plan") is critical to the success of CTO PCI. By developing a game plan, overextending an already difficult procedure and increasing the risk of complications is minimized. This plan must start with a decision as to whether the CTO is producing symptoms and/or ischemia, and, if so, whether revascularization is actually required (as opposed to medical therapy). If revascularization is chosen, it must be decided whether the patient would be better served with a coronary artery bypass graft (CABG) or PCI because CTOs typically occur in patients with multivessel disease. If PCI is chosen, the next decision is whether the complexity is within the operator's technical expertise or should be referred to a CTO expert. That being the case, the primary issues are the following:

- *Timing*: It is recommended that the routine approach of CTO PCI should be as a stand-alone procedure rather than ad hoc following a diagnostic procedure. This approach will allow decreasing contrast and radiation dose; will facilitate PCI preparation, including angiography review and developing a technical strategy; and will permit discussion with the patient and his or her family regarding the risks and benefits of the procedure. Dedicated CTO PCI days allow undivided attention to each procedure and flexibility in case a procedure takes longer to complete than expected.

- *Angiogram review*: Detailed review of the diagnostic coronary angiogram is critical to devise a procedural plan and is discussed in the following section.

- *Vascular access*: Most operators prefer bilateral femoral access and 8Fr catheters to maximize space for gear entry and exit. Long (45 cm) 8Fr sheaths that facilitate guide manipulation and enhance catheter support are frequently used. Radial access may be utilized, understanding that the guide catheter diameter is sometimes more limited. Furthermore, if in planning the technical strategy it is determined that there is not a good retrograde approach, the radial artery is a reasonable access site for retrograde angiography even with limited transradial experience.

- *Guide catheters*: Larger (e.g., 8Fr) guide catheters provide superior support and enable trapping of nearly all types of CTO PCI equipment. The most commonly used guide types are AL1 for the right coronary (RCA) and a supportive C-curved catheter (e.g., XB 3.5 or EBU 3.75) for the left coronary artery (Table 8.1). Side-hole guides may allow some antegrade flow but may provide a false sense of security with left main intubation because flow through the side holes is simply inadequate. Side-hole catheters may be considered for the RCA. Side-hole catheters do not necessarily provide protection against coronary dissection. Techniques to enhance guide catheter support, such as guide catheter extensions (Guideliner [6–8Fr], Guidezilla 6Fr]) and side-branch anchoring, may be needed during CTO PCI.

- *Anticoagulation*: Unfractionated heparin is preferred for CTO PCI because it can be reversed if a complication occurs. Glycoprotein IIb/IIIa inhibitor should be used sparingly during and after CTO PCI because any small, otherwise well-tolerated perforation may persistently bleed and produce a tamponade.

- *Contrast/Radiation limits*: These parameters should be considered prior to the procedure. The amount of contrast considered acceptable relates specifically to the risk of contrast-induced nephropathy. Radiation doses should be monitored and relative limits determined before the procedure is started.

Angiography

Pre-PCI Angiography

Pre-PCI single-vessel diagnostic angiography for planned subsequent CTO PCI should strive for the following:

1. Characterize as clearly as possible in as many views as necessary the proximal and distal cap and the likely course of the CTO. Magnification level should show the whole heart without including extraneous extracardiac structures and without panning. Typically, left anterior descending (LAD) and circumflex (LCX) CTO proximal

Table 8.1

Checklist of Equipment Needed for Chronic Total Occlusion (CTO) Interventions

Category	Equipment	Essential: "Must Have"	Desirable: "Good to Have"
1.	Sheaths		Long (45-cm) sheaths 90 cm long (for retrograde)
2.	Guides/Guide accessories	Supportive guides Examples XB/EBU 3.0, 3.5, 3.75, 4.0 AL1, AL 0.75 JR4 (particularly for radial RCA) Accessories Y-connector with hemostatic valve (Examples: Co-pilot, Guardian) Guide catheter extender examples: Guideliner, Guidezilla	Side-hole guides, especially RCA guides
3.	Microcatheters	Examples: Finecross (150 cm for retrograde/135 cm for antegrade) Corsair or TurnPike (150 cm for retrograde/135 cm for antegrade) Small (1.20, 1.25, or 1.5 mm diameter) OTW ≥145 cm length balloon catheter TwinPass (dual-lumen)	Other microcatheter-like devices Examples Venture (steerable tip) MultiCross (multiple wires) CenterCross (increase support)
4.	Guidewires*	Polymerjacketed, low tip load, tapered wire: Example, Fielder XT Penetrating wire: Example, Confianza Pro 12 Moderate tip load, hydrophilic wire: Example, Pilot 200 Very steerable wire: Examples, Gaia 1st, 2nd, 3rd Retrograde collateral crossing wire: Example, Sion, Fielder FC Retrograde externalization wire: Examples, RG3, R350	Higher tip load, non-polymer jacketed wires: Examples, Miracle Bros 3, 6, 12

#			
5.	Dissection/reentry equipment	CrossBoss catheter (for controlled dissection)	
		Stingray balloon (platform for lumen reentry)	
		Stingray wire (for lumen reentry)	
6.	Snares	Examples, Ensnare or Atrieve 18–30 mm or 27–45 mm	Amplatz Gooseneck snares
7.	Balloon "uncrossable-undilatable" lesion equipment	Small 20-mm long OTW and RX and balloon catheters	Angiosculpt
		Threader catheter	
		Tornus catheter	
		Laser	
		Rotational atherectomy	
		Turnpike Spiral	
8.	Intravascular imaging	IV ultrasound (IVUS) (any)	IVUS (solid state)
9.	Complication management	Covered stents	
		Coils with delivery microcatheters (Examples: Renegade, Progreat)	
		Pericardiocentesis tray	
10.	Radiation protection	Radiation scatter shields	
		X-ray machine with radiation-reduction protocols	

*For radial operators, 300-cm wires are required because the trapping technique cannot be used through a 6 Fr guide catheter for trapping over-the-wire balloons, the CrossBoss catheter, and the Stingray balloon. However, trapping can be performed for the Finecross and the Tornus 2.1 microcatheter through a 6 Fr guide catheter. Alternatively, guidewire extensions (for the Asahi and Abbott guidewires) may be used for most wires with the proper extension.Modified with permission from Brilakis ES, ed. *Manual of Coronary Chronic Total Occlusion Interventions. A Step-By-Step Approach.* Waltham, MA: Elsevier; 2013.

caps should be visualized in the right anterior oblique (RAO) caudal, RAO cranial, left anterior oblique (LAO) cranial, and LAO caudal views. RCA CTO proximal caps should be assessed in LAO, LAO cranial, and RAO projections.

2. The distal vessel filled by collaterals should also be displayed in appropriate views. For example, when injecting the RCA for an LAD CTO, an additional RAO cranial projection, unusually performed otherwise, may be very helpful to visualize the LAD distal to the CTO.

3. Provide clear delineation of all collateral channels. To maximize clarity, angiography should be performed using a large enough field to visualize the channels without panning. Selecting the proper views to show collateral channels is also very important. For septal channels, irrespective of whether they are coming from the LAD to the posterior descending artery (PDA) or vice versa, a straight RAO and RAO with 30-degree cranial angulation usually provide the best view as to course and angulation.

Angiography at the Beginning of CTO

The importance of dual angiography for CTO PCI cannot be overstated. It should be used in most, if not all, cases with the possible exception of all collaterals being ipsilateral. Dual injections should be performed with the retrograde injection first followed by the antegrade one after 2–3 seconds. Those injections will confirm if the previously selected strategy from single-injection angiography performed during the diagnostic procedure (usually at a separate time) is still appropriate for the CTO anatomy (please see the next section "Putting It All Together"). Often, the CTO length is overestimated with single injections, and it is not rare to find a patent microchannel with dual injections, which will substantially facilitate opening the artery.

Putting It All Together: The Hybrid Algorithm

The "hybrid algorithm" was developed to provide a means to determine the most effective, safe, and efficient approach to treat a specific CTO based on angiographic characteristics. It implies experience with all the techniques described herein. Based on the hybrid approach (Fig. 8.1), antegrade wire escalation is preferred as the initial approach in

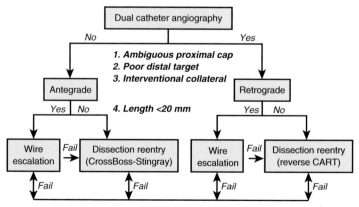

Figure 8.1 The hybrid algorithm. It provides a guide to choosing and prioritizing strategies to treat chronic total occlusions (CTO). The hybrid algorithm also recommends switching strategies should there be an impasse with one approach.

short (<20 mm long) occlusions as described later. A primary antegrade dissection/reentry approach is favored for long (≥20 mm) lesions if there is a good "landing zone" and the distal cap is not at a bifurcation. Finally, a primary retrograde approach is preferred for lesions with an ambiguous proximal cap, poor distal target vessel, proximal cap at a large bifurcation, and good interventional collaterals. Early change between strategies is encouraged if the initially selected strategy fails to achieve progress within a reasonable amount of time.

The Essential CTO Tool Box

Having the right tools is crucial for the success of CTO PCI. Equipment can be grouped into 10 categories: (1) sheaths, (2) guide catheters, (3) microcatheters, (4) guidewires, (5) dissection/reentry equipment, (6) snares, (7) equipment for "balloon uncrossable" and "balloon undilatable" lesions, (8) intravascular imaging, (9) equipment for managing complications, and (10) equipment for minimizing operator radiation exposure (Table 8.1).

These 10 categories include equipment required for wire escalation, antegrade dissection/reentry techniques, and retrograde approaches. Supportive guide catheters are important and are used routinely for antegrade and often retrograde access. There is a very large portfolio of available guidewires. In general, guidewires may be classified as hydrophilic (jacketed) and non-hydrophilic (non-jacketed). Each wire has its own unique combination of flexibility, trackability, torque transmission (or steerability), lubricity (or hydrophilicity), shaft support, wire tip load or strength, wire tip prolapsability, radiovisibility, ability to shape and retain tip configuration, tip taper and thickness, and tactile feedback. The operator should become familiar with the properties of each wire that might be applied to a lesion so that a wire plan can be developed. Antegrade and retrograde techniques typically utilize a microcatheter that allows easy guidewire exchanges, enhances guidewire support, modulates wire tip load, and facilitates wire tip movement. Antegrade dissection can be achieved either with a knuckled guidewire or with the CrossBoss catheter, and antegrade reentry can be facilitated by use of the Stingray system (Boston Scientific, Natick, MA) described below. Various guidewires and microcatheters are needed for the retrograde approach, whereas low-profile balloons, laser, and rotational atherectomy are often needed for "balloon uncrossable" and "balloon undilatable" lesions. Intravascular ultrasonography can facilitate CTO crossing and stent optimization. Availability of covered stents and coils is important for treating perforations. Practically, it is easiest to place all CTO PCI equipment in a single CTO PCI cart that expedites access to this equipment during the procedure, much of which is rarely used for a non-CTO lesion.

Technical Approaches

Antegrade Intraluminal (Intraplaque) Approach ("Wire Escalation")

The antegrade intraluminal (lumen-to-lumen through the CTO) wire escalation method (AWE) is the most commonly used CTO crossing technique and works best for short (<20 mm) occlusions or occlusions with a visible "microchannel" (a "functional" CTO). Antegrade wire escalation can be divided into seven steps:

First, a microcatheter is selected for guidewire delivery. Microcatheters are preferred to over-the-wire (OTW) balloons because they are more flexible; less likely to kink, especially when exchanging guidewires; and have a well-defined radiopaque tip. They are, however, more expensive than OTW balloon catheters.

Second, the microcatheter is advanced to the CTO proximal cap over a workhorse guidewire to minimize the risk of injuring the target vessel proximal to the occlusion.

Third, the crossing CTO guidewire tip is shaped (with the exception of the Gaia guidewires that are pre-shaped). A small (1 mm long, 30- to 45-degree) distal bend is usually created after inserting the guidewire through a guidewire introducer.

Fourth, the shaped guidewire selected to cross the CTO replaces the workhorse wire. Many operators prefer to start with a soft, tapered, polymer-jacketed wire (such as the Fielder XT, Asahi Intecc, Tokyo). If this wire fails to cross, and the course of the CTO vessel is well understood, a stiffer, highly torqueable, tapered guidewire (such as Gaia 2nd, Asahi Intecc) is used, whereas if the course of the occlusion is unclear, a stiffer, polymer-jacketed guidewire (such as the Pilot 200, Asahi Intecc) may be used. For heavily calcified proximal caps, a highly penetrating guidewire, such as the Confianza Pro 12 (Asahi Intecc) or the Hornet 14 (Boston Scientific, Minneapolis, MN) may allow entry into the occlusion, usually followed by de-escalation using a softer guidewire.

Fifth, the guidewire is advanced using sliding, drilling, or penetration or a combination of these techniques. *Sliding* is performed with the forward movement of a tapered, polymer-jacketed guidewire, aiming to track microchannels within the CTO. *Drilling* is performed by controlled rotation of the guidewire in both directions (limited to <90° in each direction). *Penetration* consists of forward guidewire advancement intentionally steering (directing) the wire, rather than nonspecific rotation, usually using a stiff wire (such as Gaia 3rd or Confianza Pro 12) aiming to penetrate the occlusion.

Sixth, the wire position is evaluated by angiography to determine the optimal next action, frequently using the contralateral catheter injection alone or sometimes with dual injections. Clear identification (e.g., by color coding) of retrograde and antegrade guides is crucial to avoid inadvertent antegrade dye injection once the proximal cap has been breached or there is a possibility of a subintimal location of the guidewire. Contralateral injection is preferred for guidewire manipulation with an antegrade attempt once the proximal cap has been modified. Forceful antegrade injections should be avoided once antegrade intervention begins because it can propagate a hydraulic dissection down the guidewire path. Antegrade injection may turn a benign guidewire perforation into an uncontrolled hydraulic perforation. If an automatic injector is used, it should be limited to the retrograde guide.

There are three potential wire positions: (a) crossing into the distal true lumen, (b) passing into the subintimal space, and (c) exiting the vessel structure (wire perforation). Wire position is most commonly assessed by contralateral injection. Accurate assessment is critical because guidewire exit is almost never dangerous, whereas passage of the larger microcatheter or balloon catheter can lead to perforation and tamponade.

Seventh, if the wire crosses into the distal true lumen, balloon angioplasty and stenting are performed as per standard practice of non-CTO lesions. If the wire enters the subintimal space, it can be redirected into the distal true lumen or a second guidewire may be introduced using the "parallel wire" technique (Fig. 8.2), occasionally through a dual-lumen microcatheter, such as the TwinPass (Vascular Solutions, Minneapolis, MN) (Fig. 8.3). Alternatively (and currently preferred by most operators where product is available) use of a dedicated reentry system is employed (Stingray balloon and guidewire; Boston Scientific).

If the wire exits the vessel "architecture" (i.e., wire perforation), it is withdrawn (without advancing the microcatheter over it) and crossing attempts are restarted, assuming there is no evidence of accumulating pericardial effusion.

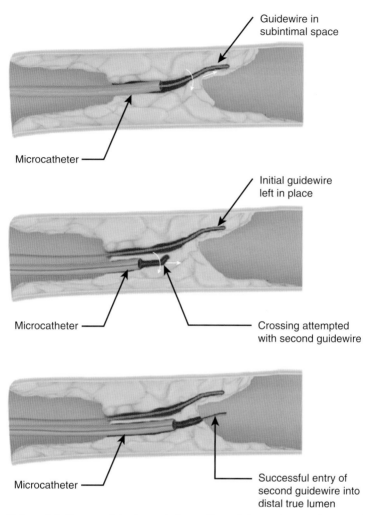

Figure 8.2 The parallel wire technique. *(From Brilakis ES, ed. Manual of Coronary Chronic Total Occlusion Interventions. A Step-By-Step Approach. Waltham, MA: Elsevier; 2013.)*

Multiple issues may arise in trying to cross the proximal cap. Some of the most common ones and possible solutions are listed in Table 8.2. Occasionally a balloon catheter cannot cross a CTO after intraluminal (intraplaque) wire passage. Multiple methods and devices have been described to overcome this problem. A few devices that may be used are the Tornus (Asahi Intec, Tokyo, Japan), the Turnpike Spiral (Vascular Solutions, Minneapolis, MN), rotational atherectomy, or laser. Rotational atherectomy mandates, however, an exchange of the CTO guidewire for a Rotawire, which can be especially challenging and sometimes not possible to pass distally. The reader is referred to the texts listed at the end of the chapter for more complete descriptions.

The J-CTO score has been used to estimate the "degree of difficulty" in passing a guidewire distally in the true lumen within 30 min. Five parameters predict wire crossing within 30 minutes and may be useful for the beginning or early stage operator in gauging technical difficulties. The five factors (each scored as 1 point) are (1) lesion length of greater than 20 mm; (2) tortuosity (i.e., lesion angulation >45%), (3) blunt proximal cap, (4) calcifications along the occluded segment, and (5) previous failed PCI attempt. An "easy" lesion has a score of 0, moderately difficult 1–2, and difficult greater than 2.

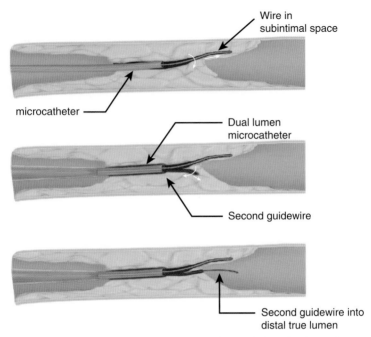

Figure 8.3 Use of a dual-lumen catheter for achieving distal true lumen entry when antegrade wire crossing attempts result in subintimal guide-wire position. *(From Brilakis ES, ed.* Manual of Coronary Chronic Total Occlusion Interventions. A Step-By-Step Approach. *Waltham, MA: Elsevier; 2013.)*

Table 8.2

Commonly Encountered Problems With the Antegrade Approach and Potential Solutions

Issue: Cannot cross proximal cap with wire
Potential Solution:
1. Use increased support guide catheter.
2. Deliver microcatheter near proximal cap to increase wire penetration force.
3. Use wire with increased tip strength or penetration power.
4. Use anchor technique.
5. Use "open sesame" technique.
6. Use "mother-and-child" technique with guide extender.
7. Consider other devices (e.g., Crosser, CrossBoss).
8. Consider retrograde approach.
Issue: Wire passes subintimally
Potential Solution:
Redirect wire into true lumen through microcatheter
Use parallel wire technique.
1. Use Stingray to re-enter lumen.
2. Use STAR/LAST techniques.
Issue: Wire does not pass through entire CTO
Potential Solution:
1. Consider different wire.
2. Increase backup support (see above).
The interested reader is referred to the texts at the end of the chapter for detailed descriptions of these techniques.

Frequent wire, catheter, and other equipment exchanges require that the operator "trap" a short wire (or alternatively use a more cumbersome 300-cm-length wire). Wires are trapped with a 3-mm rapid-exchange balloon catheter in a 7Fr or 8Fr guide and 2.5-mm balloon in a 6Fr guide. Trapping is not possible in a 6Fr guide for OTW balloons, the CrossBoss catheter, and the Stingray balloon catheter.

Antegrade Dissection/Reentry

The most frequent failure mode of antegrade wire escalation is wire tracking into the subintimal space. As lesion complexity increases, particularly in long (>20 mm), tortuous, and/or calcified lesions, there is a consequent increase in the probability of wire passage into the subintimal space. Antegrade dissection and reentry (ADR) techniques have been developed to provide a solution to dealing with this situation. The first ADR method described was called the *subintimal tracking and reentry* (STAR) technique. It involves forceful advancement of a polymeric guidewire with a curve tip (knuckled) within the subintimal space toward the distal branches of the occluded vessel to create a communication between false and true lumens. A modification of the STAR technique called the Carlino technique involved instillation of a small amount of contrast to increase the operator's confidence with this technique. Two other ADR techniques, the mini-STAR and the limited antegrade subintimal tracking (LAST) have been described with the aim of intentionally re-entering the true lumen as early as possible distal to the occlusion. In mini-STAR, reentry is achieved by advancing the loop of a hydrophilic wire (e.g., Fielder FC or XT wire; Asahi Intecc) immediately distal to the lesion and trying to re-enter, whereas, in LAST, reentry is achieved by using a stiffer-tipped wire such as a Pilot 200 (Abbott Vascular) or a Confianza Pro 12 (Asahi Intecc) guidewire with an acute distal bend (45 to 60 degrees) to puncture from the subintimal position into the intraluminal space. All these techniques are limited, however, by the unpredictability of the distal reentry site. These techniques have been associated with a relatively limited improvement in short- and long- term outcomes and are used at present primarily as "bail out" techniques when other methods have failed.

There is currently one dedicated ADR system approved by the U.S. Food and Drug Administration, the StingRay system (Boston Scientific, Minneapolis, MN). With this device, a more controlled reentry point can be achieved. The system consists of the CrossBoss catheter, designed to provide a controlled dissection of the subintimal space; the Stingray LP balloon placed at the proposed reentry site; and the StingRay wire to re-enter the true lumen (Fig. 8.4).

The CrossBoss catheter is a dissection device with a 1-mm rounded metallic hydrophilic-coated distal tip. When the CrossBoss catheter is rotated rapidly (so-called fast-spin technique), it will either track through intimal plaque and re-enter the distal true lumen itself or, alternatively, create a controlled subintimal dissection plane that allows the Stingray balloon catheter to be delivered (Fig. 8.4). The CrossBoss is spun in most cases without a leading guidewire. If its course is impeded by subintimal calcification or a sharp bend, a soft tapered polymeric wire can be advanced, knuckled, and forcefully pushed past the obstruction, whereupon the CrossBoss can be spun again forward and the wire retracted. The Stingray balloon is 2.5 mm in diameter, 10 mm in length, and has a flat shape with two side exit ports opposed 180 degrees apart; upon low-pressure (2–4 atm) inflation, it orients with one exit port facing the true lumen and one exit port pointing away from the true lumen. This configuration allows a specialized wire (the StingRay guidewire) to puncture into the distal true lumen when oriented toward the appropriate port. The 0.014-inch StingRay wire has an icepick-like prong at its tip to facilitate puncturing into the true lumen. Once the lumen has been punctured, the StingRay wire can be advanced after a contralateral contrast injection is performed to confirm the wire is in the true lumen. The StingRay balloon is then deflated, removed, and exchanged for an OTW catheter to perform subsequent dilatation and stenting of the CTO. Alternatively, the StingRay wire can be removed after sticking from the false to the true lumen and exchanged for a more steerable, more "vessel friendly," typically polymer-jacketed wire such as a Pilot 200 to track the vessel (the so-called stick-and-swap

Antegrade dissection re-entry using the Stingray system

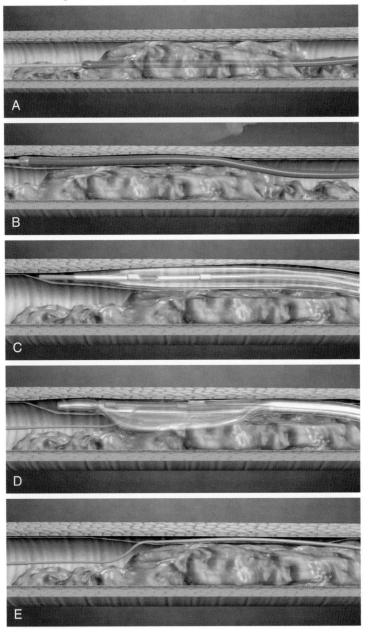

Figure 8.4 (A) CrossBoss tracking through a chronic total occlusion (CTO) and staying into distal true lumen. (B) CrossBoss creating a controlled dissection plane that allows the Stingray balloon catheter to be delivered. (C) The Stingray catheter distal end at planned reentry site prior to balloon inflation. (D) With inflation, the Stingray balloon orients one exit port toward the true lumen allowing the Stingray guidewire to puncture the tissue plane into the distal true lumen. (E) Once the StingRay wire has punctured into the true lumen, it may be removed and "swapped" for a more "vessel friendly" wire such a Pilot 200 ("stick-and-swap" maneuver) or, less frequently, left in place if reentry has been difficult. The rest of the intervention can be then be completed in the usual manner. *(Adapted with permission from Rinfret S, ed. Percutaneous Intervention for Coronary Chronic Occlusion. New York: Springer; 2016.)*

maneuver). Thus, a targeted procedure can be reliably performed to select the reentry site.

Lesions most suited for ADR are longer occlusions (>20 mm) where there is a good distal vessel to attempt reentry ("landing zone") that is proximal to major side branches; this factor is crucial to prevent the loss of significant territories after stent deployment. The place of ADR in a treatment strategy continues to evolve as experience grows (see Hybrid Algorithm [?], Fig. 8.1).

ADR techniques are relatively safe, although they remain associated with a 0.4%–5.0% risk of perforation. Side branch occlusions increase risk for periprocedural myocardial infarction with ST-segment elevation developing when there is no well-developed collateral circulation to the myocardial territory. Dissection/reentry is especially challenging in patients when the distal cap is at a bifurcation because reentry can usually be achieved in only 1 of the branches. In this case a retrograde approach (if there are interventional collaterals) may be preferable.

Retrograde Approaches

Using a retrograde approach, a CTO can be passed lumen-to-lumen, which occurs in the minority of cases (10%–20%) or by dissection-reentry as in most other cases. The definition of a satisfactory "interventional" collateral channel varies from one operator to another and depends in large part on the operator's experience. There are two primary types of retrograde conduits: collateral channels or surgical bypass grafts. Septal or epicardial collateral channels and patent and occluded grafts may be considered in individual cases. Septal collaterals are usually preferred over epicardial collaterals because septal channel perforation is usually without clinical effect whereas epicardial collateral perforation may result in cardiac tamponade. One possible exception to the use of septal collaterals is through a tortuous internal mammary graft. In this circumstance, the microcatheter may "accordion" the graft and produce profound ischemia; therefore, before attempting to cross the septal collateral in such situation, an injection into the mammary graft with the microcatheter into the donor vessel should be performed to ensure adequate flow. Bypass grafts can also be used to reconstruct diseased native vessels where the grafts were anastomosed; the rationale for this approach is related to the better outcome of recanalizing the native vessel over a degenerated bypass graft. Even occluded grafts can be used, especially if the occlusion is recent and the proximal cap of the SVG occlusion is tapered; crossing those SVG occlusions is relatively easy with the support of a microcatheter, and the retrograde approach can be performed as if done from a collateral channel.

The retrograde technique may be performed via the following steps:

Step 1: Getting to the Collateral Channels

An 85- to 90-cm guide catheter is usually necessary to allow passage of equipment to the retrograde targets. Such guides are commercially available for most shapes; alternatively, a 100-cm guide can be shortened. Once the decision is made of which collaterals will be attempted to cross, a microcatheter with a workhorse wire is used to reach the collateral and on occasion to enter the collateral. The workhorse wire is then exchanged for a collateral crossing wire.

Step 2: Crossing a Collateral Channel

Certain wires have gained favor for collateral crossing because they are highly steerable and "gentle" (i.e., have a soft tip that is less likely to perforate a fragile collateral). Availability of wires varies based on country. In the United States, as of this writing, favored wires include the Sion and Fielder FC (Asahi Intecc, Tokyo); it is likely that other wires will be available in the future that may supersede these wires.

Collateral wire passing may target a particular collateral or test several channels in search of a path of least resistance leading to the recipient vessel ("septal surfing technique"). With the surfing technique, a given septal trunk is passed with a guidewire and if it does not seem to provide any connection, a different one is selected. Wire movement should be primarily by wire rotation rather than pushing, which will increase perforation risk. Even invisible channels can sometimes be crossed with "surfing."

Epicardial collaterals are frequently extremely tortuous. They should be avoided unless the operator is very experienced because a perforation can lead to catastrophic consequences, especially in post-CABG patients in whom fluid collection may be loculated and difficult to remove without surgery. Gentle wire manipulation with microcatheter advancement and a clear understanding of the collateral's course is important to decrease the risk of perforation. The operator who uses this technique should be prepared to treat a perforation promptly to avoid tamponade and its consequences.

Step 3: Advancing the Microcatheter to the Distal CTO Cap

Once the retrograde guidewire has reached the distal cap, the micro-catheter should succeed in traversing the collateral in the vast majority of cases. For the small minority, there are a number of techniques to facilitate microcatheter passage to that point, including increased guide support by a guide extension through the retrograde guide or balloon inflation of the septal collateral channel. All microcatheters should be advanced with combinations of clockwise and counterclockwise rotations, with care not to overtorque. An overtorqued catheter can be damaged and should then be removed and exchanged if catheter movement is impaired.

Crossing a patent saphenous vein graft (SVG) can usually be performed with a workhorse wire. Occluded SVGs are more difficult to cross. A polymer-jacketed wire with a more forceful tip, such as a Pilot 200 guidewire (Abbott Vascular, Santa Clara, CA), may be particularly helpful. Attention to track structures such as clips and distal remnants of graft anastomoses are important. If there is ambiguity in the guidewire course, the wire can be removed and distal contrast injection performed through the microcatheter. Once the guidewire reaches the distal target vessel (usually confirmed from another source of collaterals from an additional retrograde catheter injection), the microcatheter is advanced to the distal cap.

Step 4: Crossing the CTO

Once the catheter is at the distal CTO cap, crossing strategy will depend in part on lesion length and presence of calcium. Longer lesions, especially when severely calcified, are unlikely to be crossed intraluminally. With such anatomy, a retrograde dissection and reentry technique, also referred to as *reverse controlled antegrade and retrograde subintimal tracking* (reverse CART) will most often be employed. In the case of a shorter noncalcified lesion, a true-to-true lumen crossing may be attempted. Choice of the guidewire will depend on the anatomy of the segment to be crossed. Very short but heavily calcified segments may be attempted with sharper guidewires, such as the Confianza Pro 12 (Asahi Intecc) or Progress 200T (Abbott Vascular). Longer and noncalcified lesions may be best approached with the Pilot 200, the Gaia 2nd, or Gaia 3rd (Asahi Intecc).

If the CTO length is longer, a dissection and reentry technique, typically reverse CART, is usually required. This technique requires guidewire crossing of the CTO segment in the subintimal space both antegrade and retrograde (Fig. 8.5). Once a retrograde guidewire is secured in the subintimal space, an antegrade guidewire is directed into the subintimal space. Enlarging the space with an antegrade balloon

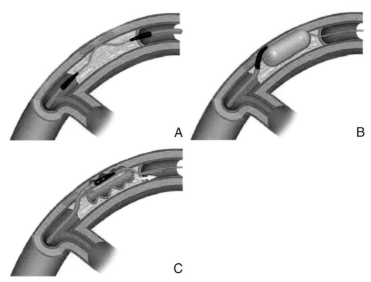

Figure 8.5 Reverse controlled antegrade and retrograde subintimal tracking (CART). (A) Antegrade and retrograde wires are in the subintimal space. (B) Antegrade ballooning using a balloon diameter approximately the size of the vessel is performed. (C) The retrograde wire is passed into the subintimal space connecting to the proximal true lumen with the microcatheter following it. The addition of a guide catheter extender through the antegrade guide catheter has improved passage into the anterograde guide (GuideLiner-assisted reverse CART). *(From Spratt JC. A guide to mastering retrograde CTO PCI. Online. Optima Education Ltd; 2015; www.ctoibooks.com.)*

will help to track the retrograde wire in the dissection plane to the proximal true lumen. The use of a guide catheter extension from the antegrade side can aid in passing the retrograde wire into the antegrade guide catheter. The antegrade balloon diameter should be selected based on the presumed size of the vessel. The size of a knuckled wire, from one adventitial border to the other, is a good indication of the size of the vessel.

Step 5: Externalization of the Retrograde Guidewire

Once the retrograde wire enters the antegrade guide or guide extender, the microcatheter is subsequently advanced into it. The short guidewire can be trapped in the antegrade guide catheter to allow the retrograde microcatheter to be advanced into the antegrade guide. The short retrograde wire may then be removed and replaced with a long guidewire (>300 cm) and externalized. The currently favored long wires include RG3 (Asahi Intecc) or the R350 (Vascular Solutions). However, if the retrograde wire fails to enter the antegrade guide extension or the guide catheter but instead floats into the aorta, the microcatheter is advanced, the short wire removed, a long guidewire advanced into the aorta, and the wire snared and externalized. Large-size snare catheters are used from the antegrade side (such as 18–30 mm triple-loop catheter). The externalized wire is pulled from the antegrade guide, the mangled snared tip is cut off, and this wire is used to perform PCI in an antegrade manner.

Step 6: Antegrade PCI on an Externalized Guidewire

When advancing the antegrade balloon and stent catheters, care should be taken not to pull on the wire because it will further intubate the retrograde guide, which may damage the donor artery ostium. The retrograde microcatheter should be maintained in the collateral throughout the PCI to protect this vessel from the shearing stress of a naked guidewire. Pulling the retrograde guide catheter into the aorta

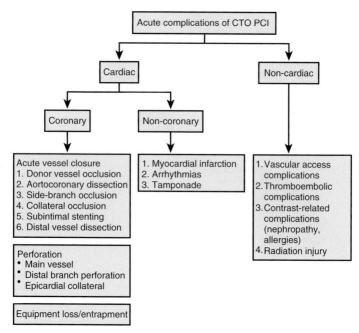

Figure 8.6 Potential complications that may occur with chronic total occlusion percutaneous coronary intervention.

when performing the antegrade maneuvers on the retrograde guidewire ensures safety of the donor artery.

Step 7: Pulling Out the Retrograde Gear

After completion of stenting, the retrograde microcatheter should be readvanced toward the antegrade guide, at least in the stented segment, and the guidewire pulled back into the microcatheter. Maintaining the retrograde guide outside the donor artery ostium is important to minimize donor vessel injury. The microcatheter is removed using continuous clockwise rotation up to reaching the donor vessel (not completely out). Then, a retrograde injection should be performed to ensure absence of donor artery dissection; if dissection has, in fact, occurred, a guidewire can easily be inserted into the microcatheter, directed distally in the donor vessel to treat the dissection.

Complications

Complications of CTO PCI can be classified according to timing (acute vs. long-term) and location (coronary, cardiac noncoronary, and noncardiac) (Fig. 8.6). Acute coronary complications include acute vessel occlusion, perforation, and equipment loss or entrapment. Although the CTO vessel is by definition chronically occluded, attempts to recanalize the CTO can result in further flow compromise (i.e., from a non-CTO vessel, that can have adverse hemodynamic consequences). The best example is donor vessel injury during retrograde crossing attempts that can lead to rapid hemodynamic compromise. Aortocoronary dissections can also occur during CTO PCI and are most often treated with ceasing further injections and stenting the vessel ostium. Occasionally compromising flow through a solitary large collateral vessel can cause ischemia leading to arrhythmias or hypotension.

There are three types of coronary perforations associated with CTO PCI: (a) main vessel perforation; (b) distal artery perforation, typically secondary to wire perforation; and (c) collateral vessel perforation in either a septal or epicardial collateral. Main vessel perforation may be treated by prolonged balloon inflation (in some cases of contained perforation) or covered stent implantation when there is clear and brisk contrast exit into the pericardial space. Distal artery perforation and collateral vessel perforation may require embolization to the small branch, such as by coiling or fat embolization. Perforations are of particular concern among patients with prior CABG surgery because pericardial adhesions (which may in turn be protective of generalized effusion and tamponade) may, however, lead to loculated pericardial effusions that can cause hemodynamic compromise, shock, and death. One example is atrial compression. Loculated hematomas in post-CABG patients are sometimes not amenable to drainage without cardiac surgery or computed tomography–guided aspiration.

Noncoronary cardiac complications include periprocedural myocardial infarction, arrhythmias, and tamponade (due to the coronary complication of perforation). Other acute general complications include vascular access complications (that may be reduced by using ultrasound-guided access, micropuncture needles, or transradial access), systemic thromboembolic complications (less likely if the activated clotting time is kept >300 seconds), contrast allergic reactions, and radiation skin injury. Using low frame per second fluoroscopy (usually 7.5 frames per sec or lower), minimizing use of cineangiography, and paying meticulous attention to the position of the image intensifier in relation to the patient (flat plate should be as close to "touching" the patient as possible) can reduce patient (and operator) radiation dose. If CTO crossing is not achieved after 5 Gray of air kerma dose, consideration for terminating the procedure should be given if the procedure is not progressing or near completion.

Long-term complications of CTO PCI are similar to non-CTO PCI and include in-stent restenosis (that is significantly reduced by use of DES, especially second-generation), stent thrombosis, and coronary aneurysm formation, a complication that, in general, has been rare. Based on current information, long-term complications with CTO and non-CTO PCI appear to be similar.

Key Points for CTO PCI

- It is important to develop a "game plan" prior to the procedure, including limits of procedure for contrast, radiation, time on cath lab table, and the technical approach, including guide catheter, wire, and stepwise strategy.

- Use bilateral coronary angiography in most cases to identify CTO characteristics, particularly length and presumed course.

- Consider all approaches to recanalize the CTO, moving nimbly from one technique to another based on the progress being made with each.

- Consider stopping if myocardial staining occurs, especially if disappearing from one injection to the next, or a small contained perforation occurs; be knowledgeable in perforation management.

- Stop if a type II or III perforation occurs, and treat a perforation as described for management of complications. Employ anticoagulation reversal, balloon tamponade, and covered stent techniques if necessary.

- If the procedure is not successful, consider a second attempt if other technical approaches may be used with a reasonable chance of success.

Suggested Reading

Brilakis ES, ed. *Manual of Coronary Chronic Total Occlusion Interventions. A Step-By-Step Approach*. Waltham, MA: Elsevier; 2013.

Carlino M, Magri C, Uretsky BF, et al. Treatment of the chronic total occlusion: a call to action for the interventional community. *Catheter Cardiovasc Interv*. 2015;85:771-778.

Rinfret S, ed. *Percutaneous Intervention for Coronary Chronic Occlusion: The Hybrid Approach*. New York: Springer; 2016.

Spratt JC, ed. *A guide to mastering retrograde CTO PCI*. Optima Education Ltd; 2015 Online: www.ctoibooks.com.

9

High-Risk Patients and Interventions ▶

ARANG SAMIM · RYAN BERG

A typical low-risk, elective coronary intervention has an in-hospital mortality rate of 0.2% compared to a 66% in-hospital mortality rate for the highest risk of interventions. It is critical for the interventional cardiologist and catheterization laboratory staff to understand the patient's clinical and anatomic risk factors that contribute to this elevated risk in order to appropriately plan for the intervention and for possible advanced therapies such as mechanical circulatory support, and to provide a truly informed consent consultation for the patient and his or her family.

The most comprehensive risk prediction tool for in-hospital mortality is the CathPCI registry. Version 4 was updated in 2009 to include extreme-risk patients, including those with cardiogenic shock and preoperative cardiac arrest. Data from 1.2 million procedures were used to develop both a full (precatheterization and postcatheterization data) and a precatheterization-only risk prediction model for percutaneous coronary intervention (PCI) in-hospital mortality. These models show that increasing clinical acuity is the strongest predictor of mortality. In the absence of cardiogenic shock, the risk of in-hospital mortality for elective, urgent, and emergent cases was 0.2%, 0.6%, and 2.3%, respectively. In the presence of transient shock but not salvage status, the risk of in-hospital mortality was 15.1%; with sustained shock or salvage, the risk was 33.8%; and, with sustained shock and salvage, the risk was 65.9%.

Table 9.1 shows the adjusted odds ratio of mortality with the various clinical predictors. In addition to clinical acuity, higher age (especially >70 years), history of renal disease, cerebrovascular disease, peripheral arterial disease, COPD, diabetes, heart failure, lower ejection fraction, cardiac arrest within 24 hours, having an ST-segment elevation myocardial infarction (STEMI), or a body mass index (BMI) of >30 kg/m^2 were all independent predictors of mortality. After diagnostic catheterization, the full model also predicts higher mortality if there was recent (<30 days) in-stent thrombosis, proximal left anterior descending (LAD) artery disease, left main disease, multivessel disease, or a chronic total occlusion. These anatomic risks correlate to increased SYNTAX scores, another anatomic risk prediction model that can assess preoperative major adverse cardiac events when treating complicated coronary anatomy.

These risk factors have also been incorporated into a simple-to-use online/app risk calculator (http://scaipciriskapp.org/) using these same variables to help calculate a bedside in-hospital mortality risk.

As detailed earlier, both the patient's clinical presentation and associated comorbidities and the severity of the underlying ischemic territory play important roles in determining what is a "high-risk PCI." From an operator's perspective, several distinct topics will be covered here that will encompass the majority of issues when faced with a

Table 9.1

NCDR Cath PCI Registry In-Hospital Mortality Risk Prediction Model (Full and Precatheterization)

	Full Model			Pre-Cath Model		
	OR	95% CI	Chi-Square	OR	95% CI	Chi-Square
Intercept			873.59			796.27
STEMI Patients	1.87	1.75–2.00	327.44	1.80	1.68–1.93	295.95
Age*						
≤70 yrs	1.35	1.30–1.40	253.97	1.37	1.32–1.42	291.68
>70 yrs	1.71	1.64–1.78	612.70	1.74	1.67–1.81	654.44
BMI						
≤30 kg/m²	0.81	0.78–0.84	121.86	0.082	0.79–0.85	113.87
>30 kg/m²	1.14	1.10–1.17	79.77	1.13	1.10–1.16	70.93
CVD	1.13	1.06–1.21	14.48	1.15	1.08–1.23	18.81
PAD	1.27	1.19–1.36	53.78	1.33	1.25–1.42	76.08
Chronic lung disease	1.42	1.34–1.50	135.89	1.39	1.31–1.47	121.19
Prior PCI	0.70	0.67–0.74	162.68	0.72	0.68–0.76	144.66
Diabetes						
Insulin diabetes vs. no diabetes	1.32	1.23–1.42	58.41	1.37	1.28–1.47	76.44
Noninsulin diabetes vs. no diabetes	1.16	1.09–1.22	23.58	1.18	1.12–1.26	32.89
GFR mL/min/1.73 m²	0.90	0.90–0.91	673.43	0.90	0.90–0.91	679.80
Renal failure, GFR <30 ml/min/1.73 m² or dialysis	1.55	1.42–1.68	104.48	1.55	1.42–1.68	105.65

EF	0.90	0.89–0.91	377.63	0.89	0.88–0.90	543.86
Cardiogenic shock and PCI status						3666.71
Sustained shock or salvage	141.36	119.74–166.87	3420.73	164.31	139.30–193.81	5131.47
Sustained shock and salvage	54.84	48.99–61.38	4842.11	60.73	54.27–67.95	3697.87
Transient shock but not salvage	31.68	28.25–35.53	3488.06	34.33	30.64–38.48	1449.09
Emergency PCI without shock/salvage	7.57	6.80–8.43	1365.59	7.99	7.18–8.89	442.23
Urgent PCI without shock/salvage	2.71	2.47–2.98	426.39	2.76	2.51–3.04	207.07
Heart failure NYHA class within 2 weeks						
IV	1.71	1.58–1.85	186.70	1.76	1.63–1.90	207.07
I/II/III	1.20	1.12–1.29	23.29	1.21	1.12–1.30	25.25
Cardiac arrest within 24 h	3.75	3.51–4.00	1553.24	3.66	3.43–3.91	1510.24
At least 1 previously treated lesion within 1 month with in-stent thrombosis	2.11	1.71–2.59	49.75			
Highest risk lesion: segment category						
PLAD vs. other	1.33	1.26–1.40	101.60			
Left main vs. other	2.06	1.85–2.28	178.36			
Number of diseased vessels: 2, 3 vs. 0, 1	1.53	1.46–1.61	294.84			
Chronic total occlusion	1.55	1.40–1.71	69.99			

*Per 10-u increase. +Per 5-u increase. Cardiogenic shock & PCI Status. Versus no heart failure within 2 weeks.

Cath, catheterization; *CI,* confidence interval; *EF,* ejection fraction; *NCDR,* National Cardiovascular Data Registry; *OR,* odds ratio; *PLAD,* proximal left anterior descending.

high-risk PCI. With experience, the operator will learn to quickly appreciate the severity of each case and to plan accordingly.

ST-Elevation Myocardial Infarction (STEMI)

STEMI is one of the highest risk clinical scenarios for the interventional cardiologist. While a complete overview of management of STEMI is beyond the scope of this chapter, a few salient points will be reviewed.

Timing of Perfusion

Reperfusion strategies have evolved with current therapies and evidence. Current guidelines dictate that first medical contact to device time should be less than 90 minutes in a PCI-capable facility. When patients present to a non–PCI-capable hospital, they should be transferred urgently for primary PCI if feasible within 120 minutes of first medical contact. Otherwise, fibrinolytic therapy should be instituted within 30 minutes. The patient should then be transferred urgently if there is evidence of failed reperfusion (less than 50% resolution in the lead with previous maximal ST-segment elevation). If fibrinolytic reperfusion was successful, the patient should still be transferred within 3–24 hours to a PCI facility as part of a pharmaco-invasive strategy.

Determination of Risk

STEMI patients reflect a heterogeneous group. To highlight the differences, a 75-year-old diabetic with anterior STEMI is at a markedly higher risk than a 45-year-old patient with inferior STEMI. Risk stratification can be done using well-validated risk tools such as the thrombolysis in myocardial infarction (TIMI) and GRACE risk scores. Use of risk scores can be done quickly with the advent of mobile phone apps and can help guide informed discussion with the patient and family and dictate the intensity of appropriate care (see Table 9.2).

Table 9.2

TIMI Risk Score for ST-Elevation Myocardial Infarction (STEMI) Summarized for Printing on Laminated Card for Clinical Use				
TIMI Risk Score for STEMI		**Risk Score**	**Odds of Death by 30***	
History		0	0.1	0.1–0.2
Age 65–74	2 points	1	0.3	0.2–0.3
≥75	3 points	2	0.4	0.3–0.5
DM,HTN or angina	1 point	3	0.7	0.6–0.9
		4	1.2	1.0–1.5
Examination		5	2.2	1.9–2.6
SBP <100	3 points	6	3.0	2.5–3.6
HR >100	2 points	7	4.8	3.8–6.1
KILLIP II–IV	2 points	8	5.8	4.2–7.8
Weight <67 kg	1 point	>8	8.8	6.3–12
Presentation				
Anterior STE or LBBB	1 point			
Time to RX >4 hrs	1 point			
Risk Score = Total	(0–14)			

*References to average mortality (95% confidence intervals).

DM, diabetes mellitus; *SBP,* systolic blood pressure; *HR,* heart rate; *RX,* treatment.

From Morrow D, Antman E, Charlesworth A, et al. TIMI risk score for ST-elevation myocardial infarction: a convenient, bedside, clinical score for risk assessment at presentation. *Circulation.* 2000;102:2031–37.

PCI of Non–Infarct-Related Artery

In STEMI patients, the clear goal is timely and efficacious reperfusion of the infarct-related artery to reduce infarct size and reduce major adverse cardiac events (MACE). Fifty percent of these patients will have obstructive disease in a non–infarct-related artery. Previous data showed worse outcomes in patients who underwent additional PCI of a non-infarct artery without hemodynamic instability or shock. Therefore, in previous guidelines, it was an American College of Cardiology (ACC)/ American Heart Association (AHA) Class III recommendation against such intervention. It was recommended to defer these lesions to a later time governed by clinical events or results of noninvasive testing. Since then, randomized controlled trials such as PRAMI, CvLPRIT, and DANAMI 3 PRIMULTI have shown improved outcomes with patients who underwent multivessel PCI as compared with culprit lesion-only PCI during the index hospitalization. Based on these findings, PCI of a noninfarct artery may be considered in STEMI patients with multivessel disease who are hemodynamically stable either at the time of primary PCI or as a planned stage procedure and is now given a class IIb recommendation in the latest STEMI guidelines.

Routine Use of Aspiration Thrombectomy

Due to the thrombotic milieu frequently encountered, aspiration thrombectomy, with its relative ease of use, had become integrated in the treatment strategy of infarct related arteries in STEMI. This was supported by the results of the TAPAS and EXPIRA trials and led initially to a class IIa recommendation for its use in PCI. Since then, the INFUSE-AMI, TASTE, and TOTAL trials did not show a clinical benefit, but did show a small but significant increase in the risk of stroke with the use of aspiration thrombectomy. The updated 2015 ACC/AHA guideline now gives a class III recommendation for the routine use of aspiration thrombectomy and adds a class IIB recommendation for selective or "bail-out" aspiration thrombectomy. On a case-by-case basis, thrombectomy can still result in a substantial reduction in thrombus burden in difficult cases, and this still remains an important adjunctive tool in these select cases. The risk of stroke underscores the importance of meticulous technique to ensure aspirated thrombus does not release prematurely, including adequate backbleeding or direct suction of 5 cc of blood to clear the guide of any thrombus. We also recommend leaving the aspiration catheter on negative suction as the catheter is pulled out of the guide and body because it is more likely to hold onto clot that might be on the edge of the aspiration catheter.

Cardiogenic Shock

Patients who present with acute MI and cardiogenic shock (CS) are at very high risk, and revascularization is the only proven mortality benefit in this population. By definition, CS is end-organ hypoperfusion secondary to cardiac failure, of which MI is the leading cause and characterized by systolic blood pressure (SBP) of less than 90 mm Hg with a cardiac index of less than 1.8 L/min/m^2 (or <2.2 L/min/m^2 when on support). CS will complicate approximately 5–8% of patients with an STEMI presentation. Since patients are usually quickly triaged in the ED and brought emergently to the cath lab, cardiac output is usually not known and thus careful attention to clinical cues such as cool extremities, lack of urine output, or altered mental status are important. It is a good rule of thumb to treat any MI patient with an SBP of less than 90 mm Hg, especially in presence of tachycardia, as a shock patient and institute appropriate resuscitation measures. If the patient does not immediately improve with one inotrope or vasopressor, up titrate therapy and plan prompt use of a mechanical circulatory support (MCS) system before the patient spirals into refractory CS. We are often preoccupied on door-to-balloon time when rushing to open the infarct-related artery when, in fact, it may be more prudent to stabilize the patient with endotracheal intubation for respiratory failure and percutaneous mechanical support in shock to prevent end-organ dysfunction and multisystem organ failure. While there is still debate over whether such advanced therapies significantly affect mortality, we have very limited data in this population to prove or refute this point. Most of the case series with newer MCS are with patients who were already in CS for an average of 2 days prior to institution of therapy, and randomized data are affected by many confounders, such as the type of MCS placed and definition of CS. Different options for MCS will be discussed later.

In an attempt to improve cardiac output in MI patients complicated by CS, several devices have been developed to either artificially add to or augment the heart's pump function. Physiologically, MCS devices can unload the left ventricle, decreasing myocardial stress and oxygen demand as well as decreasing pulmonary artery pressure. These devices vary considerably with respect to design, ease of placement, and amount of hemodynamic support generated. They are indicated for refractory CS due to MI but also other disease states such as myocarditis, structural heart disease, acute heart failure, and arrhythmias such as incessant ventricular tachycardia. The common MCS systems in use today are the intra-aortic balloon pump (IABP), Impella, TandemHeart, and extracorporeal membrane oxygenation (ECMO) systems.

Intra-Aortic Balloon Counterpulsation

The IABP has been used since the 1960s and has been widely used periprocedurally in the setting of cardiogenic shock. The device is a balloon mounted to dual-lumen catheter and is inserted percutaneously through the femoral artery under fluoroscopic guidance. One lumen is used for rapid balloon inflation and deflation, and the other is used for aspiration, flushing, and hemodynamic monitoring. The timing of balloon inflation is critical for its effect hemodynamically. The balloon inflates in early diastole to improve upstream blood flow, and the increased diastolic pressure increases coronary perfusion (blood flow in the coronary arteries is predominantly during diastole; see Fig. 9.1); it deflates during early systole, and the elastic recoil of the aorta reduces afterload. To ensure proper timing of balloon inflation, the device is connected to a bedside computer-controlled monitor and can use EKG or pressure tracings to time balloon inflation (see Fig. 9.2). It had a class IB indication in the 2004 ACC/AHA STEMI guidelines. However, data from the SHOCK II trial, which randomized acute MI and CS patients to either IABP or no IABP, show no difference in outcomes, and use of IABP has been downgraded to a class IIa recommendation in the 2013 ACC/AHA STEMI guidelines. It only augments cardiac output by roughly 0.3–0.5 L/min. Tables 9.3 and 9.4 show the common indications and contraindications for the IABP.

Sizing Recommendations

Balloon sizing (see Table 9.5) is based predominantly on the patient's height. The sheath size is generally 7–8F and usually varies by size of balloon required, and most IAB kits come with their own sheaths. The balloon can also be inserted sheathless in cases where the patient's femoral anatomy is diseased or of smaller caliber.

Proper Positioning

The balloon tip should be placed at the proximal descending aorta such that it is 1–2 cm below the origin of the left subclavian artery; distally, it should ideally be above the renal arteries to avoid hypoperfusion (see Fig. 9.3). On daily X-rays, the tip should be seen between the second and third intercostal space (Fig. 9.4).

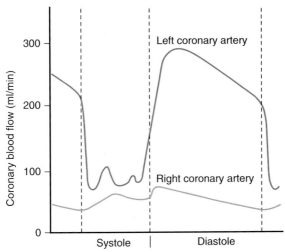

Figure 9.1 Coronary perfusion during counterpulsation. Coronary flow is predominantly diastolic and further enhanced by counterpulsation, which augments diastolic blood flow and thus coronary perfusion. In addition, aortic recoil during diastole further improves efficiency of the left ventricle. *(From Patterson T, Perera D, Redwood SR. Intra-aortic balloon pump for high-risk percutaneous coronary intervention.* Circ Cardiovasc Interv. *2014;7:712–20.)*

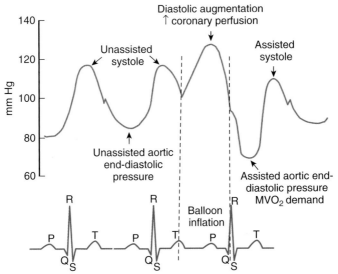

Figure 9.2 Systemic arterial pressure waveform on introduction of intra-aortic balloon pump–assisted diastolic augmentation. The intra-aortic balloon pump inflates at the dicrotic notch, leading to peak-augmented diastolic pressure. As the balloon deflates, assisted end diastolic pressure is seen to be lower than unassisted end diastolic pressure, and assisted systolic pressure is lower than unassisted systolic pressure. Peak diastolic augmentation should be greater than the unassisted systolic pressure, and both assisted pressures should be less than the unassisted pressures. *(From Patterson T, Perera D, Redwood SR. Intra-aortic balloon pump for high-risk percutaneous coronary intervention.* Circ Cardiovasc Interv. *2014;7:712–20.)*

Anticoagulation of IABP

Historically, systemic anticoagulation with heparin was recommended for all patients with IABP due to concerns of thrombus forming on the indwelling balloon and catheter. Recent literature suggests that routine use of anticoagulation resulted in increased bleeding, and patients not

Table 9.3

Indications for Intra-Aortic Balloon Pump (IABP) Counterpulsation
Cardiogenic shock from any causes (MI, severe valvular lesion, myocarditis, etc.)
With jeopardized myocardium at risk
Bridge to another assist device
Unstable angina, refractory to medical therapy
Unstable ventricular arrhythmias
High-risk PCI in setting of severely depressed LV function
High-risk PCI involving unprotected left main or last remaining patent vessel

Table 9.4

Contraindications to Use of Intra-Aortic Balloon Pump	
Absolute Contraindications	**Relative Contraindications**
Moderate or severe aortic valve insufficiency	Severe atherosclerosis
	Blood dyscrasias
Dissection or aortic aneurysm	End-stage cardiomyopathy unless bridging to VAD
Previous aortic stenting	Severe sepsis

Table 9.5

Standard Intra-Aortic Balloon Sizing Guide		
Patient Height	**IAB Volume**	**Body Surface Area**
147–162 cm	30 cc	<1.8 m^2
162–182 cm	40 cc	>1.8 m^2
>182 cm	50 cc	>1.8 m^2

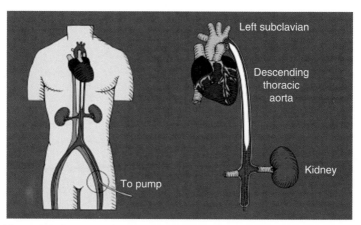

Figure 9.3 Correct placement of the intra-aortic balloon pump. *(Courtesy of Arrow International, Inc.)*

heparinized had no higher incidence of thromboembolic events. In clinical practice, the risks and benefits of systemic anticoagulation should be weighed in each patient. In those with increased bleeding risk or with bleeding complications, omission of anticoagulation appears to be safe with IABP at 1:1 counterpulsation.

Weaning of IABP

Once the patient has stabilized hemodynamically and has been weaned off most inotropic agents, the IABP can be weaned by reducing the

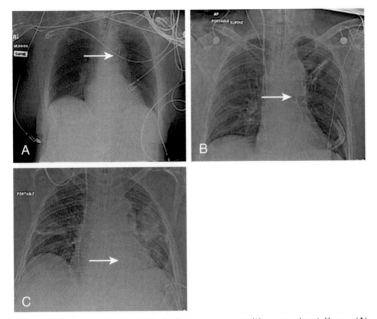

Figure 9.4 Proper intra-aortic balloon pump position on chest X-ray. (A) Acceptable tip position at the level of the carina and just below the aortic knob. (B) Malpositioned, tip at the T5–T6 level. (C) Severely malpositioned, at T7, greater than 10 cm below the aortic knob. *(From Siriwardena M, Pilbrow A, Framptom C, et al. Complications of intra-aortic balloon pump use: does the final position of the IABP tip matter? Anaesth Intensive Care. 2015;43:66–73.)*

frequency of balloon assistance to the cardiac cycle from 1:1, to 1:2, and then to 1:3. The speed of weaning depends on the patient's status and length of time on support. Patients who have been on IABP prophylactically will be weaned off much more quickly than will those who have required support for several days. ECG, vital signs, urine output, and mentation should be carefully monitored; any perturbations reflect an intolerance to withdrawal of support and weaning should be halted. Generally, if a patient has tolerated augmentation at 1:3 for an hour, the IABP can be discontinued. Of note, the current consoles have the ability to automatically change from ECG triggering to pressure triggering and thus there is no need to place the IABP on standby during CPR in the event of a cardiac arrest.

Removal of IABP

Removal of the balloon requires the following steps:

1. Remove all anchoring ties and sutures.
2. Disconnect the balloon from the console. The patient's blood pressure will collapse the balloon, but some institution protocols still require attachment of a one-way valve and 60-cc syringe for aspiration. We don't recommend this because if too much air is aspirated, the balloon will infold, creating "wings" that can make for an overall larger surface area of the balloon, and this can cause arterial injury with removal.
3. With one hand holding the sheath, the other hand pulls back the balloon until resistance is felt, indicating that the balloon has reached the end of the sheath. Do not attempt to pull the balloon through the sheath because it may cause fragmentation of the balloon. Continue removal of both catheter and sheath together. During removal, if any undue resistance is felt, the balloon may be entrapped and may require surgical removal.
4. While keeping firm pressure on the femoral artery proximal to the insertion site, pull out the balloon and sheath together.

5. Allow 1–2 seconds of bleeding to encourage extravasation of any potential thromboembolic material outside of the body. Then apply pressure to the femoral artery above the insertion site and release the pressure from below the insertion site to allow back-bleeding for 1–2 seconds.

6. Apply firm pressure to the arteriotomy site for approximately 20–30 minutes (or longer if necessary) to achieve adequate hemostasis, especially in anticoagulated patients. Some operators will use compression devices such as the FemoStop (Abbott St. Jude Medical) to aid hemostasis.

ECMO

ECMO has also been around in some fashion since the 1960s, but its use in CS in recent years has greatly increased with improvements in design and reliability and the need for greater hemodynamic support than can be achieved with the IABP. ECMO involves drainage of blood from the vascular system to outside the body, where it can be oxygenated and mechanically pumped back to the circulation. ECMO circuits can be either venous-venous (VV) or venous-arterial (VA) and either peripherally or centrally placed. VV ECMO can be done via one central cannula from the right internal jugular vein, in which case blood is extracted from the right atrium or vena cava, circulated, and then infused back to the right atrium. A two-cannula method uses a cannula inserted in the femoral vein to drain the inferior vena cava and a second cannula for perfusion either from the contralateral femoral vein or the right internal jugular vein. VV ECMO is for hemodynamically stable patients having trouble with oxygenation and thus not used in the setting of CS. VA ECMO (Table 9.6) circuits bypass both the heart and the lungs and can be placed peripherally, with the perfusion cannula inserted via the femoral artery and advanced to the abdominal aorta and the drainage cannula advanced through the femoral vein to the IVC (Fig. 9.5). Larger size cannulas for increased flow need to be placed centrally with direct right atrium and ascending aorta cannulation by a surgeon (Fig. 9.6). Systemic anticoagulation with a goal activated clotting time (ACT) of 180–220 seconds is required for the ECMO circuit.

Table 9.6

Indications for Veno-Arterial Extracorporeal Membrane Oxygenation (ECMO) Support
• Cardiogenic shock, Severe cardiac failure due to almost any cause:
• Acute coronary syndrome
• Cardiac arrhythmic storm refractory to other measures
• Sepsis with profound cardiac depression
• Drug toxicity with profound cardiac depression
• Myocarditis
• Pulmonary embolism
• Isolated cardiac trauma
• Acute anaphylaxis
• Postcardiotomy: inability to wean from cardiopulmonary bypass after cardiac surgery
• Post heart transplant: primary graft failure after heart or heart-lung transplantation
• Chronic cardiomyopathy:
• As a bridge to longer term VAD support
• Or as a bridge to decision
• Periprocedural support for high-risk percutaneous cardiac interventions
• Bridge to transplant

VA, venoarterial.

From Makdisi G, Wang IW. Extracorporeal membrane oxygenation (ECMO): review of a lifesaving technology. *J Thorac Dis*. 2015;7:E166–E176.

Peripheral veno-arterial ECMO cannulation approach

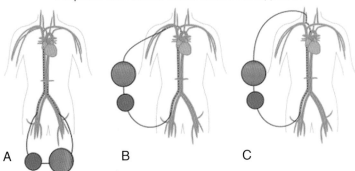

Figure 9.5 Peripheral veno-arterial extracorporeal membrane oxygenation (ECMO) cannulation approach: femoral vein (for drainage), (A) femoral, (B) axillary, (C) carotid arteries are used for perfusion. *(From Makdisi G, Wang IW. Extracorporeal membrane oxygenation (ECMO) review of a lifesaving technology.* J Thorac Dis. *2015;7:E166–E176.)*

Central veno-arterial ECMO cannulation approach

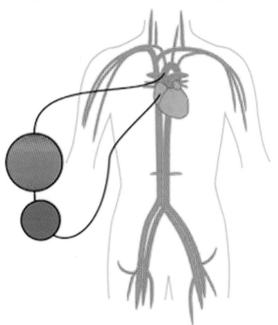

Figure 9.6 Central veno-arterial extracorporeal membrane oxygenation (ECMO) cannulation approach. *(From Makdisi G, Wang IW. Extra corporeal membrane oxygenation (ECMO) review of a lifesaving technology.* J Thorac Dis. *2015;7:E166–E176.)*

Most interventional cardiologists do not employ ECMO, and even at large institutions ECMO placement is typically done by cardiothoracic surgeons. But advancements in ECMO technology such as frictionless pumps, more efficient gas exchangers, and lower priming volumes have decreased the complexity such that these circuits are being instituted in the ED. There are now even portable devices intended for use in the field for out-of-hospital cardiac arrest patients. Interventional cardiologists will likely benefit from experience with ECMO placement and management for cases of critically ill patients in refractory shock. ECMO has the ability to fully support oxygenation as well as perfusion, providing 3–4 L/min with peripherally inserted devices and 5 L/min for central ECMO. However, unlike the other MCS devices, ECMO does not unload the heart effectively, and patients may develop left ventricular (LV) distention. To unload the LV, some institutions combine ECMO with either an Impella or IABP placement.

TandemHeart

The TandemHeart is a percutaneously placed left atrial to femoral artery bypass circuit and requires a transseptal puncture to access the left atrium (Fig. 9.7). Compared to the IABP, the TandemHeart is superior in hemodynamic support and ability to unload the LV, producing flow rates of 3–4 L/min. Systemic anticoagulation with a goal ACT of 180–220 seconds is required for the TandemHeart circuit. Two randomized trials failed to show a mortality benefit at 30 days, and, due to the time and experience required for insertion, it is infrequently used in the setting of acute MI complicated by CS.

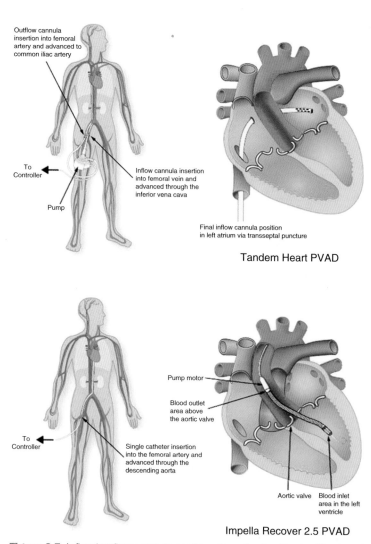

Figure 9.7 Inflow/outflow cannula configurations for the TandemHeart and Impella Recover 2.5 percutaneous ventricular assist devices (PVADs). *(From Kar B, Basra SS, Shah N, et al. Percutaneous circulatory support in cardiogenic shock. Circulation. 2012;125:1809–17.)*

Impella Ventricular Support

The Impella pump device is a catheter-based axial flow pump inserted percutaneously. The unit is advanced across the aortic valve and positioned such that the distal inlet can aspirate blood through the motor and pump it out through the proximal outlet tip into the ascending aorta (Figs. 9.7 and 9.8). The Impella comes in several configurations. The Impella 2.5 generates up to 2.5 L/min as the name implies and requires a 13F sheath, whereas the Impella CP can generate 3.5 L/min and requires a 14F sheath. The large Impella 5.0 requires a 21F sheath and surgical cutdown to the femoral artery or a vascular graft sewn to the axillary artery. The Impella RP is a right ventricular assist device that can generate 4 L/min and is inserted via a 21F catheter through the femoral vein; it is placed with the inlet tip in the right ventricle and the outlet in the main pulmonary artery in cases of right ventricular failure. The Impella device unloads the LV, thereby reducing LV end diastolic pressure (LVEDP), LV work, and myocardial oxygen demand and resulting in more favorable LV pressure volume curve characteristics (Fig. 9.8). The Impella is load dependent; its ability to pump decreases with increasing afterload and accounts for the characteristic phasic

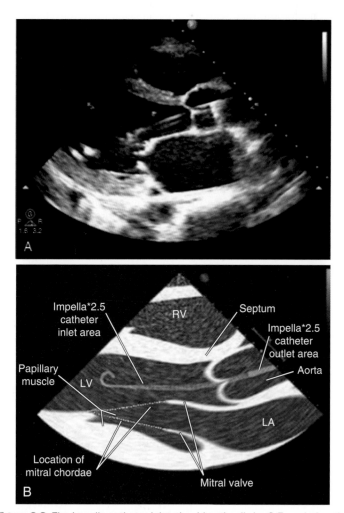

Figure 9.8 The Impella catheter inlet should optimally be 3.5 cm below the aortic valve as seen in (A) echo image and (B) schematic drawing. *(From Burzotta F, Trani C, Doshi SN, et al. Impella ventricular support in clinical practice: Collaborative viewpoint from a European expert user group.* Int J Cardiol. *2015;201:684–91.)*

motor current fluctuations during the cardiac cycle, in which the highest flow is achieved during systole. Flow is independent of cardiac rhythm, which is another advantage over the IABP.

Access site issues are a major source of complications for all MCS devices and the Impella is no exception. Careful planning on the best approach, especially in an elective situation, is important to reduce adverse events. Suitability of access site should be screened angiographically, and ultrasound-guided access may help in proper femoral arteriotomy. Femoral access can be managed with use of Perclose Proglide (Abbott Vascular, Temecula, CA) closure devices in what is referred to as "pre-close" technique. After obtaining initial access with a standard 6 or 7F sheath, the sheath is exchanged over a wire for the Perclose device. Instead of deploying the suturing needle at the 12 o'clock position, it is deployed at 10 o'clock. The sutures are harvested, and the deployment device is rewired and exchanged for a second Perclose device, which is deployed at the 2 o'clock position and again the device is removed after rewiring the vessel. It is important not to tie down the sutures but to allow for dilation of the artery to be upsized for the Impella sheath. The sutures are secured out of the way on the patient's drape with use of steri-strips or a hemostat. The wire will still be in place, and this method will allow dilation of the artery in stepwise fashion using an 8–10F dilator and then with the Impella sheath and introducer. The Impella device requires a 0.018-inch stiff wire in the LV in order for the device to be advanced across the aortic valve to the LV. Placing a curl on the tip of the wire may help prevent the wire from irritating or perforating the LV wall. With completion of the procedure, and if the patient is hemodynamically stable, the Impella can be quickly weaned off and then removed from the patient. The two Percloses can be tied down with the wire remaining in the vessel before final closure to maintain access in the case of an issue. The sutures should not be crisscrossed and should be individually tied down, beginning with the first Perclose placed (in this example, the one deployed at the 10 o'clock position).

When the Impella is placed emergently, there will not be time to use the pre-close technique. Generally, if the device is left in place more than 24 hours, hemostasis should be achieved with prolonged manual compression, given the risk for infection. Since the Impella repositioning sheath is tapered, you cannot remove the device through this sheath. However, if Impella support is needed only briefly, the access site can be closed using a "post-close" technique as follows:

Cut the Impella catheter after it has been shut down and withdrawn to the level of the descending aorta and then remove the repositioning sheath. Using the Impella as a rail, advance a mother-and-daughter 10F sheath placed in a 13F sheath (the 10F sheath acts as an introducer, large enough to go over the Impella shaft). Remove the 10F sheath (as you would with any introducer) and flush the 13F sheath. Advance a buddy wire, such as a standard 0.035-inch 180-cm J-wire into the sheath, alongside the Impella catheter shaft. Pull the Impella back until it meets the 13F sheath and then remove the two, leaving only the J-wire in place. With the J-wire maintaining vessel access, use two Perclose devices in the 10 o'clock and 2 o'clock positions, rewiring the vessel to maintain access in case of an issue. Take care during deployment not to pull the foot plate through the large-bore arteriotomy site. It is important to have an assistant holding manual pressure proximal to the arteriotomy site throughout this process to minimize blood loss.

Future Impella devices are expected to come with an updated repositioning sheath with side port to allow buddy wiring, making this process unnecessary.

Proper positioning of the Impella is essential to enable proper support. On occasion, transfer from the catheterization lab to the ICU may result in malpositioning and inadequate support. This can be minimized by ensuring excess slack is removed and that the catheter lies on the inner curve of the aorta. Also important is LV apical placement of the wire prior to advancing the Impella to avoid catheter-induced mitral valve dysfunction or papillary muscle entrainment. Bedside echocardiography should be done to ensure proper placement (Fig. 9.9). Color Doppler should reveal mosaic flow in the aortic root reflecting continuous flow through the Impella outlet. The Impella console has common alarms (Table 9.7) that can alert staff to malpositioning.

Systemic anticoagulation is required for the Impella system, and is generally achieved with heparin to an ACT of 160–180 seconds. Abiomed recommends a solution of 5%–20% dextrose with 50 units/mL of heparin to maintain patency of the purge pathway in the event of blood migrating into the motor. Usually, the purge fluid flow rate is 4–8 mL/hr. In cases of heparin-induced thrombocytopenia, both systemic and purge fluid anticoagulant can be changed to a direct thrombin inhibitor such as bivalirudin.

Like the other MCS devices, data are mixed in regards to the overall benefit of the device. One small study of patients with CS due to MI showed no survival benefit of the Impella 2.5 device compared to the IABP despite its superior hemodynamics. The PROTECT-II trial compared IABP and Impella in high-risk PCI CS patients and found no difference between major events at 30 days. Results from the USpella Registry show that in acute coronary syndrome patients complicated by CS, pre-PCI placement of an Impella device significantly improved survival compared to placement post-PCI. However, in the absence of benefit of randomized data, these registry studies can only be seen as hypothesis-generating. Critics of MCS devices will extrapolate that since randomized data have

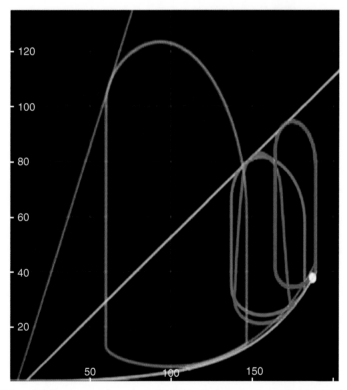

Figure 9.9 Pressure–volume loop. Verticle axis is pressure, mmHg; horizontal axis is volume, ml. Normal conditions (*brown*), acute heart failure without hemodynamic support (*blue*), with Impella CP support (*green*), and with extracorporeal membrane oxygenation (ECMO) support (*red*). The loop area is an estimate of the mechanical work performed by the ventricle. Note the area reduction (work reduction) by the Impella device and the characteristic oblique vertical lines in the latter, indicating continuous emptying of the ventricle even in the "isovolumic" phases. (*From Burzotta F, Trani C, Doshi SN, et al. Impella ventricular support in clinical practice: Collaborative viewpoint from a European expert user group. Int J Cardiol. 2015;201:684-91.*)

Table 9.7

Common Impella Console Alarms

Alarm Condition	Frequency	Interpretation	Clinical Picture	Treatment
Position wrong	Common	Inlet and outlet in the same chamber (both in LV or both in AO)	May occur during the start-up phase and transportation	Reposition under echo or fluoroscopic guidance
Position unknown	Common	Difference between max and min pressure on aortic pressure curve <20 mm Hg	Frequently due to low native heart pulsatility	Reposition under echo or fluoroscopic guidance
Suction	Common	Above-normal motor current necessary to set performance level reduction of flow due to insufficient volume	Device too deep or low-volume status; frequently due to high resistance in Impella inflow when in contact with LV wall or papillary muscle	Reposition under echo or fluoroscopic guidance
Low volume/suction	Common	Flow lower than expected for set performance level either due to suction or due to high afterload	May cause hemolysis if positioned incorrectly; check free hemoglobin (>40 ml/dL)	Optimize volume status RV failure
High purge pressures	Rare	Increased pressure (>1100 mm Hg) at purge system due to increased resistance anywhere along the purge lumen necessary to prevent blood entry in the motor compartment	After long-term support, catheter kink or blood ingress into motor. May precede to motor stop if extreme	Place a new purge cassette when longer term support is needed
Sudden pump stop	Very rare	Most likely clot ingestion	Possible systemic emboli	Exclude LV thrombus with adequate anticoagulation (ACT 180–200s)

From Burzotta F, Trani C, Doshi SN, et al. Impella ventricular support in clinical practice: collaborative viewpoint from a European expert user group. *Int J Cardiol.* 2015;201:684–91.

not shown any device to improve survival compared to IABP alone, and with recent studies showing that IABP did not improve survival compared to no IABP, then there is little evidence for these therapies. Overall, this is a subject that needs much larger studies with appropriate patient selection and early use of MCS to differentiate those who may truly benefit from these therapies. On a case-by-case basis, MCS can still be beneficial in properly selected individuals, and, for now, their use is still only a class IIb indication in the 2011 ACC guidelines. See Videos 9.1, 9.2, and 9.3 for a case where hemodynamic support proved to be a lifesaving adjunct to a patient presenting with an acute MI due to left main disease causing CS.

High-Risk Anatomic Lesions

Unprotected Left Main Disease

The left main coronary artery supplies up to 70% of the myocardium and thus treatment of unprotected left main disease is of highest risk due to the amount of myocardium in jeopardy. Complications during left main PCI will lead to hypotension, ventricular tachycardia/fibrillation, and death. The term *protected left main* is defined as the presence of at least one patent bypass graft to the LAD or the left circumflex (LCX) arteries; the absence of such is termed *unprotected left main disease*. PCI for treatment of protected left main disease is well established because these patients have already had bypass surgery, and the left main can be treated as a single coronary artery since these patients have adequate blood supply to the grafted vessel. Historically, treatment of unprotected left main disease has been largely relegated to bypass surgery. However, with improvements in PCI and advancements in stent technology, imaging modalities, and the ability to provide percutaneous hemodynamic support, unprotected left main PCI has become feasible and safe. Of the 1800 patients randomized in the SYNTAX trial comparing coronary artery bypass graft (CABG) surgery to PCI, 705 patients had left main disease. Analysis of this subgroup showed that PCI had similar rates of mortality and a lower rate of stroke but with higher rates of revascularization. In patients with lower SYNTAX scores, PCI resulted in favorable outcomes in comparison with CABG. Five-year outcomes from the PRECOMBAT trial, comparing PCI to CABG for unprotected left main disease, did not show any difference in rate of MACE, although this study was underpowered due to the lower than expected rates of primary end points in the CABG group. Distal left main bifurcation disease and more complex anatomy are predictors of poor procedural success; as such, having a SYNTAX score of less than 22 is a class IIa indication and a SYNTAX score of less than 33 is a class IIb indication for revascularization with PCI in patients who are at higher risk to undergo CABG. The ongoing EXCEL trial, which compares second-generation drug-eluting stents (DES) to CABG in unprotected left main disease in patients with low or intermediate SYNTAX scores hopes to definitively show that stenting is comparable, if not superior, to surgery. For now, CABG for left main disease remains the standard of care (class I indication), and a heart team approach should be used for the management of these patients. In the setting of an acute MI, left main disease as the culprit vessel is rare, occurring at only 4% in the GRACE registry. This is likely due to the fact that abrupt closure of the left main will usually result in sudden cardiac death, and these patients do not survive to reach the cath lab. GRACE registry data showed improved survival with either PCI or CABG compared to no revascularization. Patients with acute MI due to left main disease are generally stabilized and referred for emergency surgery. If the patient has reduced TIMI flow and is unstable, many operators will perform balloon angioplasty with aims to restore TIMI 3 flow and stabilize the patient for emergent surgery. Current ACC/AHA guidelines give a class IIa recommendation to unprotected left main PCI in ACS patients who are not candidates for CABG or for patients with STEMI due to a culprit left main lesion and reduced TIMI flow when it can be done more quickly and safely than CABG.

Aorta-Ostial Lesions

Ostial lesions (lesions within 3 mm of the ostia) pose a greater challenge due to risk of complication involving the mother branch. In the case of an aorta-ostial lesion, the difficulty lies in proper stent deployment to ensure adequate ostial coverage. The operator will need to negotiate guide management in order to place the stent, and these interventions have a higher rate of geographic miss. Also, aorto-ostial lesions may be difficult to dilate due to greater thickness of the muscular wall at the aorta, and the elasticity may increase recoil. Here we discuss some general key points in the management of these lesions:

1. Ensure that the ostial lesion is not due to catheter-induced spasm (especially with ostial right coronary artery [RCA] disease).

2. The use of intravascular ultrasound (IVUS) is very helpful in aorto-ostial lesions. IVUS can help appropriately size the artery to help pick out the proper sized stent. In the case of downstream tandem lesions, fractional flow reserve (FFR) is not useful to determine the physiologic significance of an aorto-ostial lesion and therefore IVUS anatomic correlates of physiologic significance (minimal luminal cross sectional area <6 mm^2 in a left main) can be used. Finally, IVUS can be used to evaluate stent apposition, expansion, and ostial placement after the stent is placed to verify a good result. Optical computed tomography (OCT) will be less helpful because the guide catheter needs to stay engaged in the ostium in order to deliver contrast for the blood-free lumen that OCT requires. Therefore, the guide catheter will obstruct visualization of the ostial lesion itself.

3. Choose a guide catheter that does not aggressively engage the ostium, depending on the takeoff, such as a standard Judkins catheter. Use of side-hole catheters is common in hopes that the side holes will help coronary perfusion when the guide obstructs flow. However, this likely does not provide any extra significant extra flow. The side holes are useful to see what the true aortic pressure is, but this can give a false sense of security when coronary perfusion is truly hampered, so aorto-ostial interventions should be performed as quickly as possible.

4. Preload the guide catheter with the guidewire to expedite wiring of the vessel; then, the guide can be partially disengaged to allow blood flow in cases where catheter dampening is encountered.

5. Properly prepare the lesion as necessary (predilation, cutting/scoring balloon, and/or rotational atherectomy to debulk heavily calcified lesions).

6. As in most interventions, use of a DES is preferred over a bare metal stent (BMS) if clinically appropriate.

7. Use a longer than anticipated stent length to ensure adequate coverage of the ostium. This will also reduce bobbing of the stent back and forth during each cardiac cycle.

8. Use one of 4 techniques (discussed below) to help line up the stent to the true ostium.

9. Flaring of the ostium stent struts to the aorta wall can be done with a postdilatation balloon that is only halfway advanced past the ostium. Alternatively, a specially designed ostial balloon, the Flash Ostial balloon (Cardinal Health), can be used for postdilation.

There are four standard techniques to try to line up the stent in the ostium: the conventional method, Szabo technique, the floating wire technique, and the use of the Ostial Pro system.

In the *conventional technique*, the catheter is engaged and the stent delivery system is advanced to just beyond the tip. Then the entire system is slowly withdrawn and contrast injections are done in multiple views to ensure proper positioning such that 1–2 mm of stent struts protrude into the aorta to ensure proper ostial coverage. For left main lesions, AP caudal or LAO caudal views are used; for ostial RCA lesions, LAO caudal views tend to be the most helpful for correct positioning. The disadvantages to this technique include contrast load due to frequent injections, need for optimal non-foreshortened views, and potential vessel trauma and dissection from multiple engagement and disengagements, as well as excessive strut protrusion that may make subsequent engagement of the vessel challenging.

The *Szabo technique* (Fig. 9.10) can be used for ostial stent deployment. It uses a second wire that is advanced outside the guide into the aorta. Then the distal end of this wire is passed in the proximal stent strut outside the patient before being advanced to the lesion. The wire through the proximal strut will anchor the stent at the ostium and prevent a geographic miss. Putting the guidewire in the last stent cell through the strut requires partial inflation of the stent delivery balloon (1–2 atm) to help flare the end to accommodate the second wire, which some argue may damage the stent or make it more difficult to deliver. While there was initial enthusiasm with this strategy, follow-up studies using ultrasound imaging, angiographic analysis of restenosis, and, above all, in vitro testing conclude that the Szabo technique is not a predictable and precise technique to implant a stent accurately at the level of the ostium.

The *floating wire technique* (Fig. 9.11) employs a second wire to help stabilize the guide catheter just outside the ostium such that the

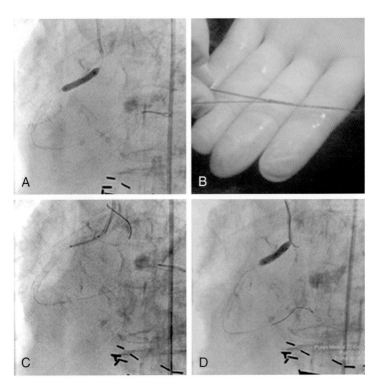

Figure 9.10 Szabo technique for aorto-ostial percutaneous coronary intervention (PCI). (A) Lesion predilatation using a noncompliant balloon. (B) Threading of anchor wire through proximal stent struts. (C) Positioning of ostial stent with anchor wire prolapsed into aortic root. (D) After low-pressure deployment, the anchor wire is retracted and the stent fully deployed. *(From Sharma A, Kovacic JC, Sharma S. The Szabo technique in a patient with ostial RCA in-stent restenosis. Cardiology Today's Intervention. http://www.healio.com/cardiology/intervention.)*

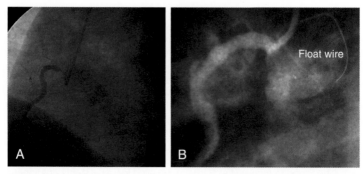

Figure 9.11 Example of a difficult aorta-ostial percutaneous coronary intervention (PCI). (A) Severe ostial right cardiac artery (RCA) lesion that resulted in pressure dampening and ST-elevation with engagement. (B) Use of a floating wire in the aorta prevented pressure dampening and assisted in proper stent positioning for successful ostial RCA intervention. *(From Chen J. Floating wire technique for treatment of aorto-ostial lesions.* http://www.cathlabdigest.com/articles/Floating-Wire-Technique-Treatment -Aorto-Ostial-Lesions.)

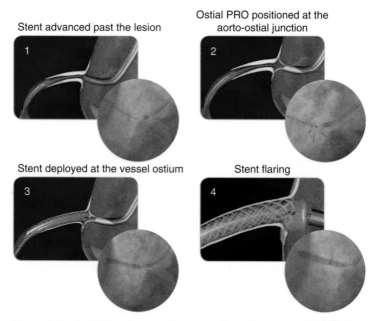

Figure 9.12 Ostial-Pro stent positioning system. *(Courtesy of Merit Medical Systems, Inc.)*

stent can be properly deployed with minimal movement or engagement of the vessel. This second guidewire is curved, with a large exaggerated loop, and is advanced outside the guide into the aorta. The guide catheter can then be advanced to the ostium, and the wire floating in the aorta will prevent catheter engagement. Using constant forward pressure to maintain this position, the stent can be deployed with the proximal stent marker just beyond the tip of the guide to ensure coverage of the ostium.

The *Ostial-Pro* (Merit Medical, South Jordan, UT) is a device specifically designed for proper stent positioning during aorto-ostial interventions (Fig. 9.12). It consists of nitinol wire with a distal cylindrical slit with four flexible, self-expanding gold-plated legs that abut the aorta when advanced out of the guide. After the lesion has been wired and the stent advanced distal to the lesion, the Ostial-Pro is advanced through the guide, and the four legs expand outside the catheter. Forward pressure on the guide catheter will position the legs against the aortic wall and stabilize guide position. The gold plating on the legs will help fluoroscopic assessment of the true plane of the ostium. From there, the stent can be withdrawn to just proximal to the guide tip and deployed in usual fashion. The Ostial-Pro can then be drawn back, and further inflation overlapping the ostium will help flare the stent against the aortic wall.

Saphenous Vein Graft (SVG) PCI

Although SVGs are widely used as a bypass conduit, these grafts fail in about 7% of patients within the first week, 15% in the first year, and by an additional 1–2% per year thereafter, resulting in about 50% or more failures at the 10-year postop mark. Early graft closure (within the first month) is usually due to technical issues and acute thrombosis. After this period, these grafts are prone to accelerated atherosclerosis when compared to native vessels. The saphenous vein lacks arterial tone, and, after exposure to arterial pressure, this leads to intimal damage with resultant smooth muscle cell proliferation, platelet aggregation, and neointimal hyperplasia. These lesions contain an abundance of thrombotic and atheromatous material and are often very friable, leading to distal embolization of atheroembolic debris. Thus, the lesions are high-risk and require careful planning and technique because their complication rate is double that of native-artery PCI. Chronic total occlusions of SVGs have a much lower procedural success and high MACE, leading to an ACC/AHA class III recommendation against PCI for chronic SVG occlusions. Make sure to review prior angiograms to determine the location and anatomy of SVGs. Prior reports may inform you on which catheters will be better at engaging the graft because adequate guide support is crucial to a smooth procedure. Consider intervention on the native vessel if feasible due to lower complication rates. Prior to intervention, ensure that your cath lab has appropriately sized (and not expired) covered stents in case there is an SVG perforation. Note that SVG perforation will not cause cardiac tamponade due to its extra pericardial course, but rather localized perforation or continued hemorrhage into the mediastinum.

Several strategies, described here, can help improve outcomes in SVG PCI including direct stenting, using relatively small DES, and using embolic protection devices. Routine adjunctive pharmacotherapy is usually not beneficial but may be used to help with no reflow situations.

Due to the amount of friable atheroembolic debris, balloon predilation risks dislodgement of such debris, distal embolization, and subsequent slow or no flow. Also, predilation may not be as important in SVG PCI due to the less calcified nature of these plaques, which would impede stent expansion. Although there are no prospective randomized data to support this, registry review of SVG interventions showed fewer non-Q MI in those patients who underwent direct stenting.

Given the amount of friable atheromatous material in SVG lesions, care must be taken not to oversize the stent, and sizing should be approximately 1:1. In an IVUS study of SVG lesions treated with DES, smaller stent diameter to reference lumen diameter showed the least amount of plaque extrusion through the stent struts, but there was no difference in target vessel revascularization at 1 year. Proponents of this technique argue that since vein grafts are oversized compared to the vessel they supply, undersizing the stent will not affect blood flow as long as the mean luminal area is greater than 6 mm^2. Long-term restenosis rates for this method are unknown, and further randomized studies are warranted.

Due to the nature of the lesions, initially, covered stents were thought to help reduce distal embolization by trapping friable atheroembolic debris. However, several randomized trials failed to show this benefit over BMS, with some studies showing high target vessel failure in the covered stent group. DES is generally preferred over BMS, although the data for this are not as robust as for native vessel PCI. The saphenous vein grafts trial (SOS) demonstrated reduced MACE in patients randomized to DES at 3 years as compared to BMS. Meta-analysis of trials comparing BMS to DES in SVG lesions has shown reduced risk of MACE and improved efficacy with the use of DES.

Embolic protection is another important adjunct to SVG intervention. Currently available devices include distal occlusion and aspiration systems, retrievable filter wire-based systems, and proximal flow interruption catheters. The SAFER study showed a 42% reduction in 30-day MACE with the GuardWire distal occlusion balloon compared to no embolic protection device. Subsequent studies have compared newer devices with the GuardWire as the reference standard, and these devices were found to be noninferior. These include the more commonly used Filterwire EZ (Boston Scientific, Marlborough, MA) and SpiderFx (Medtronic, Minneapolis, MN) systems that use a filter basket instead of a balloon. Use of embolic protection devices is given a class I recommendation in the ACC/AHA guidelines based on data supporting its role in preventing no-reflow and periprocedural myocardial infarction. For detailed techniques on these devices, see Chapter 5.

Initially hypothesized to reduce embolization, routine use of glycoprotein IIb/IIIa inhibitors has not been shown to be of benefit in SVG interventions and has received a class III indication in the ACC/AHA guidelines, based largely on a pooled analysis of five studies that did not show any benefit.

Despite using the techniques just described, dislodgement of debris from degenerated SVGs results in distal embolization, complicating 10–15% of SVG PCI. These patients have a 31% rate of periprocedural MI and increased in-hospital mortality. Plugging of the distal arterial bed by atheroemboli results in ischemia and vasospasm and further promotes platelet aggregation. Use of vasodilators is effective in treatment of no flow, including high-dose adenosine, calcium channel blockers, and nitroprusside. It is important to repeat boluses and use additional agents if flow is not improved. If adenosine is used, do not give more than 100 mcg at a time to avoid prolonged sinus pauses. Also, infusion through a microcatheter can be used to aid in delivery to the distal microvasculature. One study even showed that nicardipine pretreatment during SVG PCI prevented no reflow without the use of embolic protection devices.

SUMMARY

High-risk PCI is guided by the patient's clinical acuity and history as well as by the complexity of coronary anatomy. Advanced aged, severely depressed LV ejection fraction, and CS leave the patient in a highly vulnerable state such that any perturbation in hemodynamics during intervention may lead to catastrophic results. This risk needs to be appreciated beforehand, using clinical judgment and validated tools such as clinical and anatomic scoring systems that will help guide a thoughtful, informed consent consultation. Careful preprocedural planning, including the use of mechanical circulatory support devices when necessary, is paramount to success in these high-risk yet high-reward procedures.

Suggested Reading

Abbo KM, Dooris M, Glazier S. Features and outcomes of no-reflow after percutaneous coronary intervention. *Am J Cardiol.* 1995;75:778-782.

Baim DS, Wahr D, George B. SAFER Trial Investigators Randomized trial of a distal embolic protection device during percutaneous intervention of saphenous vein aorto-coronary bypass grafts. *Circulation.* 2002;105:1285-1290.

Brennan JM, Curtis JP, Dai D, et al. Enhanced mortality risked prediction with a focus on high risk percutaneous coronary intervention. *JACC Cardiovasc Interv.* 2013;6(8):790-799.

Brilakis ES, Lichtenwalter C, de Lemos JA. A randomized controlled trial of a paclitaxel-eluting stent versus a similar bare-metal stent in saphenous vein graft lesions: the SOS (Stenting of Saphenous Vein Grafts) trial. *J Am Coll Cardiol.* 2009;53:919-928.

Burkhoff D, Cohen H, Brunckhorst C, et al. A randomized multicenter clinical study to evaluate the safety and efficacy of the TandemHeart percutaneous ventricular assist device versus conventional therapy with intraaortic balloon pumping for treatment of cardiogenic shock. *Am Heart J.* 2006;152.

Chen J. Floating wire technique for treatment of aorto-ostial lesions. *Cath Lab Digest.* 2007;15(4).

Dangas GD, Kini AS, Sharma SK, et al. Impact of hemodynamic support with Impella 2.5 versus intra-aortic balloon pump on prognostically important clinical outcomes in patients undergoing high-risk percutaneous coronary intervention (from the PROTECT II randomized trial). *Am J Cardiol.* 2014;113:222-228.

Dishmon DA, Elhaddi A, Packard K, et al. High incidence of inaccurate stent placement in the treatment of coronary aorto-ostial disease. *J Invasive Cardiol.* 2011;23(8):322-326.

Engstrøm T, Kelbæk H, Helqvist S, et al. Complete revascularisation versus treatment of the culprit lesion only in patients with ST-segment elevation myocardial infarction and multivessel disease (DANAMI 3-PRIMULTI): an open-label, randomised controlled trial. *Lancet.* 2015;386:665-671.

Fischell TA, Subraya RG, Ashraf K, et al. "Pharmacologic" distal protection using prophylactic, intragraft nicardipine to prevent no-reflow and non–Q-wave myocardial infarction during elective saphenous vein graft intervention. *J Invasive Cardiol.* 2007;19:58-62.

Fröbert O, Lagerqvist B, Olivecrona GK, et al. Thrombus aspiration during ST-segment elevation myocardial infarction. *N Engl J Med.* 2013;369:1587-1597.

Gershlick AH, Khan JN, Kelly DJ, et al. Randomized trial of complete versus lesion-only revascularization in patients undergoing primary percutaneous coronary intervention for STEMI and multivessel disease: the CvLPRIT trial. *J Am Coll Cardiol.* 2015;65:963-972.

Goldman S, Zadina K, Mortiz T, et al. Long-term patency of saphenous vein and left internal mammary artery grafts after coronary artery bypass surgery results from a Department of Veterans Affairs Cooperative Study. *J Am Coll Cardiol.* 2004;44:2149-2156.

Hannan EL, Samadashvili Z, Walford G, et al. Culprit vessel percutaneous coronary intervention versus multivessel and staged percutaneous coronary intervention for ST-segment elevation myocardial infarction patients with multivessel disease. *JACC Cardiovasc Interv.* 2010;3:22-31.

Hindnavis V, Cho S-H, Goldberg S. Saphenous vein graft intervention: a review. *Cath Lab Digest.* 2012;20(3).

Hong YJ, Pichard AD, Mintz GS. Outcome of undersized drug-eluting stents for percutaneous coronary intervention of saphenous vein graft lesions. *Am J Cardiol.* 2010;105:179-185.

Jolly SS, Cairns JA, Yusuf S, et al. Randomized trial of primary PCI with or without routine manual thrombectomy. *N Engl J Med.* 2015;372:1389-1398.

Kar B, Basra S, Shah N, et al. Percutaneous circulatory support in cardiogenic shock. *Circulation.* 2012;125:1809-1817.

Keeley EC, Boura JA, Grines CL. Primary angioplasty versus intravenous thrombolytic therapy for acute myocardial infarction: a quantitative review of 23 randomised trials. *Lancet.* 2003;361:13-20.

Kogan A, Preisman S, Sternik L, et al. Heparin-free management of intra-aortic balloon pump after cardiac surgery. *J Card Surg.* 2012;27(4):434-437.

Lee MS, Park S-J, Kandzari DE, et al. Saphenous vein graft intervention. *JACC Cardiovasc Interv.* 2011;4(8):831-843.

Levine GN, Bates ER, Blankenship JC, et al. 2015 ACC/AHA/SCAI focused update on primary percutaneous coronary intervention for patients with ST-elevation myocardial infarction. *J Am Coll Cardiol.* 2016;67(10):1235-1250.

Maiello PC, Osterne EM, Filho WA. Ostial lesions in main coronary arteries treated with the Szabo technique. *Rev Bras Cardiol Invasiva.* 2012;20(2):173-177.

Makdisi G, Wang IW. Extra Corporeal Membrane Oxygenation (ECMO) review of a lifesaving technology. *J Thorac Dis.* 2015;7(7):E166-E176.

Montalescot G, Brieger D, Eagle KA. Unprotected left main revascularization in patients with acute coronary syndromes. *Eur Heart J.* 2009;30:2308-2317.

Morice MC, Serruys PW, Kappetein AP. Outcomes in patients with de novo left main disease treated with either percutaneous coronary intervention using paclitaxel-eluting stents or coronary artery bypass graft treatment in the Synergy Between Percutaneous Coronary Intervention with TAXUS and Cardiac Surgery (SYNTAX) trial. *Circulation.* 2010;121:2645-2653.

Morrow D, Antman E, Charlesworth A, et al. TIMI risk score for ST-elevation myocardial infarction: a convenient, bedside, clinical score for risk assessment at presentation. *Circulation.* 2000;102:2031-2037.

Motwani JG, Topol EJ. Aortocoronary saphenous vein graft disease: pathogenesis, predisposition, and prevention. *Circulation.* 1998;97(9):916-931.

O'Gara PT, Kushner FG, Ascheim DD, et al. 2013 ACCF/AHA guideline for the management of ST-elevation myocardial infarction: a report of the American College of Cardiology Foundation/American Heart Association Task Force on Practice Guidelines. *J Am Coll Cardiol.* 2013;61:e78-e140.

O'Neill WW, Kleiman NS, Moses J, et al. A prospective, randomized clinical trial of hemodynamic support with Impella 2.5 versus intra-aortic balloon pump in patients undergoing high-risk percutaneous coronary intervention: the PROTECT II study. *Circulation.* 2012;126:1717-1727.

O'Neill WW, Schreiber T, Wohns DH, et al. The current use of Impella 2.5 in acute myocardial infarction complicated by cardiogenic shock: results from the USpella registry. *J Interv Cardiol.* 2014;27:1-11.

Pappalardo A, Mamas MA, Imola F. Percutaneous coronary intervention of unprotected left main coronary artery disease as culprit lesion in patients with acute myocardial infarction. *JACC Cardiovasc Interv* 2011;4:618-626.

Park DW, Clare RM, Schulte PJ, et al. Extent, location, and clinical significance of non-infarct-related coronary artery disease among patients with ST-elevation myocardial infarction. *JAMA*. 2014;312:2019-2027.

Park SJ, Kim YH, Park DW. Randomized trial of stents versus bypass surgery for left main coronary artery disease. *N Engl J Med*. 2011;364:1718-1727.

Popma JJ, Dick RJ, Haudenschild CC, et al. Atherectomy of right coronary ostial stenoses: initial and long-term results, technical features and histologic findings. *Am J Cardiol*. 1991;67(5):431-433.

Pucher PH, Cummings IG, Shipolini AR, et al. Is heparin needed for patients with an intra-aortic balloon pump? *Interact Cardiovasc Thorac Surg*. 2012;15(1):136-139.

Roffi M, Mukherjee D, Chew DP, et al. Lack of benefit from intravenous platelet glycoprotein IIb/IIIa receptor inhibition as adjunctive treatment for percutaneous interventions of aortocoronary bypass grafts: a pooled analysis of five randomized clinical trials. *Circulation*. 2002;106(24):3063-3067.

Saltiel FS, Fischell TA. The ostial pro stent positioning system: perfecting aorto-ostial stent placement. *Cath Lab Digest*. 2008;16:3.

Sardella G, Mancone M, Bucciarelli-Ducci C, et al. Thrombus aspiration during primary percutaneous coronary intervention improves myocardial reperfusion and reduces infarct size: the EXPIRA (thrombectomy with export catheter in infarct-related artery during primary percutaneous coronary intervention) prospective, randomized trial. *J Am Coll Cardiol*. 2009;53:309-315.

Sdringola S, Assali AR, Ghani M. Risk assessment of slow or no-reflow phenomenon in aortocoronary vein graft percutaneous intervention. *Catheter Cardiovasc Interv*. 2001;54:318-324.

Serruys PW, Morice MC, Kappetein AP. Percutaneous coronary intervention versus coronary-artery bypass grafting for severe coronary artery disease. *N Engl J Med*. 2009;360:961-972.

Seyfarth M, Sibbing D, Bauer I, et al. A randomized clinical trial to evaluate the safety and efficacy of a percutaneous left ventricular assist device versus intra-aortic balloon pumping for treatment of cardiogenic shock caused by myocardial infarction. *J Am Coll Cardiol*. 2008;52:1584-1588.

Sianos G, Morel MA, Kappetein AP, et al. The SYNTAX score: an angiographic tool grading the complexity of coronary artery disease. *Euro Interv*. 2005;1:219-227.

Stone GW, Maehara A, Witzenbichler B, et al. Intracoronary abciximab and aspiration thrombectomy in patients with large anterior myocardial infarction: the INFUSE-AMI randomized trial. *JAMA*. 2012;307:1817-1826.

Teirstein PS, Price MJ. Left main percutaneous coronary intervention. *J Am Coll Cardiol*. 2012;60(17):1605-1613.

Thiele H, Sick P, Boudriot E, et al. Randomized comparison of intra-aortic balloon support with a percutaneous left ventricular assist device in patients with revascularized acute myocardial infarction complicated by cardiogenic shock. *Eur Heart J*. 2005;26:1276-1283.

Thiele H, Zeymer U, Neumann F-J, et al. Intraaortic balloon support for myocardial infarction with cardiogenic shock. *N Engl J Med*. 2012;367:1287-1296.

Vaquerizo B, Serra A, Ormison J, et al. Bench top evaluation and clinical experience with the Szabo technique: new questions for a complex lesion. *Catheter Cardiovasc Interv*. 2012;79:378-389.

Vermeersch P, Agostoni P, Verheye S. Randomized double-blind comparison of sirolimus-eluting stent versus bare-metal stent implantation in diseased saphenous vein grafts: six-month angiographic, intravascular ultrasound, and clinical follow-up of the RRISC trial. *J Am Coll Cardiol*. 2006;48:2423-2431.

Vlaar PJ, Mahmoud KD, Holmes DR Jr, et al. Culprit vessel only versus multivessel and staged percutaneous coronary intervention for multivessel disease in patients presenting with ST-segment elevation myocardial infarction: a pairwise and network meta-analysis. *J Am Coll Cardiol*. 2011;58:692-703.

Vlaar PJ, Svilaas T, van der Horst IC, et al. Cardiac death and reinfarction after 1 year in the Thrombus Aspiration during Percutaneous coronary intervention in Acute myocardial infarction Study (TAPAS): a 1-year follow-up study. *Lancet*. 2008;371:1915-1920.

Wald DS, Morris JK, Wald NJ, et al. Randomized trial of preventive angioplasty in myocardial infarction. *N Engl J Med*. 2013;369:1115-1123.

Complications of Percutaneous Coronary Interventions ▶

MICHAEL J. LIM

Percutaneous coronary intervention (PCI) is associated with rare but serious complications. Most of the complications are generic to all diagnostic coronary angiography procedures, and some are specific to coronary intervention. Events like death, myocardial infarction (MI), and bleeding occur at higher rates for interventional procedures since there is prolonged procedural time, complexity, and the use of anticoagulation (Tables 10.1 and 10.2). It is critical to understand the possible complications of PCI in order to provide proper informed consent to the patient. It is also critical to be vigilant and to recognize potential complications at an early stage to try to avoid a catastrophic outcome, as the most common cause of all post-PCI deaths is from a procedural complication rather than from a preexisting cardiac condition. Fortunately, death is very rare with diagnostic angiography (<0.1%). The mortality rate increases 13 times with the addition of the complexity of coronary intervention to 1.3% (Table 10.3).

Complications of PCI can occur at any step of the procedure, from the administration of sedation to the transfer as the patient leaves the laboratory. This chapter will discuss many of the possible complications in the order that they might be encountered during the procedure.

Vascular Access

The first part of any PCI begins with vascular access. Using the femoral access, the major complications are femoral artery dissections (Fig. 10.1), pseudoaneurysm, arteriovenous (AV) fistula, and retroperitoneal bleeding. As seen in Table 10.1, the incidence of these complications is increased compared to a strictly diagnostic procedure. All arterial complications are markedly reduced (but are not eliminated) using the radial artery access.

Femoral Access Complications

Pseudo-Aneurysm

A femoral artery pseudoaneurysm represents a failure of sealing of the initial arterial puncture site, allowing arterial blood to flow into the surrounding tissue. This forms a pulsatile hematoma that acts as the covering roof over the aneurysm (see Fig. 10.1). Pseudoaneurysms are late appearing, associated with local pain and swelling, and diagnosed with femoral ultrasound with an excellent sensitivity of 94%–97%. There are multiple risk factors for pseudoaneurysm (Box 10.1).

Small pseudoaneurysms (<2 cm) often close spontaneously within 1 month. In larger pseudoaneurysms, or in small ones that fail to close,

Table 10.1

Event Rates of Diagnostic Versus Percutaneous Coronary Intervention Complications		
Complication	Event Rate Diagnostic Procedure (%)	Event Rate Interventional Procedure (%)
Death	0.1	1.3
Significant bleed	0.5	5–12
AV fistula	0.75	1.1
Pseudoaneurysm	0.2	1–2
Contrast-induced nephropathy	5	8–57
Periprocedural myocardial infarction (>3 × ULN cardiac enzyme)	0.1	8
Air embolism	0.1–0.3	0.1–0.3
Cerebrovascular accident	0.3	0.3
Ventricular arrhythmia	0.4	0.84
Coronary dissection	0.03–0.46	29–50
Aortic dissection	<0.01	0.03
Infection/bacteremia	0.11	0.64
Anaphylactoid reaction to contrast	0.23	0.23
Cholesterol embolization	0.8–1.4	0.8–1.4

AV, arteriovenous; *MI,* myocardial infarction; *ULN,* upper limits of normal.

Table 10.2

Complications Specific to Percutaneous Coronary Intervention	
Complication	Event Rate (%)
No reflow phenomenon	2
Stent thrombosis	2
Vessel perforation	0.84
Stent embolization	0.4–2
Need for emergent bypass surgery	0.15–0.3
Wire fracture	0.1
Stent infection	<0.1 (case reports only)

Table 10.3

Modes of Death During Percutaneous Coronary Intervention	
Mode of Death	Event Rate (%)
Low output failure	66.1
Ventricular arrhythmias	10.7
Stroke	4.1
Preexisting renal failure	4.1
Bleeding	2.5
Ventricular rupture	2.5
Respiratory failure	2.5
Pulmonary embolism	1.7
Infection	1.7

Adapted from Table 1, page 633 of Malenka DJ, O'Rourke D, Miller MA et al. Cause of in-hospital death in 12,232 consecutive patients undergoing percutaneous transluminal coronary angioplasty. *Am Heart J.* 1999;137(4):632–38.

active treatment is necessary. The two most common treatment methods are ultrasound-guided compression or thrombin injection. In some hospitals, ultrasound-guided compression is not offered because of increased stress-related wrist injury to the ultrasound technician. Other advantages of thrombin injection over ultrasound compression are seen in Box 10.2.

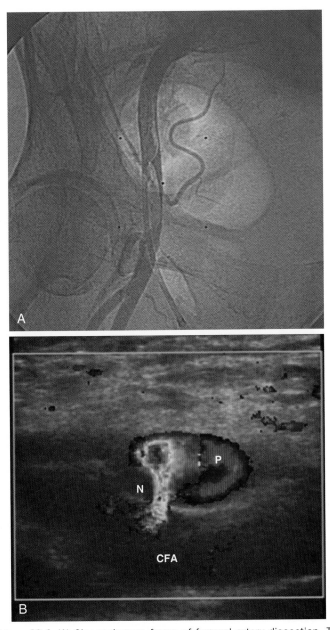

Figure 10.1 (A) Cineangiogram frame of femoral artery dissection. This problem may be associated with limb ischemia or bleeding. It may require surgery but more often can be treated by contralateral access and implantation of iliac stent. (B) Ultrasound picture of a pseudoaneurysm (*P*) arising from the common femoral artery (*CFA*). The circular color object is the hematoma which is fed by blood flow from the artery through the characteristic narrow neck (*N*). *(From Ahmad F, Turner SA, Torrie P, et al. Iatrogenic femoral artery pseudoaneurysms—a review of current methods of diagnosis and treatment. Clin Radiol. 2008;63:1310–6, fig. 1.)*

Thrombin injection can be performed by diluting 1000 U thrombin in a 1-mL syringe with normal saline (final concentration of 100 U per 0.1 mL) and injecting with direct ultrasound visualization through a long 22-gauge needle until thrombus is formed in the pseudoaneurysm cavity and Doppler-detected flow is abolished (see Fig. 10.2). Rarely, in very large pseudoaneurysms and those resistant to thrombin injection, vascular surgery is required.

> **Box 10.1** Risk Factors for Pseudoaneurysm Formation
>
> **Procedural Factors**
>
> Catheterization of both artery and vein
> Cannulation of the superficial femoral or profunda femoris rather than common femoral
> Inadequate compression postprocedure
> More anticoagulation used
>
> **Patient Factors**
>
> Obesity
> Hemodialysis
> Calcified arteries

> **Box 10.2** Advantages of Thrombin Injection Compared With Ultrasound Compression
>
> Greater technical success (96% vs. 74%)
> Less painful to the patient and technician
> No conscious sedation required
> Effective in patients on anticoagulation
> Can be used in pseudoaneurysms above the inguinal ligament

Another complication of vascular access is AV fistula formation (Fig. 10.2). This is recognized on physical examination by a palpable thrill or an audible continuous bruit. Unlike pseudoaneurysms, conservative treatment with watchful waiting is the most common treatment modality (90%). One-third of persistent AV fistulae will close during the first 12 months. Most persistent AV fistulae are asymptomatic and do not require repair. Rarely, they can be symptomatic (moderate pain) and, in large patient series, about 10% of AV fistulae will ultimately require surgical repair.

Arteriovenous Fistula

AV fistulae produce low shunt blood flow volumes (160–510 mL/min) compared to most large intracardiac (e.g., left to right) shunts or dialysis shunts (1000 mL/min). AV shunt flows must exceed 30% of the cardiac output to produce symptoms, and therefore it is quite rare to have a truly symptomatic shunt from a femoral AV fistula. The main risk factor for development of an AV fistula is a low arterial puncture, responsible for almost 85% of all AV fistulae.

Infection

A rare complication of groin access is systemic infection. The Society for Coronary Angiography and Intervention has detailed infection control guidelines for the cardiac catheterization laboratory. Proper sterile technique, including hand-washing and use of hats, masks, gown, and gloves, has limited bacterial infections to only 0.64% of interventional cases, with septic complications occurring in only 0.24% of cases. Routine antibiotic prophylaxis is *not* recommended before cardiac catheterization. However, if there is any concern for contamination of the femoral sheath (transport between rooms, patient touching site, changing out sheaths in a delayed procedure), it is standard to give 1 g cephalexin as a prophylactic measure. If the patient is allergic, 1 g of vancomycin can be given alternatively.

An equally concerning infectious complication is the exposure of the physicians or staff to the patient's potential pathogens. Universal precautions are to be followed by everyone in the catheterization laboratory. If there is an occupational exposure, proper management per

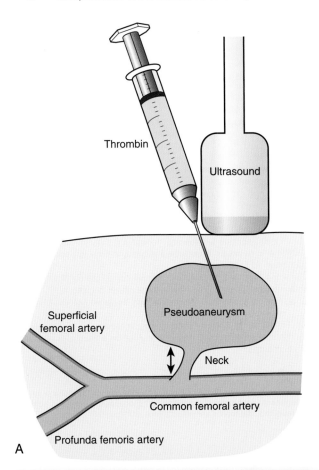

Thrombin

Ultrasound

Pseudoaneurysm

Superficial
femoral artery

Neck

Common femoral artery

Profunda femoris artery

A

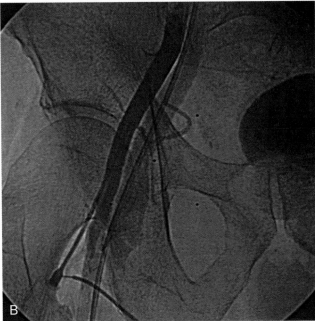

B

Figure 10.2 (A) Schematic representation of the technique utilized to inject thrombin into a pseudoaneurysm under ultrasound guidance. (B) Cineangiogram of arteriovenous fistula. Contrast visualized in the vein returning cranially indicates a communication with the artery (i.e., a fistula). Treatment is described in the text. *(A is from Ahmad F, Turner SA, Torrie P, et al. Iatrogenic femoral artery pseudoaneurysms—a review of current methods of diagnosis and treatment.* Clin Radiol. *2008;63:1310, fig. 3.)*

Box 10.3 Management of Occupational Exposure to Hepatitis B Virus, Hepatitis C Virus, and HIV

I. Definition: Direct contact with blood or body fluids (including percutaneous injury), contact of mucous membranes, or skin contact, especially if abraded.

II. Procedure
   A. Clean site of exposure with soap and copious amounts of water; flush mucous membrane with large quantities of water.
   B. Victim should report incident promptly, including patient/source information.
   C. Provide wound care and review with victim tetanus and hepatitis B prophylaxis information.
   D. Counsel and obtain consent for HIV testing from both victim and patient/source.
   E. Order the following laboratory specimen with appropriate consent obtained:
      1. Victim: hepatitis C antibody, hepatitis B surface antigen, HIV
      2. Patient: hepatitis B surface antigen and core antibody, hepatitis C antibody, ALT, RPR, HIV
   F. Review hepatitis B vaccination and response status of victim, and follow postexposure prophylaxis to hepatitis B protocol.
   G. If patient is hepatitis C positive or has elevated ALT:
      1. Follow postexposure prophylaxis to hepatitis B protocol.
      2. Follow up for anti-HIV therapy per protocol.
      3. Schedule hepatitis C and HIV testing for 6 weeks, 3 months, and 6 months.

ALT, alanine aminotransferase; *HIV,* human immunodeficiency virus; *RPR,* rapid plasma reagin.
Adapted from table 2, page 85 of Chambers C, Eisenhauer M, McNicol L, et al. Infection control guidelines for the cardiac catheterization laboratory: society guidelines revisited. *Catheter Cardiovasc Interv.* 2006;67:78–86.

Table 10.4

Significant Risk Factors for Major Femoral Bleeding	
Risk Factor	**Odds Ratio**
Age >75 vs. <55	2.59
Heparin use postprocedure	2.46
Severe renal impairment	2.25
Age 65–74 vs. <55	2.18
Female patient	1.64
Closure device use	1.58
Sheath size 7F–8F vs. <6F	1.53
GP IIb/IIIa use	1.39
Longer procedure duration	1.2

Adapted from Doyle B, Ting HH, Bell MR, et al. Major femoral bleeding complications after PCI. *JACC Cardiovasc Interv.* 2008;1(2):202–9.

your hospital guidelines should be followed. See Box 10.3 for U.S. Public Health Service guidelines.

Bleeding

The last and most dangerous complication of groin access is major femoral bleeding. Large femoral hematomas have an incidence of 2.8% compared to a 0.3% incidence of retroperitoneal bleeds. A retroperitoneal hematoma or a significant femoral hematoma (>5 cm) often requires blood transfusions and prolonged hospitalization. More significant bleeds can require surgery, and significant bleeding in relation to PCI has been shown to correlate with mortality. Significant risk factors for major femoral bleeding are listed in Table 10.4.

The bleeding complication of most concern is a retroperitoneal hematoma because large amounts of blood can fill the pelvic cavity, and shock can develop rapidly. If a retroperitoneal bleed is suspected (Box 10.4), volume (crystalloid solutions) should be given and blood should be ordered immediately for transfusion as soon as available. A vascular surgeon should also be consulted immediately. If the patient remains hemodynamically unstable despite volume resuscitation, surgery or endovascular repair (covered stent placement) may be needed; this occurs in approximately 16% of patients. However, the majority (84%) of cases can undergo a conservative "watchful waiting" strategy because the hematoma usually stabilizes from tamponade of the initial site of extravasation. A computed tomography (CT) scan will be confirmative of the clinical diagnosis and should only be ordered once the patient is stable. Vascular surgeons use the CT scan as a baseline study and as a method to localize the origin of the bleed (if radiographic contrast media is used). Most retroperitoneal hematomas are caused by bleeding from the external iliac artery above the inguinal ligament or inferior epigastric artery. Rarely, bleeding below the inguinal ligament can track between tissue planes and extend into a retroperitoneal accumulation. Bleeding might also rarely extend to the scrotum through extension along the spermatic cord. Most cases of scrotal hematoma can also be managed conservatively with elevation and ice. However, rarely, large tense scrotal hematomas can cause significant pain and may compromise the viability of the scrotal skin and/or testicle, which would require urgent surgical exploration (Fig. 10.3).

Box 10.4 Classical Signs and Symptoms of Retroperitoneal Bleed

Hypotension
Bradycardia
Back/flank pain
Groin pain
Abdominal pain
Transient response to fluid loading
Grey Turner sign (bruising along flank) [late appearing]
Cullen sign (bruising around umbilicus) [late appearing]

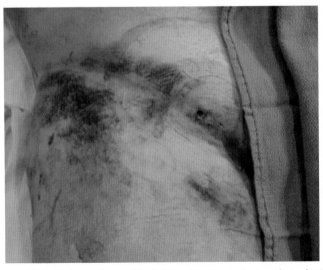

Figure 10.3 Picture of a patient following a cardiac catheterization utilizing femoral access who developed a large hematoma. *(Courtesy of Dr. Zoltan Turi.)*

Complications of Radial Access

Radial Artery Occlusion (2%–10%)

The radial artery may not be found to be patent following radial catheterization procedures; however, in most instances, the consequence of this complication is felt to be quite benign. This is mainly due to the nature of the dual circulation that exists between the radial artery and ulnar artery in supplying the hand with blood flow. When found to be intact by an Allen or Barbeau test prior to the procedure, circulation is believed to be intact from the ulnar artery through the palmar arch to supply the thumb and first finger with flow, thereby eliminating the complication of hand ischemia should the patency of the radial artery not remain following the procedure. Factors believed to be associated with radial occlusion include lack of adequate anticoagulation, too large a sheath size compared to the vessel size (e.g., consider 5F sheaths for smaller patients and women), prolonged and aggressive postprocedure compression without maintenance of forward flow, and repeat cannulations of the same radial artery.

When the radial artery has been imaged months after a radial catheterization, it has been noted that there is intimal hyperplasia within the radial artery with diffuse narrowing. This has been termed *nonocclusive radial artery injury*, but again, has not been associated with any serious complications from a patient standpoint.

Radial Artery Spasm (12%–22%)

Spasm of the vessel can occur and is frequently due to significant alpha$_1$ adenoreceptors within the medial layer of the vessel; it is overcome and minimized by the use of vasodilators (e.g., intra-arterial verapamil and/or nitroglycerin). Occasionally, it has been reported that a severe spasm entraps the catheter or long sheath so that it cannot be withdrawn. This diffuse and severe spasm has been managed by increased sedation, sometimes requiring a local nerve block or induction of general anesthesia. Care should be taken to never "force" the withdrawal of a catheter or sheath when resistance has been met because radial artery evulsion has also been reported.

Forearm Bleeding, Hematoma, and Compartment Syndrome

Bleeding within the forearm can arise if a perforation occurs anywhere within the course of the radial artery (Figs. 10.4 and 10.5). This can occur particularly with the use of hydrophilic guidewires (as opposed to nonhydrophilic J-tipped wires) that can advance into small side branches without much appreciated resistance felt by the operator. Furthermore, navigating anatomic variants such as a radial recurrent loop also increases the risk of perforation. Bertrand et al. studied this in a patient population that had all undergone radial artery catheterizations and subsequent interventions and classified the bleeding by grade. Bleeds were characterized as Grade I: superficial hematoma 5 cm or less in diameter (5.3% occurrence), Grade II: superficial hematoma 10 cm or less in diameter (2.5% occurrence), Grade III: hematoma greater than 10 cm but contained below the level of the elbow (1.6% occurrence), Grade IV: hematoma extending above the elbow (0.1%), Grade V: any bleed associated with an ischemic threat to the hand (0% occurrence). The keys to bleeding within the forearm are therefore prevention and recognition. Prevention can be achieved by avoiding hydrophilic straight guidewires for the most part. Bleeding must be recognized in the event of a hematoma or pain within the forearm after the procedure. If the sheath is still in place, angiography can demonstrate extravasation of contrast and thus the location of the

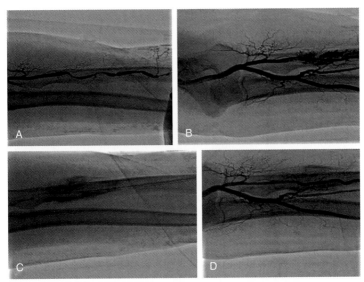

Figure 10.4 Radial artery rupture and salvage during coronary intervention through the radial artery. (A) Radial artery angiography through a 2.7F pressure arterial sheath after generous intra-arterial nitroglycerin and verapamil administration, revealing diffuse spasm of the entry site and stenosis of the middle portion of the radial artery. (B) Radial artery angiography through a 6F sheath, revealing rupture of the radial artery. (C) Prolonged balloon inflation. (D) Sealing and stenosis resolution after prolonged balloon inflation. *(From J Am Coll Cardiol Intv. 2009;2(11):1158–9, fig. 1.)*

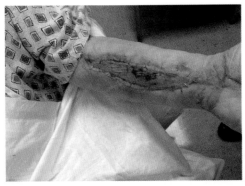

Figure 10.5 Photography of surgical repair with skin graft after compartment syndrome resulting from bleeding into the forearm.

bleed. Compression, often achieved with an ACE bandage wrapped around the entire forearm, and avoidance of further anticoagulation are often enough to avoid further complication.

However bleeding into the forearm can result in increased pressure within the fascial planes and resultant compartment syndrome. This would be the most serious complication from radial artery catheterization because it threatens the entire hand and must be recognized and treated emergently. Measurement of interfascial pressure with a manometer confirms the diagnosis, and fasciotomy with hematoma evacuation remains the only treatment available. Fortunately, this is a very rare occurrence.

Complications of Vascular Access Closure Devices

Many arterial access sites are closed in the laboratory with percutaneous vascular closure devices. Hemostasis success rates are less than 100%. Each device has failure modes particular to its mechanism of action. Suture fractures or failure to deliver a knot (Prostar, Perclose), clip failure (StarClose), collagen introduction or emboli into the vessel (Angio-Seal), or any failure to seal the puncture site can cause femoral or retroperitoneal bleeding. All vascular complications, including pseudoaneurysm, bleeding and hematoma, infection, arterial stenosis or occlusion, and venous thrombosis, can occur with an incidence of approximately 1%–5%.

Compared to manual compression, percutaneous closure device complications tend to have a greater incidence of pseudoaneurysms not amenable to ultrasound compression therapy, a greater loss of blood and need for transfusions, a greater incidence of arterial stenosis or occlusion, the need for more extensive surgical repair, and a greater incidence of groin infections. Thus, patients treated with vascular closure devices merit as much if not more attention to vascular complications than those treated with manual compression.

Atheroembolism

After vascular access is obtained, the guide catheter is advanced over a guidewire along the aorta to finally seat in the coronary artery of interest. The guidewire protects the vessels from the guide catheter scraping against the aortic wall and causing atheroembolism. This is even more common in larger diameter guide catheters. The guidewire itself can also cause atheroembolism. To minimize atheroembolism, always aspirate blood from the catheter to clear any debris that might have been picked up in transit. If a guide catheter is connected to a Y-connector during advancement, the valve should be cleared before proceeding.

Peripheral atheroembolism with obstruction of small arteries and arterioles by cholesterol crystals is known to produce the cholesterol embolization syndrome (CES), a rare occurrence (incidence of 0.75%–1.4%) using the preceding precautions. Cholesterol emboli are diagnosed by one of three cutaneous signs (see Box 10.5 and Fig. 10.6) and an elevated eosinophil count. In-hospital mortality is as high as 16% in those patients with definite CES because multiorgan embolization often can lead to multiorgan failure.

Atheroembolism can also cause a cerebral vascular accident (CVA) or transient ischemic attack (TIA). The overall incidence of TIA (0.04%) or CVA (0.25%) is quite low after PCI. There are various multivariate predictors of in-hospital CVA (see Table 10.5).

The most common indicator of a periprocedural TIA or CVA is motor or speech deficits. In-hospital death can occur in up to 25% of those with a CVA, but increased mortality is not expected with a TIA. Management follows recommendations of the neurologic consultation. If a stroke occurs during the procedure, consideration should be given for an emergent neurointervention with resultant cerebral angiography and intervention if an ischemic stroke with arterial occlusion is found.

Box 10.5 Cutaneous Signs of Cholesterol Embolization Syndrome

Livedo reticularis
Blue toe syndrome (also known as *purple toe syndrome or trash foot*)
Digital gangrene

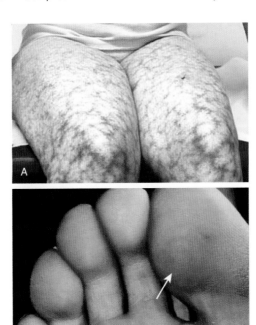

Figure 10.6 (A) Picture showing a patient with livedo reticularis on both legs secondary to the "showering" of emboli after a cardiac catheterization. (B) Picture of a patient's foot depicting the typical findings of cholesterol emboli to the great toe (*arrow*) following cardiac catheterization. *(A is from Kauke T, Reininger A. N Engl J Med. 2007;356:284. B is from Venzon R, Bromet D, Schaer G. Use of corticosteroids in the treatment of cholesterol crystal embolization after percutaneous transluminal coronary angioplasty.* J Invas Cardiol. *2004;16(4):222–3.)*

Table 10.5

Independent Predictors of In-Hospital Cardiovascular Accident (CVA)	
Predictor of CVA	**Odds Ratio**
Thrombolytics prior to PCI	4.7
Creatinine clearance <40 mL/min	3.1
Urgent or emergent PCI	2.7
Unplanned intra-aortic balloon pump	2.3
IV heparin prior to PCI	1.9
Hypertension	1.9
Diabetes	1.8

CVA, cerebrovascular accident; PCI, percutaneous coronary intervention.
Adapted from Dukkipati S, O'Neill WW, Harjai KJ, et al. Characteristics of cerebrovascular accidents after percutaneous coronary interventions. *J Am Coll Cardiol.* 2004;43(7):1161–7.

If a stroke occurs postprocedure, confirmed by advanced imaging (Fig. 10.7), then thrombolysis can be considered (after hemorrhagic stroke has been ruled out).

Complications Related to Guide Catheters, Balloons, Stents, and Intravascular Devices

The guide catheter itself can cause coronary dissection with or without extension to the aortic root. Guide catheter–related dissection is a rare

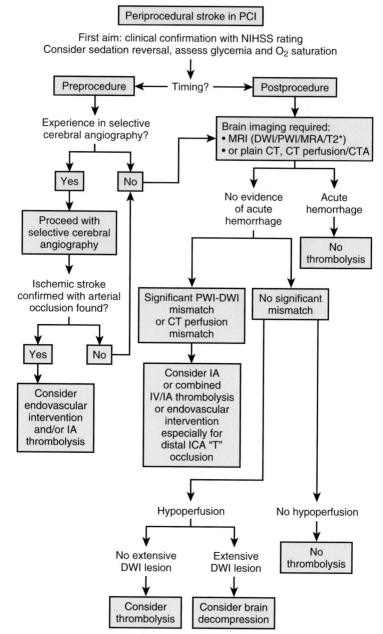

Figure 10.7 Suggested algorithm for the workup and treatment of an ischemic stroke following a catheterization procedure. *CT,* computed tomography; *CTA,* computed tomography angiography; *DWI,* diffusion-weighted imaging; *IA,* intra-arterial; *ICA,* internal carotid artery; *IV,* intravenous; *MRA,* magnetic resonance angiography; *MRI,* magnetic resonance imaging; *PWI,* perfusion-weighted imaging. *(Adapted from Hamon M, Baron JC, Viader F, et al. Periprocedural stroke and cardiac catheterization. Circulation. 2008;118:678–83.)*

event with a reported incidence of 0.03%–0.3%. The mechanism of the dissection is likely due to mechanical trauma to the intima of the vessel (either normal or with plaque) from a catheter that is wedged into the wall rather than lying coaxial in the vessel lumen. A jet of contrast from an abnormally seated catheter can aggravate or produce a coronary dissection. Dissection of the right coronary artery (RCA) from guide catheter trauma is more common than left main dissection because of relative size differences in the ostia. The Amplatz left guide catheters are the most likely to dissect the coronary artery; this is due to its predilection to dive deeply into the artery. Stenting the dissected area remains the standard of treatment. A guide catheter ostial or proximal dissection should be fixed before proceeding to the intended PCI lesion. The rationale is that if the dissection is not fixed, it can propagate forward and cause abrupt vessel closure or propagate backward and cause aortic dissection.

More commonly, coronary dissection is caused by balloon angioplasty trauma. Although microscopic dissections occur with every balloon angioplasty procedure, larger angiographically visible dissections are present in only 30%–50% of all angioplasty procedures. In the era before stenting, coronary dissection was a significant risk factor for acute or abrupt vessel closure, a rare phenomenon in modern PCI procedures with stents easily sealing the tissue flaps. The classifications of coronary dissections are provided in Table 10.6 and Fig. 10.8.

The incidence of aortic dissection caused by guide catheter trauma is very rare (0.02%–0.07%) (Fig. 10.9). Table 10.7 shows a classification scheme for extension of an aortic dissection. Almost all cases of retrograde extension of dissection are from the RCA although there are a couple of case reports of similar dissection from the left main. Class I and II lesions have a good prognosis and can be treated by stenting of the coronary dissection with close clinical follow-up. It is reasonable

Table 10.6

Classification of Coronary Dissection	
Type of Dissection	**Description**
Type A	Luminal haziness
Type B	Linear dissection
Type C	Extraluminal contrast staining
Type D	Spiral dissection
Type E	Dissection with reduced flow
Type F	Dissection with total occlusion

Dissection type	Description	Angiographic appearance
A	Minor radiolucencies within the coronary lumen during contrast injection with minimal or no persistence after dye clearance.	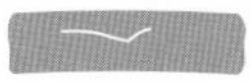
B	Parallel tracts or double lumen separated by a radiolucent area during contrast injection with minimal or no persistence after dye clearance.	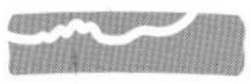
C	Extraluminal cap with persistence of contrast after dye clearance from the coronary lumen.	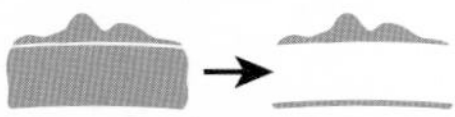
D	Spiral luminal filling defects.	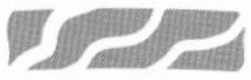
E+	New persistent filling defects.	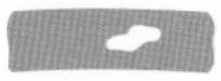
F+	Those non-A–E types that lead to impaired flow or total occlusion.	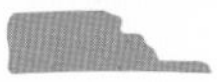
+ May represent thrombus.		

Figure 10.8 Types of coronary artery dissections: NHLBI classification system. *(From Safian R, Freed M, eds.* The Manual of Interventional Cardiology, *3rd ed. Birmingham, MI: Physicians' Press, 2001:389.)*

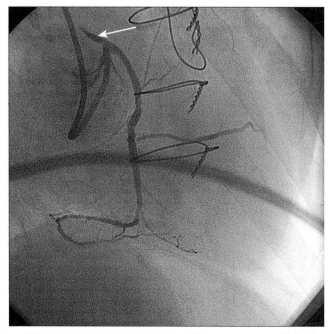

Figure 10.9 Angiogram of an anomalous right coronary artery following the placement of a stent. The arrow is pointing to a contrast stain extending upward from the ostium of the artery representing a dissection of the aorta caused by the guide catheter.

Table 10.7

Classification of Coronary Dissection With Retrograde Extension Into the Aortic Root	
Classification	**Extent of Aortic Involvement in the Dissection**
Class I	Involving the ipsilateral cusp
Class II	Involving cusp and extending up the aorta <40 mm
Class III	Involving cusp and extending up the aorta >40 mm

to follow the evolution of the dissection with imaging modalities (computed tomography [CT] or transesophageal echocardiogram [TEE]). If the patient remains stable over the next 24–48 hours of hospitalization, he or she can be safely discharged without the expectation for further complication. To reduce the chance of extension, the systolic blood pressure must be optimally controlled. However, antiplatelet therapy should not be suspended with a recently placed coronary stent. Class III lesions generally should be treated surgically and are associated with a high mortality rate.

Contrast Media Complications

Intravascular radiographic contrast media (RCM) can be associated with anaphylactoid reactions and acute renal failure. Fortunately, anaphylactoid reactions are rare, occurring in only 0.23% of procedures. Table 10.8 lists the severity classification for contrast-induced anaphylactoid reactions.

Anaphylactoid Reaction

An anaphylactoid reaction is different from an anaphylactic reaction. An anaphylactic reaction is an IgE-mediated hypersensitivity reaction

Table 10.8

Severity Classification for Contrast-Induced Anaphylactoid Reactions		
Minor	**Moderate**	**Severe**
Urticaria (limited)	Urticaria (diffuse)	Cardiovascular shock
Pruritus	Angioedema	Respiratory arrest
Erythema	Laryngeal edema	Cardiac arrest
	Bronchospasm	

requiring prior sensitization of the patient to a given antigen. An anaphylactoid reaction does not require prior sensitization and is not antibody mediated. Rather, it is an immediate hypersensitivity reaction caused by direct mast cell activation and/or activation of the kinin and complement cascades. As seen from Table 10.8, the symptoms of the reactions can be similar. Risk factors for an allergic reaction to RCM include prior RCM reaction (up to 60% chance of repeat reaction) and a history of atopy (asthma, allergic rhinitis, drug allergies, food allergies). Shellfish allergy simply is a marker for an atopic individual and therefore is a slightly higher risk of a RCM allergic reaction. Patients are no more likely to have an anaphylactoid reaction than patients with other food allergies. Shellfish allergy involves tropomyosin proteins as the antigen, having nothing to do with iodine content in various shellfish.

Individuals at risk of an anaphylactoid reaction require premedication. Prednisone 60 mg should be given the night before the procedure and the morning of the procedure. Benadryl 50 mg IV should also be given up to 1 hour before the procedure. If the first prednisone dose is missed, the glucocorticoid regimen loses its effectiveness. H_1 antihistamines have not been shown conclusively to reduce the risk of contrast-mediated reactions. Low osmolar or iso-osmolar contrast agents are used, which will further decrease the chance of an anaphylactoid reaction as compared to the obsolete high osmolar contrast agents.

Treatment of an anaphylactoid reaction depends on the severity of the reaction (see Table 10.9). For the most severe reactions, bolus epinephrine is prepared by mixing 0.1 mL of a 1 : 1000 solution or 1 mL of a 1 : 10,000 solution diluted in a 10-mL syringe with saline, producing a final concentration of 10 mcg/mL. If a patient has recently taken beta blockers, he or she might not have an adequate response to epinephrine. In this case, glucagon 1–2 mg IV over 5 minutes, then an infusion of 5–15 mcg/min, can be given to help reverse the effect of the beta blockade (by activating cyclic adenosine monophosphate [AMP] at a site independent from beta adrenergic agents).

Contrast-Induced Nephropathy (CIN)

Intravascular contrast media also can put the patient at risk for acute renal failure following PCI. This contrast-induced nephropathy (CIN) is likely caused by acute tubular necrosis. Mehran et al. developed a validated risk scoring system in order to predict the likelihood of developing CIN (see Fig. 10.10). CIN is typically defined as a relative increase in serum creatinine of greater than 25% or an absolute increase of greater than 0.5 mg/dL. While it is not uncommon to develop transient increases in serum creatinine, it is rare to need temporary dialysis and even rarer to need permanent dialysis following CIN. The time course of CIN demonstrates an increase in creatinine starting in 12–24 hours for most patients, but it may take as long as 48–96 hours to peak. Most cases show a return to baseline creatinine by days 3–5 but can take up to 7–10 days. Serum creatinine should be routinely obtained at 48–72 hours following contrast administration in a high-risk patient.

In high-risk patients, CIN prevention consists of two principles: adequate hydration and limitation of the volume of contrast administered.

Table 10.9

Treatment of Anaphylactoid Reactions in the Cardiac Catheterization Laboratory

Urticaria	Bronchospasm	Facial/Laryngeal Edema	Hypotension/Shock
Diphenhydramine 25–50 mg IV	Oxygen Albuterol Inhaler/nebulizer Diphenhydramine 50 mg IV Hydrocortisone 200–400 mg IV or methylprednisolone 125 mg IV *For severe reaction* Epinephrine bolus 10 mcg/min as needed. An infusion of 1–4 mcg/min might be needed as well.	Oxygen Emergent anesthesia consult for potential intubation. Tracheostomy tray should be available. Diphenhydramine 50 mg IV Epinephrine bolus/drip (as described under bronchospasm)	Epinephrine bolus until blood pressure (BP) is maintained; then start infusion (as described previously) 1 L normal saline bolus rapidly (pressure bag). Repeat as necessary. Diphenhydramine 50–100 mg IV Hydrocortisone 400 mg IV or methylprednisolone 125 mg IV

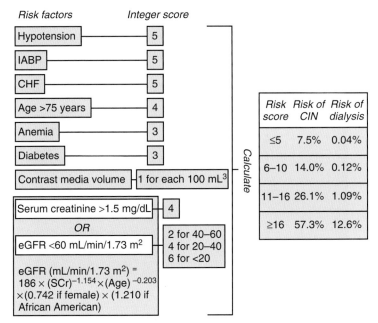

Figure 10.10 Risk score developed by Mehran et al. to predict the likelihood of developing postprocedural contrast-induced nephropathy (CIN). *CHF,* congestive heart failure; *eGFR,* estimated globular filtration rate; *IABP,* intra-aortic balloon pump.

The use of iso-osmolar contrast agents, sodium bicarbonate intravenous fluids, or *N*-acetylcysteine (600–1200 mg PO bid × 4 doses) are also purported to be effective, but the supporting data for each are weak. All other potential therapies, including diuretics, mannitol, dopamine, fenoldopam, or theophylline, have not been consistently proved to work for preventing CIN and should *not* be used.

Air Embolization

Another potential complication of coronary angiography and contrast media injection is air embolization (Fig. 10.11). This is always an iatrogenic complication due to failure to clear the air from the injection manifold system. Automatic contrast injection systems have a much lower rate of air embolism because of built-in air detection sensors. However, these systems do not fully eliminate the incidence of air embolism despite their inherent safety mechanisms and are not a replacement for a good manifold technique of aspiration and visual inspection for bubbles. Treatment of coronary air embolism consists of immediate initiation of 100% oxygen by facemask. The oxygen helps to minimize ischemia and produces a diffusion gradient favoring reabsorption of the air. If large bubbles persist, the air can be aspirated by various aspiration catheters.

Arrhythmias

Another general complication of PCI that might occur at any time during the procedure is arrhythmia (either tachycardia or bradycardia). Unstable tachycardias like ventricular tachycardia or ventricular fibrillation are more commonly seen in the setting of an acute MI. Bradycardia is most often seen in RCA occlusions; use of rotational atherectomy, especially in the RCA; or use of rheolytic thrombectomy catheters. Treatment of arrhythmias should follow standard advanced cardiovascular life support (ACLS) protocols. In general, for unstable patients,

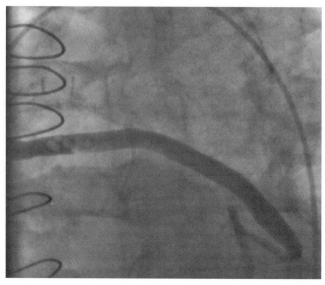

Figure 10.11 Angiogram obtained during a diagnostic catheterization depicting the injection of contrast into a vein graft to the obtuse marginal branch. On close inspection, several round objects can be seen in the proximal portion of this graft that represent air bubbles injected from the guide catheter.

it is always good practice to electrically cardiovert tachycardic arrhythmias. For unstable bradycardia, atropine can be given and transcutaneous pacing can be initiated. These measures can buy time to set up for temporary transvenous balloon flotation pacemaker placement. Transvenous pacemakers should be placed prophylactically for cases of rotational atherectomy in the RCA and in all cases of rheolytic thrombectomy. If transvenous pacing is not readily available, guidewire pacing (connecting the negative lead to guidewire and positive lead to patient) may be used, as it has been shown to be effective.

No Reflow

An acute cessation of coronary flow during PCI can occur as a result of abrupt occlusion or a consequence of distal failure of outflow. This observation, termed the *no reflow phenomenon* is used by some authors only in conjunction with microembolization, whereas others reserve the term for myocardial blush grades of 0 or 1 (regardless of coronary thrombolysis in myocardial infarction [TIMI] flow) in the setting of a primary PCI.

Regardless, the differential diagnosis of no reflow includes severe spasm, dissection, in situ thrombus, plaque rupture, or distal micro-embolization. If no reflow is due to thrombus or new plaque rupture, then manual catheter aspiration is appropriate. Additional anticoagulation with IIb/IIIa inhibitors should be started. Rechecking activated clotting time (ACT) levels is prudent. Additional angioplasty and stenting might be necessary.

If no reflow is due to dissection, additional stenting is necessary. If no reflow is due to severe spasm, intracoronary nitroglycerin doses at a concentration of 100 mcg/mL are given until the vasospasm is relieved. Although intracoronary nitroglycerin can help relieve vaso-spasm, it has not been shown to be effective in relief of the no reflow phenomenon from distal microembolization. See Table 10.10 for a list of medications that are effective in the no reflow phenomenon. Often, several grams of these agents given in small 100-mcg intracoronary boluses will be necessary.

Table 10.10

Pharmacologic Management of No Reflow Microembolization Syndrome	
Medicine	**Dose**
Adenosine	100 mcg/mL 1–2 mL bolus, reassess flow and hemodynamics
Nitroprusside	100 mcg/mL 1–2 mL IC bolus, reassess
Verapamil	100 mcg/mL 1–2 mL IC bolus, reassess

Table 10.11

Classification of Coronary Perforations	
Class	**Description**
I	Intramural crater without extravasation
II	Pericardial or myocardial blush/staining
III	Perforation >1 mm in diameter with contrast streaming or cavity spilling

No reflow from embolization to the microvasculature is most commonly seen in interventions on saphenous vein grafts and acute MIs. Prophylactic distal filters or proximal protection with the Proxis device can help reduce the embolic burden and prevent no reflow.

Coronary Perforation

The incidence of coronary perforation is 0.84% of PCI cases. Coronary perforation can be caused by a wire "exiting" the vessel or by a tear (dissection) in the vessel from balloon angioplasty, stenting, or rotational atherectomy. Table 10.11 shows the classification of coronary perforations.

Class I and II perforations are usually managed conservatively without any specific treatment. Class III perforations are associated with rapid development of tamponade (63%), the need for urgent bypass surgery (63%), and a high mortality rate (19%). To minimize the chance of wire perforation, hydrophilic tipped or stiff wires that are used to get through difficult lesions should be exchanged for workhorse wires with softer hydrophobic tips. If a *distal* perforation from a wire tip occurs, the first step should be balloon tamponade of the vessel at the perforation site. Prolonged (several minutes) inflations with test deflations can be tried over an hour. After every balloon inflation, a puff of contrast should be given to evaluate the status of the perforation. If balloon tamponade is not successful, the operator must consider distal coil placement. Anticoagulation should *not* be immediately reversed with the wire and balloon in the vessel during the attempted perforation occlusion. Immediate reversal could lead to thrombosis throughout the whole vessel, an event that leads to a higher degree of mortality than the perforation itself. Reversal of anticoagulation should be performed after the equipment is removed from the coronary vessel. Discontinue glycoprotein IIb/IIIa inhibitor after a perforation is visualized.

Covered stents are usually not helpful for distal wire perforations because of the tapered vessel size at their end. However, if a branch of a main vessel is leaking, the perforation can be excluded with a covered stent. For larger perforations, a covered stent placement with a polytetrafluoroethylene (PTFE)-covered stent is the standard of care.

If the perforation occurred after balloon and stent placement, the balloon should be immediately reinflated to stop further extravasation of blood into the pericardial space. At this point, a pericardial drain can be placed to relieve or protect against tamponade while definitive measures are taken to treat the perforation. Bivalirudin should be discontinued because it will take up to 2 hours to decrease the anticoagulation status to a normal level.

To place a covered stent, obtain contralateral access and, using a second guide catheter, intubate the perforated artery. The first guide catheter can be slightly backed out to allow intubation by the new guide. A 7F guide is recommended by the package insert to deliver the covered stents, although anecdotally, they have been delivered through 6F guiding catheters as well. Once the second guide is in place, a second guidewire should be used and placed up to the proximal edge of the inflated balloon. The balloon is then briefly deflated as the wire passes down to the distal vessel, and then the balloon is immediately reinflated. Next, a covered stent is placed over the second guidewire to the proximal edge of the inflated balloon. The balloon is deflated, and the balloon and first wire are removed as the covered stent is positioned and immediately deployed. Deployment should be done at higher atmospheres to ensure good apposition of the covered stent. If additional access is not available, a quick exchange of balloon for covered stent can be used as well. However, this allows at least 30–60 seconds of free coronary flow into the pericardial space, so a pericardial drain must already be in place. As little as 100 mL of an acute effusion can cause chamber compression and hemodynamic collapse. Once the covered stent is deployed and the coronary wire removed, heparin can be immediately reversed. The pericardial drain should be left in place overnight as a precautionary measure.

Retained PCI Equipment Components

Rarely, fragments of interventional equipment may break off and remain in a coronary artery. This may occur with guidewire tips from both fixed-wire and movable, over-the-wire balloon systems, or with distal fragments of various other catheters. These retained intravascular fragments carry the risk of coronary artery occlusion, distal embolization of clot, vessel perforation, infection, and ischemic complications. Dislodgement of stents from the delivery balloons has also been a source of retained interventional equipment.

Removal of intravascular fragments and foreign bodies should be done immediately to avoid the complications just mentioned, as well as incorporation of this material after several days during which the objects become coated and interred within the vessel. There are several techniques for removal of retained intravascular foreign bodies. Baskets, forceps, and snares are available and are manufactured in sizes appropriate for placement within the coronary arteries. Guidewire fracture has an incidence of 0.1%. Most cases of wire fracture have been reported with the rotational atherectomy wires.

There are multiple options for dealing with a retained wire fragment. A small wire fragment may be left in place and allowed to endothelialize, as a stent would. Dual antiplatelet therapy should be given if a wire is simply left in place.

For a wire fragment more centrally located in the vessel lumen, a stent can be deployed to trap the wire in place and avoid any possibility of further migration.

For a very long wire fragment extending into the guiding catheter, a balloon can be advanced to the end of the guide catheter and inflated, thereby trapping the wire against the side of the guide. At this point, the guide, balloon, and retained wire can be removed together.

For a longer wire fragment that does not extend into the guide, removal with a microsnare catheter may be the best choice. An over-the-wire balloon can be delivered next to a visible end of a retained guidewire (usually only the distal end is visible). A microsnare is then placed through the lumen of the over-the-wire balloon and is used to

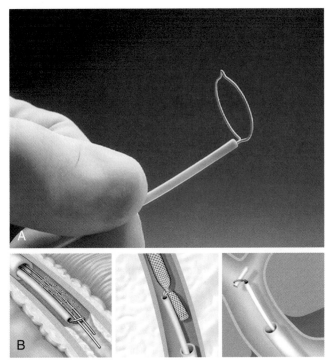

Figure 10.12 (A) Microvena snare for retrieval of intracoronary equipment fragments. (B) *Left panel:* Loop snare is used to capture a stent on second wire. *Middle:* Loop snare can be used to capture free stent. *Right panel:* Loop snare can capture catheter fragments. *(Courtesy Microvena Company, Minneapolis, MN.)*

lasso the retained wire. It can then be pulled into the guiding catheter and subsequently removed. If a microsnare (Fig. 10.12) is not readily available, using a two-wire technique, you can effectively ensnare a retained wire. This method is accomplished by placing two new guidewires next to the retained fragment. A single torquing device is placed over both wires, and the Y-connector is left slightly open as the torquing device is spun in one direction. This allows the two wires to form a double helix around each other; this helix will propagate distally and eventually ensnare the retained wire. All wires are then pulled back into the guide together (see Fig. 10.13).

Another rare complication is stent dislodgement and embolization, which occurs with an incidence of approximately 0.4%. Stent dislodgement most often occurs in tortuous, calcified vessels. Management options include retrieval, deployment in place, or crushing against the wall of the vessel with a balloon or new stent. Ideally, retrieval should be tried first so that the stent is not placed in an unintended position. Mortality rates as high as 17% have been reported for stent embolizations that are unsuccessfully managed (usually requiring emergent surgery), but they are as low as 0.9% in patients who have successful retrieval of a stent.

Retrieval methods are similar to those discussed with fractured wire retrieval. Microsnares or dual wires can be used to ensnare and remove the loose stent. Additional methods include advancing a small balloon over the same wire that the undeployed stent is floating on, inflating the balloon past the stent, and then pulling back the balloon, which should shift the free stent into the guide. If the stent is dislodged in a large proximal vessel, retrieval with myocardial biopsy forceps can be considered as well. If retrieval is not possible, then "playing the stent where it lies" (i.e., deploying or crushing the stent at that site) is the best option. To attempt to place the stent in its position, a small

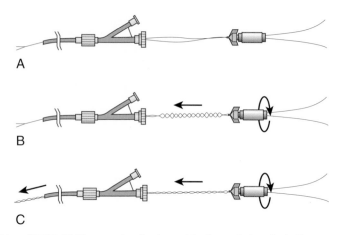

Figure 10.13 (A) Diagram showing two guidewires entering single Y-connector through a single torquing device. (B) The wires are torqued together forming a helix. (C) The helix propagates distally and can be used to ensnare a trapped wire fragment. *(From Gurley J, Booth D, Hixon C, et al. Removal of retained intracoronary percutaneous transluminal coronary angioplasty equipment by a percutaneous twin guidewire method.* Cathet Cardiovasc Diagn. *1990; 19:251–6.)*

balloon of similar or longer length than the stent is positioned across the profile of the stent. Initially, this can be attempted with a small 1.5-mm balloon blown up to 1–2 atm; this might be enough to capture the stent and move the system as a whole to a more desirable spot (to the initial lesion or at least out of the left main). If it cannot be moved, the balloon should be deployed at full atmospheres to dilate the stent as much as possible. A second undeflated balloon equal to the vessel diameter can then be placed to ensure adequate stent apposition. Rarely, a small-diameter balloon will not recross the stent. In this case, a second wire is placed down next to the embolized stent, and another stent is placed adjacent to the embolized stent and is used to crush the loose stent against the arterial wall. In more than 50% of cases of embolization, the stent might be embolized to the peripheral arteries. In these cases, snares or forceps can be used to retrieve the stent if it can be visualized in the periphery.

Stent Thrombosis

Stent thrombosis is a rare but devastating complication of PCI. Mortality rates are reported from 25% to 40%. Stent thrombosis is defined as acute (<24 hours), subacute (within 30 days), late (between 1 month and 1 year), or very late (>1 year). In an attempt to standardize the definition of stent thrombosis, the academic research consortium divided the criteria for stent thrombosis into definite, probable, or possible (see Table 10.12).

Both bare metal stent (BMS) thrombosis and drug-eluting stent (DES) thrombosis occur most commonly in the acute or subacute time frame. DES, however, also have a higher risk of thrombosis in the late and very late period due to incomplete endothelialization; this provides a strong argument for continuing dual antiplatelet therapy for at least 1 year after DES implantation. Premature discontinuation of dual antiplatelet therapy is the greatest risk factor for stent thrombosis. Other risk factors are listed in Box 10.6.

Almost one-third of patients in whom antiplatelet therapy is discontinued prematurely are at risk of stent thrombosis. Because DES require a longer duration of dual antiplatelet therapy, it is crucial to decide before the diagnostic angiogram if the patient is an appropriate

Table 10.12

Academic Research Consortium Criteria for Stent Thrombosis	
Definition	**Criteria**
Definite stent thrombosis	Angiographic confirmation of thrombus that originates inside or within 5 mm of the stent which is associated with symptoms, electrocardiogram (ECG) changes, or biomarker elevation, or pathologic confirmation of stent thrombosis determined at autopsy, or from tissue obtained following thrombectomy
Probable stent thrombosis	Unexplained death occurring within 30 days after the index procedure, or a myocardial infarction occurring at any time after the index procedure that was documented by ECG or imaging to occur in an area supplied by the stented vessel in the absence of angiographic confirmation of stent thrombosis or other culprit lesion
Possible stent thrombosis	Unexplained death occurring more than 30 days after the index procedure

---

Box 10.6 Risk Factors for Stent Thrombosis

Premature discontinuation of antiplatelet therapy
Incomplete stent expansion
Greater stent length
Subtherapeutic periprocedural anticoagulation
Cocaine use
Prior brachytherapy
Postprocedure TIMI flow grade <3
Treatment of bifurcation lesion

TIMI, thrombolysis in myocardial infarction.

---

candidate for long-term dual antiplatelet therapy. If a patient cannot afford or cannot take long-term dual antiplatelet therapy, or if the patient requires surgery in the next 12 months that would necessitate discontinuation of antiplatelet therapy, consider BMS use. Similarly, if the patient currently requires long-term Coumadin, or if the patient has a history of major bleeding episodes, he or she may not be a candidate for long-term dual antiplatelet therapy, and BMS placement should be employed.

Stent Infection

The rarest complication of PCI is stent infection. There are fewer than 20 case reports of intracoronary stent infection in the literature, which include both DES and BMS. In some cases mycotic aneurysms are formed at the site of stenting, but other cases present with persistent bacteremia. *Staphylococcus aureus* is the most common microorganism implicated. Stent infection presents within 4 weeks after stent implantation with fever and bacteremia. Typical findings of chest pain, ECG changes, and troponin elevation might be absent. A high degree of suspicion should accompany any fever occurring within 1 month of PCI. Confirmation of the diagnosis may be difficult with imaging. In addition to antibiotic therapy, most cases (>60%) will require surgery. In general, there is up to a 40% mortality rate with stent infection. Strict infection control measures (as discussed in *The Cardiac Catheterization Handbook*, 5e) must be adhered to in the catheterization laboratory.

Box 10.7 Risk Factors for Bacteremia After Cardiac Catheterization

Avoidable Risk Factors

Difficult vascular access
Multiple skin punctures
Repeated catheterization at the same vascular access site
Extended duration of the procedure
Use of multiple PTCA balloons
Deferred removal of the arterial sheath

Unavoidable Risk Factors

Presence of congestive heart failure
Patient's age >60

PTCA, percutaneous transluminal coronary angioplasty.
Adapted from Kaufman B, Kaiser C, Pfisterer M et al. Coronary stent infection: a rare but severe complication of percutaneous coronary intervention. *Swiss Med Wkly.* 2005;135:483–7.

Risk factors for bacteremia associated with cardiac catheterization are shown in Box 10.7.

Suggested Readings

Aggarwal B, Ellis SG, Lincoff AM, et al. Cause of death within 30 days of percutaneous coronary intervention in an era of mandatory outcome reporting. *J Am Coll Cardiol.* 2013;62(5):409-415.

Ahmad F, et al. Iatrogenic femoral artery pseudoaneurysms – a review of current methods of diagnosis and treatment. *Clin Radiol.* 2008;63(12):1310-1316.

Al-Lamee R, Ielasi A, Latib A, et al. Incidence, predictors, management, immediate and long-term outcomes following grade III coronary perforation. *J Am Coll Cardiol.* 2011;4:87-95.

Amin AP, Caruso M, Artero PC, et al. Reducing bleeding complications in the cathlab: a patient-centered approach. *J Am Coll Cardiol.* 2016;67(13S):84-84.

Bashore TM, Gehrig T. Cholesterol emboli after invasive cardiac procedures. *J Am Coll Cardiol.* 2003;42:217-218.

Chambers C, et al. Infection control guidelines for the cardiac catheterization laboratory: society guidelines revisited. *Catheter Cardiovasc Interv.* 2006;67:78-86.

Chan YC, et al. Management of spontaneous and iatrogenic retroperitoneal haemorrhage: conservative management, endovascular intervention or open surgery? *Int J Clin Pract.* 2008;62(10):1604-1613.

Doyle B, et al. Bleeding, blood transfusion, and increased mortality after percutaneous coronary intervention: implications for contemporary practice. *J Am Coll Cardiol.* 2009;53:2019-2027.

Dukkipati S, O'Neill WW, Harjai KJ, et al. Characteristics of cerebrovascular accidents after percutaneous coronary interventions. *J Am Coll Cardiol.* 2004;43(7):1161-1167.

Dunning DW, et al. Iatrogenic coronary artery dissections extending into and involving the aortic root. *Catheter Cardiovasc Interv.* 2000;51:387-393.

Frank JJ, Kamalakanna D, Kodenchery M, et al. Retroperitoneal hematoma in patients undergoing cardiac catheterization. *J Interv Cardiol.* 2010;23:569-574.

Fuchs S, Stabile E, Kinnaird TD, et al. Stroke complicating percutaneous coronary interventions: incidence, predictors, and prognostic implications. *Circulation.* 2002;106(1):86-91.

Fukumoto Y, et al. The incidence and risk factors of cholesterol embolization syndrome, a complication of cardiac catheterization: a prospective study. *J Am Coll Cardiol.* 2003;42:211-216.

Gavlick K, et al. Snare retrieval of the distal tip of a fractured rotational atherectomy guidewire: roping the steer by its horns. *J Invasive Cardiol.* 2005;17(12):E55-E58.

Grines CL, et al. Prevention of premature discontinuation of dual antiplatelet therapy in patients with coronary artery stents: a science advisory from the AHA, ACC, SCAI, ACS, ADA, with representation from the ACP. *J Am Coll Cardiol.* 2007;49:734-739.

Gurm GS, Seth M, Kooiman J, et al. A novel tool for reliable and accurate prediction of renal complications in patients undergoing percutaneous coronary intervention. *J Am Coll Cardiol.* 2013;61(22):2242-2248.

Hamon M, et al. Periprocedural stroke and cardiac catheterization. *Circulation.* 2008;118:678-683.

Han C, Strauss C, Garberich R, et al. Prospective decision support tool guides usage of vascular closure devices that reduce bleeding complications, length of stay, and variable costs in high bleed risk patients. *J Am Coll Cardiol.* 2016;67(13S):73.

Holmes DR, et al. Iatrogenic pericardial effusion and tamponade in the percutaneous intracardiac intervention era. *JACC Cardiovasc Interv.* 2009;2(8):706-718.

Holmes DR, et al. Stent thrombosis. *J Am Coll Cardiol.* 2010;56:1357-1365.

Mamas MA, Anderson SG, Carr M, et al. Baseline bleeding risk and arterial access site practice in relation to procedural outcomes after percutaneous coronary intervention. *J Am Coll Cardiol.* 2014;64(15):1554-1564.

Mathias W, Tsutsui JM, Tavares BG, et al. Diagnostic ultrasound impulses improve microvascular flow in patients with STEMI receiving intravenous microbubbles. *J Am Coll Cardiol.* 2016;67(21):2506-2515.

Mehran R, et al. A simple risk score for prediction of contrast-induced nephropathy after percutaneous coronary intervention. *J Am Coll Cardiol.* 2004;44(7):1393-1399.

Mixon TA, et al. Temporary coronary guidewire pacing during percutaneous coronary intervention. *Catheter Cardiovasc Interv.* 2004;61:494-500.

Nayak KR, et al. Anaphylactoid reactions to radiocontrast agents: prevention and treatment in the cardiac catheterization laboratory. *J Invasive Cardiol.* 2009;21:548-551.

Ndrepepa G, et al. Predictive factors and impact of no reflow after primary percutaneous coronary intervention in patients with acute myocardial infarction. *Circ Cardiovasc Interv.* 2010;3:27-33.

Niccoli G, et al. Myocardial no-reflow in humans. *J Am Coll Cardiol.* 2009;54(4):281-292.

Parsh J, Seth M, Green J, et al. The deadly impact of coronary perforation in women undergoing PCI: insights from BMC2. *J Am Coll Cardiol.* 2016;67(13S):179-179.

Patel V, Michael T, Mogabgab O, et al. Clinical, angiographic and procedural predictors of periprocedural complications in coronary chronic total occlusion PCI. *J Am Coll Cardiol.* 2013;61(10S).

Patterson MS, Kiemeneij F. Coronary air embolism treated with aspiration catheter. *Heart.* 2005;91(5):e36.

Prasad A, Banerjee S, Brilakis ES. Hemodynamic consequences of massive coronary air embolism. *Circulation.* 2007;115:51-53.

Prasan A, Brieger D, Adams M, et al. Stent deployment within a guide catheter aids removal of a fractured buddy wire. *Catheter Cardiovasc Interv.* 2002;56:212-214.

Rezkalla SH, Kloner RA. Coronary no-reflow phenomenon: from the experimental laboratory to the cardiac catheterization laboratory. *Catheter Cardiovasc Interv.* 2008;72:950-957.

Sankaranarayanan R, Msairi A, Davis GK. Review: stroke complicating cardiac catheterization: a preventable and treatable complication. *J Invasive Cardiol.* 2007;19:40-45.

Seshadri N, Whitlow PL, Acharya N, et al. Emergency coronary artery bypass surgery in the contemporary percutaneous coronary intervention era. *Circulation.* 2002;106(18):2346-2350.

Stankovic G, Orlic D, Corvaja N, et al. Incidence, predictors, in-hospital, and late outcomes of coronary artery perforations. *Am J Cardiol.* 2004;93(2):213-216.

Subherwal S, Peterson ED, Dai D, et al. Temporal trends in and factors associated with bleeding complications among patients undergoing percutaneous coronary intervention: a report from the National Cardiovascular Data CathPCI Registry. *J Am Coll Cardiol.* 2012;59(21):1861-1869.

van Werkum JW, Heestermans AA, Zomer AC, et al. Predictors of coronary stent thrombosis: the Dutch Stent Thrombosis Registry. *J Am Coll Cardiol.* 2009;53(16):1399-1409.

11

Peripheral Vascular Intervention

ANDREW J. KLEIN · AMMAR NASIR ·
PRANAV M. PATEL

Peripheral arterial disease (PAD) refers to stenotic, occlusive, and aneurysmal diseases of the aorta and branch arteries that include the lower extremity, upper extremity, renal, mesenteric, and carotid arterial beds. PAD is a common manifestation of atherosclerosis, and its prevalence increases with age and concurrent cardiovascular risk factors such as diabetes and tobacco use. PAD also encompasses aneurysms and vasculitic processes. As with coronary artery disease (CAD), PAD has a natural history, progression pattern, and susceptibility for developing vulnerable and complex plaques with a strong positive correlation to cardiovascular events and mortality.

This chapter will focus exclusively on peripheral arterial intervention excluding endovascular aneurysm repair (EVAR) and other large vessel aneurysm treatment as well as vasculitides, given these topics are broad and require distinct review of their own. Regardless, interventional cardiologists who wish to perform peripheral vascular intervention (PVI) need to be familiar with all systemic diseases that impact every aspect of the vascular system. This requires specialized training in both vascular and endovascular medicine, which is separate and distinct from training in coronary intervention. In addition, PVI incorporates venous intervention, which also requires additional training and expertise.

Cardiologists are perfectly positioned to treat patients with PAD based on their expertise in the foundations of care for patients with atherosclerotic vascular disease including PAD. Given that patients with PAD are at marked risk of cardiovascular morbidity and mortality—primarily due to stroke (from cerebrovascular atherosclerosis) and myocardial infarction (MI; from coronary atherosclerosis)—risk factor reduction/modification of atherosclerosis and concomitant comorbidities that increase cardiovascular morbidity and mortality including tobacco use, hypertension, dyslipidemia, and diabetes is paramount. Cardiovascular disease is the major cause of death in patients with intermittent claudication. Patients with newly diagnosed PAD are 6 times more likely to die within the next 10 years when compared with patients without PAD.

When assessing patients with possible PAD, an accurate history and physical is most important. One must assess PAD risk factors, optimize medical therapy, and address foot care. The American College of Cardiology/American Heart Association (ACC/AHA) developed guidelines to aid in the diagnosis and management of patients with PAD. These guidelines suggest that the following individuals would be at risk from PAD:

- Age less than 50 years, with diabetes and one other atherosclerosis risk factor (smoking, dyslipidemia, hypertension, or hyperhomocysteinemia)

- Age 50–69 years and history of smoking or diabetes
- Age 70 or older
- Symptoms with exertion involving the lower extremities (suggestive of claudication) or ischemic rest pain
- Abnormal lower extremity pulse examination
- Known atherosclerotic coronary, carotid, or renal artery disease

It is essential to assess PAD risk factors, perform CAD screening tests for cardiovascular disease and optimize medical therapy. The key component to the diagnosis of PAD is the presence of symptoms. However, fewer than 20% of PAD patients report the typical symptoms of intermittent claudication which include:

1. A history of walking impairment, claudication, ischemic rest pain, and/or nonhealing wounds is recommended as a required component of a standard review of symptoms for adults 50 years and older who have atherosclerosis risk factors and for adults 70 years and older.

2. Individuals with asymptomatic lower extremity PAD should be identified by examination and/or measurement of the ankle-brachial index (ABI) so that therapeutic interventions known to diminish their increased risk of MI, stroke, and death may be offered.

3. Smoking cessation, lipid lowering, and diabetes and hypertension treatment according to current national treatment guidelines are recommended for individuals with asymptomatic lower extremity PAD.

4. Antiplatelet therapy is indicated for individuals with asymptomatic lower extremity PAD to reduce the risk of adverse cardiovascular ischemic events.

   Patients with symptoms of intermittent claudication should undergo a vascular physical examination, including measurement of the ABI and if the resting index is normal with exercise.

   Before undergoing evaluation for revascularization, patients with intermittent claudication should have significant functional impairment with a reasonable likelihood of symptomatic improvement and absence of other disease that would comparably limit exercise even if the claudication was improved (e.g., angina, heart failure, chronic respiratory disease, or orthopedic limitations).

   Individuals with intermittent claudication who are offered the option of endovascular or surgical therapies should:

   (a) be provided information regarding supervised claudication exercise therapy and pharmacotherapy;

   (b) receive comprehensive risk factor modification and antiplatelet therapy;

   (c) have a significant disability, either being unable to perform normal work or having serious impairment of other activities important to the patient; and

   (d) have lower extremity PAD lesion anatomy such that the revascularization procedure would have low risk and a high probability of initial and long-term success.

The key component to the diagnosis of PAD is the presence of symptoms or a screening ABI performed in the appropriate population. Patients may present with classical claudication, which is muscle cramping from lack of oxygen upon exertion due to an upstream occlusion/stenosis that is relieved with rest. Intermittent claudication is the most classic manifestation of PAD. The sensitivity of the Rose claudication questionnaire approaches approximately 10%–30%; however, similar questions (and modifications to the Rose questionnaire) are still very helpful in diagnosing intermittent claudication.

True vascular claudication must be distinguished from "pseudo-claudication" caused by severe venous obstructive disease, chronic compartment syndrome, lumbar disease and spinal stenosis, osteoarthritis, and inflammatory muscle diseases. The characteristic features of pseudoclaudication that distinguish it from claudication and questions on intermittent claudication are summarized in Table 11.1 and Box 11.1.

Symptoms of intermittent claudication classically start distally within a muscle group (below the stenosis) and then ascend with continued activity. Rest pain that occurs with leg elevation and is relieved paradoxically by walking may suggest severe PAD (because the effects of gravity increase arterial perfusion of muscle groups). Critical PAD may present as tissue ulceration and gangrene. The ACC/AHA guidelines suggest that individuals with PAD present in clinical practice with distinct syndromes (Box 11.2).

However, 10%–30% of PAD patients may report atypical symptoms. Additionally, despite numerous studies demonstrating a poor quality of life in patients with PAD secondary to limited functionality, many patients with atherosclerosis of the lower extremities often underreport

Table 11.1

Distinguishing Characteristics Between Claudication and Pseudoclaudication

	Claudication	Pseudoclaudication
Characteristic of discomfort	Cramping, tightness, aching, fatigue	Same as claudication plus tingling, burning, numbness
Location of discomfort	Buttock, hip, thigh, calf, foot	Same as claudication
Induced by exercise	Yes	Variable
Reproducible with distance walked	Consistent	Variable
Occurs with standing	No	Yes
Actions which provide relief	Standing	Sitting, change position
Time to relief	<5 minutes	≤30 minutes

Box 11.1   Rose Questionnaire: Symptoms of Classic Intermittent Claudication

Calf pain caused by exertion that:
1. Does not occur at rest
2. Does not resolve during walking
3. Stops the patient from continuous walking
4. Resolves within 10 minutes of rest

Box 11.2   Clinical Syndromes of patients with PAD

Asymptomatic: Without obvious symptomatic complaint (but usually with a functional impairment)
Classic claudication: Lower extremity symptoms confined to the muscles with a consistent (reproducible) onset with exercise and relief with rest
"Atypical" leg pain: Lower extremity discomfort that is exertional but that does not consistently resolve with rest, consistently limits exercise at a reproducible distance, or meets all "Rose questionnaire" criteria
Critical limb ischemia: Ischemic rest pain, nonhealing wound, or gangrene
Acute limb ischemia: The five P's, defined by the clinical symptoms and signs that suggest potential limb jeopardy: Pain, Pulselessness, Pallor, Paresthesias, Paralysis, and Polar cool or cold limb (as a sixth "P")

symptoms. For those with symptoms of claudication or atypical symptoms (fatigue, numbness, pain, loss of power), a careful review of functional status over time is essential because this disease process also progresses in a large subset of patients, despite teaching to the contrary. At each clinic visit, a careful review of symptoms must be obtained and should include the following:

- Any exertional limitation of the lower extremity muscles or any history of impaired ambulation. This limitation may be described as cramping, fatigue, aching, numbness, or pain. The primary site(s) of discomfort in the buttock, thigh, calf, or foot should be documented, along with the relation of such discomfort to rest or exertion.
- Any poorly healing or nonhealing wounds of the legs or feet
- Any pain at rest localized to the lower leg or foot and its association with the upright or recumbent positions
- Postprandial abdominal pain that is provoked by eating and associated with weight loss
- Family history of a first-degree relative with an abdominal aortic aneurysm (AAA)

The physical exam defines the location, severity, and etiology of PAD and its symptoms. Arterial pulse intensity should be assessed and should be recorded numerically as shown in Table 11.2. Physical examination for PAD must include assessment of blood pressure in both arms (to assess for upper extremity arterial disease) and careful evaluation of all pulses (Box 11.3). All pulses should be assessed (with Doppler if needed for strength and character—diffuse versus normal), as well as presence of bruits (carotid, supraclavicular, abdominal, femoral). Careful examination of the musculoskeletal system is imperative to document muscle atrophy and any joint effusions that may imply a potential systemic inflammatory process leading to the presenting symptoms. The legs should be examined for any evidence of impaired circulation such as hair loss and/or smooth/shiny skin. Careful inspection of the feet for wounds, dystrophic nails, coolness,

Table 11.2

Gradation of Arterial Pulse	
Numerical Gradation	**Clinical Assessment**
0	Absent
1	Diminished
2	Normal
3	Bounding

Box 11.3 Physical Examination Findings of PAD

Limb examination (and comparison with the opposite limb) includes:
1. Absent or diminished femoral or pedal pulses (especially after exercising the limb)
2. Arterial bruits
3. Hair loss
4. Poor nail growth (brittle nails)
5. Dry, scaly, atrophic skin
6. Dependent rubor
7. Pallor with leg elevation after 1 minute at 60 degrees (normal color should return in 10–15 seconds; longer than 40 seconds indicates severe ischemia)
8. Ischemic tissue ulceration (punched-out, painful, with little bleeding), gangrene

pallor, or cyanosis of the foot must be made at every visit. Dry, cracking skin, which can be a nidus for cellulitis, as well as tinea, must be evaluated and treated.

Diagnostic Testing

Ankle-Brachial Index

Determining the ABI both at rest and after exercise is very useful especially in individuals at risk of developing PAD. The toe-brachial index (TBI) should be used in individuals with noncompressible pedal pulses (e.g., the elderly). Exercise ABI may be even more useful than resting ABI, serving to unmask PAD when resting ABI is normal. Exercise ABI testing will also assess the functional severity of claudication and aid differentiation of intermittent claudication from pseudoclaudication. Performing segmental ABI and pulse volume recordings together with the ABI can indicate presence of multilevel occlusive lower extremity PAD.

Duplex Ultrasound

Arterial duplex ultrasound of the extremities identifies the anatomic location and degree of stenosis of PAD. This imaging modality is technologist dependent but, when coupled with ABIs, can provide useful information without the need for contrast or radiation. Duplex is often used to monitor for restenosis after lower extremity revascularization.

Magnetic Resonance Angiography

Magnetic resonance angiography (MRA) of the extremities is also useful to diagnose anatomic location and degree of stenosis of PAD. The MRA should be performed with gadolinium enhancement. Although it must be noted that gadolinium use in individuals with an estimated glomerular filtration rate (eGFR) of less than 60 mL/min has been associated with nephrogenic systemic fibrosis (NSF)/nephrogenic fibrosing dermopathy. MRA of the extremities is useful in selecting patients with lower extremity PAD as candidates for endovascular intervention, however, it can often overestimate the degree of stenosis and fails to show the degree of vessel calcification.

Computerized Tomographic Angiography

Computed tomography angiography (CTA) of the extremities also diagnoses the anatomic location and presence of significant stenosis in patients with lower extremity PAD. CTA may be considered as a substitute for MRA for those patients with contraindications to MRA (claustrophobia, presence of non-MRI compatible pacemaker/implantable cardioverter-defibrillator) but does require the use of intravenous contrast and some radiation exposure.

Peripheral Vascular or Endovascular Intervention

Patient Selection for Peripheral Endovascular Intervention

When considering patients for PVI, an accurate history and physical is most important. Current ACC guidelines suggest that a vascular history and physical exam are essential prior to any intervention:

1. Individuals at risk for lower extremity PAD should undergo a vascular review of symptoms to assess walking impairment, claudication, ischemic rest pain, and/or the presence of nonhealing wounds.
2. Individuals at risk for lower extremity PAD should undergo comprehensive pulse examination and inspection of the feet.
3. Individuals over 50 years of age should be asked if they have a family history of a first-order relative with an AAA.

Endovascular procedures or *percutaneous catheter-based revascularization techniques* is the group name for techniques used to achieve the nonsurgical revascularization of PAD patients. Endovascular therapy offers several distinct advantages over surgical revascularization:

1. Performed using local anesthesia, enabling the treatment of patients who are at high risk for general anesthesia
2. Lower morbidity and mortality compared to surgical revascularization
3. Earlier ambulation on the day of treatment and earlier return to normal activity within 24–48 hours
4. Endovascular therapies may be repeated if necessary, generally without increased difficulty or increased patient risk compared to the first procedure.
5. Prior angioplasty does not preclude surgery if required at a later date.

Problems secondary to endovascular intervention are generally related to bleeding and vascular access.

The evaluation prior to performing endovascular intervention is identical to that for a patient undergoing cardiac catheterization and includes a complete blood count, serum electrolytes, coagulation panel (activated partial prothromboplastin time, prothrombin time, international normalized ratio), serum creatinine, glomerular filtration rate, stool Hemoccult, and fasting glucose.

Premedication

The standard premedication for endovascular intervention includes aspirin therapy (81–325 mg/day). Other antiplatelet agents (clopidogrel, ticagrelor, prasugrel) have been used prior to carotid artery and cerebrovascular intervention. There are no data to suggest that the use of these additional antiplatelet agents increases the procedural success rate or decreases the rate of complications. Their use is optional.

Vascular Access

Successful endovascular intervention requires appropriate choice of vascular access. In most cases access is obtained using a 21-gauge needle and 0.18-inch wire (4F micropuncture set). The retrograde approach to the common femoral artery (CFA) is the most frequently used vascular access. The inguinal crease is highly variable in relation to the CFA bifurcation in up to 75% of patients. Identifying the femoral head under fluoroscopy is very helpful (Fig. 11.1) because this will help ensure puncture of the vessel above the CFA bifurcation and below the inguinal ligament. Vascular access with the use of ultrasound imaging is also safe and effective because this allows direct imaging of the vessel.

The majority of PVIs can be performed from several access sites (Box 11.4). Box 11.5 suggests some of the most useful angiographic views for different vascular territories. On most occasions the location of the lesion (to be intervened upon) will determine the most appropriate access site. Retrograde CFA access permits selective angiography and intervention of the contralateral pelvic and lower extremity vessels.

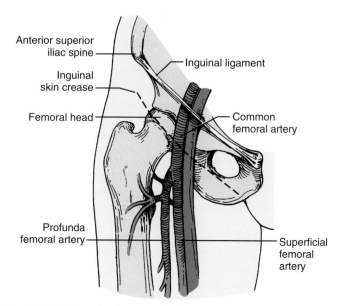

Anterior superior iliac spine

Inguinal skin crease

Femoral head

Profunda femoral artery

Inguinal ligament

Common femoral artery

Superficial femoral artery

Figure 11.1 Schematic diagram showing vascular supply in right femoral area.

Box 11.4   Arterial Access for Different Vascular Territories

Vascular Access	Artery to Revascularize
Retrograde CFA	Arch vessels, renal, and mesenteric
Contralateral CFA	Contralateral iliacs, CFA, PFA, SFA, popliteal
Antegrade CFA	Mid-distal femoral, popliteal, infrapopliteal
Brachial/radial artery	Renal (caudal takeoff), mesenteric, iliac arteries
Retrograde popliteal artery	SFA and iliac artery
Retrograde pedal	Infrapopliteal, popliteal, SFA

CFA, common femoral artery; *PFA,* profunda femoral artery; *SFA,* superficial femoral artery.

Box 11.5   Most Useful Angiographic Views for Different Vascular Territories

Artery or Vascular Territory	Angiographic View
Aortic arch	30–60-degree LAO (with slight cranial angulation)
Brachiocephalic vessels (origin)	30–60-degree LAO
Subclavian	AP, ipsilateral oblique with caudal angulation
Vertebral origin	AP, ipsilateral oblique with cranial angulation
Carotid extracranial	Lateral, AP, ipsilateral oblique
Renal arteries (origin)	AP to LAO 10–15 degrees
Mesenteric arteries (origin)	Lateral or steep RAO
Iliac artery	Contralateral 20- to 45-degree oblique and 20-degree caudal
CFA, SFA, and PFA arteries	Ipsilateral 30–60-degree oblique
Femoropopliteal	AP
Infrapopliteal trifurcation and runoff	AP

AP, anteroposterior; *CFA,* common femoral artery; *LAO,* left anterior oblique; *PFA,* profunda femoris artery; *SFA,* superficial femoral artery; *RAO,* right anterior oblique.

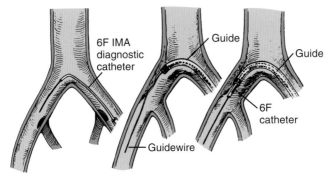

Figure 11.2 Schematic diagram of contralateral femoral access.

After gaining retrograde access (Fig. 11.2) to the CFA, the contralateral iliofemoral system is reached by placing a diagnostic catheter with an acute bend at the tip (usually an internal mammary artery, rim, omniflush, or Simmons catheter) at the aortic bifurcation. The catheter is manipulated so that the tip "engages" the ostium of the contralateral common iliac artery (CIA). A stiff, angled 0.035-inch Glidewire (Terumo Medical Corp, Somerset, NJ) is then carefully steered to the femoral artery and the diagnostic catheter is advanced over the Glidewire into the CFA. The Glidewire is then exchanged through the diagnostic catheter for a stiff guidewire (Amplatz extra-stiff, Cook, Bloomington, IN), which is advanced into the distal femoral artery. The diagnostic catheter is then removed, leaving the extra-stiff wire in place. A crossover sheath (6–8F) may then be advanced over the stiff guidewire and positioned in the contralateral CFA. This allows contrast injection during lesion dilation and backup support for crossing lesions. This type of sheath manipulation may be very difficult with individuals who have an acute angle between the origin of the CIAs or those who have aortofemoral bypass grafts.

Antegrade CFA access allows for easy treatment of distal superficial femoral artery (SFA), popliteal, and below-the-knee lesions, especially for total occlusions of the popliteal, antegrade femoral access is preferred. Antegrade femoral artery access is technically more difficult and has higher complication rates (hemorrhage and dissection) than retrograde femoral access. It is more technically demanding than retrograde CFA access, particularly in obese patients. Antegrade CFA access may carry a higher complication rate than retrograde CFA access. When entering the CFA in an antegrade fashion, it is helpful to identify the femoral head under fluoroscopy. Needle entry into the CFA should be caudal to the inguinal ligament since a higher puncture location may result in intraperitoneal bleeding and difficult postprocedural hemostasis. The appropriate skin entry site will be 1–2 centimeters above (cephalad to) the inguinal crease. This location may be difficult to identify in obese individuals. Ultrasound guidance is strongly recommended, along with use of micropuncture technique. Once access is obtained with the micropuncture sheath, an injection of contrast is recommended to ensure that the sheath enters into the SFA and not the profunda. Separating out the bifurcation of these vessels is best done using an ipsilateral oblique (20–30 degrees) contrast injection. Given the angulation of the antegrade access and potential for sheath kinking, advancement of a supportive 0.035-inch wire (Amplatz 180 cm) into the SFA for sheath placement is recommended. Additionally, if the lesion is in the popliteal, one can place a longer (23–30 cm) sheath, which will also provide excellent support. Often predilatation of the track and CFA is required with a smaller dilator prior to placement of the definitive sheath. After sheath placement, the patient should receive unfractionated heparin with a goal ACT of greater than 225 seconds.

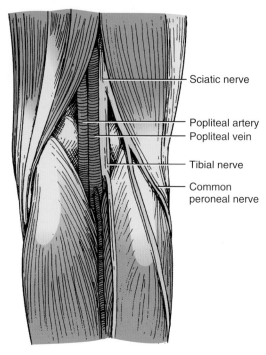

Figure 11.3 Schematic diagram of the right popliteal fossa.

Retrograde popliteal artery access can be useful when trying to cross an occluded SFA. It is important to be aware of the anatomic relationship between the popliteal artery and vein. At the level of the joint space, the artery courses anterior to the vein, whereas, at approximately 6 cm cephalad to the joint space, the artery is medial to the vein (Fig. 11.3). For popliteal arterial puncture, the vessel should be free of significant disease and larger than 4 mm in diameter. Prior angiography and/or color-flow duplex imaging may provide useful information regarding puncture of this vessel. The first step is to gain contralateral CFA access in order to provide contrast injections to help visualize the target popliteal artery. The CFA sheath is secured in place, and the patient is turned to the prone position. Contrast injections performed through the contralateral CFA sheath allow fluoroscopic visualization of the popliteal artery. In this way a micropuncture needle is directed obliquely from medial to lateral so that the artery is entered approximately 5–6 cm above the joint space. A 0.035-inch floppy guidewire is then advanced into the popliteal artery, and a 4–6F sheath is then inserted.

A more contemporary approach for SFA and popliteal occlusions that are occluded at the ostium (flush to wall) and not approachable from an antegrade approach is pedal access. The occlusion is then crossed in a retrograde fashion, which often is easier to cross than antegrade due to a softer distal than proximal cap of these occlusions. Access via the posterior tibial (PT) and dorsalis pedis (DP) is best obtained using ultrasound guidance and is similar to radial access. Careful management of these alternative access points is required to preclude vessel thrombosis, dissection, hematoma, and compartment syndrome as well as nerve injury.

Nonselective Abdominal Angiography

Vascular access for initial aortoiliac intervention may be performed via radial, brachial, axillary, or femoral artery access. After insertion of a 4–6F sheath, a pigtail or other "flush" angiographic catheter can be advanced to the level of the mesenteric or renal arteries (approximately lumbar level L1 at the spine) to perform nonselective angiography. The "flush" catheters have multiple side holes and include the tennis racket, pigtail, omniflush straight, and universal catheters. These catheters should generally be advanced over a 0.035-inch wire with a gentle, floppy tip such as a Wholey or other type of steerable wire. This type of 0.035-inch wire is more maneuverable and ultimately more forgiving in patients with severely stenotic or calcified vessels. If there is some difficulty navigating past severely stenotic lesions with these wires, then a 0.035-inch angled and tapered Glidewire may be able to perform this task. Because angiographic contrast is delivered under force, using end-hole catheters during nonselective power injection may damage more fragile, smaller side branch arteries or atherosclerotic plaque, increasing the risk of vessel dissection and trauma. Operators should not inject into small branches of the aorta and should position their catheters safely (below T12) and not directly against the aortic wall. Positioning of catheters above T12 can result in accidental power injection into the artery of Adamkiewicz, which may cause paralysis. The operator should also be aware of the catheter's maximal flow tolerance, number of side holes, tapering of the tip, and internal diameter of the catheter. Effective catheter length is reduced by the number of side holes present.

Abdominal angiography is performed to evaluate the abdominal aorta, mesenteric vessels, renal arteries, and other visceral vessels. Digital subtraction angiography (DSA) may be preferred over standard cineangiography. The angiogram can be performed in an anterior-posterior (AP) projection. If there is a specific interest in the renal arteries and the aorto-renal junction, then a left anterior (LAO) projection of approximately 5–30 degrees may provide better visualization of the origin of both renal arteries. In this particular case, the universal and tennis racket catheters may be preferred because they deploy contrast dye in a caudal direction (rather than the cephalad direction of the pigtail catheter) and so prevent the dilution that may occur with illumination of the celiac trunk and superior mesenteric artery.

Nonselective angiography requires knowledge of image angulations and vascular anatomy to better define disease involving the aorto-visceral vessel junction and other ostial disease.

Selective Angiography

Selective angiography is the direct injection of contrast into a target vessel via a catheter. Prior to contrast injection, the catheter tip should be moving freely, and the fidelity of the hemodynamic waveform should be normal without any attenuation or "dampening," which may correlate with thrombus or atheroma within the catheter. The dampened waveform may suggest that the catheter tip is against the vessel wall or against an atherosclerotic plaque. Injection of contrast when the waveform is dampened may result in vessel dissection or embolus of the clot or atheroma.

Selective angiography also requires gentle torque movements of the catheter tip. Any type of aggressive catheter movement (without the use of guidewires) may also result in atheroemboli and vessel dissection. In some cases (especially cannulation of the renal and mesenteric vessels), a "no-touch" or minimal touch technique may be recommended. Catheters (in most cases) will be easier to manipulate than sheaths. The use of a braided catheter may be preferred for very tortuous anatomy because the metal braid within the catheter provides excellent catheter support, strength, and kink resistance. Many catheters used in selective angiography also have an outer hydrophilic layer that provides better tracking through tortuous vessels, extra lubricity, and less thrombogenicity.

Iliac Artery Intervention

Iliac artery intervention is very important, not only for improving flow to the lower extremities, but also for cardiovascular therapies such as coronary artery intervention, insertion of an intra-aortic balloon pump or other cardiac output assist devices, or for treatment of vascular access site complications. Retrograde common femoral artery access is the most frequently used access for percutaneous angiography and intervention for both coronary and noncoronary vessels. Percutaneous revascularization for iliac obstructive disease rivals that of surgical intervention with respect to long-term patency, and surgery should really be only considered when concomitant aneurysmal disease is present or for failure of previous endovascular therapy. The Trans-Atlantic Inter-Society Consensus (TASC) lesion guidelines are often used to describe the complexity of lesions and not necessarily to drive the technique of revascularization, given advances in endovascular technique and newer devices. Guidelines regarding the appropriateness of aorto-iliac intervention have been published and detail various clinical scenarios to help guide operators. For patients undergoing endovascular revascularization of the iliac vessels, it is imperative to have preprocedural noninvasive imaging in order to plan vascular access and treatment options. This imaging permits the optimal selection of arterial access.

Indications

The indication to perform an intervention of the iliac arteries includes vascular access and symptomatic lower extremity ischemia. Iliac intervention may also be appropriate in patients with severe stenosis or occlusion of the femoropopliteal or infrapopliteal arteries and concomitant moderate iliac artery disease in whom revascularizing the moderately stenosed iliac artery may improve the arterial inflow and lead to symptomatic improvement or salvage of the limb.

Endovascular treatment of significant iliac artery stenosis with claudication is indicated as follows:

- Provisional stent placement is indicated for use in iliac arteries as salvage therapy for suboptimal or failed result from balloon dilation (e.g., persistent gradient, residual diameter stenosis >50%, or flow-limiting dissection).
- Stenting is effective as primary therapy for CIA stenosie and occlusions.
- Stenting is effective as primary therapy in external iliac artery stenosis and occlusions.

Techniques

The retrograde ipsilateral CFA access is the most commonly used vascular access for revascularization of the common and external iliac artery. Occasionally, contralateral, axillary, or brachial access may be necessary when the distal portion of the external iliac and/or CFA artery is involved. The preferred site for arterial access depends on the location of the target lesion(s), any associated lesions in the contralateral iliac, and/or if any runoff vessels have to be treated at the same time. For CIA as well as proximal/mid external iliac (EIA) lesions, ipsilateral retrograde access is usually adequate. For distal EIA and CFA lesions, contralateral CFA access and crossover is preferred. Bilateral ostial CIA disease in which kissing stents/percutaneous transluminal angioplasty (PTA) is planned requires bilateral CFA access. At times, upper extremity access (left brachial or left radial) may be required in cases of chronic total occlusions (CTO) in order to facilitate both antegrade and retrograde crossing and also for better visualization of the extent of occlusion.

After gaining vascular access, heparin is administered (and maintained to a therapeutic ACT). In many cases direct thrombin inhibitors such as bivalirudin are also acceptable for anticoagulation (especially in patients with or at risk for heparin-induced thrombocytopenia and thrombosis syndrome [HIT/HITTS]). Bivalirudin is not recommended in occlusions, given the irreversible nature of this medication and the higher risk of vessel perforation.

After the target lesion has been identified, the reference vessel diameter (RVD) is determined. Peripheral balloon or stent oversizing may lead to tear or rupture of the external iliac artery, and so the use of quantitative angiography or intravascular ultrasound (IVUS) to measure vessel diameter is encouraged. Visual estimation of vessel diameter is discouraged.

Given the size, calcification, and tortuosity of the iliac vessels, 0.035-inch guidewires are often exclusively used in the iliac vascular bed. Smaller wires (0.018/0.014 inch) can be used but often lack the support needed, given the size of the balloons and stents used in this arena. Steerable hydrophilic wires (Glidewire Advantage, Stiff-angled Glidewire, Terumo, Inc., Somerset, NJ) are often required for tortuous vessels whereas supportive 0.035-inch wires (Supracore, Lunderquist, or Amplatz) are needed in calcific vessels to deliver balloons and stents. The use of longer sheaths (23–30 cm) should be considered in CIA lesions in order to visualize the lesions as well as deliver balloons and stents through potentially challenging anatomy. Sheath size should depend on the size of the vessel being intervened upon. All iliac interventions carry a risk of vessel perforation that can be fatal in minutes, and the minimal sheath size to deliver a covered stent to the area of intervention should always be placed. In cases of chronic total occlusion where the risk of rupture is higher, all patients should have adequate intravenous access and be typed and screened for blood prior to the procedure. Operators must be familiar with the location and operation of covered stents as well as have aortic occlusion balloons present (Coda balloons). Various techniques and crossing devices are available, and, in the hands of experienced operators, iliac CTOs can be successfully revascularized in 85%–95% of cases.

Once the lesion has been crossed with a steerable wire such as a Wholey wire or Glidewire, a catheter such a hydrophilic Glidecatheter (Terumo Medical Corp., Somerset, NJ) is positioned immediately above the lesion. Universal or pigtail catheters may also be used because distal abdominal aortograms will also provide excellent bilateral pelvic vessel angiograms. When the lesion is located in the distal common iliac or proximal external iliac artery, retrograde injections of contrast through the femoral sheath may also be used. One particular angiographic view, which separates the origin of the internal and external iliac arteries, is the contralateral caudal oblique view (20 degrees lateral oblique and 20 degrees caudal).

Next, the soft-tip guidewire can be exchanged for an extra-stiff guidewire (0.035-inch Amplatzer wire, Cook, Bloomington, IN) to provide support and trackability for stent placement. The lesion is dilated with a balloon sized 1:1 with the RVD or using the lowest pressure that will fully expand the balloon. The balloon may also be sized smaller than the RVD. The results are assessed by reinserting the catheter above the lesion or using a hand injection of contrast through the sheath. Although provisional stent placement is indicated for use in iliac arteries as salvage therapy for suboptimal or failed result from balloon dilation (e.g., persistent gradient, residual diameter stenosis >50%, or flow-limiting dissection), most experts believe that stenting is effective as primary therapy for common and external iliac artery stenosie and occlusions.

Balloon-expandable stents are preferred when a precise stent placement is required (ostial lesions), and self-expanding stents are preferred when precision is not a critical factor and the vessel tapers in size (Fig. 11.4). Balloon-expandable stents also offer greater radial

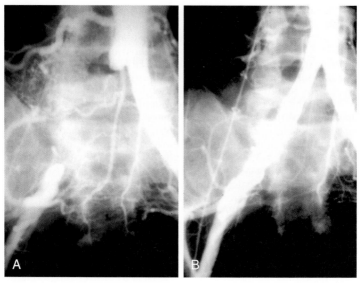

Figure 11.4 (A) Baseline angiogram with occlusion of right common iliac artery. (B) Following successful angioplasty and stent placement.

force in heavily calcified and bulky iliac vessels. In cases where the risk of perforation or vessel rupture is considered high (calcified stenosis/chronic total occlusions), some operators prefer covered stents. Atrium ICAST (Atrium, Hudson, NH) stents are covered balloon-expandable stents and have been demonstrated to be advantageous in CTOs. Given the ability to precisely place these stents, they are often used in the distal aorta and common iliac. The covered VIABAHN (W. L. Gore & Associates, Flagstaff, AZ) stents are also used in iliac arteries. These self-expanding stents feature a heparinized surface for a localized anticoagulation effect. They are durable and reinforced with a polytetrafluoroethylene (ePTFE) liner attached to an external nitinol stent structure but lack any radial strength. For balloon-expandable stents, it is reasonable to use an arterial sheath long enough to cross the lesion to avoid having the undeployed stent strut catch on the lesion, thus risking embolization or dislodgment of the stent. With the sheath and stent across the lesion, the sheath is then withdrawn and contrast is injected to confirm the correct position of the stent. The stent is then deployed using at least 6–8 atm of pressure to ensure adequate stent expansion and apposition to the vascular wall. Repeat balloon inflation using higher pressure can be performed if there are any questions regarding adequate stent expansion. Simultaneous translesional pressures gradients using a catheter or pressure measuring guidewire proximal and the distal vascular sheath should ensure a final gradient of is 5 mm Hg or less. It should be noted that a perfect angiographic result is not mandatory, and residual stenosis of up to 30% may result in a translesional gradient of <5 mm Hg. This fact needs to be weighed against the greater risk of complications (vessel perforation) from very aggressive postdilatation.

Either balloon-expandable or self-expanding stents can be used in the iliac bed. With the characteristic tortuosity of the iliac vessels and tapering vessel size (especially of the EIAs), nitinol-based self-expanding stents have the advantage of better flexibility and conformability. These stents should always be oversized by 1–2 mm at least, and IVUS may be useful for vessel sizing. Deployment of these stents is subject to the stent moving forward during deployment, and operators must adjust the delivery sheath appropriately. Shortening of the stent in the EIA is also common because one often underappreciates the tortuosity of this vessel as it proceeds ventrally from deep in the retro-peritoneum.

Common Femoral Artery

The CFA crosses the inguinal ligament, is subject to marked compression, and is traditionally felt to be a "no-stent" zone. Given the low-risk nature and excellent long-term patency of endarterectomy, the CFA is best treated with an open surgical approach. Sometimes CFA intervention is required in patients who are not surgical candidates and is typically performed from the contralateral approach using standard techniques. Given the desire to avoid stenting in this area, endovascular revascularization of the CFA is often accomplished using a variety of non-stent techniques (atherectomy and PTA, whether in combination or alone; Fig. 11.5). These techniques possess the potential for distal embolization, which can lead to acute limb ischemia if not performed in conjunction with the use of embolic protection devices. The most important component of the CFA is the origin of the profunda femoris artery. The profunda is considered by many to be "the sacred vessel of the leg" and must be preserved under all circumstances given the collaterals it supplies to the lower leg. This fact precludes the use of subintimal dissection for the treatment of CFA disease and requires operators to carefully observe for any dissections in the CFA that may compromise flow to the profunda. For these reasons, the optimal therapy for obstructive disease of the CFA is surgical.

Femoropopliteal Artery Intervention

Atherosclerotic occlusive disease is more common in the femoropopliteal arterial bed than in the iliac artery. When the femoropopliteal artery is involved in symptomatic lower extremity PAD, complete occlusions are three times more frequent than stenosis. In contrast to the iliac arterial bed, the superficial femoral and popliteal arteries (femoropopliteal segment) have proved resistant to durable endovascular results. This is most likely secondary to the nature of atherosclerosis in this segment (i.e., diffuse, calcific, and often occlusive). This type of atherosclerosis, when coupled with the extreme length of this segment and all of the complex biophysical forces to which the vessel is exposed with daily movement, contributes to the challenges of endovascular therapy for the SFA/popliteal. Long segments of heavily calcified plaque can impair stent expansion and result in higher rates of restenosis as well as the potential for stent fracture. However, new stent technologies and devices are now producing long-term data that argue for an endovascular-first strategy for revascularization in this segment, dependent on numerous factors including patient, disease, and operator experience. Box 11.6 demonstrates the morphologic stratification of femoropopliteal lesions according to the TASC group.

Indications

Revascularization of the femoral or popliteal arteries is reserved for patients with lifestyle-limiting claudication, ischemic rest pain, and limb-threatening ischemia. Treatment of short (<5 cm) occlusions yields better results than treatment of long (>10 cm) occlusions or stenosis. The presence of patent runoff vessels correlates with long-term benefits, reflected in the improved outcome in patients with milder symptoms. Significant residual stenosis after angioplasty correlates with a poor long-term outcome, whereas the absence of diabetes correlates with an improved patency rate.

Endovascular intervention is not indicated if there is no significant pressure gradient across a stenosis despite flow augmentation with

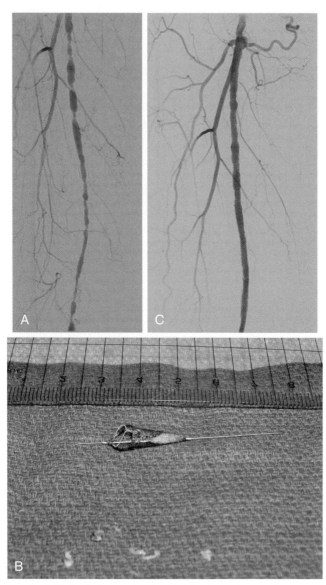

Figure 11.5 (A) Angiogram of serial lesions in superficial femoral artery (SFA). (B) Atherectomy of serial SFA lesions with subsequent collection of plaque (some in distal protection device/basket). (C) Angiogram of SFA after successful atherectomy.

vasodilators. Stenosis of 50%–75% diameter by angiography may or may not be hemodynamically significant, and intravascular pressure measurements have been recommended to determine whether these lesions are significant and also to predict patient improvement if the lesion is treated. However, there is no consensus on a diagnostic trans-stenotic pressure criterion or on methods to measure these pressures. One criterion suggests a mean gradient of 10 mm Hg before or after vasodilators; another has suggested use of a mean gradient of 5 mm Hg, or 10, 15, or 20 mm Hg peak systolic. A third criterion uses a 15% peak systolic pressure gradient after administration of a vasodilator. Pressure measurements may be obtained with two separate pressure transducers or by obtaining pullback pressures with a single transducer. Pressures obtained with the catheter positioned across the stenosis may artifactually increase the pressure gradient by reducing the residual

> **Box 11.6** Morphologic Stratification of Femoropopliteal Lesions
>
> TASC type A femoropopliteal lesions:
> - Single stenosis <10 cm in length
> - Single occlusion <5 cm in length
>
> TASC type B femoropopliteal lesions:
> - Multiple lesions (stenosis or occlusions), each <5 cm
> - Single stenosis or occlusion <15 cm not involving the infrageniculate popliteal artery
> - Single or multiple lesions in the absence of continuous tibial vessels to improve inflow for a distal bypass
> - Heavily calcified occlusion <5 cm in length
> - Single popliteal stenosis
>
> TASC type C femoropopliteal lesions:
> - Multiple stenosis or occlusions totaling >15 cm with or without heavy calcification
> - Recurrent stenosis or occlusions that need treatment after two endovascular interventions
>
> TASC type D femoropopliteal lesions:
> - Chronic total occlusions of CFA or SFA (>20 cm, involving the popliteal artery)
> - Chronic total occlusion of popliteal artery and proximal trifurcation vessels

CFA, common femoral artery; *SFA*, superficial femoral artery.

lumen with the catheter. No studies have been performed to assess the safety and efficacy of treating asymptomatic but hemodynamically significant lesions to prevent progression of disease. Primary stent placement is not recommended in the femoral, popliteal, or tibial arteries. Endovascular intervention is not indicated as prophylactic therapy in an asymptomatic patient with lower extremity PAD.

Technique

The most commonly used vascular access for the treatment of femoropopliteal arterial disease is the contralateral CFA access. The crossover technique involves engaging the contralateral CIA with a catheter and wire. The more catheter there is across the bifurcation, the greater the support. Particularly challenging bifurcations require the use of shapeable catheters such as the Simmons catheter, which can be brought down to engage the iliac and anchor across the bifurcation. Support is also gained by the wire that is used, and operators have a bevy of options from which to choose including some that are hydrophilic on the front end and stiff on the back to permit the use of one wire. Once the wire is successfully advanced to the contralateral CFA, the catheter should then be advanced to the CFA, the wire exchanged for a stiff supportive wire (Amplatz or Supracore), and the catheter removed. The sheath is then exchanged for a 45-cm sheath, which is advanced carefully around the aortoiliac bifurcation to the contralateral CFA. One technique to use when the sheath will not advance, secondary to calcification and tortuosity is balloon-assisted tracking wherein a 6–7 mm × 40 mm balloon is advanced over the wire to just outside the sheath and inflated to 2–4 atm and then rapidly deflated while forward pressure is put on the sheath and back pressure on the balloon. In this fashion, the balloon acts as a dilator to keep the sheath off the arterial wall, and it permits the sheath to track through tortuous segments. Following placement of a crossover sheath, unfractionated heparin to achieve an ACT greater than at least 225 seconds is recommended. The SFA and popliteal lesions can then be tackled using whatever techniques are required. It is imperative to note what size sheath is required. Antegrade vascular access cannot be used for the treatment of CFA or ostial SFA disease. Brachial and retrograde popliteal access is occasionally used; in particular, popliteal access may prove useful to recanalize SFA occlusions when antegrade approaches have failed. In cases of limb salvage, a retrograde posterior tibial approach can also be used.

As for iliac interventions, the operator obtains vascular access and administers antithombin medications. All patients should be pretreated with 325 mg of aspirin at least 24 hours before the procedure (if no contraindications). For total occlusions, hydrophilic guidewires (Glidewire) are very useful when other guidewires frequently fail to cross. On occasion, 0.011 to 0.018-inch wires can be used to cross subtotal occlusions. When a hydrophilic guidewire or 0.014- to 0.018-inch wires are used to cross a lesion, it is usually preferable to exchange these wires for a nonhydrophilic wire prior to intervention. This will provide better support and traction for the balloon catheters and stents. After the RVD is measured with quantitative angiography, the lesion is dilated with a balloon sized 1:1 with the reference vessel using the lowest pressure that will fully expand the balloon.

If the postprocedural angiogram shows a satisfactory angiographic result (a residual diameter stenosis of <30%) and no flow-limiting dissection, the procedure is terminated (Fig. 11.6). However if there is significant residual stenosis, flow-limiting dissection, or abrupt occlusion, the operator should proceed with stent placement (Fig. 11.7). In general

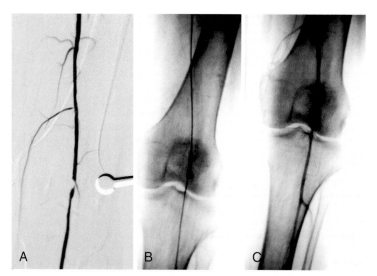

Figure 11.6 (A) Baseline angiogram of lesion in popliteal artery. (B) Balloon inflation. (C) Post-balloon angiogram.

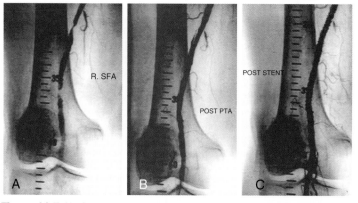

Figure 11.7 (A) Right femoral and popliteal artery stenosis. (B) Following balloon dilation with dissection present. (C) Following stent placement.

terms, balloon-expandable stents are not used in this vascular bed, and the preferred stent is a self-expanding nitinol stent. The stent should be oversized by 1 mm to the reference lumen diameter. Finally, when a stent is needed, we add to the pharmacologic regimen Clopidogrel 75 mg for 1–3 months, after a loading dose of 300–600 mg, although no consensus data/guidelines exist regarding optimal duration of dual antiplatelet therapy post PVI.

Stent grafts (Viabahn, Gore) are stents with an ePTFE covering also approved for use in the SFA/popliteal segment. These are excellent for covering perforations and aneurysms and can be used to cover and treat in-stent restenosis because the ePTFE is impermeable to tissue in-growth. However restenosis can occur at the inlet and outlet of ePTFE stent grafts, and these grafts—under low-flow conditions—can thrombose, leading to acute limb ischemia. Viabahn occlusion can be challenging because it is resistant to solely thrombolytic therapy given the nidus is inflow/outflow disease and often requires mechanical and/or rheolytic thrombectomy and/or expeditious surgical revascularization.

In response to the suboptimal results of stenting for the femoro-popliteal artery, there has been a movement to using non-stent technologies such as atherectomy. Atherectomy devices can be divided into either excisional (removal of the plaque) (TurboHawk, Jetstream, Phoenix) or ablative (disintegration or fragmentation of the plaque: Laser, Diamondback). These devices are particularly useful in "no stent" zones where vessels cross joint spaces and are subject to extreme biophysical forces. Each device has advantages and disadvantages as well as limitations and potential complications. All these devices are expensive and are rarely used as stand-alone therapy and hence raise the cost of each procedure significantly.

Balloon angioplasty is plagued by high rates of restenosis. In order to enhance patency rates without having to leave a stent in place, drug-coated balloons (DCBs) have been developed. Although stents are very similar, DCBs are not, and operators must familiarize themselves with each balloon with respect to drug, dose, and excipient. The trials involving DCBs all vary regarding their use as stand-alone or adjunctive therapy, if the disease is de novo or restenosis, and what drug/dose was present. Technically speaking, inflation of DCBs is no different than other balloons except for duration. Most DCBs need to be inflated for at least 3 minutes to permit transfer of the drug to the vessel. Also, without a scaffold to treat dissections or elastic recoil, there are limitations of this technology.

Infrapopliteal Interventions

Intervention to the infrapopliteal arteries, which are often diffusely diseased, small and/or occluded, and prone to high restenosis rates, is often reserved only for nonhealing wounds or rest pain. These vessels are similar in size to the coronaries except considerably longer. For this reason, long, low-profile balloons have been developed to aid in the treatment of these vessels. Coupled with the use of advanced techniques such as retrograde access, dissection/re-entry, and smaller re-entry devices borrowed from the coronary realm, successful endovascular intervention to these vessels is now possible.

Technique

The preferred vascular access to perform percutaneous intervention of the infrapopliteal vessels is the ipsilateral antegrade CFA access, which enables an almost direct approach to the infrapopliteal vessels. The contralateral CFA access using a crossover approach is also useful, particularly when planning simultaneous revascularization of the iliac arteries, CFA, or proximal SFA. When using the contralateral crossover approach, the operator must bear in mind that catheter length is an issue and that long (150 cm) catheters are usually necessary to reach the infrapopliteal vessels. On occasion, a retrograde ipsilateral PT artery approach can be plausible, especially in the cases of limb salvage. All patients are pretreated with 325 mg of aspirin at least 24 hours prior to the procedure. After contralateral CFA vascular access has been obtained, the patient is anticoagulated with 50–60 units/kg of heparin. Initially a soft-tipped 0.035-inch guidewire (e.g., Wholey wire) is advanced to the distal popliteal artery. A 6F multipurpose guiding catheter or 4–5F Glidecatheter is then advanced over the guidewire and positioned at the mid- or distal popliteal artery. Baseline angiography of the infrapopliteal vessels is obtained using injection of contrast through the catheter or sheath. After the stenosis has been identified, the lesion is usually crossed with a 0.014- or 0.018-inch guide wire. After the lesion is crossed, online quantitative angiography is obtained for a more accurate measurement of the RVD. A balloon catheter is chosen for a 1:1 balloon-to-RVD ratio. The balloon is inflated usually at 6–8 atm of inflation pressure, or to allow complete expansion of the balloon. Multiple inflations are performed as necessary to attain a satisfactory angiographic result. Suboptimal angiographic result, more than 30% residual stenosis, dissection, or slow flow may require stent deployment. Post-stenting angiography is obtained, and special attention must be paid to rule out dissection or perforation (Fig. 11.8).

The treatment modalities for infrapopliteal lesions are limited and mainly involve PTA alone. Although the long-term patency of angioplasty is limited, there is often sufficient vessel patency to heal the wound. The initial studies using DCBs have failed to show a benefit, but this may be related to the technique of drug coating. Ongoing studies using other DCBs are anticipated in the coming year. Another treatment modality used for infrapopliteal intervention is the placement of drug-eluting coronary stents (DES). Several studies have demonstrated a benefit of this approach for focal disease of the infrapopliteal segment, flow-limiting dissections, and/or abrupt closure.

When coronary stents are deployed in the infrapopliteal vessels, patients are treated with Clopidogrel, with a loading dose of 300–600 mg given at the end of the procedure followed by 75 mg/day for at least 4 weeks. Glycoprotein IIb/IIIa inhibitors may have some benefit in selected cases of infrapopliteal intervention. The postprocedural sheath management is similar to revascularization in other vascular territories. However gentle manual compression for hemostasis is likely superior to other techniques in the setting of calcified, stenotic, and small lumen arterial vessels.

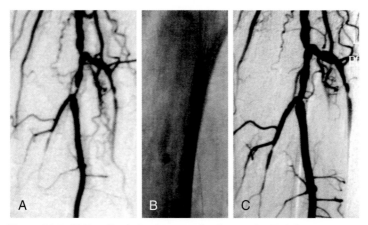

Figure 11.8 (A) Baseline below-knee popliteal stenosis. (B) 3.5-mm coronary balloon inflation. (C) Post-angioplasty result.

Peripheral Vascular Intervention Complications

PVIs have complications common to other vascular procedures. Complications can occur intra-procedurally as well as postprocedure. Access-related complications include trauma to the accessed artery (dissection, perforation) (Fig. 11.9) leading to retroperitoneal bleeding, femoral pseudoaneurysm (Fig. 11.10), or the creation of an arteriovenous (AV) fistula. With balloon angioplasty of any vessel, there is a risk of complications at that site including dissection, perforation, and embolization (cholesterol, particulate, air, or thrombus). Instrumentation of any vascular structure and the use of contrast can lead to stroke, MI, or contrast-induced nephropathy. All potential complications should be reviewed with the patient prior to the procedure for proper informed consent.

Operators should always attempt to minimize the chances of complications by careful preprocedural planning as well as meticulous technique with access and wire management. Patients undergoing peripheral vascular procedures have extensive vascular disease and are at markedly elevated risk of complications. The best approach to complications is to be prepared for them and have an array of devices on hand that can treat each potential complication. Dissections can be treated with prolonged balloon inflation or stent placement. Most wire perforations seal on their own or with balloon tamponade proximal to the occlusion

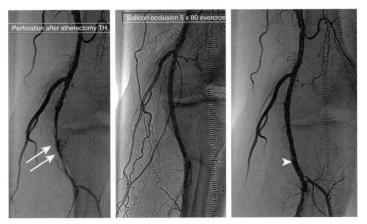

Figure 11.9 Angiogram showing perforation of popliteal artery with salvage by covered stent.

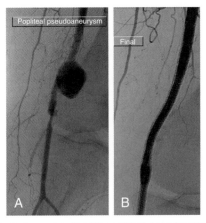

Figure 11.10 Angiogram showing (A) popliteal pseudoaneurysm and (B) its repair by stenting.

with or without reversal of the anticoagulant. For large perforations, covered stents and coils can be used. When large vessels (iliacs) are perforated, large aortic occlusion balloons for balloon tamponade and the large sheaths by which these are delivered must be available.

Thrombus formation either in situ or from a complication that occludes flow to a vascular bed must be treated expeditiously. Devices to treat thrombosis and embolization are critical to have available, and familiarity with each of these devices is essential. Thrombus can be treated with medications (tissue plasminogen activator [tPA]) or mechanically using aspiration/rheolytic thrombectomy. There are devices that permit both the administration of tPA followed by mechanical thrombectomy to remove the clot. Another management option for thrombus is low-pressure balloon angioplasty and/or stenting to push the clot to the side of the vessel and restore flow. These are similar to techniques used in the coronary circulation. Most complications can be managed endovascularly; however surgical back-up is required to perform any of these procedures in the situation that the complication cannot be controlled endovascularly or if there is concomitant compartment syndrome requiring fasciotomy.

Postprocedural Management of Patients

Patients undergoing peripheral intervention often have a high burden of systemic arteriosclerosis and thus are prone to adverse outcomes. Careful monitoring of access sites for hematomas and/or RP bleeding is advised. Although most of these procedures can be safely performed on an elective basis, patients should be given explicit instructions of when to call and/or re-present to the hospital.

Antiplatelet therapy post-peripheral intervention is controversial. As these patients have PAD, which is a CAD equivalent, they should be at least on daily aspirin. Some have advocated clopidogrel in place of aspirin, and most will advocate dual-platelet therapy postintervention for 1–12 months, based on few or no data.

Patient post-peripheral interventions need to be monitored closely for reoccurrence and/or restenosis. This requires baseline studies to be obtained immediately (within 2 weeks of the procedure), and these usually consist of ABIs with duplex imaging. In this fashion one can monitor closely for evidence of restenosis, which is easier to treat than occlusion. There are no formal guidelines on the frequency or duration of surveillance. Of note, it is import to monitor stent grafts because these have a tendency to occlude rapidly, and thrombotic occlusion of the graft can present with dramatic symptoms including acute limb ischemia. For renal interventions, a new baseline duplex is essential, given this will have higher velocities from the stent being in place, and it is these velocities that must be followed over time. For below-the-knee interventions in the setting of critical limb ischemia, clinical observation of wound healing is most often done as a surrogate for patency. These patients must be carefully seen at frequent intervals to monitor for any signs of a plateau in wound healing that most likely represents restenosis and thus the need for repeat intervention. A deterioration in ABI/TBI measurements may also indicate restenosis.

Training Standards for Peripheral Angioplasty

Body of Knowledge

As described by the ACC/AHA Committee on Peripheral Vascular Disease, physicians should have extensive clinical training in the diagnosis and treatment of patients with peripheral vascular disease. The body of knowledge necessary includes the anatomy, natural history, and clinical manifestations of peripheral vascular disease; noninvasive assessment of peripheral vascular disease; indications and contraindications for angioplasty; risks and benefits of angioplasty; recognition of complications; alternative therapies; principles of thrombolytic techniques; and technical aspects and usage of x-ray equipment needed for diagnostic peripheral angiography and PTA.

Every cardiology fellowship training program must provide COCATS 4 level I training in vascular medicine, which should impart the basic knowledge to provide care to patients with vascular disease. Completion of level II or III training allows trainees to be eligible to obtain the Registered Physician in Vascular Interpretation (RPVI) certification, which is required by most institutions to bill for reading diagnostic studies. This level requires the supervised interpretation of at least 500 diagnostic vascular studies across various modalities. Level III training in vascular medicine requires a dedicated year of training beyond general cardiology.

There is a board certification in Vascular Medicine administered by the American Board of Vascular Medicine (ABVM). There are two pathways through which one can become eligible for this exam: the Training Pathway and the Practice Pathway (available through 2016). For those in training, one must complete a cardiology fellowship that includes level II COCATS training or complete a dedicated vascular medicine fellowship of at least 12 months that meets the requirements as endorsed by the Society of Vascular Medicine Board. The practice pathway permits a practicing physician to sit for the board if board certified in medicine/cardiology, has devoted him- or herself to the practice of vascular medicine or to vascular medicine research, and has documentation by a local chair or physician colleague regarding the applicants expertise in vascular medicine.

Vascular medicine requirements are somewhat different from those required to perform PVI. For those physicians who wish to perform PVI, it is recommended that they receive at least COCATS II training in vascular medicine in addition to a dedicated year of training in PVI. Interventional fellowships alone may not meet the prerequisites for the RPVI certification. The ABVM offers an Endovascular Board Certification, which also has two pathways. Trainees must complete an interventional cardiology fellowship that includes training in PVI. They are required to perform 300 diagnostic coronary angiograms (200 as primary operator), and 100 diagnostic and 50 therapeutic peripheral interventions, at least half as the primary operator. Counting of cases and procedures should follow the COCATS document. Fellows may apply for this within the first 3 years out of fellowship when using their cases from training; otherwise, additional documentation that meets the practice pathway must be attained. Certification letters are naturally required from program directors as well. Practicing physicians who wish to attain the Endovascular certification can do so for now through the practice pathway. This requires active privileges to perform PVI and the performance of 100 diagnostic angiograms with at least 50 as primary operator. Cases that were performed during training do not count toward this number. These cases must be performed within 1–2 years of the application with 50% in the 12 months prior to the application. Additionally, operators must demonstrate the completion of 50 PVIs with at least 25 as primary operator within the same time requirements.

The aforementioned requirements are not the same as hospital privileges, which often incorporate specifics for PVI and carotid intervention. Most hospitals will also require that the applicant have training and experience in the use of thrombolytic therapy in peripheral arteries, having participated in at least 10 such cases. These requirements are normally met during a formal subspecialty training program of at least 1 year in duration, completed after at least one of the basic training requirements listed in the previous paragraph has been met. However they may be met in part or in total during initial residency or fellowship. In all instances, complete and detailed documentation of the afore-mentioned procedural training should be available.

Maintenance of Privileges

Maintenance of PTA privileges requires ongoing experience in performing these procedures, with acceptable success and complication rates. The determination of a minimum number of procedures per year is at the discretion of the credentialing or clinical privileges committee of each hospital. Whether or not a minimum number is specified, main-tenance of privileges is also dependent on the physician's active participa-tion in the institution's quality improvement program that monitors indications, success rates, and complications. These data may be used within the individual institution in considering renewal of clinical privileges. All physicians performing these procedures must participate in the quality improvement program and will be evaluated using the same criteria.

Physicians who were granted privileges before the implementation of this standard should not necessarily have their status altered if they do not meet the qualifications outlined in this statement. However, if they do not meet the qualifications, they should acquire the necessary training or experience to do so within 3 years. They must also participate in the institution's quality improvement program and will be evaluated using the same standards for indications, success rates, and complications.

Suggested Reading

Carter SA, Tate RB. The value of toe pulse waves in determination of risks for limb amputation and death in patients with peripheral artery disease and skin ulcers or gangrene. *J Vasc Surg.* 2001;33(4):708-714.

Creager MA, Goldstone J, Hirshfeld JW Jr, et al.; American College of Cardiology/American Heart Association/American College of Physician Task Force on Clinical Competence. CC/ACP/SCAI/SVMB/SVS clinical competence statement on vascular medicine and catheter-based peripheral vascular interventions: a report of the American College of Cardiology/American Heart Association/American College of Physician Task Force on Clinical Competence (ACC/ACP/SCAI/SVMB/SVS Writing Committee to develop a clinical competence statement on peripheral vascular disease). *J Am Coll Cardiol.* 2004;44(4):941-957.

Creager MA, Gornik HL, Gray BH, et al. COCATS 4 Task Force 9: training in vascular medicine. *J Am Coll Cardiol.* 2015;65(17):1832-1843.

Diehm C, Schuster A, Allenberg H, et al. High prevalence of peripheral arterial disease and comorbidity in 6880 primary care patients: cross sectional study. *Atherosclerosis.* 2004;172:95-105.

Dormandy JA, Rutherford RB. Management of peripheral arterial disease (PAD). TASC Working Group. TransAtlantic Inter-Society Consensus (TASC). *J Vasc Surg.* 2000;31(1 Pt 2):S1-S296.

Dorros G, Jaff MR, Dorros AM, et al. Tibioperoneal (outflow lesion) angioplasty can be used as primary treatment in 235 patients with critical limb ischemia—five-year follow-up. *Circulation.* 2001;104:2057.

Feiring AJ, Wesolowski AA, Lade S. Primary stent-supported angioplasty for treatment of below-knee critical limb ischemia and severe claudication. *J Am Coll Cardiol.* 2004;44:2307-2314.

Gey DC, Lesho EP, Manngold J. Management of peripheral artery disease. *Am Fam Physician.* 2004;69:525-533.

Gray BH, Diaz-Sandoval LJ, Dieter RS, et al. SCAI expert consensus statement for infra-popliteal arterial intervention appropriate use. *Catheter Cardiovasc Interv.* 2014;84(4):539-545.

Hirsch AT, Criqui MH, Treat-Jacobson D, et al. Peripheral arterial disease detection, awareness, and treatment in primary care. *J Am Med Assoc.* 2001;286:1317-1324.

Hirsch AT, et al. ACC/AHA 2005 Guidelines for the management of patients with peripheral arterial disease (lower extremity, renal, mesenteric, and abdominal aortic). *J Am Coll Cardiol.* 2006;47:e1-e192.

Kakkar AM, Abbott JD. Percutaneous versus surgical management of lower extremity peripheral artery disease. *Curr Atheroscler Rep.* 2015;17(2):479.

Kasirajan K, O'Hara PJ, Gray BH, et al. Chronic mesenteric ischemia: open surgery versus percutaneous angioplasty and stenting. *J Vasc Surg.* 2001;33:63-71.

Kinlay S. Management of critical limb ischemia. *Circ Cardiovasc Interv.* 2016;9(2):e001946.

Klein AJ, Feldman DN, Aronow HD, et al. SCAI expert consensus statement for aorto-iliac arterial intervention appropriate use. *Catheter Cardiovasc Interv.* 2014;84:520-528.

Klein AJ, Pinto DS, Gray BH, et al. SCAI expert consensus statement for femoral-popliteal arterial intervention appropriate use. *Catheter Cardiovasc Interv.* 2014;84:529-538.

Krajcer Z, Howell MH. Update on endovascular treatment of peripheral vascular disease: new tools, techniques, and indications. *Tex Heart Inst J.* 2000;27(4):369-385.

McDermott MM, Liu K, Greenland P, et al. Functional decline in peripheral arterial disease: associations with the ankle brachial index and leg symptoms. *JAMA.* 2004;292:453-461.

Norgren L, Hiatt WR, Dormandy JA, et al. Inter-society consensus for the management of peripheral arterial disease (TASC II). *Eur J Vasc Endovasc Surg.* 2007;33:S1-S70.

Norgren L, Hiatt WR, Dormandy JA, et al. Inter-society consensus for the management of peripheral arterial disease (TASC II). *J Vasc Surg.* 2007;45(suppl S):S5-S67.

O'Hare AM, Glidden DV, Fox CS, et al. High prevalence of peripheral arterial disease in persons with renal insufficiency: results from the National Health and Nutrition Examination Survey 1999–2000. *Circulation.* 2004;109:320-323.

Pasternak RC, Criqui MH, Benjamin EJ, et al. Atherosclerotic Vascular Disease Conference: Writing Group I: epidemiology. *Circulation.* 2004;109:2605-2612.

Rooke TW, Hirsch AT, Misra S, et al. 2011 ACCF/AHA focused update of the guideline for the management of patients with peripheral artery disease (updating the 2005 guideline): a report of the American College of Cardiology Foundation/American Heart Association Task Force on Practice Guidelines: developed in collaboration with the Society for Cardiovascular Angiography and Interventions, Society of Interventional Radiology, Society for Vascular Medicine, and Society for Vascular Surgery. *Catheter Cardiovasc Interv.* 2011;79:501-531.

Selvin E, Erlinger TP. Prevalence of and risk factors for peripheral arterial disease in the United States: results from the National Health and Nutrition Examination Survey, 1999–2000. *Circulation.* 2004;110:738-743.

Thukkani AK, Kinlay S. Endovascular intervention for peripheral artery disease. *Circ Res.* 2015;116(9):1599-1613.

Aortic, Renal, Subclavian, and Carotid Interventions

JOSE D. TAFUR · CHRISTOPHER J. WHITE

Introduction

The technical skills necessary to perform coronary angioplasty are transferable to the peripheral vasculature. The difficult task is learning the indications for revascularization (patient selection) among other treatment options and managing complications unique to peripheral vascular disease (PVD) interventions. Appropriate preparation and training, including understanding the value of a team approach that includes vascular surgeons, neurologists, and vascular medicine physicians, are necessary and should be encouraged.

Abdominal Aortic Interventions

Abdominal Aortic Aneurysm

The word "aneurysm" refers to a local dilatation of an artery with a diameter at least 1.5 times the normal measurement. An abdominal aortic aneurysm (AAA) should be determined by formulas that adjust for age and/or body surface area or by calculating the ratio between normal and dilated aortic segments.[1,2] AAA is present when the diameter of the aorta reaches 3.0 cm[3]. The size of the aorta can be measured in any plane that is perpendicular to the aortic axis, but, in practice, the anteroposterior diameter is measured most easily and reproducibly.

Epidemiology

The incidence of AAA is much higher in men than women. The prevalence in men is 41–49 per 100,000 men and 7–12 per 100,000 women.[4,5] The risk factors for development of AAA include smoking, older age, hyperlipidemia, hypertension, and family history (Table 12.1).

Pathogenesis

The pathophysiology of AAA is multifactorial. Most aortic aneurysms represent a manifestation of aortic medial degeneration, which denotes complex biological mechanisms.

Detection

Most aortic aneurysms are diagnosed incidentally on abdominal imaging performed for unrelated indications. Physical examination is not accurate, identifying less than 75% of AAA of greater than 5 cm in diameter.[4] Bidimensional abdominal ultrasonography is the most commonly used imaging modality for diagnosis and follow-up.

Table 12.1

A: Risk Factors for the Development of Abdominal Aortic Aneurysm	
Risk Factor	**Odds Ratio (OR)**
History of smoking	3.59 (3.0–4.28)
Family history	1.88 (1.58–2.24)
Age	1.52 (1.44–1.62)
Hyperlipidemia	1.46 (1.29–1.65)
Hypertension	1.14 (1.02–1.26)

B: Rates of Rupture Based on Aneurysm Diameter	
Maximal Diameter	**5-Year Rupture Rate**
<4.0 cm	2%
4.0–4.9 cm	3%–12%
5.0–5.9 cm	25%
6.0–6.9 cm	35%
>7.0 cm	75%

Adapted from Lederle FA, Johnson GR, Wilson SE, et al. Relationship of age, gender, race, and body size to infrarenal aortic diameter. The Aneurysm Detection and Management (ADAM) Veterans Affairs Cooperative Study Investigators. *J Vasc Surg.* 1997;26:595–601.

Table 12.2

U.S. Preventive Services Task Force (USPSTF) Recommendations for Abdominal Aortic Aneurysm Screening	
Population	**Recommendation**
Men aged 65–75 years who have ever smoked	The USPSTF recommends one-time screening for abdominal aortic aneurysm (AAA) with ultrasonography in men aged 65–75 years who have ever smoked.
Men aged 65–75 years who have never smoked	The USPSTF recommends that clinicians selectively offer screening for AAA in men aged 65–75 years who have never smoked rather than routinely screening all men in this group.
Women aged 65–75 years who have ever smoked	The USPSTF concludes that the current evidence is insufficient to assess the balance of benefits and harms of screening for AAA in women aged 65–75 years who have ever smoked.
Women who have never smoked	The USPSTF recommends against routine screening for AAA in women who have never smoked.

Ultrasonography is a noninvasive, low-risk, inexpensive diagnostic tool. However ultrasound typically underestimates the size of AAA compared to computed tomography angiography (CTA) by 2–4 mm. When using serial imaging to follow up the progression of disease, it is important to use a consistent imaging modality. CTA is the modality of choice for planning an endovascular or a surgical intervention because it provides low interobserver variability and helps determine the anatomic eligibility for endovascular repair, but it is less attractive for serial follow-up due to the ionizing radiation and radiographic contrast exposure.

For asymptomatic patients, the U.S. preventive task force recommends one-time screening for AAA with abdominal ultrasonography in men older than 65 with a smoking history (Table 12.2). Screening is not recommended in men who have never smoked or in women.

Indications for Intervention

Symptomatic AAA

There are three main clinical presentations of AAA: (1) Rupture or impending rupture, (2) embolic or thrombotic complications, and (3) compression of adjacent structures due to mass effect.

The classic clinical triad of AAA rupture includes sudden onset of abdominal or lower back pain, pulsatile abdominal mass, and hypotension; however, this triad is present in less than 40% of patients. The prognosis of ruptured AAA is very poor, with most patients not surviving to the hospital and an in-hospital mortality of around 40–50%. It is estimated that 80% of the mortality from AAA is secondary to rupture, thus highlighting the importance of early detection and intervention.

Asymptomatic AAA

The decision to treat an asymptomatic AAA should include the risk of rupture, the procedural risk, and the patient's life expectancy. The maximum aneurysmal diameter is currently accepted as the most primary determinant of the risk of rupture. In general terms, the risk of rupture increases substantially when the diameter is greater than 5 cm (Fig. 12.1). Additionally, rapidly expanding aneurysms, defined as a greater than 1 cm increase in diameter over 1 year or 0.5 cm diameter over 6 months, represent a higher risk of rupture and constitute an indication for intervention.[6] The operative mortality of elective open AAA repair is reported to be between 5% and 8%.

Endovascular Aneurysm Repair. Conceptually, during endovascular aneurysm repair (EVAR), an endoluminal stent graft connects the proximal "normal" nondilated portion of the aorta to the aneurysm to the distal nondilated arteries, therefore excluding the aneurysm from the circulation. Excluding the aneurysm decreases the pressure on the wall and eliminates the risk of rupture. The EVAR-1 and DREAM trials randomized patients who were suitable for both EVAR and open repair, showing similar 2-year all-cause mortality but lower aneurysm-related deaths for the EVAR group (4% vs. 7%; $p = 0.04$ in EVAR-1 and 2% vs. 6% in DREAM). Since then, EVAR has gained significant acceptance as the treatment of choice for most asymptomatic aortic aneurysms requiring repair.

Not all patients are anatomically suitable for EVAR. Preprocedural planning is the cornerstone of a successful procedure, and CTA is the

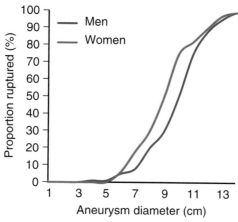

Figure 12.1 Cumulative distribution of rupture repair as a function of aortic diameter. *(Adapted from Lo et al., Relative importance of aneurysm diameter and body size for predicting abdominal aortic aneurysm rupture in men and women. J Vasc Surg. 2014 May;59(5):1209–16.)*

modality of choice for anatomic evaluation prior to endovascular repair. The critical anatomic elements that determine the patient's suitability for EVAR are:

1. A patent superior mesenteric artery (SMA) or celiac trunk: The inferior mesenteric artery is usually excluded with the graft. One of the worse complications of EVAR is ischemic colitis, which occurs in fewer than 2% of elective cases. The risk of colon necrosis is higher if the patient has had previous abdominal surgery that interrupts the collateral circulation from the SMA and celiac arteries or if there is significant pre-existing stenosis of these arteries.

2. An infrarenal neck diameter of <32 mm and >10–15 mm in length is needed to appropriately land the proximal end of the graft and create a complete seal. The most common reason for a patient with AAA to be considered unsuitable for EVAR is the anatomy of the proximal aortic neck. In a series of 526 patients, EVAR performed in subjects with a hostile neck—defined as length of less than 10 mm, angle of greater than 60 degrees, diameter of greater than 28 mm, or more than 50% circumferential thrombus or calcification—was associated with higher rates of intraprocedural type I endoleak (poor edge sealing).

3. No more than 90 degrees of circumferential calcification or mural thrombus in the infrarenal neck: This would interfere with appropriate anchoring and sealing of the device.

4. The minimal diameter of the external iliac arteries is large enough to allow the passage of the device (currently, 14F).

5. Distal fixation requires 10–15 mm in length of normal vessel in the common iliac segment, similar to that required for proximal fixation.

6. The diameter of the common internal iliac artery should be less than 20 mm; if this is not the case, an additional cuff is required to extend the graft into the external iliac artery with coiling of the internal iliac artery.

Available Devices. Presently, several devices have received U.S. Food and Drug Administration (FDA) approval for the treatment of AAA in the United States (Table 12.3). The basic EVAR system includes three main components: A delivery system, a stent graft, and a fabric sleeve for exclusion of the aneurysm. Earlier devices used either an aorto-aortic or aorto-unifemoral design that required a subsequent femoral-femoral bypass and embolization of the contralateral iliac artery. Modern grafts currently rely on distal fixation in both common iliac arteries.

Table 12.3

Currently Available Endovascular Aneurysm Repair (EVAR) Devices in the United States				
Company	Device	Largest Main Body Diameter (mm)	Delivery System Profile	Fixed Location
Cook Medical	Zenith Flex	36	20, 23, 26 F	Suprarenal
Endologix	Powerlink	28	21 F	Infrarenal
W.L. Gore & associates	Excluder AAA endoprothesis	28.5	18 F	Infrarenal
Medtronic Vascular	AneuRx AAA Advantage	28	21 F	Infrarenal
	Talent abdominal	36	22, 24 F	Suprarenal
TriVascular	Ovation Prime	30	15 F	Suprarenal

Technique. There is some variation in technique depending on the type of endograft used. However there is a common workflow for most EVAR procedures:

1. *Aortogram*: After bilateral femoral access is obtained, a marked pigtail is inserted through the contralateral side to the main graft and positioned just above the level of the renal arteries. A digital subtraction angiogram is performed, and the level of the lowest renal artery is identified.

2. *Embolization of internal iliac artery when necessary*: If the common iliac arteries are aneurysmal, the distal limb of the device can be anchored in the external iliac artery. However, collateral flow into the ipsilateral internal iliac artery can result in a type II endoleak (see later discussion). Prophylactic embolization with coils of the internal iliac artery can be performed during EVAR or in a staged manner prior to the procedure.

3. *Introduction and deployment of the endograft*: Once the lowest renal artery is identified, the sheath containing the endograft is positioned just below it. It is important to adjust the angulation of the x-ray camera to be perpendicular to the plane of the infrarenal aorta for appropriate positioning (Fig. 12.2). The pigtail used for aortography should be removed prior to deployment. Post-positioning ballooning is often required, and it depends on the device used.

4. *Deployment of the contralateral limb*: For modular endografts, one needs to deploy a separate iliac limb graft in the contralateral side. A wire should be introduced into the main limb of the endograft via the contralateral femoral artery. Once the wire is successfully placed in the suprarenal aorta through the already deployed endograft, the sheath with the iliac endograft is advanced into the main body of the endograft. The final step is to deploy the contralateral limb.

5. *Dilation of the endograft*: Although stent grafts are self-expanding, balloon expansion of the proximal and distal attachment sites should be performed, as well as the junction of the modular components.

6. *Completion angiogram*: A completion angiogram with a power injector is performed at completion of the procedure and identifies endoleaks (Fig. 12.3 and Table 12.4).

Surveillance After EVAR

EVAR offers the advantage of lower perioperative morbidity but carries the cost of device-related complications like endoleaks, device migration, and graft thrombosis. Because of these potential complications, lifelong surveillance is mandatory. Current standard of care includes serial studies at 1, 6, 12 months and yearly thereafter (Table 12.5).[7] Since the advent of EVAR, this has largely been accomplished with serial CTA. There is, however, increasing awareness of the risks and costs of a lifelong CT imaging mandate, which has led to several cohort analyses comparing CT using color duplex ultrasonography with contrast-enhanced ultrasound for the evaluation of the endograft and aneurysm sac post-EVAR. Identifying endoleaks by ultrasound requires the use of color Doppler. The reported specificity of endoleak identification by Doppler is high (89%–97%). Color Doppler has a great advantage over CTA for the identification of endoleaks' flow direction because this parameter is difficult to be assessed by CTA. Ultrasound's results are influenced by the examiner, bowel gas, possible patient obesity, and presence of a large hernia in the abdominal wall. Technological advances in ultrasound imaging have reduced the impact of these limitations and increased the diagnostic value of color Doppler. Typical post-EVAR CT and magnetic resonance (MR) scans cost approximately US$1500–$2000 and $2000–$2600, respectively. A typical

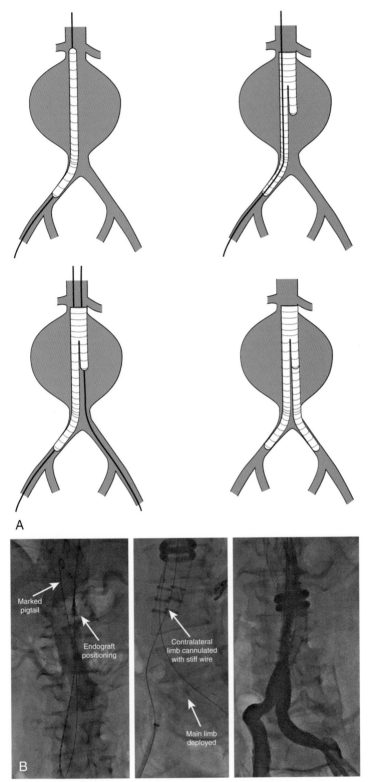

Figure 12.2 (A) Procedural steps for endovascular aneurysm repair (EVAR). (B) Example of EVAR with Ovation device. *(Courtesy of Stephen Jenkins.)*

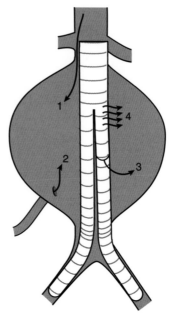

Figure 12.3 Classification of endoleaks.

Table 12.4

Classification of Endoleaks

Type	Definition	Causes	Treatment
1	Arises from the distal and proximal attachment sites	Undersizing of the stent, poor sealing, neck dilatation and stent migration	Postdilatation of the stent
2	Retrograde filling of the aneurysmal sac from lumbar or internal iliac arteries that were excluded with the endograft	Collateral circulation	Benign course. If needing treatment, trans-lumbar embolization or surgical ligation
3	Limb separation or fabric wear	Mainly occur with modular grafts at the sites of attachment	Regrafting
4	Extravasation through graft material	Due to porosity of the fabric material	Benign course, usually aneurysmal sac thrombosis without clinical consequence
5	Endotension: Space between aortic graft and the native aorta has elevated pressure without demonstrable endoleak	Missed endoleaks, thrombosed endoleaks, hygroma, infection	Unknown

Table 12.5

Appropriate Use Criteria for Noninvasive Surveillance Imaging After Endovascular Aneurysm Repair (EVAR)			
Baseline (within 1 month of implant) New or worsening symptoms	**Appropriate Use Score (1–9)**		
First year	At 3–6 months	At 6–8 months	At 9–12 months
No endoleak, stable size	I (3)	U (5)	U (6)
Endoleak or growing aneurysm	U (6)	A (8)	A (7)
After 1st year	Every 6 months	Every 12 months	Every 24+ months
No endoleak, stable size	I (3)	A (7)	U (5)
Endoleak or growing aneurysm	A (6)	A (7)	U (5)

A, appropriate; *I*, inappropriate; *U*, uncertain.

post-EVAR surveillance duplex, in comparison, costs approximately $600–$800.

Renal Artery Interventions

Renal artery stenosis (RAS) is the single largest cause of secondary hypertension, affecting 25–35% of patients with secondary hypertension,[8,9] is associated with progressive renal insufficiency, and causes cardiovascular complications such as refractory heart failure and flash pulmonary edema. An understanding of the underlying pathophysiologic mechanisms, clinical manifestations, and medical and interventional treatment strategies is paramount in optimizing the care of patients with RAS. A critical issue is appropriate patient selection for interventional procedures.

Clinical Syndromes Associated With RAS

Renovascular Hypertension

Resistant hypertension is defined as blood pressure above goal on three different classes of antihypertensive medications, ideally including a diuretic drug. Patients with resistant hypertension should be evaluated for secondary causes of hypertension. In patients older than 50 years of age who were referred to a hypertension center, 13% had a secondary cause of hypertension, the most common of which was renovascular disease.

RAS is a common finding in hypertensive patients undergoing cardiac catheterization to assess coronary artery disease. In a series of 1089 renal arteries in 534 patients undergoing angiography with either uncontrolled hypertension or flash pulmonary edema, 19% were found to have significant RAS at the time of coronary angiography that required revascularization (Table 12.6).[10]

Ischemic Nephropathy

RAS is a potentially a reversible form of renal insufficiency. As many as 11–14% of patients starting dialysis from end-stage renal disease (ESRD) are attributable to RAS.[11] Favorable predictors of improvement with intervention include a rapid recent increase in serum creatinine concentration, decrease in GFR during angiotensin-converting enzyme inhibitor (ACEI) or angiotensin receptor blocker (ARB) treatment, absence of glomerular or interstitial fibrosis on kidney biopsy, and kidney pole-to-pole length of greater than 8.0 cm and the absence of proteinuria. In 73 patients with chronic renal failure (estimated glomerular filtration rate [eGFR] <50 mL/min) and clinical evidence of RAS, renal stenting demonstrated a renal function improved in 34 of 59 patients (57.6%). The most important predictor of improvement was

Table 12.6

Prevalence of Renal Artery Stenosis (RAS) in Patients Undergoing Angiography With Either Uncontrolled Hypertension or Flash Pulmonary Edema ($n = 1089$).			
	Diseased Vessels (>70% Diameter Stenosis)	Patients Treated	Prevalence
Bilateral	26	26	
Unilateral	74	74	
Solitary renal arteries	2	1	
Complete occlusions	4	0	
Total		101	19%

the slope of the reciprocal serum creatinine plot before revascularization, suggesting that rapidly progressive renal failure is associated with a more favorable response after revascularization.[12]

Current American College of Cardiology/American Heart Association (ACC/AHA) guidelines recommend renal artery stenting for patients with ischemic nephropathy if they have progressive chronic kidney disease (CKD) with bilateral RAS (class IIa, LOE B), progressive CKD with RAS to a solitary functioning kidney (class IIa, LOE B), and CKD with unilateral RAS (class IIb, LOE C).

Cardiac Destabilization Syndromes

The most widely recognized example of a cardiac destabilization syndrome is "flash" pulmonary or Pickering syndrome. Renovascular disease may also complicate the treatment of patients with heart failure or coronary artery disease.

In patients with either CHF or an acute coronary syndrome, successful renal stent placement resulted in a significant decrease in blood pressure and symptom improvement in 88% (42 of 48) of patients. For those patients who presented with unstable angina, renal artery stenting improved the Canadian Class Society (CCS) symptoms at least by one class level regardless of concomitant coronary intervention (Fig. 12.4).

Current ACC/AHA guidelines recommend renal artery stenting for RAS with recurrent, unexplained heart failure decompensation or sudden unexplained pulmonary edema (class I, LOE B) and for hemodynamically significant RAS and medically refractory unstable angina (class IIa, LOE B).

Diagnostic Testing

Doppler Ultrasound Evaluation

Renal artery Doppler ultrasound (DUS) carries a sensitivity of 97%, specificity of 81%, and negative predictive value of 95% for the detection of significant RAS. The success of this technology is highly dependent on the skill of the technician performing the examination. A peak systolic velocity (PSV) of greater than 180 cm/sec has a 95% sensitivity and 90% specificity for significant RAS. When the ratio of the PSV of the stenosed renal artery to the PSV in the aorta is greater than 3.5, DUS predicts more than 60% RAS with a 92% sensitivity.[13,14] Duplex also allows follow-up of stent patency in patients who have undergone renal artery stenting; however, criteria for native renal artery stenosis overestimates the degree of angiographic in-stent restenosis (ISR). Surveillance monitoring for renal stent patency should take into account that PSV and renal artery ratio (RAR) obtained by DUS are higher for any given degree of arterial narrowing within the stent. PSV of greater than 395 cm/s or a RAR of greater than 5.1 were the most predictive of angiographically significant ISR in more than 70% of cases.[15]

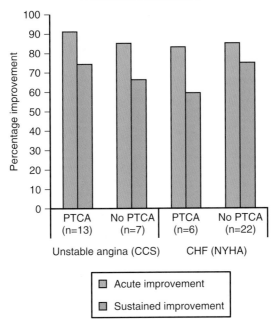

Figure 12.4 Improvement in cardiac destabilization syndromes after renal artery revascularization. *(From Khoshla et al. Effects of renal artery stent implantation in patients with renovascular hypertension presenting with unstable angina or congestive heart failure. Am J Cardiol. 1997;80:363–66.)*

DUS can be performed without risk to the patient because there is no iodinated contrast or ionizing radiation required. The main limitations for DUS include unsatisfactory exams due to overlying bowel gas or large body habitus. DUS is not useful in detecting accessory renal arteries. There is a requirement for a capable sonographer who is allowed enough time to perform the examination.

Computed Tomographic Angiography

CTA can provide high-resolution cross-sectional imaging of RAS while supplying three-dimensional angiographic images of the aorta, renal, and visceral arteries that allow localization and enumeration of the renal arteries, including accessory branches. Sensitivity (59%–96%) and specificity (82%–99%) of CTA for detecting significant RAS compare well with invasive angiography.[16] CTA requires the administration of 100–150 mL of iodinated contrast and therefore carries the potential risk of contrast-induced nephropathy (CIN). Additionally, CT requires the use of ionizing radiation. However as CTA scanner technology advances, spatial resolution will improve, scanning time will decrease, the administered contrast load may be reduced, and the amount of radiation will be decreased. Additionally, iso-osmolar contrast media are now available with decreased potential for nephrotoxicity. CTA can be used to follow patients with prior stents to detect ISR, an advantage over MR angiography (MRA) in which metallic stents generate artifact.

Magnetic Resonance Angiography

This imaging modality allows localization and enumeration of the renal arteries and characterization of the stenosis. When compared to invasive angiography, it has a sensitivity between 92% and 97% and a specificity between 73% and 93% for detection of RAS.[17,18] MRA does not require the use of ionizing radiation. Limitations for MRA include the association of gadolinium with nephrogenic systemic fibrosis when administered to patients with an eGFR of less than 30 mL/1.73 m^2 and the fact that metal causes artifacts on MRA, renders it unusable as a test for patients with prior renal stents.

Treatment Strategies

Medical Management of RAS

Medical management of atherosclerotic vascular disease involves blood pressure control, lipid-lowering therapy, an antiplatelet agent, and lifestyle advice, including dietary counseling, smoking cessation, and increased physical activity. Historically, the use of renin angiotensin aldosterone system (RAAS) antagonists (ACEIs or ARBs) was contraindicated in this patient group owing to concerns of worsening renal function. Concerns with RAAS antagonists in this patient group are probably overstated. When utilized prospectively, RAAS antagonists were tolerated in 357 of 378 patients (92%), even in 54/69 (78.3%) patients with bilateral RAS (>60%) or occlusion.[19] Despite the lack of randomized trials, there is consensus that RAAS antagonists should be used in patients with RAS; however, they should be carefully monitored and introduced slowly.

Lipid-lowering therapy is widely accepted as one of the main treatments for all atherosclerotic vascular disease. Additionally, the use of antiplatelet agents and smoking cessation in patients with RAS has the same benefits as in other forms of atherosclerotic disease, including peripheral and coronary artery disease.

The Cardiovascular Outcomes in Renal Atherosclerotic Lesions (CORAL) trial defined poorly controlled hypertension as a systolic blood pressure of 155 mm Hg or higher while receiving two or more antihypertensive medications. This trial found that the primary composite end point (death from cardiovascular or renal causes, myocardial infarction, stroke, hospitalization for congestive failure, progressive renal insufficiency, or the need for renal replacement therapy) in patients with renal artery stenosis (>60% diameter stenosis) did not differ comparing an initial strategy of medical therapy versus medical therapy plus renal artery stenting in patients with hypertension and RAS. All patients received, unless contraindicated, the angiotensin II type-1 receptor blocker candesartan with or without hydrochlorothiazide, and the combination agent amlodipine–atorvastatin, with the dose adjusted on the basis of blood pressure and lipid status.[20] CORAL confirms the guideline recommendations that first-line therapy for patients with RAS and hypertension is a trial of optimal medical therapy. For those who fail optimal medical therapy (resistant hypertension), renal intervention remains an appropriate strategy.

In the treatment of resistant hypertension, one of the three agents should be a diuretic, and all agents should be prescribed at optimal dose amounts. Resistant hypertension includes patients with uncontrolled hypertension with less than optimal medical therapy if they do not tolerate their medications. Resistant hypertension also includes patients whose blood pressure is controlled with the use of more than three medications. That is, patients whose blood pressure is controlled but who require four or more medications to do so should be considered resistant to treatment. It is important to note that the CORAL trial does not apply to patients with resistant or refractory hypertension. CORAL did not investigate patients in whom medical therapy had failed to control blood pressure, and therefore it will be unlikely to change the ACC/AHA recommendations for renal artery revascularization. Current ACC/AHA guidelines recommend renal artery stenting for patients with RAS and accelerated or resistant hypertension or in patients with hypertension with medication intolerance (class IIa, LOE B).

Renal Artery Surgery

Surgical repair of RAS was the only available revascularization option before renal artery angioplasty. In an observational series of 500 patients with RAS and hypertension managed with surgical revascularization and followed for up to 10 years, 12% of patients were cured of their hypertension and 73% were improved. Importantly, 30-day mortality ranged from 4.6% to 7.3%. Complications of surgery include surgical infections, surgery-related bleeding, urinary tract infection, and pseudomembranous colitis. Today, percutaneous catheter-based therapy has largely replaced surgical renal revascularization for RAS because of the increased morbidity and mortality associated with surgery.

Renal Artery Stenting

Renal artery stenting is the standard of care for patients with hemodynamically significant renal artery stenosis (>70% angiographic diameter renal artery stenosis or 50–70% stenosis with a significant translesional gradient) and (1) resistant or uncontrolled hypertension and the failure of three antihypertensive drugs, one of which is a diuretic, or hypertension with intolerance to medication; (2) ischemic nephropathy; and (3) cardiac destabilization syndromes. This population was not addressed by the CORAL trial.

Despite excellent angiographic outcomes achieved with renal stenting, there is a mismatch between angiographic (>97%) and clinical (~70%) success for controlling hypertension and renal dysfunction. Technically, renal artery stent placement is highly successful and safe. In a meta-analysis of 14 studies (678 patients) evaluating renal artery stenting for either hypertension or CKD, the procedure success rate was 98% (95% CI; 95–100%).[21] However, the clinical response rate for hypertension was only 69%, with a cure rate of 20% and improvement in blood pressure in 49% (Fig. 12.5A). Renal function improved in 30% and stabilized in 38% of patients with an overall favorable response rate of 68% (Fig. 12.5B).[21] The mismatch between angiographic success and clinical response may be explained by (1) treatment of nonobstructive RAS lesions (visually overestimating the stenosis severity), or (2) symptoms (hypertension or CKD) were not caused by renal artery stenosis (i.e., essential hypertension). The key to successful clinical outcomes is to identify which patients are likely to benefit from intervention.

Several recent randomized clinical trials have attempted to determine the clinical benefit of renal artery stenting. The STAR and ASTRAL trials were flawed by poor design and the inability to objectively assess the severity of the RAS. They failed to select patients with hemodynamically significant RAS lesions that would cause renal hypoperfusion and included inexperienced operators, thus resulting in an unusually high complication rate.[22,23]

Selecting Patients Likely to Benefit From Revascularization

The "Achilles heel" of renal artery revascularization is that angiography is a very uncertain and unreliable "gold standard" for determining the hemodynamic severity of moderate RAS. When a single operator performed visual estimation of angiographic diameter stenosis in patients with moderate RAS (50%–90% diameter stenosis), the correlation was poor between the angiographic diameter stenosis and resting mean translesional pressure gradient ($r = 0.43$; $p = 0.12$), hyperemic mean translesional pressure gradient ($r = 0.22$; $p = 0.44$), and renal fractional flow reserve (FFR) ($r = 0.18$; $p = 0.54$) (Fig. 12.6).[24] Therefore physiologic assessment should always be performed in patients with moderate RAS lesions.

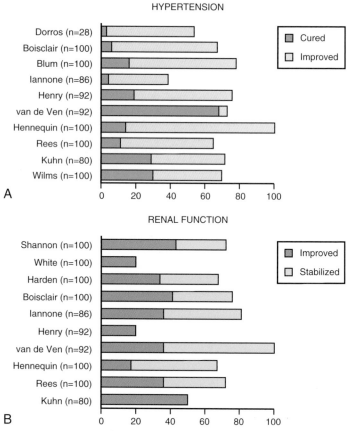

Figure 12.5 Summary of initial reported series in terms of improvement of (A) hypertension and (B) renal function after renal artery revascularization. Despite a technical success of >95%, clinical outcomes did not match technical success. This suggests that selection of patients is crucial to obtaining clinical benefit.

Translesional Pressure Gradients

A translesional resting pressure ratio of less than 0.90 (P_d/P_a) or a hyperemic systolic gradient of greater than 20 mm Hg correlated with a significant rise in renin concentration in the ipsilateral renal vein. Based on these observations, an expert consensus panel recommended that a peak systolic gradient of at least 20 mm Hg or a mean pressure gradient of 10 mm Hg be used to confirm the severity of lesions with 70% or greater diameter stenosis in symptomatic patients with RAS. Because the catheter itself can introduce an artificial gradient, measurements should be done with either a 4F or smaller catheter or a 0.014-inch pressure wire.

Renal Artery Fractional Flow Reserve

Another method to determine the severity of angiographic RAS is to quantify the FFR. This hemodynamic assessment of flow, which is widely used in the coronary circulation, is based on the principle that flow across a conduit artery is proportional to pressure across the vascular bed and inversely proportional to the resistance of the vascular bed. Under conditions of maximum hyperemia, the flow through the conduit artery is maximal while the resistance of the vascular bed is at a minimum and constant. Any reduction in flow under these conditions is caused by a stenosis and is proportional to the ratio of pressure distal to the stenosis (P_d) and the pressure proximal to the stenosis (P_a).

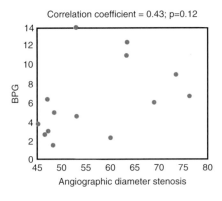

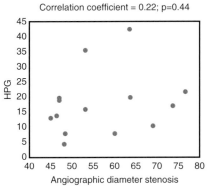

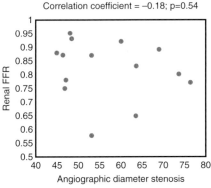

Figure 12.6 Correlations among angiographic diameter stenosis and resting or basal pressure gradient (BPG), hyperemic pressure gradient (HPG), and renal fractional flow reserve (FFR). *(From Subramanian et al. Renal fractional flow reserve: A hemodynamic evaluation of moderate renal artery stenoses. Catheter Cardiovasc Interv. 2005;64:480–6.)*

FFR is measured after induction of maximum hyperemia. Renal hyperemia can be achieved with papaverine, dopamine, or acetylcholine (see Table 12.7). Translesional pressure gradients are measured, and FFR (P_d/P_a) is calculated using a 0.014-inch pressure guidewire. Renal artery FFR correlates well with other hemodynamic parameters of lesion severity[25,26] (Fig. 12.7) and in some series has been proved to be a better predictor of clinical response. In one study, renal FFR was measured after renal stent placement in 17 patients with refractory hypertension and moderate to severe (50–90%) stenosis, unilateral RAS. Ten patients had normal baseline renal FFR (defined as FFR ≥0.80), whereas an abnormal baseline renal FFR (<0.80) was recorded in seven patients. At 3 months after intervention, 86% of patients with an abnormal renal FFR experienced improvement in their BP, compared

Table 12.7

Medications Used to Induce Pharmacologic Renal Hyperemia			
Agent	**Dose**	**Maximum Dose**	**Drug Considerations**
Papaverine	32 mg	40 mg	Hypotension, crystallization with heparin
Acetylcholine	100 µg	1000 µg	Hypotension, tachyarrhythmias
Dopamine	50 µg/kg	200 µg/kg	Tachyarrhythmias

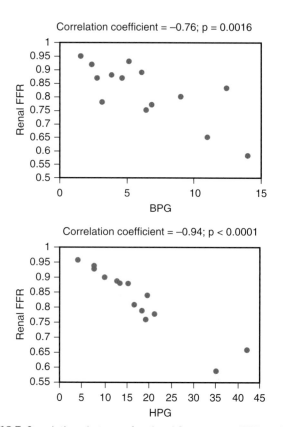

Figure 12.7 Correlations between fractional flow reserve (FFR) and resting or basal pressure gradient (BPG) *(top)* and hyperemic pressure gradient (HPG) *(bottom)*. *(From Subramanian et al. Renal fractional flow reserve: A hemodynamic evaluation of moderate renal artery stenoses. Catheter Cardiovasc Interv. 2005;64:480–6.)*

with only 30% of those with normal renal FFR ($p = 0.04$) (see Fig. 12.8). In this small series, baseline systolic, mean, or hyperemic translesional pressure gradients were not different between patients whose blood pressure improved and those in whom it did not.[27]

Technical Aspects of Revascularization

There are several important technical and procedural considerations to prevent complications during renal stenting. Selective renal angiography should be preceded by nonselective abdominal aortography. The catheter-in-catheter or no-touch techniques should be used to minimize contact with the aortic wall and injury to the renal ostium during guiding catheter engagement (Fig. 12.9). Aggressive preprocedure

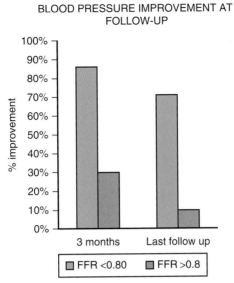

BLOOD PRESSURE IMPROVEMENT AT FOLLOW-UP

Figure 12.8 Blood pressure improvement at follow-up stratified by baseline renal FFR (<0.8 vs. ≥0.80). *(From Mitchell et al. Predicting blood pressure improvement in hypertensive patients after renal artery stent placement: renal fractional flow reserve.* Catheter Cardiovascular Interv. *2007;69:685–9.)*

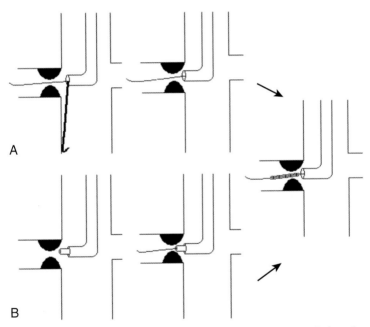

Figure 12.9 (A) No-touch technique. (B) Catheter-in-catheter technique for renal artery stenting from radial access.

hydration and limiting contrast volume are helpful to prevent the development of CIN.

Radial Access

The radial approach for renal stenting represents a valuable tool to reduce access-site complications and improve patient comfort. However the operator needs specific technical skills as well as knowledge of device compatibility. Both radial arteries are suitable for renal intervention. Depending on the configuration of the aortic arch, the left radial access allows a shorter distance to renal arteries. The right radial

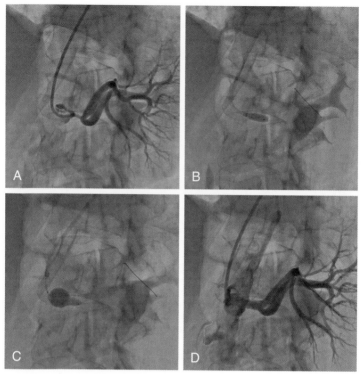

Figure 12.10 Renal intervention via right radial access. (A) Diagnostic angiogram. (B) A 6-mm Herculink stent deployment. (C) Ostial postdilation with Flash balloon. (D) Final result.

approach is more comfortable for the operator, and radiation exposure is less compared to the left. The use of 125-cm-long guiding catheters with 150-cm balloon/stent shafts is appropriate for almost all patients, whereas the 100-cm-long catheters and 135-cm-long balloon/stent shafts may not reach the renal arteries in taller patients or in patients with excessive aortic arch tortuosity.[28] Fig. 12.10 shows an example of renal artery stenting via right radial access.

Embolic Protection Devices

Atheroembolism has been associated with an increase in morbidity and a dramatic reduction in 5-year survival compared with patients who had no evidence on biopsy of renal atheroembolization (54% vs. 85%, $p = 0.011$).[29] Since atheroembolism is a potential complication of renal artery stenting, investigators have looked for the role of embolic protection devices (EPDs) in optimizing outcomes after renal intervention. However distal protection may be complicated by a proximal bifurcation of renal arteries, which would require two EPD devices and a 0.035-inch lumen balloon/stent catheter. In a randomized controlled study, 100 patients undergoing renal artery stenting were assigned to an open-label EPD or use of abciximab in a 2×2 factorial design. A positive interaction was observed between treatment with abciximab and embolic protection. Renal artery stenting alone, stenting with EPD, and stenting with abciximab were associated with similar and modest declines in eGFR at 1-month follow-up (−10, −12, −10 mL/min/1.73 m^2 eGFR change, respectively); however, the group treated with both EPD and abciximab was protected from a decline in eGFR and had results superior to the other three groups (+9 mL/min/1.73 m^2 eGFR change; $p < 0.01$).[30] At present, we reserve the use of EPDs with renal stenting for patients with impaired renal function.

Stent Sizing With IVUS

IVUS can provide precise anatomic characterization of the atherosclerotic plaque. IVUS guidance during renal artery stent placement resulted in additional lumen enlargement not considered necessary at angiography.[31] In a series of 363 renal artery interventions, follow-up angiography was available in 102 patients (34%) at an average of 303 days. Larger diameter arteries were associated with a significantly lower incidence of angiographic restenosis. The restenosis rate was 36% for vessels with a reference diameter of less than 4.5 mm compared with 16% in vessels with a reference diameter of 4.5–6 mm ($p = 0.068$) and 6.5% in vessels with reference diameter greater than 6 mm ($p < 0.01$).[32] IVUS allows a more accurate way to measure vessel diameter than two-dimensional angiography, allowing the operator to safely maximize the stent size. Visual estimation tends to underestimate the size of the vessel, which can translate to higher rates of ISR.

Drug-Eluting Stent Versus Bare Metal Stent

Restenosis after stent angioplasty of atherosclerotic RAS is a limitation, especially in small-diameter renal arteries. Recent reports suggest that with optimal deployment techniques, restenosis rates of less than 11% can be achieved when followed up to 60 months when using bare metal stents (BMS).[33,34]

The GREAT study (Palmaz Genesis Peripheral Stainless Steel Balloon Expandable Stent, comparing a Sirolimus-Coated with an Uncoated Stent in REnal Artery Treatment)[35] was a prospective, multicenter study of angiographic patency of renal artery stents placed in 105 patients with atherosclerotic RAS. The binary restenosis rate was 6.7% for sirolimus-eluting stents (SES) versus 14.6% for the BMS ($p = 0.30$). At 1-year follow-up, the clinical patency was 88.5% in the BMS and 98.1% in the drug-eluting stent (DES) group ($p = 0.21$). There is no substantial difference between BMS and DES for RAS at this time.

Restenosis Lesions

The durability of renal artery interventions is limited by the development of ISR and the need for secondary or tertiary renal interventions. Two meta-analyses of renal artery intervention have demonstrated mean restenosis rates after stent placement of 16% and 17% at 2 and 5 years follow-up, respectively.[21,36] Renal stents have excellent long-term patency rates, with cumulative primary patency of 79–85% and a secondary patency of 92–98% at 5 years.[33,34] A larger RVD and larger acute gain (post-stent minimal lumen diameter) after stent deployment are associated with a lower incidence of restenosis: the restenosis rate for smaller renal arteries (RVD ≤4.5 mm) was 36% compared with a restenosis rate of 6.5% for larger renal arteries (RVD >6.0 mm).[32]

The optimal treatment of renal artery ISR is uncertain.

The use of covered stents in the renal arteries has been reported in the management of complications including perforation.[37] Polytetrafluoroethylene (PTFE)-covered stents and DESs may offer a way to treat recurrent renal artery stenosis. In a series of patients diagnosed having their at least second ISR following renal artery stenting, covered stents had 17% (1/6) ISR at a mean follow-up of 36 months whereas DES were free of ISR (0/10).[38,39]

Follow-Up

Patients should be followed clinically in terms of blood pressure control with laboratory results to monitor renal function and with surveillance DUS imaging at 1 month, 6 months, and 1 year and annually thereafter recommended to evaluate stent patency.[7] DUS is the recommended imaging technique to screen for ISR. DUS surveillance monitoring for renal stent patency should take into account that a stented artery is less compliant than a native artery and that PSV and RAR obtained by DUS are higher for any given degree of arterial narrowing within the stent[15]; therefore, obtaining a postprocedure DUS is reasonable to establish a new baseline PSV.

Subclavian Interventions

Subclavian and innominate artery (S/IA) obstruction is an important cause of symptomatic extracranial cerebrovascular disease and may be associated with significant morbidity.[40] Symptoms include those associated with posterior cerebral ischemia (vertebrobasilar insufficiency [VBI]) due to reversal of flow in the vertebral artery (subclavian steal syndrome), angina pectoris due to reversal of flow in an internal mammary arterial graft (coronary-subclavian steal syndrome), and arm ischemia due to claudication related to exercise or distal embolization.[41]

Although the technical success of surgical revascularization is high, major complications include stroke in 0.5–5%, perioperative death in 2–3%, and an overall complication rate of 13–19%.

Catheter-based revascularization with stents for S/IA obstruction was introduced a decade later to treat failures and complications of PTA. In a series of 170 consecutive patients, stent placement improved overall technical success (98%), target lesion revascularization (TLR) (14.6%), primary patency (83% at 66 months), and secondary patency (96% at 54 months). Complications occurred in 5.9% ($n = 10$) of patients with no procedure-related deaths and one embolic stroke, which compares favorably with surgical series. Stent placement provided immediate relief of symptoms in 93% of the patients, of which more than 80% remained symptom-free at last follow-up.[42]

Diagnosis of Subclavian/Innominate Artery Stenosis

Screening for S/IA disease is easily performed by obtaining bilateral arm blood pressure in the office. A systolic blood pressure difference of 15 mm Hg or greater is highly ($\geq$90%) specific for diagnosing subclavian stenosis, and this physical finding has proved to be an independent predictor of adverse cardiovascular events, including mortality.[43,44] Noninvasive studies include DUS, CTA and MRA.

DUS is an inexpensive and useful method of evaluating S/IA stenosis. The subclavian artery can be visualized on ultrasound; additionally, Doppler can measure velocities and direction of flow in the subclavian artery as well as the vertebral artery, therefore providing information about the underlying pathophysiologic process. Reversal of flow in the vertebral artery is seen in cases of subclavian steal syndrome. CTA and MRA can provide more anatomic detail, including the aortic arch anatomy, and can give precise determinations of anatomic relations of the diseased segments to the ostia of the vertebral and internal mammary arteries.

Indications for Revascularization

Subclavian steal syndrome (SSS): This term refers to the clinical syndrome that results after the development of flow reversal in the ipsilateral vertebral artery with a hemodynamically significant subclavian artery stenosis or occlusion. Subclavian steal syndrome implies the presence of symptoms due to arterial insufficiency in the brain, specifically, posterior circulation symptoms. The diagnosis of SSS requires the presence of neurologic symptoms usually triggered by arm exercise with all of the following: (1) evidence of subclavian or innominate artery occlusion or marked stenosis, (2) retrograde vertebral flow, and (3) patency of both vertebral and the basilar arteries.

Coronary-subclavian steal syndrome: Coronary-subclavian steal phenomenon is seen in patients with prior coronary artery bypass surgery (CABG) using the internal mammary artery (IMA). In the presence of a hemodynamically significant subclavian stenosis proximal to the origin of the IMA, flow through the IMA may reverse and "steal" flow from the coronary vasculature during upper extremity exercise. Coronary and graft angiography can demonstrate retrograde flow in the involved IMA during selective angiography of the grafted coronary artery. Simultaneous coronary and cerebrovascular ischemia have also been reported. Identification of significant subclavian artery stenosis prior to CABG can prevent this important problem. Those patients with a high-grade subclavian artery stenosis should be treated prior to placement of an internal mammary graft. Grafting the IMA to the left anterior descending (LAD) coronary artery during CABG operations has been proved to have the highest patency rate and is associated with the highest survival and lower complications when compared to other conduits.[45] Therefore, any interruption in the hemodynamic integrity of this conduit, which includes S/IA stenosis, may jeopardize the clinical benefit and result in coronary-subclavian steal syndrome.

Arm claudication: Upper extremity claudication is far less common than lower extremity claudication. However, lifestyle-limiting exertional symptoms, especially in the dominant hand, can be successfully treated with subclavian stent placement.

Technical Considerations

Vascular Access

Access site selection depends on the nature of the obstructive lesion. Femoral access offers an advantage in better visualizing the ostium at the aortic arch. For occlusions, a dual approach may be necessary. In such circumstances, femoral access helps identify the ostium of the artery, and a wire placed in the ipsilateral upper extremity can help identify the target. Radial access is a good alternative to brachial access; however the placement of large stents (average 6 mm) often requires 6F or 7F systems, which limits the use of the radial artery to a select group of patients.[46]

Angiography

Selective angiography of the innominate or left subclavian artery from a femoral approach can be accomplished most of the times with a JR4 or a Berenstein diagnostic catheter. For patients with type III aortic arch, alternative "shepherd's crook" catheters like the Vitek or Simmons may be required (Fig. 12.11). After selective engagement of the subclavian or innominate artery, at least two orthogonal views are recommended. The bifurcation of the right subclavian artery and right common carotid artery is best evaluated in the right anterior oblique (RAO) projection;

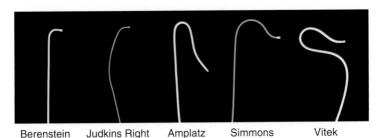

| Berenstein | Judkins Right | Amplatz | Simmons | Vitek |

Figure 12.11 Catheter shapes most used for engagement of the great vessels.

the origins of the right IMA and the right vertebral artery are better visualized in the left anterior oblique (LAO) projection. On the left side, the origin of the left IMA and the left vertebral artery can be visualized in the antero-posterior (AP) projection. Digital subtraction angiography (DSA) can be used to better delineate the vascular anatomy without overlying bony structures; however, it requires adequate breath-holding to prevent motion artifacts.

Stenting

The choice of guiding catheter and/or sheath is largely dependent on the aortic arch anatomy. A coronary guiding catheter may allow easier access to the ostia of the subclavian artery in patients with challenging anatomy or ostial lesions; however, it requires at least an 8F lumen in order to deliver equipment necessary for subclavian stenting and a larger sheath in the femoral artery. On the other hand, a guide-sheath like a Shuttle sheath will require a smaller arterial puncture to deliver the same equipment (6/7F) but is less steerable in engaging the ostium of the subclavian artery.

A 0.035-inch wire is preferred for delivery of interventional equipment; however, in some circumstances, when the lesion is heavily calcified with severe stenosis or there is an occlusion, a 0.014- or 0.018-inch wire can be used. In some cases of occlusion or severe stenosis, a femoral approach can be challenging, and the operator may not be able to cross the lesion. A retrograde approach via the brachial or radial access can be considered. On some occasions, it is necessary to use both antegrade and retrograde routes in order to cross the lesion.

Once the lesion is crossed, balloon angioplasty is usually performed prior to stenting to facilitate stent delivery and to provide some information about the size of the vessel. The subclavian artery usually ranges from 6 to 8 mm in diameter. Balloon angioplasty alone is rarely performed because the use of BMSs achieves patency rates of 97% at 12 months and 75% at 10 years compared to restenosis rates of 15%–20% with balloon angioplasty alone. Covered stents may be necessary to treat complications like vessel rupture or subclavian artery aneurysms.

When the stenosis is proximal to the vertebral and internal mammary arteries, balloon-expandable stents are preferred over self-expanding stents for precision in placement and the need for stronger radial force in this vascular structure. It is important to know that the proximal subclavian artery is an intrathoracic structure and its rupture may manifest with intrathoracic hemorrhage. An example of subclavian stenting is shown in Fig. 12.12.

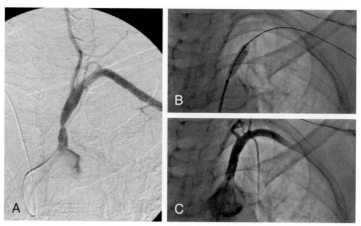

Figure 12.12 (A) Diagnostic angiography via right radial access using Simmons 2 catheter. (B) Stent deployment in left subclavian artery through a shuttle sheath. (C) Final result.

In-Stent Restenosis

The management of ISR largely depends on the presumed etiology. Geographic miss is a common cause of ISR, especially when the lesion involves the true ostium. Re-stenting with appropriate ostial coverage is required in those situations. When there is suspected underexpansion based on angiography or intravascular ultrasound, aggressive stent dilation with high-pressure balloons is recommended and provisional restenting is preserved for unsatisfactory results. When neither of these situations is present, repeated angioplasty with vascular brachytherapy or drug-eluting balloons is an available option, although there is no current evidence to support its use.

Complications

The major risk of S/IA intervention is distal embolization. Embolization may occur in the ipsilateral digits or in the posterior circulation via the vertebral artery. During innominate artery intervention, potential embolization to the anterior cerebral circulation may occur via the right common carotid artery. Additionally, a challenging arch is a risk factor for embolic complications because it requires more manipulation.

Carotid Interventions

Epidemiology and Natural History

Atherosclerotic carotid artery disease is responsible for 80% of new noncardioembolic strokes. Carotid plaque most often causes cerebrovascular events due to plaque rupture with atheroembolization, rather than carotid artery occlusion (<20% of ischemic strokes) with thrombosis (Fig. 12.13).[47]

The natural history of carotid artery stenosis depends on the presence of symptoms (transient ischemic attack [TIA], stroke, amaurosis

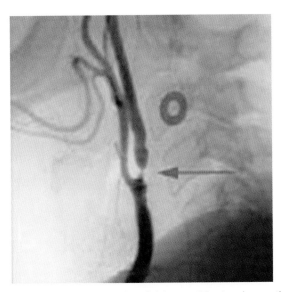

Figure 12.13 Catheter angiography of right carotid artery in a patient with recent transient ischemic attack. There is severe stenosis the origin of the internal carotid artery (arrow). The washer is placed as a reference for size. *(Courtesy of Dotter Interventional Institute, Portland, Oregon. http://www.ohsu. edu/dotter/carotid_stenting.htm)*

fugax). Symptomatic patients have a 5- to 10-fold risk of stroke when compared to asymptomatic patients. Asymptomatic patients with carotid artery stenosis outnumber symptomatic patients by 4:1. Because the majority (≥80%) of ischemic strokes have no warning symptoms, the management of asymptomatic carotid atherosclerosis with revascularization or medical therapy is important.

Transient focal neurologic symptoms are associated with a 30% risk of stroke within 6 months.[48] *TIA* is currently defined as a transient episode of neurologic dysfunction caused by focal brain, spinal cord, or retinal ischemia and without acute infarction, based on pathologic imaging, other objective evidence, and/or clinical evidence. *Stroke*, central nervous system (CNS) infarction, is defined by neuropathologic, neuroimaging, and/or clinical evidence of permanent injury.[49] However many of the initial studies that illustrated the natural history of this disease as well as our current standards of practice predated this updated definition and included only a clinical definition of infarction.

Asymptomatic Patients

Two randomized controlled trials (Asymptomatic Carotid Atherosclerosis Study [ACAS] and the Asymptomatic Carotid Surgery Trial [ACST]) showed that carotid endarterectomy (CEA) reduced the incidence of ipsilateral stroke in patients with asymptomatic carotid artery stenosis by 60% or more when compared to 50% reduction by medical therapy (e.g., aspirin) alone. However CEA did not reduce overall stroke and death and did not show any benefit in women or in patients older than 75 years of age. It is important to note that the medical therapy provided in these trials (aspirin) has significantly improved nowadays. Currently, the risk of progression of an asymptomatic carotid artery stenosis to occlusion with modern medical therapy is very low. In a cohort of 3681 patients with yearly duplex follow-up, 316 (8.6%) asymptomatic patients had occlusion that occurred during observation. Of these, 80% (254) of the occlusions occurred before the initiation of modern intensive medical therapy[50] (Fig. 12.14).

Symptomatic Patients

The natural history of symptomatic carotid artery stenosis was reflected in the medical arm of the randomized North American Symptomatic Carotid Endarterectomy Trial (NASCET). The 5-year risk of ipsilateral stroke in those medically managed was 18.7% among those with lesions

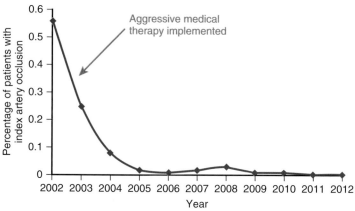

Figure 12.14 Percentage of patients with index carotid artery occlusion in a 10-year cohort.

of less than 50% in severity.[51] In those with 50%–69% stenosis, the risk over the same time period was 22.2%. In those with a 70%–99% stenosis, the 2-year risk of ipsilateral stroke was 26%.[52] The risk of stroke increases with severity of stenosis, and the 3-year risk of ipsilateral stroke in symptomatic patients with stenosis greater than 80% was 26.5%; however, as the stenosis approaches total occlusion (95%–99%), the risk of ipsilateral stroke goes down to 17.2%.[47]

Clinical Presentation

Symptoms of carotid artery stenosis include ipsilateral transient visual defects (amaurosis fugax) from retinal emboli; contralateral weakness or numbness of an extremity or the face or a combination of these; visual field defect; dysarthria; and, in the case of dominant hemisphere involvement, aphasia. The National Institutes of Health Stroke Scale (NIHSS) should be performed in all symptomatic patients to quantify the neurologic deficit, which correlates with outcome.[53]

Anatomic Imaging

DSA is the gold standard for defining carotid anatomy, with the NASCET method of stenosis measurement the most widely accepted methodology (Fig. 12.15). Invasive cerebral catheter–based angiography carries a risk of cerebral infarction of 0.5%–1.2%; therefore, noninvasive imaging should be the initial strategy for evaluation. Carotid duplex imaging, transcranial Doppler imaging, CTA, and MRA are the noninvasive methods of assessment. Duplex imaging is the best initial choice given its safety profile, low cost, and wide availability. Cerebral and cervical imaging should define the aortic arch and the circle of Willis (Fig. 12.16).

Medical Therapy

Medical therapy for carotid atherosclerosis should focus on preventing stroke and stabilizing atherosclerotic lesions to prevent plaque rupture and atheroembolization. Blood pressure control is of paramount importance since it is a primary risk factor for stroke; it is also a risk factor for atrial fibrillation and myocardial infarction, both of which increase the likelihood of stroke.[54] ACEIs and ARBs seem to be of particular benefit in stroke prevention, particularly in those at higher risk for cardiovascular disease.

Cholesterol lowering with statin drugs and antiplatelet medications including aspirin and clopidogrel has a significant role in both primary and secondary prevention of stroke in patients with carotid artery disease (Table 12.8).

There is uncertainty regarding the best therapy for asymptomatic carotid artery disease, a question to be addressed by the CREST 2 study.

Surgical Therapy to Prevent Stroke

Asymptomatic Patients

The purpose of carotid revascularization is to prevent ischemic stroke. Although there have been three large randomized studies comparing CEA to antiplatelet (aspirin) therapy in the treatment of at least moderate (≥50%–60%) carotid stenosis in patients without focal neurologic symptoms, the benefit of surgery was significant across varying degrees of stenosis (60%–90% stenosis). However, CEA did not reduce overall stroke and death and did not show any benefit in women or in patients older than 75 years of age.

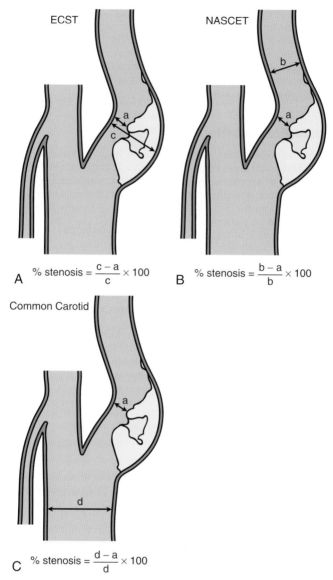

A   % stenosis = $\dfrac{c - a}{c} \times 100$

B   % stenosis = $\dfrac{b - a}{b} \times 100$

C   % stenosis = $\dfrac{d - a}{d} \times 100$

Figure 12.15 Methods of grading carotid artery stenosis in different trials.

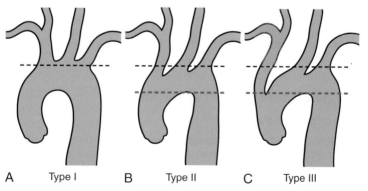

A   Type I   B   Type II   C   Type III

Figure 12.16 Aortic arch types. A, Type I arch: all vessels originate at the superior margin of the arch. B, Type II arch: at least one vessel originates between the superior and inferior margins of the aortic arch. C, Type III arch: at least one vessel originates below the inferior margin of the aortic arch.

Table 12.8

Classification of Statin Drugs Based on Their Ability to Lower LDL		
High-Intensity Statin Therapy	**Moderate-Intensity Statin Therapy**	**Low-Intensity Statin Therapy**
Lowers cholesterol by ≥50%	Lowers cholesterol by 30%–50%	Lowers cholesterol by <30%
Atorvastatin 40–80 mg/day	Atorvastatin 10–20 mg/day	Simvastatin 10 mg/day
Rosuvastatin 20–40 mg/day	Rosuvastatin 5–10 mg/day	Pravastatin 10–20 mg/day
	Simvastatin 20–40 mg/day	Lovastatin 20 mg/day
	Pravastatin 40–80 mg/day	Fluvastatin 20–40 mg/day
	Lovastatin 40 mg/day	Pitavastatin 1 mg/day
	Fluvastatin XL 80 mg/day	
	Fluvastatin 40 mg twice a day	
	Pitavastatin 2–4 mg/day	

Symptomatic Patients

Three large randomized controlled studies have evaluated the benefit of CEA compared to medical therapy in symptomatic patients with moderate to severe carotid artery disease. Early results from NASCET and ECST confirmed the significant benefit of CEA. At a mean follow-up of almost 1 year, there was a reduction in ipsilateral stroke or TIA from 19.4% in the medical treatment arm to 7.7% in the surgical arm, an absolute reduction in risk of 11.7%. The benefit of surgery was most profound in patients with stenosis of greater than 70% (absolute risk reduction of 17.7%).

Current American Heart Association/American Stroke Association (AHA/ASA) guidelines recommend CEA in symptomatic patients with stenosis of 50–99% if the risk of perioperative stroke or death is less than 6%. In asymptomatic patients, guidelines recommend CEA for stenosis of 60–99% if the perioperative risk of stroke is less than 3% and life expectancy is at least 5 years. Some have recommended delaying revascularization in asymptomatic patients until the stenosis has reached 80%, but the evidence from ACST demonstrated equal benefit for moderate and severe stenosis.

Carotid Artery Stenting

Clinical Evidence

For carotid artery stenting (CAS) to become a routine and commonly used procedure, clinical trial data must justify its performance relative to the standard, CEA. When interpreting data on carotid stenting, it is important to realize that a patient who is at high risk for surgery is not necessarily at increased risk for stenting (and vice versa). Features that place a patient at increased risk for complications from CEA and CAS are summarized in Table 12.9.

High Surgical Risk Patients

The Stenting and Angioplasty with Protection in Patients at High Risk for Endarterectomy (SAPPHIRE) trial is the only randomized trial comparing high surgical risk (HSR) patients treated with CEA to those treated with CAS.[55] In that trial, 334 patients with a symptomatic stenosis of 50% or greater or an asymptomatic stenosis of 80% or greater (~30% were symptomatic) were randomized to either CEA or CAS. The primary end point of death, stroke, or myocardial infarction (MI) at 30 days plus ipsilateral stroke or death from neurologic cause between day 31 and 1 year occurred in 12.2% of patients in the stenting group and 20.1% in the CEA group ($p = 0.004$ for noninferiority). The 30-day stroke

Table 12.9

High-Risk Features of Carotid Artery Stenting (CAS) and Carotid Endarterectomy (CEA)			
High-Risk Features for CAS		**High-Risk Features for CEA**	
Clinical Features	**Angiographic Features**	**Comorbidities**	**Anatomic Features**
Age ≥75–80	≥2 acute (90-degree) bends	Age ≥80	Lesion C2 or higher; below clavicle
Dementia	Circumferential calcification	Class III/IV CHF or Angina	Prior neck surgery (including ipsilateral CEA) or radiation
Bleeding disorder	Intracranial microangiopathy	Left main or ≥2 vessel CAD	Contralateral carotid occlusion
Multiple lacunar strokes	Evidence of thrombus	Urgent heart surgery	Tracheostoma
Renal failure	Poor vascular access	LVEF ≤30% MI within 30 days Severe chronic lung disease Severe renal disease	Contralateral laryngeal nerve palsy

Adapted from Bates ER, Babb JD, Casey DE, Jr., et al. ACCF/SCAI/SVMB/SIR/ASITN 2007 clinical expert consensus document on carotid stenting: a report of the American College of Cardiology Foundation Task Force on Clinical Expert Consensus Documents (ACCF/SCAI/SVMB/SIR/ASITN Clinical Expert Consensus Document Committee on Carotid Stenting). *J Am Coll Cardiol.* 2007;49:126–70; and Roubin GS, Iyer S, Halkin A, Vitek J, Brennan C. Realizing the potential of carotid artery stenting: proposed paradigms for patient selection and procedural technique. *Circulation.* 2006;113:2021–30.

and death rate among the asymptomatic patients was 4.6% for the CAS group and 5.4% for the CEA group. At 3 years, there were no differences between the CEA or CAS groups[56] (Fig. 12.17).

Most of the contemporary registry data focuses on HSR patients, and data from more than 10,000 HSR patients have been published. These registries generally include symptomatic patients with 50% or greater stenosis and asymptomatic patients with 70–80% or greater stenosis. Data from many of these studies are summarized in Fig. 12.18.

Average Surgical Risk Patients

Four large randomized studies in average or usual surgical risk patients have compared CAS to CEA. Three of these trials were conducted in Europe and were compromised by allowing very inexperienced CAS operators to participate in the trials and not requiring EPDs to be used.

The Carotid Revascularization Endarterectomy versus Stenting Trial (CREST) is the largest ($n = 2502$) randomized trial published comparing CAS with EPD to CEA in patients at average risk for surgery and including both symptomatic ($n = 1321$) and asymptomatic ($n = 1181$) patients.[57] The primary outcome of periprocedural stroke, death, or MI or follow-up ipsilateral stroke was not significantly different between the two groups (7.2% for CAS and 6.8% for CEA). The 30-day risk of all stroke was higher for CAS (4.1% vs. 2.3%, $p = 0.01$), whereas CEA was associated with a higher 30-day risk of MI (2.3% vs. 1.1%, $p = 0.03$) (Fig. 12.19).

For average surgical risk asymptomatic carotid stenosis patients enrolled in the Asymptomatic Carotid Trial (ACT-1), stenting was noninferior to endarterectomy with regard to death, stroke, or MI within 30 days after the procedure or ipsilateral stroke within 1 year (3.8% vs. 3.4%) (Fig. 12.20).

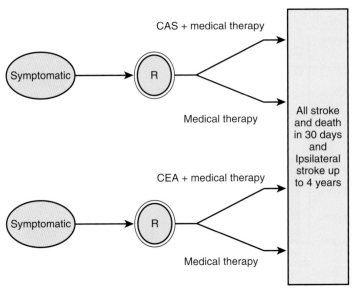

Figure 12.17 CREST-2 trial design. *R*, randomized,

HIGH SURGICAL RISK CAS

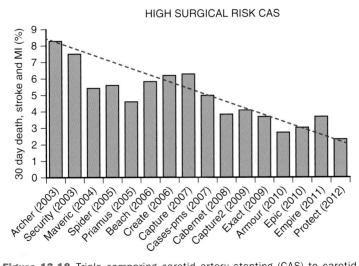

Figure 12.18 Trials comparing carotid artery stenting (CAS) to carotid endarterectomy (CEA) in high surgical risk patients.

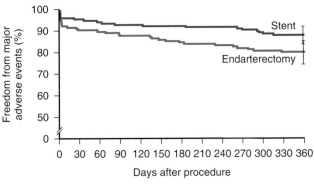

Figure 12.19 Results of the CREST trial.

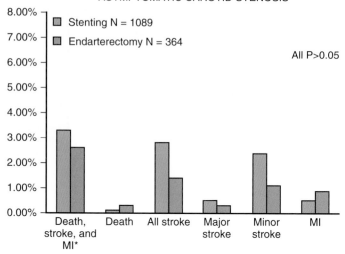

Figure 12.20 Results of ACT-1 trial.

When taken together, the message from these five large randomized controlled trials is that CAS with EPD is a reasonable alternative to CEA for average surgical risk patients but, as with CEA, only when performed by experienced operators.

Technical Aspects

Baseline Aortography and Cerebral Angiography

Vascular access is most commonly obtained from the femoral artery although brachial or radial access may be used. Prior to selective angiography, an arch aortogram is performed with a pigtail catheter placed in the proximal ascending aorta to define the anatomy of the aortic arch, which is critical to the success of the stent procedure. This is done in the 45-degree LAO position with a large-format image intensifier (12- to 16-inch) using DSA and a power injector (15 cc per second for 3 seconds).

Once the morphology of the aortic arch is determined, catheters are chosen for selective angiography of the cervical arteries supplying the brain (right and left carotid and vertebral arteries) and the cerebral vasculature. For a type I arch, Berenstein or Judkins Right (JR) catheters are often used. For type II or III arch morphologies, shepherd's crook–shaped catheters (i.e., Simmons or Vitek catheters) may be best (Fig. 12.11).

Angiograms are obtained to delineate the anterior and posterior circulation supplying the brain. The intracranial and extracranial portions of each vessel are studied. Generally, two orthogonal views of each are obtained, one in the AP projection and one in the lateral projection. Alternatively, some operators use rotational angiography. It is important to demonstrate the circle of Willis to define any baseline abnormalities. DSA may be performed with a 50-50 mix of saline and contrast. An external reference object is used with carotid angiograms in order to accurately measure the diameter of the artery.

Internal Carotid Intervention

The steps for internal carotid intervention are summarized in Fig. 12.21. A diagnostic catheter is used to engage the common carotid artery (CCA), and a roadmap angiogram is made of the carotid bifurcation. A 0.035-inch stiff angled hydrophilic glidewire is advanced into the external carotid artery, and the diagnostic catheter is advanced over the wire into the common carotid artery. The glidewire is exchanged for a 0.035-inch

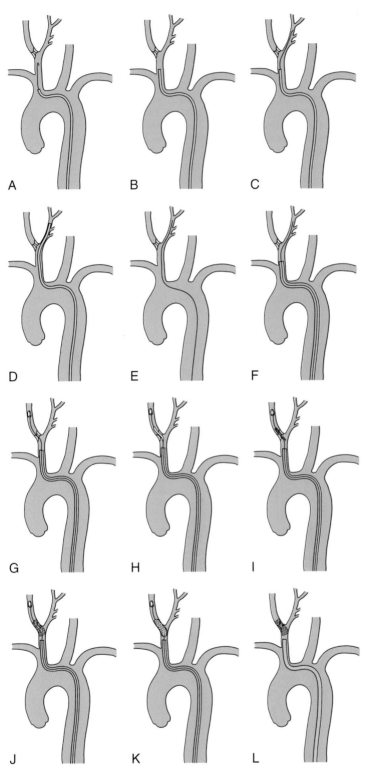

Figure 12.21 Internal carotid artery stenting, step by step. Stenting of the internal carotid artery (ICA). (A) The common carotid artery (CCA) is accessed with a diagnostic catheter and standard 0.035-inch J wire. (B) The catheter is advanced over the J wire but remains in the CCA. (C) The J wire is exchanged for a hydrophilic stiff-angled 0.035″ wire. (D) The catheter is advanced to the ECA and the hydrophilic wire is removed. (E) A stiff Amplatz wire is advanced to the ECA and the catheter is removed. (F) A long 6F sheath is advanced over a dilator to the CCA. (G) After removing the Amplatz wire and dilator, the lesion is crossed with a wire/filter device. (H) Predilation. (I) Stent placement. (J) Stent deployment. The ostium of the ECA is often "jailed". (K) postdilation. (L) Final result.

stiff Amplatz wire over which an 8F guiding catheter or a 6F sheath may be advanced to the CCA. Care must be taken to avoid plaque disruption with wires and catheters, and, at this point in the procedure, the plaque in the internal carotid artery should remain untouched.

Because of the very low incidence of stroke complicating CAS, demonstrating clinical benefit for any EPD in a randomized clinical trial is difficult. Two meta-analyses support the use of EPDs (215). The risk-to-benefit assessment intuitively favors using a protection device.[58,59] One simply has to retrieve a filter full of debris to realize the empirical benefits relative to the rare complications associated with an EPD. At present, optimal practice should include the use of an EPD, one that the operator is most comfortable using.

EPDs are standard of care in the United States, and several types exist (Fig. 12.22). If the distal EPD will not cross the lesion, the stenosis may be crossed with a conventional 0.014-inch guidewire and subsequently predilated with a small (2.5 mm) balloon. Then the EPD may be placed. After distal EPD deployment, the lesion is often predilated with an undersized coronary balloon, typically 3–4 mm in diameter. A self-expanding stent is then placed across the lesion. The stent is typically sized to fit the CCA. There is no demonstrated benefit for

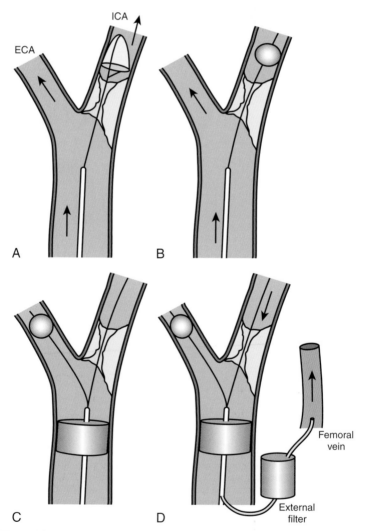

Figure 12.22 Types of embolic protection devices. Embolic protection devices (EPDs). (A) Filter-type device. (B) Balloon occlusion of internal carotid artery (ICA). (C, D) Proximal protection with flow reversal. *ECA,* external carotid artery.

using tapered stents. It is common practice, when treating an internal carotid bifurcation lesion to place the stent across the ostium of the external carotid artery.

There are two types of self-expanding stents: closed-cell and open-cell. *Open-cell stents* are more flexible and may better navigate tortuous vessels. *Closed-cell stents* are more rigid but may better "cover" atherosclerotic plaque. While some evidence suggests that the frequency of embolic complications in symptomatic patients is lower with closed-cell stents, others have found no significant correlation between stent design and outcomes.[60,61] Typical stent sizes are 6–10 mm in diameter and 2–4 cm in length. Gentle postdilation with a 5 mm or smaller balloon is often performed to improve stent apposition with the vessel wall. There is no benefit to aggressive postdilation since restenosis and late loss are very low in the carotid artery. Balloons are conservatively sized (≤1 : 1) to minimize vessel trauma/dissection, plaque embolization, and stimulation of the carotid sinus. A poststent carotid diameter stenosis of 50% or less is an acceptable result.

An alternative to distal embolic protection is proximal protection. Two devices are available: the Gore flow reversal system (W L Gore, Flagstaff, AZ) and the Mo.Ma system (Medtronic, Minneapolis, MN). Both are positioned in a similar fashion. With the Gore device, the external carotid artery is accessed as above and a balloon-tipped sheath is advanced over the 0.035-inch stiff wire into the CCA. This sheath has a port for an occlusion balloon to be placed in the external carotid artery. The external and common carotid balloons are inflated, arresting antegrade flow. The Mo.Ma system is similar but consists of a single sheath with two balloons: a proximal balloon in the CCA and a distal balloon in the external carotid artery. When the balloons are inflated, blood flow is arrested. In either system, once patient tolerance of balloon occlusion is confirmed, the internal carotid lesion is crossed with a 0.014-inch wire, dilated, and stented as described previously. With the Mo.Ma system, blood is manually aspirated after the stenting procedure to clear the debris distal to the common carotid balloon. The Gore system, however, provides continuous flow reversal by having the arterial sheath connected to a venous sheath (Fig. 12.22).[62] While experience with these devices is limited, data indicate that they can provide excellent results. A 1300-patient single-center prospective registry reported 99.7% procedural success with the Mo.Ma device and a 30-day death and stroke rate of 1.38%.[63]

Following the procedure, if a filter-type EPD is used, the EPD is retrieved and final carotid and cerebral angiography is performed (Fig. 12.23). If a proximal protection device is used, the balloons are deflated and final angiography is performed. It is important to confirm that the carotid artery is free of dissection and that the cerebral vasculature is intact. Prior to removal of equipment, a neurologic examination assessing speech, movement, and mental status should be performed. If a neurologic deficit is found, a culprit lesion is sought and neurovascular rescue attempted.

Aorto-Ostial and Common Carotid Interventions

Femoral access is obtained with a 6 to 9F sheath depending on the diameter of the balloon and stent that will be used. After anticoagulation

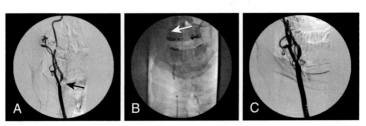

Figure 12.23 Example of carotid artery stenting using distal embolic protection device.

(activated clotting time [ACT] ≥250 sec) and appropriate diagnostic imaging of the target lesion, a 5F diagnostic catheter is advanced through a guide catheter (i.e., JR 4 or multipurpose guide) to the ostium of the target CCA. The ostial lesion is crossed with a steerable 0.035-inch hydrophilic glidewire. The diagnostic catheter is then advanced across the lesion into the distal vessel. The glidewire is exchanged for a stiff 0.035-inch Amplatz wire, and the guide catheter is carefully advanced over the diagnostic catheter until it engages the ostium of the CCA. The diagnostic catheter is then slowly removed.

The lesion is predilated with a balloon sized 1:1 with the CCA. As the balloon deflates, the guide is gently advanced or "telescoped" over the balloon and across the lesion (Fig. 12.24). This will protect

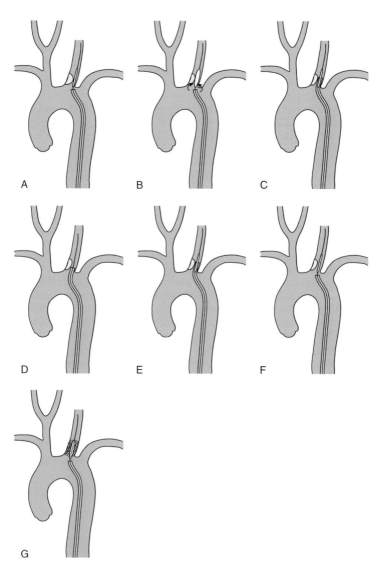

Figure 12.24 Common carotid intervention, step by step. Dilating and stenting aorto-ostial lesions. (A) The lesion is crossed with a 0.035-inch wire and pre-dilation balloon is placed. (B) The lesion is predilated and as the balloon deflates, the guide catheter is advanced, thus "swallowing" the balloon. (C) The guide is now distal to the lesion. (D) The balloon is removed. (E) a balloon-expandable stent is placed, although a portion of it remains within the guide. (F) The guide is withdrawn, uncovering the stent and leaving it in contact with the lesion. (G) The stent is deployed. If a stent is required distally, the stent balloon is "swallowed".

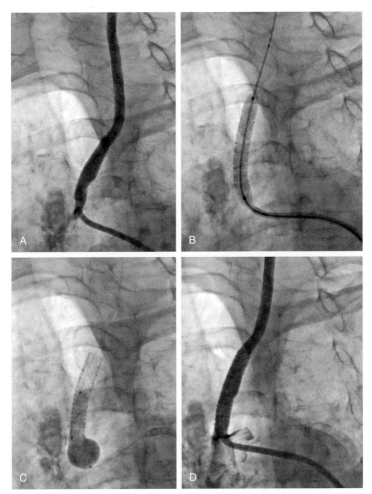

Figure 12.25 Angiography of the common carotid intervention. (A) Aorto-ostial common carotid stenosis. (B) Sent inflation with stent partially protruding into the aorta. (C) Post-dilation with Ostial flash balloon. (D) Final result.

the stent as it is delivered to the lesion. The predilation balloon is removed, and a balloon-expandable stent is placed (in arteries protected by the axial skeleton, balloon-expandable stents are more often used). After positioning the stent at the target lesion, the guide catheter is withdrawn, uncovering the stent and placing it in contact with the target lesion. The proximal stent should protrude very slightly into the aorta (≤1 mm) to ensure lesion coverage. After verifying adequate placement with contrast injections through the guide catheter, the stent is deployed at nominal pressure. As the balloon deflates, the guide is again gently telescoped over the balloon to allow further stents to be delivered distally if needed. A larger semi-compliant balloon may be used to flare the protruding portion of the stent in order to facilitate future angiography. Final angiography and neurologic assessment are performed (Fig. 12.25). The access site is managed similarly to other interventional procedures. Sheath removal is performed when the ACT is 170 seconds or less if a closure device is not used.

Complications and Troubleshooting

Stroke

In a review of more than 54,000 patients, the 30-day risk of stroke during or after CAS was 3.9%.[59] Symptomatic patients were twice as likely to have an adverse event as asymptomatic patients. While providing a good general idea of the stroke risk, this review found significant heterogeneity between studies, and stroke risk differs among patients depending on lesion severity, symptomatic status, and other factors such as renal function.

Most events occur within 24 hours of the procedure. If the patient develops a focal neurologic deficit *during* the procedure, an embolic event is assumed. Immediate cerebral angiography should be performed and rescue intervention should be attempted. Typically these emboli are plaque elements and not amenable to thrombolytic agents. Attempts at revascularization with angioplasty and stenting and/or thrombectomy are recommended. Mental status changes *after* the procedure warrant CT evaluation to rule out intracranial bleeding or hyperperfusion syndrome (see later discussion).

Hemodynamic Instability

Stimulation of the carotid sinus baroreceptor is common during carotid interventions and can cause hypotension and bradycardia. Typically patients who are most sensitive will react negatively to predilation of their lesion. Acute hypotension can lead to brain hypoperfusion and neurologic symptoms due to impaired cerebral autoregulation.

Atropine (0.4–1 mg) may be used to treat acute bradycardia. A prophylactic dose may be considered before stent deployment if the patient was sensitive to predilation, but there is a risk of urinary retention in men. The dose may be repeated if necessary. Aggressive fluid administration is important in treating hypotension, but vasopressor medications may be needed to maintain a systolic blood pressure of 100 mm Hg or higher. We use repeated boluses, as needed, of 25–50 mcg of phenylephrine. A continuous infusion may be required if hypotension persists. In most patients, however, phenylephrine can be weaned within several hours of the procedure, and the patient can ambulate in preparation for discharge the next day. Midodrine 2.5–10 mg three times daily (and then titrated downward as tolerated) can be useful to support blood pressure in the setting of prolonged hypotension. Adjusting the patient's antihypertensive regimen will be necessary over the short term. Keep in mind that access site bleeding is a common cause of hypotension and should be ruled out in these patients.

Hyperperfusion Syndrome and Intracranial Hemorrhage

The opening of a stenotic carotid artery can lead to significant increases in cerebral blood flow, sometimes to levels more than twice the pre-procedure flow. Hyperperfusion syndrome occurs in fewer than 1% of carotid stent patients and is defined clinically by the presence of an ipsilateral throbbing headache, a seizure, or a focal neurologic deficit. A chronically stenotic carotid artery can cause the cerebral vasculature to remain in a state of constant maximal vasodilation. When the stenosis is suddenly alleviated, cerebral autoregulatory mechanisms fail to control blood flow, a problem exacerbated by hypertension. The resulting elevated cerebral perfusion pressure can lead to cerebral edema or, worse, intracranial hemorrhage.

Neurologic symptoms from cerebral edema are usually transient but must be addressed. A neurology consultation and head CT should be obtained if this diagnosis is entertained. When diagnosed, strict control of blood pressure is critical, and consideration of mannitol, diuretics, or antiepileptic medications (depending on presentation) is warranted. Medications that cause cerebral arterial vasodilation (i.e., hydralazine) should theoretically be avoided. Intracranial bleeding is life-threatening. If it occurs, antiplatelet medications should be stopped and a neurosurgical team consulted. Strict blood pressure control (goal systolic pressure of 120–140 mm Hg) may decrease the risk of hyperperfusion syndrome and intracranial bleeding.

Follow-Up

After intervention, patients should be followed to ensure continuation of best medical therapy and to monitor the patency of the stent with DUS, and the development of focal neurologic symptoms. DUS studies are recommended immediately after the procedure, at baseline (or within 1 month of intervention), at 6 and 12 months and yearly thereafter.[64] It is important to remember that carotid DUS velocities are altered after stenting and that overestimation of stenosis is very common.[65]

References

1. Sonesson B, Resch T, Lanne T, et al. The fate of the infrarenal aortic neck after open aneurysm surgery. *J Vasc Surg.* 1998;28:889-894.
2. Pearce WH, Slaughter MS, LeMaire S, et al. Aortic diameter as a function of age, gender, and body surface area. *Surgery.* 1993;114:691-697.
3. Hirsch AT, Haskal ZJ, Hertzer NR, et al. ACC/AHA 2005 guidelines for the management of patients with peripheral arterial disease (lower extremity, renal, mesenteric, and abdominal aortic): executive summary a collaborative report from the American Association for Vascular Surgery/Society for Vascular Surgery, Society for Cardiovascular Angiography and Interventions, Society for Vascular Medicine and Biology, Society of Interventional Radiology, and the ACC/AHA Task Force on Practice Guidelines (Writing Committee to Develop Guidelines for the Management of Patients With Peripheral Arterial Disease) endorsed by the American Association of Cardiovascular and Pulmonary Rehabilitation; National Heart, Lung, and Blood Institute; Society for Vascular Nursing; TransAtlantic Inter-Society Consensus; and Vascular Disease Foundation. *J Am Coll Cardiol.* 2006;47:1239-1312.
4. Lederle FA, Johnson GR, Wilson SE, et al. Prevalence and associations of abdominal aortic aneurysm detected through screening. Aneurysm Detection and Management (ADAM) Veterans Affairs Cooperative Study Group. *Ann Intern Med.* 1997;126:441-449.
5. Lederle FA, Johnson GR, Wilson SE, et al. Relationship of age, gender, race, and body size to infrarenal aortic diameter. The Aneurysm Detection and Management (ADAM) Veterans Affairs Cooperative Study Investigators. *J Vasc Surg.* 1997;26:595-601.
6. Cronenwett JL. Variables that affect the expansion rate and rupture of abdominal aortic aneurysms. *Ann N Y Acad Sci.* 1996;800:56-67.
7. American College of Cardiology Foundation, American College of Radiology, American Institute of Ultrasound in Medicine, et al. (ACCF/ACR/AIUM/ASE/ASN/ICAVL/SCAI/SCCT/SIR/SVM/SVS/SVU) [corrected] 2012 appropriate use criteria for peripheral vascular ultrasound and physiological testing part I: arterial ultrasound and physiological testing: a report of the American College of Cardiology Foundation appropriate use criteria task force, American College of Radiology, American Institute of Ultrasound in Medicine, American Society of Echocardiography, American Society of Nephrology, Intersocietal Commission for the Accreditation of Vascular Laboratories, Society for Cardiovascular Angiography and Interventions, Society of Cardiovascular Computed Tomography, Society for Interventional Radiology, Society for Vascular Medicine, Society for Vascular Surgery, [corrected] and Society for Vascular Ultrasound. [corrected]. *J Am Coll Cardiol.* 2012;60:242-276.
8. Benjamin MM, Fazel P, Filardo G, et al. Prevalence of and risk factors of renal artery stenosis in patients with resistant hypertension. *Am J Cardiol.* 2014;113:687-690.
9. Crowley JJ, Santos RM, Peter RH, et al. Progression of renal artery stenosis in patients undergoing cardiac catheterization. *Am Heart J.* 1998;136:913-918.
10. Khosla S, Kunjummen B, Manda R, et al. Prevalence of renal artery stenosis requiring revascularization in patients initially referred for coronary angiography. *Catheter Cardiovasc Interv.* 2003;58:400-403.
11. Preston RA, Epstein M. Ischemic renal disease: an emerging cause of chronic renal failure and end-stage renal disease. *J Hypertens.* 1997;15:1365-1377.
12. Muray S, Martin M, Amoedo ML, et al. Rapid decline in renal function reflects reversibility and predicts the outcome after angioplasty in renal artery stenosis. *Am J Kidney Dis.* 2002;39:60-66.
13. Strandness DE Jr. Duplex imaging for the detection of renal artery stenosis. *Am J Kidney Dis.* 1994;24:674-678.
14. Olin JW, Piedmonte MR, Young JR, et al. The utility of duplex ultrasound scanning of the renal arteries for diagnosing significant renal artery stenosis. *Ann Intern Med.* 1995;122:833-838.
15. Chi YW, White CJ, Thornton S, et al. Ultrasound velocity criteria for renal in-stent restenosis. *J Vasc Surg.* 2009;50:119-123.
16. Kim TS, Chung JW, Park JH, et al. Renal artery evaluation: comparison of spiral CT angiography to intra-arterial DSA. *J Vasc Interv Radiol.* 1998;9:553-559.
17. Turgutalp K, Kiykim A, Ozhan O, et al. Comparison of diagnostic accuracy of Doppler USG and contrast-enhanced magnetic resonance angiography and selective renal arteriography in patients with atherosclerotic renal artery stenosis. *Med Sci Monit.* 2013;19:475-482.
18. Tan KT, van Beek EJ, Brown PW, et al. Magnetic resonance angiography for the diagnosis of renal artery stenosis: a meta-analysis. *Clin Radiol.* 2002;57:617-624.

19. Chrysochou C, Foley RN, Young JF, et al. Dispelling the myth: the use of renin-angiotensin blockade in atheromatous renovascular disease. *Nephrol Dial Transplant.* 2012;27:1403-1409.

20. Cooper CJ, Murphy TP, Cutlip DE, et al. Stenting and medical therapy for atherosclerotic renal-artery stenosis. *N Engl J Med.* 2014;370:13-22.

21. Leertouwer TC, Gussenhoven EJ, Bosch JL, et al. Stent placement for renal arterial stenosis: where do we stand? A meta-analysis. *Radiology.* 2000;216:78-85.

22. Investigators A, Wheatley K, Ives N, et al. Revascularization versus medical therapy for renal-artery stenosis. *N Engl J Med.* 2009;361:1953-1962.

23. Bax L, Woittiez AJ, Kouwenberg HJ, et al. Stent placement in patients with atherosclerotic renal artery stenosis and impaired renal function: a randomized trial. *Ann Intern Med.* 2009;150:840-848, W150-1.

24. Subramanian R, White CJ, Rosenfield K, et al. Renal fractional flow reserve: a hemo-dynamic evaluation of moderate renal artery stenoses. *Catheter Cardiovasc Interv.* 2005;64:480-486.

25. Kapoor N, Fahsah I, Karim R, et al. Physiological assessment of renal artery stenosis: comparisons of resting with hyperemic renal pressure measurements. *Catheter Cardiovasc Interv.* 2010;76:726-732.

26. White CJ, Olin JW. Diagnosis and management of atherosclerotic renal artery stenosis: improving patient selection and outcomes. *Nat Clin Pract Cardiovasc Med.* 2009;6:176-190.

27. Mitchell JA, Subramanian R, White CJ, et al. Predicting blood pressure improvement in hypertensive patients after renal artery stent placement: renal fractional flow reserve. *Catheter Cardiovasc Interv.* 2007;69:685-689.

28. Trani C, Tommasino A, Burzotta F. Transradial renal stenting: why and how. *Catheter Cardiovasc Interv.* 2009;74:951-956.

29. Olin JW. Atheroembolic renal disease: underdiagnosed and misunderstood. *Catheter Cardiovasc Interv.* 2007;70:789-790.

30. Cooper CJ, Haller ST, Colyer W, et al. Embolic protection and platelet inhibition during renal artery stenting. *Circulation.* 2008;117:2752-2760.

31. Leertouwer TC, Gussenhoven EJ, van Overhagen H, et al. Stent placement for treatment of renal artery stenosis guided by intravascular ultrasound. *J Vasc Interv Radiol.* 1998;9:945-952.

32. Lederman RJ, Mendelsohn FO, Santos R, et al. Primary renal artery stenting: charac-teristics and outcomes after 363 procedures. *Am Heart J.* 2001;142:314-323.

33. Blum U, Krumme B, Flugel P, et al. Treatment of ostial renal-artery stenoses with vascular endoprostheses after unsuccessful balloon angioplasty. *N Engl J Med.* 1997;336:459-465.

34. Henry M, Amor M, Henry I, et al. Stents in the treatment of renal artery stenosis: long-term follow-up. *J Endovasc Surg.* 1999;6:42-51.

35. Zahringer M, Sapoval M, Pattynama PM, et al. Sirolimus-eluting versus bare-metal low-profile stent for renal artery treatment (GREAT Trial): angiographic follow-up after 6 months and clinical outcome up to 2 years. *J Endovasc Ther.* 2007;14:460-468.

36. Isles CG, Robertson S, Hill D. Management of renovascular disease: a review of renal artery stenting in ten studies. *QJM.* 1999;92:159-167.

37. Rasmus M, Huegli R, Jacob AL, et al. Extensive iatrogenic aortic dissection during renal angioplasty: successful treatment with a covered stent-graft. *Cardiovasc Intervent Radiol.* 2007;30:497-500.

38. Patel PM, Eisenberg J, Islam MA, et al. Percutaneous revascularization of persistent renal artery in-stent restenosis. *Vasc Med.* 2009;14:259-264.

39. Zeller T, Sixt S, Rastan A, et al. Treatment of reoccurring instent restenosis following reintervention after stent-supported renal artery angioplasty. *Catheter Cardiovasc Interv.* 2007;70:296-300.

40. Fields WS, Lemak NA. Joint Study of extracranial arterial occlusion. VII. Subclavian steal–a review of 168 cases. *JAMA.* 1972;222:1139-1143.

41. Elian D, Gerniak A, Guetta V, et al. Subclavian coronary steal syndrome: an obligatory common fate between subclavian artery, internal mammary graft and coronary circula-tion. *Cardiology.* 2002;97:175-179.

42. Patel SN, White CJ, Collins TJ, et al. Catheter-based treatment of the subclavian and innominate arteries. *Catheter Cardiovasc Interv.* 2008;71:963-968.

43. Aboyans V, Kamineni A, Allison MA, et al. The epidemiology of subclavian stenosis and its association with markers of subclinical atherosclerosis: the Multi-Ethnic Study of Atherosclerosis (MESA). *Atherosclerosis.* 2010;211:266-270.

44. Aboyans V, Criqui MH, McDermott MM, et al. The vital prognosis of subclavian stenosis. *J Am Coll Cardiol.* 2007;49:1540-1545.

45. Khot UN, Friedman DT, Pettersson G, et al. Radial artery bypass grafts have an increased occurrence of angiographically severe stenosis and occlusion compared with left internal mammary arteries and saphenous vein grafts. *Circulation.* 2004;109:2086-2091.

46. Brountzos EN, Malagari K, Kelekis DA. Endovascular treatment of occlusive lesions of the subclavian and innominate arteries. *Cardiovasc Intervent Radiol.* 2006;29:503-510.

47. Inzitari D, Eliasziw M, Gates P, et al. The causes and risk of stroke in patients with asymptomatic internal-carotid-artery stenosis. North American Symptomatic Carotid Endarterectomy Trial Collaborators. *N Engl J Med.* 2000;342:1693-1700.

48. Kleindorfer D, Panagos P, Pancioli A, et al. Incidence and short-term prognosis of transient ischemic attack in a population-based study. *Stroke.* 2005;36:720-723.

49. Easton JD, Saver JL, Albers GW, et al. Definition and evaluation of transient ischemic attack: a scientific statement for healthcare professionals from the American Heart Association/American Stroke Association Stroke Council; Council on Cardio-vascular Surgery and Anesthesia; Council on Cardiovascular Radiology and Intervention;

Council on Cardiovascular Nursing; and the Interdisciplinary Council on Peripheral Vascular Disease. The American Academy of Neurology affirms the value of this statement as an educational tool for neurologists. *Stroke*. 2009;40:2276-2293.

50. Yang C, Bogiatzi C, Spence JD. Risk of stroke at the time of carotid occlusion. *JAMA Neurol* 2015;72:1261-1267.
51. Barnett HJ, Taylor DW, Eliasziw M, et al. Benefit of carotid endarterectomy in patients with symptomatic moderate or severe stenosis. North American Symptomatic Carotid Endarterectomy Trial Collaborators. *N Engl J Med*. 1998;339:1415-1425.
52. North American Symptomatic Carotid Endarterectomy Trial Collaborators. Beneficial effect of carotid endarterectomy in symptomatic patients with high-grade carotid stenosis. *N Engl J Med*. 1991;325:445-453.
53. Bates ER, Babb JD, Casey DE Jr, et al. ACCF/SCAI/SVMB/SIR/ASITN 2007 clinical expert consensus document on carotid stenting: a report of the American College of Cardiology Foundation Task Force on Clinical Expert Consensus Documents (ACCF/SCAI/SVMB/SIR/ASITN Clinical Expert Consensus Document Committee on Carotid Stenting). *J Am Coll Cardiol*. 2007;49:126-170.
54. Blood pressure, cholesterol, and stroke in eastern Asia. Eastern Stroke and Coronary Heart Disease Collaborative Research Group. *Lancet*. 1998;352:1801-1807.
55. Yadav JS, Wholey MH, Kuntz RE, et al. Protected carotid-artery stenting versus endarterectomy in high-risk patients. *N Engl J Med*. 2004;351:1493-1501.
56. Gurm HS, Yadav JS, Fayad P, et al. Long-term results of carotid stenting versus endarterectomy in high-risk patients. *N Engl J Med*. 2008;358:1572-1579.
57. Mantese VA, Timaran CH, Chiu D, et al. The Carotid Revascularization Endarterectomy versus Stenting Trial (CREST): stenting versus carotid endarterectomy for carotid disease. *Stroke*. 2010;41:S31-S34.
58. Garg N, Karagiorgos N, Pisimisis GT, et al. Cerebral protection devices reduce periprocedural strokes during carotid angioplasty and stenting: a systematic review of the current literature. *J Endovasc Ther*. 2009;16:412-427.
59. Touze E, Trinquart L, Chatellier G, et al. Systematic review of the perioperative risks of stroke or death after carotid angioplasty and stenting. *Stroke*. 2009;40:e683-e693.
60. Hart JP, Peeters P, Verbist J, et al. Do device characteristics impact outcome in carotid artery stenting? *J Vasc Surg*. 2006;44:725-730, discussion 30–1.
61. Schillinger M, Gschwendtner M, Reimers B, et al. Does carotid stent cell design matter? *Stroke*. 2008;39:905-909.
62. Kelso R, Clair DG. Flow reversal for cerebral protection in carotid artery stenting: a review. *Perspect Vasc Surg Endovasc Ther*. 2008;20:282-290.
63. Stabile E, Salemme L, Sorrropago G, et al. Proximal endovascular occlusion for carotid artery stenting: results from a prospective registry of 1300 patients. *J Am Coll Cardiol*. 2010;3:298-304.
64. American College of Cardiology Foundation, American College of Radiology, American Institute of Ultrasound in Medicine, et al. (ACCF/ACR/AIUM/ASE/ASN/ICAVL/SCAI/SCCT/SIR/SVM/SVS) 2012 appropriate use criteria for peripheral vascular ultrasound and physiological testing part I: arterial ultrasound and physiological testing: a report of the American College of Cardiology Foundation Appropriate Use Criteria Task Force, American College of Radiology, American Institute of Ultrasound in Medicine, American Society of Echocardiography, American Society of Nephrology, Intersocietal Commission for the Accreditation of Vascular Laboratories, Society for Cardiovascular Angiography and Interventions, Society of Cardiovascular Computed Tomography, Society for Interventional Radiology, Society for Vascular Medicine, and Society for Vascular Surgery. *J Vasc Surg*. 2012;56:e17-e51.
65. Chi YW, White CJ, Woods TC, et al. Ultrasound velocity criteria for carotid in-stent restenosis. *Catheter Cardiovasc Interv*. 2007;69:349-354.

13

Mitral Stenosis

PAUL SORAJJA

Rheumatic heart disease remains the most common cause of native mitral stenosis. The pathophysiologic abnormality in these patients is obstruction to inflow caused by fusion of the valve commissures. Progressive rheumatic mitral stenosis, which may occur over decades before clinical manifestation, leads to left atrial hypertension, atrial arrhythmias, pulmonary hypertension, and congestive heart failure. This chapter discusses the evaluation of patients with rheumatic mitral stenosis and the selection and technical considerations for balloon mitral valvuloplasty.

Clinical Evaluation

Patients with mitral stenosis require a comprehensive history and physical examination. Details on symptomatology, functional limitation, arrhythmias, right-sided decompensation, and the presence of co-existent lesions serve as the basis for determining the appropriateness of interventional therapy. For all patients, a complete two-dimensional, Doppler echocardiogram should be performed. Goals of the echocardiographic evaluation in these patients are (1) to determine the severity of the mitral stenosis through examination of the mitral gradient, mitral valve area, right ventricular function, and estimated pulmonary pressures; (2) to determine the suitability for balloon mitral valvuloplasty by examining morphology of the mitral leaflets, subvalvular apparatus, and degree of regurgitation; and (3) to determine the presence of co-existent lesions that may require additional surgical or interventional therapy (e.g., aortic stenosis).

Doppler echocardiography is highly accurate for calculation of the mitral gradient because the transducer can be easily aligned with the mitral inflow in nearly all patients. For patients in whom Doppler echocardiography is either inadequate or insufficient, and in whom interventional or surgical therapy is being considered, cardiac catheterization should be performed to assess the severity of mitral stenosis. The most accurate method requires transseptal puncture with direct measurement of left atrial (LA) and left ventricular (LV) pressures. Significant overestimation of the mitral gradient can occur with use of the pulmonary capillary wedge pressure (PCWP) as a surrogate for LAP, even though the *mean levels* of these two pressure measurements are typically congruent. A minimal PCWP-LV diastolic gradient may be considered indicative of the absence of significant mitral stenosis; however, elevated PCWP-LV diastolic gradients do not accurately reflect the true mitral gradient. The inaccuracy of the PCWP as a surrogate for LAP in the measurement of the mitral gradient occurs due to damping of its waveform as well as its temporal delay in relation to the LV diastolic filling period and thus cannot be completely corrected through phase shifting (Fig. 13.1). In all invasive assessments, right heart catheterization for measurement of pulmonary pressures and

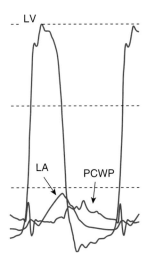

Figure 13.1 Invasive assessment of the mitral gradient. Use of the pulmonary capillary wedge pressure (PCWP) can lead to an inaccurate estimation of the mitral gradient, even though the PCWP is an accurate reflection of the mean left atrial pressure (LAP). This occurs because of temporal delay and damping of the PCWP tracing. The temporal delay can be seen in differences in timing of the V waves in the PCWP and LAP curves. While phase shifting can be used to correct the temporal delay, correction for the damping cannot be performed. LV, left ventricle.

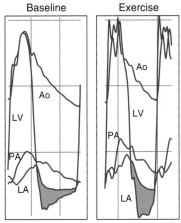

Figure 13.2 Hemodynamic assessment of mitral stenosis with exercise. *Left*: At rest, the mitral gradient is mild (mean, 4 mm Hg). *Right*: With arm ergometry, the mitral gradient becomes severe (mean, 12 mm Hg), and there also is an accompanying rise in the pulmonary artery pressure. Ao, ascending aorta; LA, left atrium; LV, left ventricle; PA, pulmonary artery.

cardiac output should be performed, followed by calculation of the mitral valve area.

It is important to note that the severity of the mitral gradient is directly proportional to the square of the transvalvular flow rate. Thus, when the resting hemodynamics are disproportional to the patient's exertional symptoms, assessments should be performed with exercise or elevation in the heart rate (e.g., arm ergometry, temporary pacing, isoproterenol administration) (Fig. 13.2).

The definitions for severity of rheumatic mitral stenosis have been recently revised (Table 13.1). These definitions reflect the levels of severity where symptoms and clinical consequences (i.e., pulmonary

Table 13.1

Stages of Mitral Stenosis

Stage	Definition	Anatomy	Hemodynamics	Consequences	Symptoms
A	At risk	Mild diastolic doming of valve	Normal flow velocity	None	None
B	Progressive	Commissural fusion, diastolic leaflet doming	Increased flow velocity PHT <150 ms MVA >1.5 cm^2	Mild-mod LAE Normal pulmonary pressure at rest	None
C	Asymptomatic severe	Commissural fusion, diastolic leaflet doming	MVA ≤1.5 cm^2 PHT ≥150 ms	Severe LAE PASP >30 mm Hg	None
D	Symptomatic severe	Commissural fusion, diastolic leaflet doming	MVA ≤1.5 cm^2 PHT ≥150 ms	Severe LAE PASP >30 mm Hg	Decreased exercise tolerance Exertional dyspnea

hypertension) typically occur and where interventional therapy may be beneficial.

Patient Selection for Balloon Mitral Valvuloplasty

Successful balloon valvuloplasty relieves mitral stenosis by splitting the commissures without disruption of the leaflets or supporting apparatus. Procedural success therefore is heavily dependent on the proper assessment of the valve morphology, which should include the mechanism of commissural fusion, the pliability of valve, and the state of the subvalvular apparatus (Fig. 13.3). Severe retraction and fusion of the chordae and papillary muscles may prevent a satisfactory result from balloon mitral valvuloplasty.

A common method for echocardiographic assessment is the Abascal or Wilkins score, in which points (1–4) are assigned according to the physical characteristics of the valve and summated (Table 13.2). A score of 8 or less is generally considered to be favorable for balloon mitral valvuloplasty. In addition to calculating this score, the presence of commissural calcification should be determined because the dominant mechanism of valvuloplasty that leads to relief of mitral stenosis is commissural splitting. Calcification of the commissures therefore increases the risk of valve leaflet tearing due to the differential stress effects of the inflated balloon. Moreover, commissural calcification has been shown to be more predictive of adverse events than the Abascal score (Fig. 13.4). While the Abascal score is predictive of postprocedural valve area and long-term outcome, patients with a high Abascal score can still be considered for balloon valvuloplasty if there is not significant calcification of the commissures.

For patients with nonpliable valves, balloon mitral valvuloplasty is associated with higher complication rates (principally due to severe regurgitation) and poorer long-term outcome (principally due to a high rate of restenosis). Contraindications for balloon valvuloplasty are left

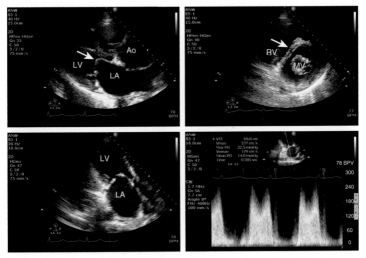

Figure 13.3 Echocardiography of a pliable valve in a patient with rheumatic mitral stenosis. *Top left*: Parasternal long-axis view showing a pliable mitral valve with the typical "hockey-stick" appearance of the anterior leaflet. *Top right*: Short-axis view demonstrating commissural fusion. The ventricular septum is flat due to severe pulmonary hypertension, secondary to the mitral stenosis (*arrow*). *Bottom left*: Apical long-axis view showing absence of significant subvalvular fusion or calcification. *Bottom right*: Doppler echocardiogram showing a mean mitral gradient of 14 mm Hg.

Table 13.2

| | | Subvalvular | Leaflet | |
Grade	Mobility	Thickening	Thickening	Calcification
Calculation of the Wilkins or Abascal Score				
1	Highly mobile valve with only leaflet tips restricted	Minimal thickening just below the mitral leaflets	Leaflets near normal in thickness (4–5 mm)	Single area of increased echo brightness
2	Leaflet mid and base portions have normal mobility	Thickening of chordal structures extending up to one third of the chordal length	Mid-leaflets normal, considerable thickening of margins (5–8 mm)	Scattered areas of brightness confined to leaflet margins
3	Valve continues to move forward in diastole, mainly from the base	Thickening extending to the distal third of chords	Thickening extending through the entire leaflet (5–8 mm)	Brightness extending into the mid-portion of the leaflets
4	No or minimal forward movement of the leaflets in diastole	Extensive thickening and shortening of all chordal structures extending down to the papillary muscles	Considerable thickening of all leaflet tissue (8–10 mm)	Extensive brightness throughout much of the leaflet tissue

The grade for each of the four characteristics (mobility, subvalvular thickening, leaflet thickening, and calcification) is assigned and the summated. A score of less than 8 is generally considered to be favorable for balloon mitral valvuloplasty.

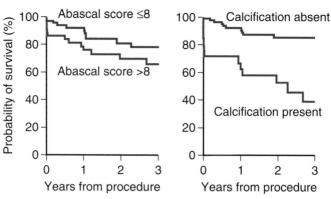

Figure 13.4 Survival free of death, repeat balloon mitral valvuloplasty, or surgical mitral valve replacement according to valve morphology. *Left*: Comparison of survival for the Abascal score. *Right*: Comparison of survival for the presence of calcification in the commissures. *Reprinted with permission from Cannan CR, Nishimura RA, Reeder GS, Ilstrup DR, Larson DR, Holmes DR, Tajik AJ. Echocardiographic assessment of commissural calcium: a simple predictor of outcome after percutaneous mitral balloon valvotomy. J Am Coll Cardiol 1997;29:175–80.*

atrial thrombus and moderate or severe mitral regurgitation. A transesophageal echocardiogram is required in all patients to evaluate for the possibility of left atrial thrombus regardless of history of atrial arrhythmias.

Indications for Balloon Mitral Valvuloplasty

Balloon mitral valvuloplasty was first introduced in 1984. With improvement in techniques and equipment, balloon mitral valvuloplasty now is the procedure of choice for selected patients with severe mitral stenosis. Patients with symptoms due to severe mitral stenosis (valve area ≤1.0 cm^2) and a pliable valve may be considered for balloon valvuloplasty. Asymptomatic patients with hemodynamically significant stenosis also may be considered when the valve morphology is pliable, particularly in the presence of severe pulmonary hypertension or new-onset atrial fibrillation. Balloon mitral valvuloplasty also has been used successfully to treat heart failure in pregnant patients. Specific clinical indications for balloon mitral valvuloplasty are:

- Symptomatic patients with severe mitral stenosis (MVA ≤1.0 cm^2, stage D) and favorable valve morphology in the absence of contraindications (class I; LOE, A)
- Asymptomatic patients with very severe mitral stenosis (MVA ≤1.0 cm^2, stage C) and favorable valve morphology in the absence of contraindications (class IIa; LOE, C)
- Asymptomatic patients with severe mitral stenosis (MVA ≤1.0 cm^2, stage C) and favorable valve morphology who have new onset of atrial fibrillation in the absence of contraindications (class IIb; LOE, C)
- Symptomatic patients with MVA of greater than 1.5 cm^2 if there is evidence of hemodynamically significant mitral stenosis during exercise (class IIb; LOE, C)
- Symptomatic patients (NYHA class III/IV) with severe mitral stenosis (MVA ≤1.0 cm^2, stage D) who have suboptimal valve anatomy and are not candidates for surgery or at high risk for surgery (class IIb; LOE, C)

The Inoue Balloon

The Inoue balloon is constructed of two layers of compliant latex that sandwich a layer of nylon mesh. The nylon mesh provides the unique shape, facilitates the three-stage inflation, and limits the maximum diameter of the balloon (Fig. 13.5). The Inoue balloon has different compliance in its sections, leading to inflation of the distal segment first (similar to a flotation catheter), followed by the proximal segment, with further inflation that creates an hourglass shape. This shape facilitates self-positioning of the balloon in the mitral valve orifice. With full inflation, the center portion of the balloon expands, resulting in splitting of the mitral commissures. The distensibility of the latex material allows each balloon to be inflated over a 4-mm range of diameter sizes (i.e., between 26 and 30 mm diameter for the largest available model). A single balloon can thus be used for sequential dilatation of the mitral valve with serially larger diameters, without removal of the balloon from the patient.

Once the transseptal puncture and a hemodynamic assessment have been completed, the Inoue balloon catheter can be prepared. The balloon catheter comes packaged with all the components necessary for the dilatation procedure (Fig. 13.6):

- A balloon-stretching metal tube
- A calibrated inflation syringe specifically matched to each balloon
- A rigid 12–14F plastic dilator

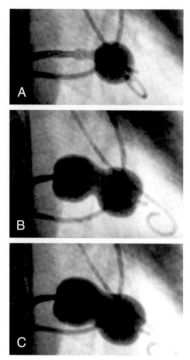

Figure 13.5 The Inoue balloon. (A) The distal segment of the balloon is inflated and passed across the mitral valve orifice. This is analogous to the manner in which a balloon flotation catheter is maneuvered from the right atrium to the right ventricle during right heart catheterization. The partially inflated balloon is pulled back until it engages the mitral valve. (B) Proximal and distal segments of the balloon are inflated, creating hourglass shape that self-positions the balloon in the mitral orifice. (C) Nearly full inflation of the balloon to open the commissures.

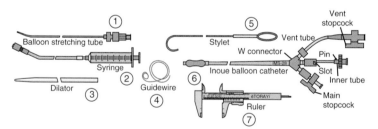

Figure 13.6 Equipment for balloon mitral valvuloplasty. The components of the equipment box supplied by Toray include (1) a long metal hypotube, the balloon-stretching tube, used to pass through the inner tube of the Inoue balloon catheter to elongate and slenderize the balloon. (2) A calibrated syringe used for inflation of the balloon. The syringe provides calibration marks so that predetermined diameters of the balloon can be achieved driven by the volume rather than pressure. (3) A dilator used to dilate the subcutaneous tissue at the femoral venous puncture site and to dilate the septum as well. (4) A 0.025-inch stainless steel spring guidewire. (5) A steering stylet that is introduced through the inner tube after the balloon is in the left atrium to help guide it across the mitral valve. (6) The balloon catheter itself, which has a W-connector from which arise a vent tube, an inner tube used for introduction of the balloon-stretching tube and stylet and for stretching the balloon, and a main stopcock for balloon inflation via the syringe. (7) A ruler or caliper, which is used to confirm that the graduations on the syringe used to inflate the balloon result in the desired inflation diameters.

- A 0.025-inch spring-tipped exchange guidewire
- A stylet
- The Inoue balloon
- Calipers for measuring the balloon diameter

The balloon catheter lumen is flushed with saline. Diluted contrast (3:1) is injected with the vent lumen raised and open to purge air, followed by closure of the vent. The calibrated balloon inflation syringe is filled slightly more than the desired inflation diameter. This slight overfilling allows air to be purged through the vent port when connected. The balloon is then fully inflated and checked with calipers for sizing. If the balloon does not inflate to the desired diameter, small amounts of diluted contrast are added or subtracted to achieve proper calibration. The balloon is allowed to deflate passively in a bath of flush solution. Small bubbles will escape from within the mesh layer of the balloon. Over a guidewire, the balloon-stretching tube is inserted to elongate the balloon catheter and advanced until it locks into the metal hub at the proximal end of the balloon catheter. The balloon and stretching tube are then advanced into the balloon catheter shaft until they engage the plastic slot on the balloon catheter Luer lock. This leaves the balloon in its elongated, slenderized form to ease percutaneous insertion and delivery across the interatrial septum.

Procedural Technique

The most common technique for balloon mitral valvuloplasty is a transvenous, antegrade approach through the fossa ovalis with use of an Inoue balloon. Transseptal puncture is performed using standard techniques under fluoroscopic or echocardiographic guidance. Of note, punctures superior or inferior to the fossa ovalis can lead to difficulty in crossing the mitral valve with the balloon catheter. Once a transseptal sheath has been placed into the left atrium, a second catheter, typically a pigtail, is placed retrograde into the left ventricle for invasive assessment of the mitral gradient at rest and, if indicated, with exercise. Right heart catheterization is performed for measurement of pulmonary pressures and cardiac output, followed by calculation of the mitral valve area.

Through the transseptal sheath, a heavy-duty spring coil guidewire is placed into the left atrium. The transeptal sheath is then exchanged for a 14F long dilator, which is used to dilate the femoral access site and the interatrial septum (Figs. 13.7 and 13.8). The size of the Inoue balloon catheter is determined by the patient's height [size in mm = (height in cm ÷ 10) + 10] (Table 13.3). This formula is used for maximal balloon sizing; consideration should be given to starting with smaller sizing in all patients followed by stepwise increases in the balloon size (1–2 mm increments). This stepwise approach should especially be undertaken when the valve pathology is less than ideal. Each Inoue balloon catheter is examined for accuracy of inflation size prior to insertion. The Inoue balloon is elongated, passed over the guidewire into the left atrium, and then shortened. Of note, to avoid inadvertent balloon tearing, elongation should only be performed with a guidewire in place.

With a thick atrial septum, the balloon catheter may need to be rotated while being passed into the left atrium. The spring coil guidewire is exchanged for a J-tipped stylet, which is then used to guide the balloon through the valve orifice using care to avoid entanglement with the subvalvular apparatus. Withdrawals of the stylet are slight and result in advancement of the catheter into the left ventricle through counterclockwise, anterior maneuvers. The distal end of the Inoue balloon is first inflated in the left ventricle using care to avoid entanglement in the subvalvular apparatus. Once position and freedom of the catheter are confirmed on echocardiography, the stylet is used to fix

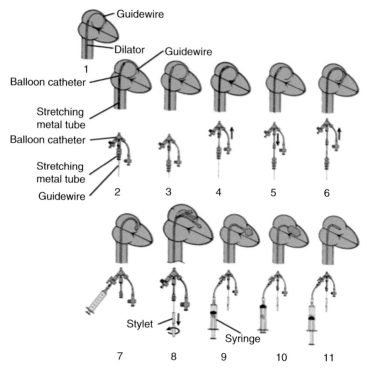

Figure 13.7 Balloon mitral valvuloplasty. (*1*) After a spring guidewire is introduced via a Mullins sheath into the left atrium, the interatrial septum is dilated using a rigid 14F plastic dilator. (*2*) The elongated balloon catheter is advanced over the wire through the interatrial septum. (*3*) The stretching metal tube is partially withdrawn, allowing the balloon to shorten and curl within the left atrium. (*4*) The balloon is advanced through the interatrial septum. (*5*) The stretching metal tube and balloon-straightening device are withdrawn further. (*6*) The balloon is advanced beyond the mitral orifice. (*7*) The distal portion of the balloon is partially inflated with a contrast-saline mixture. (*8*) With counterclockwise rotation of the stylet, slight advancement of the catheter shaft, and withdrawal of the stylet, the balloon is directed through the mitral orifice and left ventricle. (*9*) The partially inflated balloon is withdrawn against the mitral orifice. (*10*) The balloon is fully and rapidly inflated and allowed to deflate. (*11*) After deflation, in most instances, the balloon passively returns to the left atrium from the left ventricle.

the balloon across the mitral valve, followed by inflation of the proximal segment. Under echocardiographic guidance, the balloon is then fully inflated to expand its center, thus facilitating commissural splitting and valve dilatation.

During the procedure, repeat assessment of the mitral gradient, severity of mitral regurgitation, and pulmonary pressures with echocardiography and invasive monitoring is performed. When no contraindications are present, repeat dilatation with increasing inflation sizes can be performed in a stepwise fashion (1–2 mm increments) until satisfactory hemodynamic results are achieved. For invasive measurement of the mitral gradient, the LAP can be measured via the Inoue balloon catheter with the stylet removed. When rises in pulmonary pressure occur, acute, severe mitral regurgitation should be suspected.

Echocardiography should demonstrate splitting of the mitral commissures after valvuloplasty. This splitting also can be used as an end point for the procedure in patients when the preprocedural gradient is not severe and where changes in the hemodynamics are difficult to determine. Following successful dilatation, the balloon is elongated in the left atrium to minimize risk of atrial septal tears during withdrawal of the balloon into the right atrium. This is accomplished by reintroducing

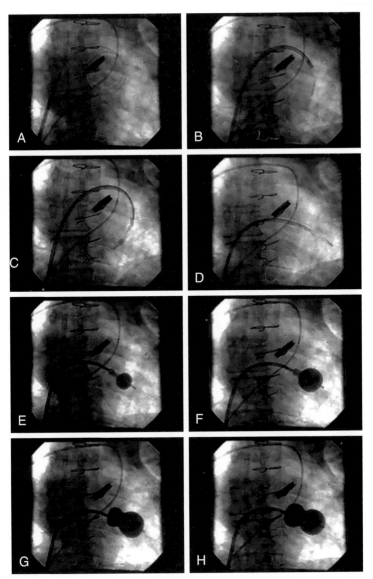

Figure 13.8 Balloon valvuloplasty in a patient with mitral stenosis. (A) A 14F dilator is advanced over a spring-coiled guidewire. The guidewire has been introduced into the left atrium via a transseptal puncture. The 14F dilator dilates both the subcutaneous tissue at the groin catheter insertion site and the left atrial puncture. A prosthetic aortic valve marks the location of the aortic root. A pulmonary artery catheter traverses the right atrium, right ventricular outflow, and pulmonary artery. (B) The uninflated balloon catheter has been introduced over the course of the spring wire. The wire has been removed. The tip of the catheter overlays the mitral orifice. (C) The tip of the balloon catheter is partially inflated so that it may be manipulated across the mitral valve using a steering stylet. (D) The uninflated balloon is now in the left ventricular apex. (E) The front portion of the balloon has been inflated and pulled back until it engages the mitral valve orifice. (F) The balloon is inflated further. (G) Additional inflation of the balloon causes the proximal portion to inflate, leaving a waist in the middle. (H) Full inflation of the balloon results in expansion of the center of the balloon, splitting the fused mitral commissures.

Table 13.3

Inoue Balloon Sizing for Mitral Valvuloplasty		
Patient Height (cm)	Balloon-Dilating Area (cm²)	Balloon Diameter Range (mm)
<160	5.13	22–26
160–179	6.16	24–28
≥180	7.07	26–30

the stretching tube, which has been preloaded with the 0.025-inch spring-tipped guidewire. The guidewire is advanced and curled in the left atrium. The balloon-stretching tube is then locked to the gold metal hub, followed by approximation of these two metal units together with the plastic Luer lock. The balloon and wire can then be withdrawn from the left atrium. An oxygen saturation run then is performed to exclude significant left-to-right shunting, and residual mitral regurgitation is assessed by either echocardiography or left ventriculography.

Left atrial thrombus is a contraindication for balloon mitral valvuloplasty. Thrombus usually responds to anticoagulation (>3 months), which thereby facilitates performance of the procedure. In some instances where the thrombus is persistent despite anticoagulation, the procedure may be performed; however, extreme care must be taken due to the risk of stroke. One option is to cross the mitral valve from the left atrium with a 7F balloon-tipped catheter, pass the Inoue exchange wire through the balloon catheter into the left ventricle, and then pass the Inoue balloon over this wire. This approach helps to minimize manipulation of the Inoue balloon in the left atrium.

Technical Considerations

- To facilitate crossing the mitral valve with the balloon, it is useful to change the x-ray projection to a shallow right anterior oblique.
- Inflation of the tip of the balloon can facilitate antegrade crossing.
- The stylet may be gently bent to accentuate its curve to facilitate passage of the balloon across the mitral valve if initial crossing is difficult.
- As the balloon deflates, it usually falls back into the left atrium. If it does not, gentle clockwise rotation of the balloon catheter will move the balloon back into the left atrium.
- If the interatrial septum is crossed in a relatively superior or anterior location, passing the balloon across the mitral valve may be difficult. In this circumstance, clockwise rotation will "bank" the balloon off the posterior atrial wall, creating a loop to allow it to cross into the left ventricle (Fig. 13.9).
- In the event the balloon is withdrawn across the septal puncture during manipulations, the coiled-spring–tipped guidewire can be reinserted to advance it back into the left atrium.
- During balloon removal, special care must be taken not to stretch and stiffen the balloon through the roof of the left atrium. This is best accomplished by withdrawing the balloon onto the stretching metal tube and then withdrawing the plastic Luer lock onto the assembled metal hub apparatus. The balloon catheter is thus pulled back across the atrial septum as it is stretched and elongated, rather than pushing the stretching metal tube forward through the septum.

Clinical Outcomes

The predominant determinant of outcome and complications with the procedure is valve morphology. Other predictors of success are age,

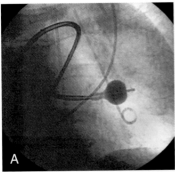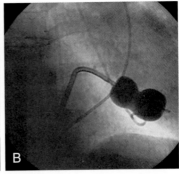

Figure 13.9 Approach for addressing a superior or anterior transseptal puncture during balloon mitral valvuloplasty. When the balloon catheter will not cross the mitral valve using the conventional method, the catheter may be rotated clockwise and manipulated across the mitral valve using an alternative approach. The balloon is introduced into the left atrium in the usual manner and guided past the mitral orifice. (A) With clockwise rotation of the stylet and catheter shaft, a loop is made directing the balloon off the posterior left atrial wall. (B) Withdrawal of the stylet and advancement of the catheter shaft direct the balloon catheter across the mitral valve into the left ventricle.

functional class, ventricular diastolic-pressure, severity of mitral stenosis, and cardiac output. In general, balloon mitral valvuloplasty leads to a doubling of the valve area (usually 1.0 cm^2 to 2.0 cm^2) and a 50%–60% reduction in the transmitral gradient (Fig. 13.10). Procedure success, defined as a final mitral valve area of greater than 1.5 cm^2 and decrease in left atrial pressure to less than 18 mm Hg in the absence of complications, occurs in 70%–95% of patients, according to the baseline morphology of the valve. Complications include acute severe mitral regurgitation (2%–10%), ventricular perforation (0.5%–4%), large atrial septal defect (<5%; larger if double balloon system used), myocardial infarction (0.3%–0.5%), systemic embolization (0.5%–3.0%), and death (<2%). Because of the complexity of the procedure, acute outcomes also directly correlate with operator experience. Overall, in patients with favorable valve morphology, the success rate of balloon valvuloplasty for mitral stenosis is greater than 90% with a complication rate of less than 3% when performed in experienced hands.

Survival free from death, repeat valvuloplasty, or mitral valve replacement over 3–7 years is 50%–70% overall but is greater than 90% in patients with favorable valve morphology. Randomized, albeit small, investigations of selected patients with mitral stenosis have demonstrated comparable outcomes of balloon mitral valvuloplasty and surgical commissurotomy. Notably, these investigations enrolled primarily young patients (mean age <30 years) with favorable valve morphology.

The two most serious complications of balloon mitral valvuloplasty are cardiac tamponade and acute mitral regurgitation. There should be a high degree of suspicion for pericardial tamponade during the entire procedure, with continuous monitoring of chest, shoulder, or back pain, as well as ventricular filling pressures, systemic pressures, and cardiac borders visible on fluoroscopy. Operators who perform balloon mitral valvuloplasty should also be skilled in pericardiocentesis, with a pericardiocentesis tray and equipment readily available. Some operators also prefer to have the chest and subxiphoid prepped in the event pericardiocentesis is required. Acute, severe mitral regurgitation occurs in 1%–2% of procedures. Vasodilator therapy (e.g., nitroprusside) and intra-aortic balloon pump therapy can be utilized to stabilize patients with hemodynamic compromise. In some instances, emergency mitral valve surgery is required.

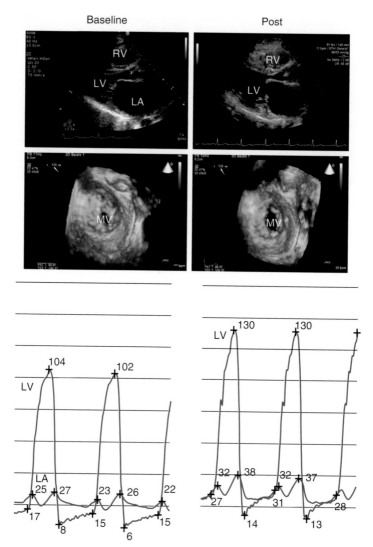

Figure 13.10 Effects of balloon mitral valvuloplasty. *Left*: Baseline evaluation shows rheumatic mitral stenosis with a pliable valve (*top*) and commissural fusion (*middle*). The mean mitral gradient is 11 mm Hg on hemodynamic catheterization. *Right*: Following balloon mitral valvuloplasty, diastolic opening of the mitral valve is augmented (*top*) with splitting of the commissures. The mean mitral gradient at the conclusion of the procedure is 3 mm Hg.

Key Points

1. Balloon mitral valvuloplasty is indicated for symptomatic patients with severe mitral stenosis (MVA ≤1.5 cm², stage D) and favorable valve morphology in the absence of contraindications. Considerations for therapy also include those with very severe mitral stenosis, new-onset atrial fibrillation, or exercise-associated mitral stenosis.

2. Patient selection is the key to success with valvuloplasty for mitral stenosis. Patients without commissural calcium and low Abascal scores (<8) have superior acute and long-term outcomes.

3. For appropriately selected patients, the results of balloon valvuloplasty for mitral stenosis are comparable to that of surgical commissurotomy.

Suggested Readings

Abascal VM, Wilkins GT, O'Shea JP, et al. Prediction of successful outcome in 130 patients undergoing percutaneous balloon mitral valvotomy. *Circulation*. 1990;82:448-456.

Bouleti C, Iung B, Himbert D, et al. Long-term efficacy of percutaneous mitral commissurotomy for restenosis after previous mitral commissurotomy. *Heart*. 2013;99:1336-1341.

Bouleti C, Iung B, Laouenan C, et al. Late results of percutaneous mitral commissurotomy up to 20 years: development and validation of a risk score predicting late functional results from a series of 912 patients. *Circulation*. 2012;125:2119-2127.

Cannan CR, Nishimura RA, Reeder GS, et al. Echocardiographic assessment of commissural calcium: a simple predictor of outcome after percutaneous mitral balloon valvotomy. *J Am Coll Cardiol*. 1997;29:175-180.

Iung B, Cormier B, Ducimetiere P, et al. Functional results 5 years after successful percutaneous mitral commissurotomy in a series of 528 patients and analysis of predictive factors. *J Am Coll Cardiol*. 1996;27:407-414.

Nishimura RA, Otto CM, Bonow RO, et al. The 2014 AHA/ACC Guideline for the Management of patients with valvular heart disease. *J Am Coll Cardiol*. 2014.

Nishimura RA, Rihal CS, Tajik AJ, et al. Accurate measurement of the transmitral gradient in patients with mitral stenosis: a simultaneous catheterization and Doppler echocardiographic study. *J Am Coll Cardiol*. 1994;24:152-158.

Song H, Kang DH, Kim JH, et al. Percutaneous mitral valvuloplasty versus surgical treatment in mitral stenosis with severe tricuspid regurgitation. *Circulation*. 2007;116:1246-1250.

Wilkins G, Weyman AE, Abascal VM, et al. Percutaneous balloon dilatation of the mitral valve: an analysis of echocardiographic variables related to outcome and the mechanism of dilatation. *Br Heart J*. 1988;60:299-308.

14

Mitral Regurgitation ▶

GAGAN D. SINGH · JASON H. ROGERS

Mitral Valve and Regurgitation Overview

The mitral valve (MV) apparatus is comprised of multiple interdependent structures (left atrium, mitral annulus, leaflets, chordae, papillary muscles, and left ventricle [LV]) actively working in synchrony to open the valve leaflets in diastole and to close them in systole. MV disease is heterogeneous and may result from pathologic changes of any, and often more than one, component of the MV apparatus. Transcatheter MV repair or replacement requires an in-depth understanding of the MV apparatus and its components (Fig. 14.1).

The landscape of transcatheter MV interventions is currently dominated by the MitraClip system and transcatheter mitral valve-in-valve (ViV) or valve-in-ring (ViR) procedures. The focus of this chapter will be to provide an overview of the MV anatomy, methods for invasive hemodynamic assessment of MV pathology, and guidance for procedural success for MitraClip and valve-in-valve and valve-in-ring procedures. Finally, investigational devices on the horizon for transcatheter MV repair/replacement will be discussed.

Anatomy

The MV (Fig. 14.1) consists of anterior and posterior leaflets that are attached at their bases to a fibromuscular annulus, and the leaflets are suspended by numerous chordae tendineae. These two leaflets are separated by the anterolateral and posteromedial commissures, which bracket the MV orifice. The posterior leaflet is divided into three major scallops, named P1, P2, and P3 from lateral to medial. The anterior leaflet does not have formal scallops, and the anterior leaflet sections are named A1, A2, and A3 based on their adjacent positions to the posterior scallops. The mitral annulus has a three-dimensional "saddle" shape with the highest (farthest from the LV apex) portions located anteriorly and posteriorly and the lowest portions located near the commissures. As seen from above, the annulus has an elliptical "D" shape with the minor axis (septal-lateral dimension) being normally less than 30 mm. The anterior portion of the mitral annulus contains the right and left fibrous trigones, two collagenous structures that demarcate the intersection of the aortic root with the mitral annulus. Between these fibrous trigones, the anterior mitral leaflet is in direct continuity with portions of the left and noncoronary aortic valve leaflets, forming the aortomitral curtain. This intimate aortic-mitral relationship has implications for percutaneous and surgical interventions on either valve since interventions that alter the geometry of one valve may affect the other. The chordae tendineae arise from two papillary muscles that are anchored in the LV wall. The anterolateral papillary muscle

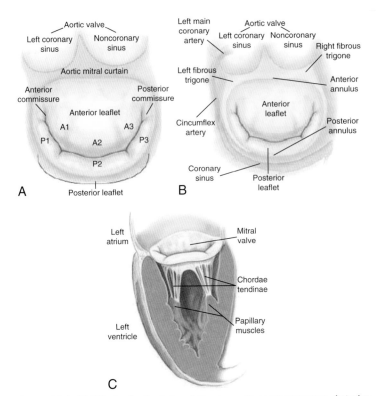

Figure 14.1 (A) Mitral valve leaflets relative to aortic coronary cusps. Anterior leaflet is divided into 3 segments (A1, A2, A3) and posterior leaflet segments (P1, P2, P3). (B) Mitral valve position relative to coronary sinus, circumflex artery, fibrous trigone, anterior mitral annulus, right fibrous trigone. (C) Cross section of mitral apparatus showing chordal attachments to the papillary muscles. *(Model-driven physiological assessment of the mitral valve from 4d TEE. Voigt I, et al. Proc. SPIE 7261, Medical Imaging 2009: Visualization, Image-Guided Procedures, and Modeling, 72610R)*

has a single head, whereas the posterior papillary muscle often has two or more subheads. The anterior papillary muscle has dual coronary perfusion (from the left anterior descending and left circumflex arteries), whereas the posterior papillary muscle is supplied from the posterior descending branch most often from the right coronary artery alone, thus making the posterior papillary muscle susceptible to rupture in the setting of acute inferior myocardial infarction—a consideration all operators must take into account if a patient remains in cardiogenic shock despite adequate coronary revascularization. Both papillary muscles give rise to chordae tendineae that are attached to both mitral leaflets. The papillary muscles are aligned parallel to the intercommissural axis of the MV. With LV enlargement or regional infarction, the papillary muscle position and function can change, applying traction to the leaflets that results in secondary mitral regurgitation (MR). The chordae that originate from the papillary muscle heads are known as first-order chordae, which then progressively divide into second- and third-order chordae. These chordae then insert either onto the free edge or body of the mitral leaflets.

Classification of Mitral Regurgitation

Etiologies of MR fall into several basic categories, with classification schema proposed by Carpentier in 1972 describing three classic mechanisms of MR (Fig. 14.2). Type I dysfunction describes the apparatus

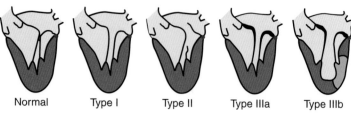

Normal   Type I   Type II   Type IIIa   Type IIIb

Figure 14.2 Carpentier classification of mitral valve regurgitation. *Type I*: Normal leaflet motion with annular dilation. *Type II*: Increased leaflet motion (leaflet prolapse or flail). *Type IIIa*: Restricted leaflet motion in systole and diastole, usually associated with leaflet and subvalvular thickening (rheumatic). *Type IIIb*: Restricted leaflet motion in systole, often seen in ischemic cardiomyopathy with history of infarct (light region in left ventricle) *(Reproduced from Lasala JM, Rogers JH, ed. Interventional Procedures for Adult Structural Heart Disease. Philadelphia: Saunders; 2014.)*

with *normal* leaflet motion but with MR due to annular dilation or leaflet perforation. Type II dysfunction is due to *excessive* leaflet motion from degenerative changes of the leaflets or chordae tendineae. Finally, type III dysfunction is a result of *restricted* leaflet motion either due to leaflet thickening (IIIa: rheumatic) or tethering of leaflets from papillary muscle or LV dysfunction (IIIb).

More commonly, MR etiologies are differentiated into primary (degenerative) or secondary (functional). Primary MR (Carpentier type II) is often due to dysfunction of one or more of the apparatus components preventing normal leaflet coaptation. Myxomatous MV disease, MV prolapse or flail leaflet, chordal rupture, fibroelastic deficiency, and/or endocarditis are a few of the potential underlying etiologies of primary MR. Surgical repair or replacement, or transcatheter therapies for those deemed high risk for surgery, is recommended for severe symptomatic primary MR. Secondary MR (Carpentier type I or type IIIb) is often due to compromised leaflet coaptation in the setting of structurally normal leaflets and supporting structures. Instead, the malcoaptation occurs as a result of tethering or restriction of leaflet motion due to dilatation of the LV, MV annulus, or left atrium. Severe symptomatic secondary MR is managed primarily with medical therapy, coronary revascularization, and cardiac resynchronization therapy (if indicated). Surgical ring annuloplasty or MV replacement can be performed, but indications for surgery lack robust clinical outcome data. The role of transcatheter MV repair in additional to standard medical practice for secondary MR is currently actively being investigated (COAPT trial).

Hemodynamic and Angiographic Assessment of Mitral Regurgitation

In the current era, many structural heart patients have complex multivalvular heart disease. Noninvasive echocardiographic assessment is currently the first-line diagnostic modality. However there are challenges with assessing MR using only the extent of color flow into the left atrium on two-dimensional transthoracic echocardiography (TTE). Quantitative measurement of MR requires the use and understanding of proximal isovelocity surface area (PISA), which in many instances can provide accurate measurement of regurgitant volume and effective orifice area. However many caveats and limitations exist, especially in patients with multiple jets or multivalvular heart disease. As such, invasive hemodynamic assessment remains an important component in the evaluation of patients with symptomatic valvular heart disease.

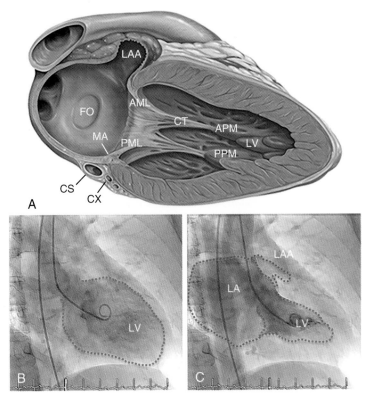

Figure 14.3 (A) Schematic diagram of the left ventricle (LV) and left atrium (LA) in the RAO projection. (B) Left ventriculogram from a patient with severe primary mitral regurgitation at end-diastole. Red dotted line outlines the LV cavity. (C) The same patient's left ventriculogram with contrast refluxing and outlining the entire LA (*green dotted line*) and the left atrial appendage (*blue dotted line*). Also see Video 14.1. LAA, left atrial appendage; FO, interatrial fossa; CS, coronary sinus; CX, circumflex artery; MA, mitral annulis; PML, posterior mitral leaflet; AML, anterior mitral leaflet; CT, chordae tendinae; APM, anterior papillary muscle; PPM, posterior papillary muscle.

In the cardiac catheterization laboratory, a formal quantitative assessment of MR can be performed by subtracting forward flow (i.e., cardiac output) from total LV output (as assessed by angiographic volume change). However this process is fraught with technical limitations and is more of historical interest. More commonly, the semi-quantitative method of left ventriculography (an "LV gram") is performed. The time and density of contrast going back into the left atrium are used to grade valve regurgitation (Fig. 14.3, Table 14.1, Video 14.1).

Technique/Tips

- Use a large bore (5–6F) angled pigtail catheter with a slight "counterclockwise" torque.
  - The counterclockwise torque pulls the pigtail catheter away from the septum and toward the center of the ventricular cavity.
  - The angled pigtail catheter allows the catheter to sit in the center of the LV instead of against the inferior wall.
  - Collectively this prevents ventricular ectopy and entanglement within the papillary muscles, thereby minimizing the chances

Table 14.1

Sellers Angiographic Classification of Mitral Regurgitation	
Grade (Severity)	**Description**
1+ (Mild)	Regurgitant contrast that clears with every beat and never opacifies the entire left atrium. Video 14.1.
2+ (Moderate)	Regurgitant contrast faintly opacifies the left atrium after several beats but the opacification never equals that of the left ventricle.
3+ (Moderately Severe)	Regurgitant contrast completely opacifies the left atrium after several beats and the density of opacification equals that of the left ventricle.
4+ (Severe)	Regurgitant contrast opacifies the entire left atrium after a single beat, with the opacification becoming denser with subsequent beats. Additionally, contrast can be seen opacifying the left atrial appendage and pulmonary veins. Video 14.1.

of the so-called "V-tach-o-gram," generally not useful in assessing MR severity.

- Be wary of diastolic contrast regurgitation post-PVC, which may overestimate MR severity.
- Do not hesitate to repeat ventriculography because an inadequate ectopy-filled ventriculography may result in over- or underestimation of true MR severity.
- A generous amount of contrast (10–12 cc/s for 3 s) is needed to completely opacify the ventricular cavity.
  - Inadequate contrast load may result in poor opacification and hence underestimation of regurgitant severity.
- The primary fluoroscopic view used is a right anterior oblique (RAO) of 30 degrees, which will lay out the left atrium to the left of the ventricular cavity (Fig. 14.3).
  - In cases where the spine or descending aorta is superimposed on the left atrium, concomitant cranial projection may be needed.
  - In the RAO projection, in addition to regurgitant severity, operators can also evaluate for the prolapsed or flail scallop in select cases (Video 14.2).
- In cases where the superimposed spine or descending aorta makes it difficult to assess MR, an orthogonal projection (left anterior oblique [LAO] with slight cranial angulation) will help better visualize the entire left atrium and flow into pulmonary veins, if present (Video 14.3).

Right Heart Catheterization

We also strongly advocate right heart catheterization in all patients with severe MR undergoing angiography and catheterization. Particular attention should be paid to the pulmonary artery and wedge (or left atrial) pressure tracings. The finding of prominent V waves in the wedge pressure (WP) or left atrial pressure (LAP) is the *sine qua non* for the presence of severe MR (Fig. 14.4A and B). Grossman's text identifies a V wave greater than twice the mean LAP or mean WP as suggestive of severe MR. However operators need to be cautious regarding the presence or the absence of V waves. Patients with either LV failure, long-standing hypertensive heart disease, or severe mitral annular calcification with functional mitral stenosis, can have enlarged and noncompliant left atria (Fig. 14.5). In these situations, a V wave in the absence of regurgitant disease can be visualized. Whether these V waves tend to be less than twice the mean LAP has not been

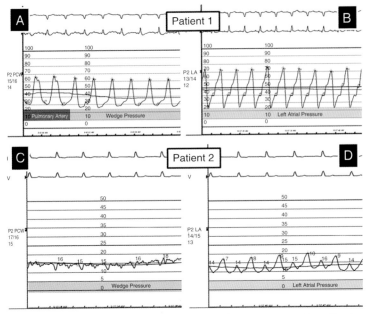

Figure 14.4 Intracardiac pressure tracings from two separate patients. Patient 1 had severe functional mitral regurgitation with pulmonary artery wedge tracing shown in the top left panel (A). Notice the progression of the waveform from one that peaks prior to the T wave and with a dicrotic notch to one that peaks after the T wave and without a dicrotic notch (A). In patients with severe MR, the peak V wave can be difficult to discern from the PA waveform. In such cases, fluoroscopy will confirm "angiographic wedge" with absence of motion of the distal tip of the wedged catheter. Other clues to help identify the source is to identify the location of the peak deflection in relation to the T wave (peak deflection is after T wave in a wedge with tall V waves and vice versa with a PA waveform) and the absence or presence of a dicrotic notch (present in a PA waveform). (B) The left atrial (LA) waveform in the same patient with functional MR with a mean LA pressure of approx. 40 mm Hg and a peak V wave of nearly 75 mm Hg. In this patient, both wedge pressure and LA pressure V waves are substantially elevated. Patient 2 also had severe long-standing functional MR. However the patient's wedge pressure tracings (C) demonstrated no significant V wave and a left atrial V wave of 20 mm Hg (D).

systematically evaluated. On the other hand, even in patients with chronic severe (4+) MR, many may not have prototypical large V waves. Progressive and slowly developing MR leads to increased compliance and enlargement of the left atrium over many years. A compliant and dilated left atrium can tolerate large regurgitant volumes without necessarily having large rises in the V waves. Additionally, a major contributor to the presence of absence of V waves can be the systemic afterload, particularly in the setting of secondary MR. One final point of caution is that the presence or absence of V waves with WP does not necessarily translate to similar findings when LAP is measured directly. We have noted an absence of large WP V waves, only to find prominent V waves when transseptal puncture is ultimately performed and direct LAP is measured in patients with severe MR (Fig. 14.4C and D). The patient or anatomic characteristics that lead to this discrepancy are unknown and currently an active area of investigation.

Transcatheter Mitral Valve Repair

There are numerous transcatheter MV repair strategies under varying stages of development and investigation. These include leaflet repair, direct and indirect annuloplasty, and ventricular and annular remodeling

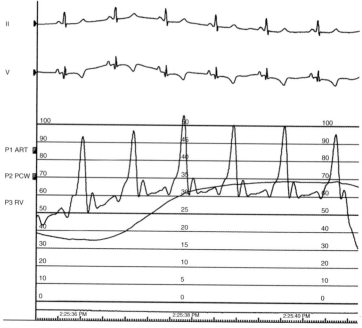

Figure 14.5 This pressure tracing is from a patient with only mild mitral regurgitation (Video 14.1; *left panel*) but with concomitant severe rheumatic mitral stenosis with a mean transmitral gradient of 15 mm Hg. This patient's end-expiratory V waves are approximately 50 mm Hg in the absence of significant mitral regurgitation.

devices, all in varying stages of development (see Table 14.2). The MitraClip (Abbott Vascular, Santa Clara CA) system currently represents the most widely used percutaneous repair technique and will be the focus of the remainder of the chapter. However readers should be aware of alternative and/or complementary technologies on the horizon.

In 1991, Dr. Alfieri performed a MV repair without annuloplasty using a stitch "edge-to-edge" technique to create a double-orifice valve. The durability of this procedure (>1500 patients) led to the development of a percutaneous technique using a clip to approximate the valve leaflets instead of a suture. The MitraClip system has been evaluated in numerous clinical trials, but the landmark studies are the safety and feasibility EVEREST I and pivotal randomized EVEREST II studies.

Clinical Results

The published clinical experience with the MitraClip in the United States includes EVEREST I, a feasibility nonrandomized trial ($n = 55$); EVEREST II, prerandomization ($n = 60$); EVEREST II, high-risk registry ($n = 78$); EVEREST II, pivotal, 2:1 randomization to MitraClip versus surgery ($n = 279$); REALISM, continued Access High Risk & Non High Risk ($n = 266$); and, more recently, commercial registry data.

EVEREST I

- Twenty-seven patients with a mean age of 69 years were enrolled.
- Of the 24 patients in whom the MitraClip was successfully deployed, 67% had less than 2+ MR upon discharge.
- At 30 days, MR severity grade decreased from 3.7 to 1.6.
- One patient experienced a stroke, and three others developed clip detachment without embolization.
- There were no cases of emergent cardiac surgery, myocardial infarction, cardiac tamponade, or septicemia.

Table 14.2

Past and Present Percutaneous Therapies for Mitral Valve Regurgitation

Target of Therapy	Device Name (Manufacturer)	Mechanism of Action/Comments	Phase of Development
Leaflet Repair	MitraClip (Abbott)	Clip-based edge-to-edge repair	FDA approved for primary MR. RCT for secondary MR
	MitraFlex	Transapical Edge-to-edge repair	Preclinical development
	Percu-Pro (Cardiosolutions)	Regurgitant orifice space-occupying	Phase I trials
Chordal Implant	Harpoon	Transapical artificial chordae	Clinical trials
	NeoChord (Neochord)	Synthetic chordae tendineae via transapical route	Clinical trials
Neoleaflet Implant	Middle Peak Medical	Synthetic neoleaflet	Clinical trials
Indirect Annuloplasty	Carillon (Cardiac Dimensions)	Coronary sinus reshaping	CE Mark approved (2011). RCT enrolling
	Mitral Cerclage	Coronary sinus-right atrial encircling	Clinical trials
	ARTO System (MVRx)	Transatrial coronary sinus-atrial septal shortening	Clinical trials
Direct Annuloplasty	Mitralign (Mitralign)	2 × 2 plicating anchors through posterior annulus	CE Mark approved 2016
	AccuCinch (Guided Delivery Systems)	Plicating anchors in ventricular side of mitral annulus	FIM reported
	Cardioband (Valtech)	Plicating anchors on atrial side of mitral annulus	CE Mark approved (2015)
	Millipede (Millipede)	Semi-rigid circumferential annular ring	Clinical trials
Mitral Annular Anchor	M-Valve	Percutaneous anchor to allow fixation of transcatheter valve	Clinical trials
Mitral Valve Replacement (Implant)	Tendyne (Abbott)	Transapical access and anchoring	Preclinical and FIM clinical trials
	CardiAQ (Edwards)	TF/TA access	
	Intrepid-12 (Medtronic)	TA access	
	Cardiovalve (Valtech)	Access TBD	
	Tiara (Neovasc)	D-shaped valve. No TF access	

FDA, Food and Drug Administration; MR, mitral regurgitation; RCT, randomized control trial; CE, "Conformité Européene"; FIM, First-In-Man; TF, transfemoral; TA, transapical.

- Ability to undergo surgical repair was preserved in those who, at the 30-day follow-up, had inadequate MR control.

EVEREST II, Randomized

- Enrolled 279 patients at 37 sites in a 2:1 fashion to the MitraClip procedure versus MV surgery.
- Major adverse event rate in the MitraClip arm was 9.6% versus 57.0% in the surgery arm ($p < 0.0001$).
- Safety benefit with device closure was largely driven by higher blood transfusion requirements (>2 units) in the surgery arm (53.2% vs. 8.8%).
- Noninferiority hypothesis was met with the clinical success rate in the MitraClip arm being 72.4% versus 87.8% in the surgery arm ($p_{NI} = 0.0012$).
- At 12 months:
  - MR reduction was greater in the surgery arm, with 97% of patients with less than 2+ MR versus 81.5% in the device arm.
  - More patients in the device arm had New York Heart Association (NYHA) functional class I or II versus the surgical arm (97.6% vs. 87.9%; $p < 0.0001$).
- At 5 years:
  - After 1 year of treatment with MitraClip, there was no difference in the composite end point (freedom from death, no new MV surgery, and MR lower than pretreatment minimum of 3+) than the surgical arm.
- Five-year mortality was similar between the two treatment arms.

EVEREST I and II Substudy of Secondary MR Patients

- MitraClip not only reduces the severity of MR but also stimulates reverse LV remodeling.
- LV chamber size decreased significantly at the 1-year follow-up.
- Acute procedural success was 89%.
- In the 12 of 19 patients for whom the 1-year follow-up was complete, freedom from death, surgery for valve dysfunction, and MR >2+ was 79%.
- NYHA class and measures of reverse remodeling showed significant improvement in the follow-up period.

The long-term data from EVEREST II suggest that although MV surgery is superior to transcatheter MV repair using MitraClip in reducing severity of MR, the device reduces symptoms, produces durable reduction in MR, and promotes favorable reverse remodeling of the LV 5 years after intervention. Hence percutaneous MV repair with the MitraClip system is a viable alternative to surgery in those patients with MV anatomy amenable to mechanical coaptation.

Indications and Clinical Evidence

Patients with a class I indication for MV surgery according to the American College of Cardiology/American Heart Association (ACC/AHA) 2006 guidelines for valvular heart disease were eligible for the EVEREST (Endovascular Valve Edge-to-Edge Repair Study) studies (Box 14.1). MV surgery is indicated in all symptomatic patients with severe MR in the absence of severe LV dysfunction and/or LV end-systolic dimension of greater than 55 mm (class I recommendation, level of evidence: B). In asymptomatic patients with severe MR, MV surgery is indicated if LV dysfunction is present (class I recommendation, level of evidence: B). Additionally patients with severe MR and new

> **Box 14.1** Inclusion Criteria for MitraClip EVEREST Trials
>
> Although the MitraClip was originally studied with strict anatomic boundaries, many studies to date have shown that MitraClip therapy can be applied to other pathologies such as noncentral, commissural, wide flail, or severe functional mitral regurgitation (MR).
> - Candidates for mitral valve repair or replacement surgery
> - Moderate to severe (3+) or severe (4+) chronic mitral valve regurgitation
> - New York Heart Association (NYHA) functional class II or greater symptoms with ejection fraction (EF) of >25% and left ventricular (LV) end-systolic dimension <55 mm
> - If asymptomatic, evidence of left ventricular dysfunction (EF < 60% but >25% and/or LV end-systolic dimension ≥40–50 mm)
> - Appropriate valve anatomy
> - Exclusion criteria included recent myocardial infarction, any interventional or surgical procedure within 30 days, mitral valve orifice area <4 cm², renal failure, and endocarditis

onset of atrial fibrillation or pulmonary hypertension were also candidates.

The original randomized EVEREST II trial and a subsequent EVEREST II high-risk study of patients with symptomatic primary MR led to the U.S. Food and Drug Administration (FDA) approval of percutaneous MV repair with the MitraClip device. In October 2013, the FDA approved percutaneous MV repair as follows:

- "[The MitraClip Clip Delivery System] is indicated for the percutaneous reduction of significant symptomatic MR (MR ≥3+) due to primary abnormality of the mitral apparatus [degenerative (primary) MR] in patients who have been determined to be at prohibitive risk for mitral valve surgery by a heart team, which includes a cardiac surgeon experienced in mitral valve surgery and a cardiologist experienced in mitral valve disease, and in whom existing comorbidities would not preclude the expected benefit from reduction of the [MR]."

The ACC/AHA guidelines for the treatment of valvular heart disease (2014):

- Class IIb (level of evidence B) recommendation for transcatheter MV repair for severely symptomatic patients (NYHA class III to IV) with chronic severe primary MR (stage D) who have favorable anatomy for the repair procedure and a reasonable life expectancy but who have a prohibitive surgical risk because of severe comorbidities and remain severely symptomatic despite optimal goal-directed medical therapy for heart failure.

Despite European registry data and EVEREST suggesting favorable benefits of percutaneous MV repair in patients with secondary MR consisting of positive LV remodeling and improved functional class, there remains no current FDA approval for this indication. A randomized controlled trial (Clinical Outcomes Assessment of the MitraClip Percutaneous Therapy [COAPT]) will determine the role of MitraClip in patients with heart failure and associated secondary MR.

MitraClip NT Procedure

Patient Setup

The procedure is performed with the patient under general anesthesia and using fluoroscopy and transesophageal echocardiography (TEE) for device guidance. Fig. 14.6 highlights the patient setup and positioning of the providers. TEE elements to note at the beginning of the procedure are presence/absence of pericardial effusion, appearance of interatrial septum (floppy, fibrous, lipomatous hypertrophy, etc.), and evaluation

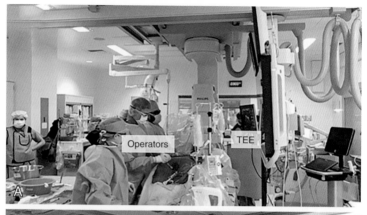

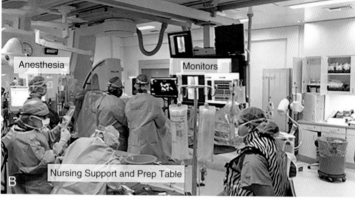

Figure 14.6 (A) A view of the room setup from the foot of the bed. The echocardiographer and transesophageal echocardiography (TEE) machine are located at the head of the bed on the patient's left. (B) A view of the room while facing the patient. The nursing support and prep table are positioned behind the operators. The anesthesiologist and the anesthesia console is located at the head of the bed on the patient's right.

of jet characteristics and potential site(s) of grasping. Some operators advocate for use of right heart catheterization pre- and intraprocedurally.

Femoral Vein Access

After fluoroscopy of the right femoral head, ultrasound guidance is used to ensure a single front-wall puncture using the standard modified Seldinger technique. Once the guidewire is in place, the skin is incised to allow for later advancement of the 24F guide catheter. After the skin is incised, the needle is withdrawn and the track is dilated with an 8F dilator. We next partially deploy two ProGlide devices in a "preclose" technique at the 11 o'clock and 1 o'clock positions. The sutures are externalized with each deployment and secured to the patient for later procurement. We next insert an 8F sheath into place, followed by 2000 units of IV heparin. Often the guidewires and catheters used for transseptal penetration (the next step) can be thrombogenic, and the initial heparin dose helps to prevent such thrombus formation from occurring.

Transseptal Anatomy

The transseptal puncture is one of the key elements to the MitraClip procedure because an "off target" transseptal access may result in difficulty maneuvering the MitraClip system and may result in suboptimal transcatheter repair.

Successful transseptal puncture mandates a three-dimensional understanding of the interatrial septal/fossa anatomy and its relationship to the surrounding structures. Under most normal anatomic conditions, the right atrium lies anterior to the LA. Furthermore, the interatrial septum is not in an exact midcoronal plane; rather, it lies off-axis, with the septum proceeding from the patients' left to the right in the antero-posterior direction. This natural orientation of the interatrial septum is the rationale for having the initial position of the transseptal needle at the 4- or 5-o'clock position (see step-by-step instructions later) so the needle (and the tenting) is perpendicular to the fossa. For purposes of transseptal puncture, the interatrial septum is initially visualized on TEE in a superior-inferior view (i.e., bicaval view) in which both the superior vena cava (SVC) and the inferior vena cava (IVC) are aligned in conjunction with the interatrial septum (Fig. 14.7). The second view used is the short-axis view in which the interatrial fossa is viewed in the anteroposterior projection with the aortic valve and the posterior wall aligned in conjunction with the interatrial septum (Fig. 14.7). It is important to appreciate that the bicaval and short-axis views are not perpendicular to each other. Instead, the short axis is often obtained with the omniplane of the TEE probe rotated to 30–60 degrees. In the short-axis view, rotation of the transseptal needle *clockwise (posterior)* not only moves the intended puncture site away from the aorta but also allows the puncture site to move away from the mitral annular plane, allowing one to gain transseptal height.

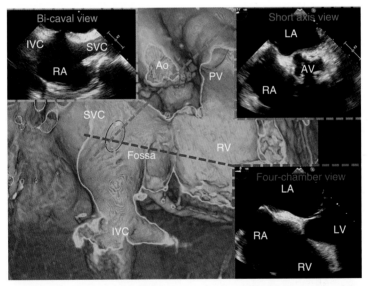

Figure 14.7 *Larger image:* Computed tomography (CT) reconstruction of the interatrial septum in place with the inflow and outflow. The top left inset shows the bicaval transesophageal echocardiography (TEE) view in which the interatrial septum is visualized with the superior and inferior vena cavae (SVC/IVC) in the same plane. The top right inset shows the "short axis" view, in which the interatrial septum is in the same plane as the aortic valve and the posterior wall of the atria. The bottom right inset shows the "four-chamber" view, in which the interatrial septum is in plane perpendicular to all four cardiac chambers. IVC, inferior vena cava; SVC, superior vena cava; RA, right atrium; LA, left atrium; AV, aortic valve; LV, left ventricle; RV, right ventricle; PV, pulmonic valve, Ao, Aorta. *(Reproduced from Singh et al. Targeted transseptal access for MitraClip percutaneous mitral valve repair.* Intervent Cardiol Clin. *2016;5:57.)*

Transseptal Technique

The traditional catheter and needle combinations include the Mullins sheath and standard Brockenbrough (BRK, St. Jude Medical, St. Paul, Minnesota) needle.

Other commonly used components include the SL1 sheath (St. Jude Medical) and radiofrequency NRG needle (Baylis Medical).

Using a multipurpose A (MPA) catheter, a 0.032-inch wire is advanced to the SVC under fluoroscopic guidance.

The MPA catheter and the venous sheath are removed over the wire; the transseptal sheath and dilator are advanced into the SVC.

The wire is then removed, and the transseptal needle is advanced to near the distal tip of the sheath and under fluoroscopic guidance (usually to ~1 cm from the tip of the dilator).

The orientation of the needle and sheath must be maintained by matching the metal arrow on the needles hub to the direction of sheaths sidearm.

It is helpful to then move the needle and sheath together with one hand grasping both as a single unit (Fig. 14.8).

This technique also maintains a constant and safe needle distance from the tip of the dilator.

The sheath, dilator, and needle are oriented such that the system is pointing toward a 4- or 5-o'clock position.

For reasons discussed earlier, this particular positioning of the transseptal system allows the needle to be perpendicular to the septum on initial engagement.

- Under fluoroscopic and TEE guidance, the sheath and needle are slowly and carefully pulled back to the junction of the SVC and right atrium.

  - On fluoroscopy, most operators may note a two-step drop or a sudden downward movement of the needle.

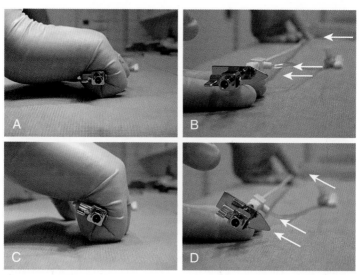

Figure 14.8 The transseptal (TS) sheath and needle are moved as one system by rotating the hand. The arrow on the TS needle should be aligned with the sidearm of the sheath, which is oriented toward the curve of the TS sheath (arrows). (A, B) The system in the horizontal (3-o'clock) position (arrows). (C, D) The system in the 4-o'clock position (arrows), which is the preferred angle of crossing for most structurally normal hearts. Note that this angle will change with right or left atrial enlargement. (Reproduced from Lasala JM, Rogers JH, ed. Interventional Procedures for Adult Structural Heart Disease. Philadelphia: Saunders; 2014.)

- The first drop occurs as the needle drops from the SVC into the right atrium (one may note a premature atrial contraction at this point).
- The next drop occurs as the needle falls into the fossa ovalis from the right atrium.
- The operator can often estimate the location of the fossa by the position of the TEE probe, which is focused on the interatrial septum.
- At this time, attention is focused almost completely on the TEE. The first view is the bicaval view in which the superior-inferior orientation of the puncture needed is determined (Video 14.4).
  - The ideal position in a routine endovascular valve edge-to-edge repair study (EVEREST) II–type patient is the *superior and posterior* fossa.
- Once the bicaval position is satisfactory, the TEE is used to display the short-axis view at the level of the aortic valve.
  - This view provides an anterior-posterior perspective on the transseptal location.
- To manipulate the transseptal needle and sheath posteriorly, the entire system is torqued clockwise.
  - The ideal position is slightly posterior of the midline (Video 14.4).
- The next view is the four- or five-chamber view in which the perpendicular (vertical) height of the transseptal tenting from the MV is measured (Fig. 14.9).
  - In general, this distance should be between 4.0 cm–4.5 cm with the MitraClip NT system, although this height may need to be

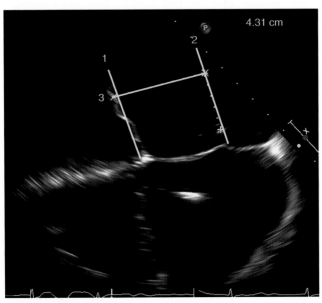

Figure 14.9 Height assessment: Once the supero-posterior fossa is engaged, then switch to the four-chamber view. First (1), a horizontal line is drawn on the mitral annular plane. Next (2), an additional line (parallel to the mitral annular plane) is drawn at the site of transseptal tenting (referred to as the transseptal plane). Finally (3), the transseptal height is determined by measuring the distance from the transseptal plane down to the coaptation plane.

adjusted for nontraditional pathology (e.g., commissural MR, large left atrium, and so forth).

- The MV reference point is either the MV annular plane or the point of coaptation of the MV leaflets.

- Once the suitability of the proposed transseptal puncture site has been confirmed by the views described, puncture across the septum is performed.

  - The transseptal needle is attached to a slow infusion of saline from the manifold.

  - Transseptal puncture is performed in the short axis of the interatrial septum in efforts to avoid hitting vital structures (e.g., posterior atrial wall, aorta, etc.).

- Once appropriate positioning is confirmed, the needle is advanced just beyond the tip of the dilator and gentle forward pressure is exerted.

  - It is important for operators not to apply excessive force because only a small amount of forward force is required.

  - Once a tent is formed, let each heartbeat "do the work."

  - The forward momentum coupled with the heart motion will ultimately result in successful puncture (Video 14.5).

  - Operators will feel a small "pop," and the actual puncture can be seen simultaneously on TEE as the needle traverses the interatrial septum.

- Once the tip of the needle enters the left atrium, bubbles in the left atrium will be seen (from the slow infusion of saline); finally, as the manifold is then converted to pressure, LAP waveforms should be noted.

- Once transseptal puncture is confirmed, the needle and sheath should be rotated slightly counterclockwise (anterior) to avoid inadvertent puncture of the posterior wall of the left atrium.

  - The dilator and sheath (as a system) are then advanced over the needle into the left atrium, preferably under TEE guidance.

  - The sheath is then advanced over the needle and dilator; finally the needle and dilator are carefully removed, and the transseptal sheath is aspirated and flushed to avoid any air entry or thrombus formation, then connected to pressure to determine preprocedural LAP and waveform.

- Additional IV heparin is administered to achieve an activated clotting time (ACT) greater than 250 s.

  - From here on, ACT levels should be routinely checked to maintain therapeutic ACT.

MitraClip NT System

The entire MitraClip NT system has several major components: the clip, steerable guide and delivery catheter, guide catheter handle, clip delivery system (CDS), and the delivery catheter (DC) handle. Procedural steps (Box 14.2) require a thorough understanding of the device components. See Figs. 14.10 and 14.11 for detailed terminology and function of all components.

MitraClip Guide Catheter Insertion Technique

If the transseptal procedure is successful, the MitraClip guide catheter can be prepped on the back table.

Box 14.2 MitraClip Procedural Steps

1. Right femoral venous access made with two ProGlides in "preclose" technique.
2. Advance transseptal sheath and needle into superior vena cava (SVC).
3. Transseptal sheath and needle aligned in the superior and posterior fossa.
4. Transseptal puncture.
5. Advance "stiff" wire into the left upper pulmonary vein.
6. Femoral vein tract dilatation.
7. Insert MitraClip Guide Catheter and dilator through the interatrial septum.
8. Remove the dilator and "stiff wire."
9. Clip delivery system (CDS) insertion into left atrium (cradling the CDS).
10. Apply "M" knob and position the CDS over the mitral valve with posterior guide torque.
11. Open the clip to 180 degrees.
12. Position the clip in bicommissural view over the intended grasp area.
13. Check alignment in transesophageal echocardiographic (TEE) three-dimensional view and make appropriate adjustments to the CDS.
14. Advance the clip into the left ventricle in biplane view (bicommissural and grasping view).
15. Recheck subvalvular three-dimensional alignment.
16. Close clip arms to 120 degrees.
17. Retract CDS in efforts to engage the anterior and posterior leaflets.
18. Drop grippers and close clip to 60%–70%.
19. Interrogate leaflet insertion and, if appropriate, close clip to 100% in bicommissural view with color Doppler.
20. Interrogate residual mitral regurgitation, pulmonary vein flow, and residual transmitral gradient.
21. Deploy clip and remove CDS.
22. Remove guide catheter.
23. Secure venous access site (preclose or "figure-of-eight" stitch).

- A 7F multipurpose catheter (oriented *superiorly and posteriorly*) is advanced through the transseptal sheath to direct a stiff 0.035-inch guidewire into the left upper pulmonary vein.
  - Alternately, a commercial preshaped spiral wire (Protrack, Baylis) can be placed in the left atrium and the guide advanced.
- The 7F multipurpose catheter and transseptal sheath are then removed "over the wire."
  - The guide catheter, with its dilator in place, is then advanced.
- The first point of resistance will be the skin as the tip of the guide catheter engages the femoral vein.
  - A gentle rocking motion of the guide catheter and forward pressure will allow the system to advance into the vein.
  - The echocardiographer now focuses on the interatrial septum as the dilator and guide catheter approach the septum.
- The guide catheter dilator has echogenic coils alerting the operator that the septum is now engaged (Video 14.6).
  - It is important not to apply excessive force to cross the septum.
  - Rather, gentle forward pressure is applied and the septum will stretch with the guide catheter dilator.
  - Sometimes gentle rocking motion of the guide catheter or applying some "negative" (Fig. 14.10D) knob to straighten the guide tip will also allow it to pass through the septum, all while steady gentle forward pressure is applied.
- Once the septum is crossed by the tip of the guide catheter, the operator will feel a "pop," and tenting of the septum on TEE will no longer be visualized.

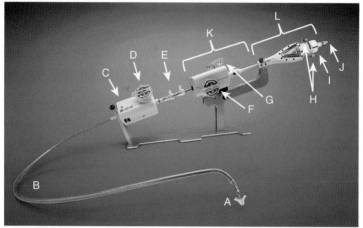

Figure 14.10 MitraClip System. (A) MitraClip. (B) Guide catheter (GC) steerable sheath. (C) GC control. (D) Plus/Minus knob. (E) GC hemostatic guide valve. (F) "M" knob. (G) Anterior/Posterior knob. (H) Gripper and lock lines. (I) Arm positioner. (J) Actuator knob. (K) Steerable sleeve handle. (L) Delivery cable (DC) handle. The guide catheter is 22F as it crosses the interatrial septum but 24F at the skin as it crosses into the femoral vein. Outside the body, the guide catheter (Fig. 14.10C) sits in its cradle and can be torqued to move the guide catheter in anterior (counterclockwise) and posterior (clockwise) rotation. This movement is involved in two important steps: insertion of the clip delivery system (i.e., cradling the clip delivery system) into the left atrium, and, finally, at the time of grasping, to allow the operator to move the clip in the antero-posterior dimension for adequate leaflet insertion. The guide catheter also has an important "Plus/Minus" knob (D). Rotating this knob in the "plus" direction flexes the guide catheter at its tip and creates a more acute bend. This maneuver can be useful when the original transseptal puncture is too anterior and moves the trajectory of the clip delivery system (CDS) away from the aorta and more perpendicular alignment with the mitral valve. CDS = A + K + L.

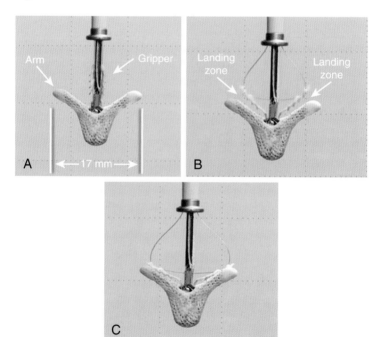

Figure 14.11 (A) The MitraClip NT in the grasping position, in which the clip arms are opened to 120 degrees with grippers retracted. (B) The "landing zone" for the mitral leaflets once the grippers are released. (C) Note that the grippers drop all the way down to clip arms when they are fully released. The grippers will drop all the way down to approximately 150 degrees.

- The dilator is withdrawn into the guide catheter, then the wire into the dilator, and then the dilator and wire are removed as a system.
  - As the dilator and wire are withdrawn from the back of the guide catheter, the flush port is being aspirated in efforts to maintain an air-free environment.

Clip Delivery System Insertion and Grasping Technique

- Once the guide catheter has successfully been placed, the clip is prepped on the back table per manufacturer specifications.
- The hemostatic valve of the guide catheter (Fig. 14.10E) is flushed with saline while a second operator/assistant advances the tip of the clip delivery system (CDS) into the guide catheter.
- The CDS is advanced into the guide catheter until the tip of the CDS and guide catheter are aligned on fluoroscopy.
  - The remainder of the advancement is done in conjunction with TEE.
  - The CDS is advanced into the left atrium with the ultimate goal of aligning a radiopaque tip ring marker on the CDS between two alignment markers on the guide catheter (Fig. 14.12).
  - The latter step is performed on fluoroscopy.
- At this point, the CDS and guide catheter are in appropriate alignment and any movement outside of the body with the control knob will have reproducible results inside the body.
- The next step is to apply "M" knob (Fig. 14.10F) until the knob approaches "3 o'clock," which allows for the CDS to be flexed down on top of the mitral leaflet.
  - In some cases, a little more or less "M" knob may be needed and will be determined on a case-by-case basis.

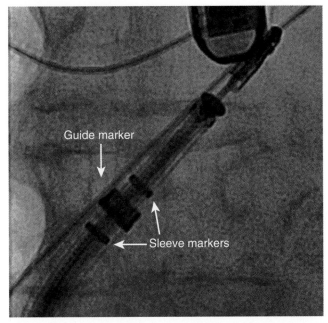

Figure 14.12 Adequate "straddling." The goal for an adequate straddle is to align the guide marker between the two sleeve markers located on the clip delivery system. "Straddling" is important because it ensures that movement outside the body on the control knobs translates into intended movements inside the body.

- Other fine-tuning adjustments (usually posterior torque; see Fig. 14.10C) with the guide catheter may be needed to center the clip over the areas of coaptation (Video 14.7).
- Next, the clip arms are opened (Fig. 14.10I) to 180 degrees and positioned over the area of intended grasp.
  - We generally prefer to locate the intended area in the bicommissural view and the LV outflow tract view with appropriate adjustments on the control knobs outside the body as needed.
- Using three-dimensional TEE, the clip is aligned exactly perpendicular to the coaptation plane in efforts to maximize leaflet grasp (Video 14.8).
- Using biplane two-dimensional TEE views (commissural and grasping), the clip is advanced into the LV just beneath the leaflets.
  - Once below the leaflets, the clip arms are closed to 120–140 degrees to allow a "crevice" for the leaflets to sit into without falling off (Fig. 14.13).
- Subannular three-dimensional alignment is again confirmed.
- The TEE is now switched over to a dedicated grasping view in which the anterior and posterior leaflet grasping/landing zones are parallel to the clip arms (Figs. 14.11B and 14.13).
- The CDS is retracted until both the anterior and posterior leaflets engage the clip arms.
  - Slight adjustments in multiple planes (A/P torque of the guide catheter, Plus/Minus knob of the guide catheter) may be needed to appropriately align the clip arms to the leaflets.
- Once both the anterior and posterior leaflets are fully engaged with the clip arms, the grippers (Fig. 14.10H) are released into the

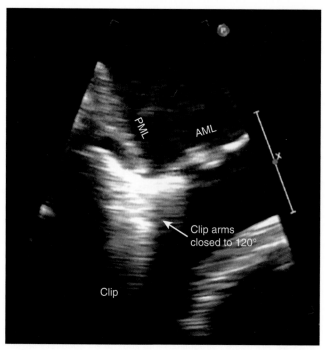

Figure 14.13 Grasping transesophageal echocardiography (TEE) view that shows the two leaflets of the mitral valve engaging the MitraClip arms, which are at 120 degrees. AML, anterior mitral valve leaflet; PML, posterior mitral valve leaflet.

> **Box 14.3** Systematic Approach to Alignment, Grasping, and Leaflet Insertion
>
> **Alignment**
>
> Once the clip has been opened above the leaflet, switch to bicommissural view with color.
>
> Ask anesthesia to change ventilation to low tidal volume (150 cc) ventilation.
>
> Assess location of intended grasp with color Doppler, and move clip to center of jet.
>
> In two-dimensional grasping view (LVOT), assess leaflet anatomy for grasp.
>
> Check three-dimensional supra-annular orientation and make appropriate adjustments.
>
> Advance clip into left ventricle (LV) in two-dimensional biplane view and make adjustments (lateral vs. medial, anterior vs. posterior) while advancing into the LV.
>
> Check three-dimensional subannular orientation and make appropriate adjustments.
>
> **Grasping**
>
> Close clip to 120–180 degrees and then retract back to engage leaflets, making adjustments as needed (e.g., anterior/posterior torque, +/−knob, etc.).
>
> Drop grippers at end-systole (allows grippers to fall as leaflets are falling onto clip).
>
> Close clip to 60%–70% closed.
>
> **Assessment of Leaflet Insertion**
>
> Check leaflet insertion in grasping, bicommissural, and 0-degree view (the latter for posterior leaflet primarily).
>
> If leaflet insertion is not adequate, release grasp and try again.
>
> If leaflet insertion is adequate, switch to two-dimensional bicommissural view with color, close the clip to 90%–100%.
>
> If expected result is achieved, check (a) residual color jet, (b) pulmonary vein flow pattern, and (c) transmitral gradients.
>
> Determine fate of clip (deploy vs. ungrasp).

leaflets followed by clip closure to 60%–70% (Video 14.9).

- It is important not the rush the grasping steps.
- Failure to adequately perform all the steps without careful attention to alignment and leaflet engagement will result in failure to adequately capture both leaflets or, worse, leaflet detachment.
  - For all aspects of this procedure, the patient is hemodynamically stable, which should allow the operator to take his or her time and follow all steps in a systematic manner (Box 14.3).
- Once grasping has occurred, the echocardiographer assesses leaflet insertion.
  - Leaflet insertion is carefully interrogated in multiple TEE views (grasping, bicommissural, and in four-chamber view) to assess appropriate insertion of both the anterior and posterior leaflets.
- If the grasp is deemed to have appropriate leaflet insertion, the clip is tightened in the bicommissural view with color Doppler.
  - This evaluates the effect, if any, this particular grasp may have on MR reduction.
- If appropriate MR reduction is achieved, the echocardiographer now assesses resultant jet(s), pulmonary vein flows, and transmitral gradient.
- If the operator/echocardiographer deems an inadequate grasp (e.g., due to inadequate leaflet insertion, inadequate MR

reduction, etc.), the leaflets are ungrasped and an alternate position is sought.

- If the alternate grasp location is immediately adjacent, then the entire system outside the body can be moved in (for more lateral grasp) or retracted (for more medial grasp).
- It is important to perform this maneuver in the bicommissural view with two-dimensional color Doppler.
- If, however, the decision is made to regrasp in a location not immediately adjacent, then it is important to open the clip until it is everted and then retract the clip back into the left atrium and start the process again.

- This latter step ensures that the clip does not get tangled in the extensive array of the subvalvular chordal apparatus.

Clip Deployment Technique

- Once an appropriate grasp with MR reduction is achieved, it is now time to deploy and disengage the clip from the CDS.
- First, the "arm angle" is confirmed.
  - The arm positioner (Fig. 14.10I) is turned counterclockwise to confirm that the clip arms do not open.
  - Once this is confirmed, the clip arm is retightened to "tight side of neutral."
- Next, the "gripper line" cap is unscrewed and confirmation is made that the gripper line is free of friction.
- Next, unscrew the "lock-line" cap and remove the "lock-line" from the body.
- "Arm angle" is again confirmed, and now the actuator knob (Fig. 14.10J) is removed.
  - The arm positioner is turned counterclockwise until the release crevice is seen, and now the actuator knob is rotated counterclockwise until the CDS disengages from the clip (generally eight turns).
  - The latter step is performed on fluoroscopy.
  - At this point, the clip remains attached externally via the "gripper line."
  - This is the last remaining contact with the entire system. In scenarios where immediate clip detachment (e.g., from both clips) is noted, the gripper line prevents the clip from embolizing to a vital vascular bed and efforts can be undertaken to retrieve and remove the clip.
  - If, however, the clip remains in adequate position with preserved leaflet insertion and MR reduction, then the gripper line is now slowly retracted and removed, and the clip is fully disengaged from the CDS.
- The CDS is retracted in the exact same manner that it was inserted.
  - Generally, this requires releasing the "M" knob while paying careful attention (by echo) to the distal tip and ensuring freedom from important structures of the LA.
  - As the M knob is released, the CDS is retracted and the guide catheter is torqued anteriorly.
- Before the CDS is fully retracted into the guide catheter and out of the body, the echocardiographer shows the short axis interatrial septal view to ensure that at least 1 cm of the guide catheter remains in the left atrium.
  - As the CDS is retracted from the guide catheter, an assistant or second operator is generally aspirating from the guide

catheter side arm port to ensure that air does not entrap into the system.

- Once fully removed, the guide catheter is flushed.

At this point, the operators and echocardiographer assess resultant hemodynamic (LAP) and echocardiographic data (residual MR, pulmonary vein flow, transmitral gradient). If additional clips are needed and tolerable, then the preceding steps are repeated.

End of Procedure and Achieving Hemostasis

- If further clips are not needed, the guide catheter is retracted back into the right atrium and ultimately removed over the wire.
- If a "preclose" technique was initially used, the ProGlide sutures are cinched down and residual bleeding is assessed.
  - If adequate hemostasis has not been achieved, options to place a "figure-of-eight" stitch or an additional ProGlide at the 12 o'clock position are considered.
- Ultimately, the wire is removed from the body, and the patient is extubated and transferred to the recovery unit for observation.

Periprocedural Care

Preprocedure, patients are pretreated with aspirin and clopidogrel (load of 300 or 600 mg is acceptable). If they are on systemic anticoagulation (e.g., for atrial fibrillation), it is halted 2–5 days prior the procedure; however the patients are still treated with aspirin and Plavix immediately prior to the procedure. Patients are also treated with preprocedural antibiotic prophylaxis at the discretion of the operator. Due to the common occurrence of postanesthesia urinary retention, we also insert urinary (e.g. Foley) catheters in these patients.

Postprocedure, patients will remain on aspirin and clopidogrel for at least 30 days. This is done to prevent device-related thrombus formation. If patients were on systemic anticoagulation prior to the procedure, they are ultimately discharged on the same anticoagulant with or without low-dose aspirin alone based on the patient's individualized bleeding risk. The patient also receives an additional two doses of antibiotic prophylaxis postprocedure. Finally, all patients receive a two-view chest x-ray and an echocardiogram prior to discharge home.

Transcatheter Mitral Valve-in-Valve and Mitral Valve-in-Ring

Repair or replacement of MV disease with bioprostheses or rings is increasingly performed over use of mechanical valves in efforts to avert lifelong systemic anticoagulation, especially with improved long-term survival and aging of the population. Overall, durability of newer generation surgical repair/replacement of the MV is felt to be anywhere from 10 to 20 years. If these patients do develop symptomatic degeneration of their initial repair or replacement, redo sternotomy with re-replacement can be considered but carries substantial morbidity and mortality, especially in this frequently morbid and aged population. Hence, for these patients, transcatheter ViV or ViR repairs are an attractive option to consider owing to reduced morbidity of these procedures compared to the surgical alternative.

The potential etiology of bioprosthetic degeneration can include valve leaflet degeneration (i.e., torn leaflets) from wear and tear, leaflet calcification leading to mitral stenosis, pannus formation leading to stenosis or the pannus impinging on the leaflet architecture resulting in regurgitation, thrombosis, leaflet perforation from endocarditis, and/

or valve frame dehiscence resulting in paravalvular leak (PVL). Leaflet tissue deterioration is overwhelmingly the main cause of bioprosthetic valve failure. In patients with prior mitral annuloplasty rings, failure can occur either due to degeneration of the native leaflets resulting in MR, valve leaflet calcification leading to stenosis, or ring dehiscence resulting in PVL.

Clinical Evidence

The clinical evidence for ViV and ViR procedures is derived primarily from the Valve-in-Valve International Data (VIVID) registry.

- A global registry currently consists of 70 sites with more than 765 patients.
- Of these, 190 patients underwent ViV or ViR mitral procedures (n = 157 for ViV, n = 33 for ViR).
- Overall age of this patient subset was 74 years, with 65% female, and an average Society of Thoracic Surgeons (STS) score of 14.
- The median time from initial surgery to transcatheter procedure was 9 years (IQR 7–12).
- The mechanism of failure was combined (regurgitation and stenosis) in 38%, regurgitation only in 37%, and stenosis in 25%.
- The most common surgical bioprosthesis (53%) and ring (70%) failure was from the Edwards Perimount Valve and Edwards Physio ring, respectively.
- The primary mode of delivery was the transapical route (85%), followed by transseptal delivery in 12%.
- An Edwards Sapien device was used for the ViV and ViR procedure for 94% of the cases.
- Thirty-day outcomes reported consist of all cause of death of 9% and a median hospital stay of 8 days.
  - Of the patients who survived to 30 days, 86% reported functional status to be NYHA class I or II.
- The 1-year overall survival was 78%.

Initial Evaluation

The initial evaluation of these patients consists of standard invasive and noninvasive hemodynamic evaluation with particular assessment of TEE and computed tomography (CT) to determine mode of prosthesis failure and sizing of the internal diameter. Most patients will carry their initial device card from the time of implant, and obtaining the exact manufacturer and model will be key in determining the appropriate sizing and device needed for the ViV or ViR procedure. TEE will not only help determine the mode of prosthesis failure, but will also inform you of the presence or absence of concomitant PVL, which will modify the ultimate transcatheter procedure. In such a case, the PVL may need to be addressed prior to the ViV and ViR procedure (Fig. 14.14). A comprehensive source of prosthesis dimensions and proposed trans-catheter valve to be used is the iPhone Valve-In-Valve (Mitral) app, which has listed commonly available bioprosthetic valves and rings used in the United States and Europe. Also provided are in vitro and fluoroscopic appearances of the prosthesis *en-face* and side views. Importantly, the internal dimensions from the manufacturer are also provided, as is the proposed size of transcatheter valve that would fit within the prosthesis. Finally, the app also provides a fluoroscopic image of what the valve would look like inside the prosthesis once it is ultimately delivered in the appropriate position. Our practice is to

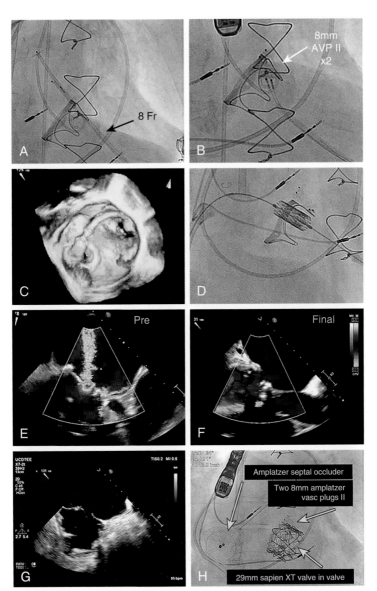

Figure 14.14 A patient with prior bioprosthetic mitral valve replacement now presents with severe symptomatic central and paravalvular leak. Initial transapical access (A) was achieved to target the paravalvular leak, which was successfully treated with two 8 mm Amplatzer Vascular Plug IIs (B). Next, after transseptal access, a 0.035-inch glidewire from the transseptal sheath was snared in the left atrium and externalized via the transapical access we then created the rail for valve-in-valve delivery. Ultimately, a 29 mm Edwards Sapien XT was deployed under rapid pacing (C,D) with postprocedure echocardiography (F) demonstrating complete reduction in central and paravalvular leak. After withdrawal of the delivery sheath, a significant interatrial defect was created (G), which was successfully closed with an Amplatzer Septal Occluder device (H).

Table 14.3

Valve-in-Valve (ViV) and Valve-in-Ring (ViR) Delivery Approaches		
Frequency	**Approach**	**Comments**
Most common	Transapical	Distal wire is in upper pulmonary vein.
	Transseptal with left ventricular (LV) rail	Stiff wire sits in LV cavity.
	Transseptal with aortic rail	Stiff wire is snared in the LV and retracted back into the descending aorta.
Least common	Transseptal with apical rail	Stiff wire is snared in the LV and externalized via a small transapical sheath.

additionally obtain a gated CT of the chest in all these patients and size the internal dimensions again to confirm the appropriate valve to be deployed. A considerable amount of time is spent on sizing because oversizing leads to underexpansion of the transcatheter valve and results in increased transvalvular gradients. Undersizing can lead to embolization, PVL, and patient–prosthesis mismatch.

ViV or ViR Approach

For transapical approaches to a ViV or ViR procedure, a small antero-lateral thoracotomy in the fifth or sixth intercostal space is used to access the LV apex (see Table 14.3). After puncture, a wire is advanced through the MV and into the left atrium. Ultimately, the transcatheter delivery system is advanced via this approach. This access route is the most common because it allows direct access to the mitral apparatus, and achieving coaxiality is relatively easy and facilitates rapid deployment. In the transseptal approach, after femoral venous access is achieved, transseptal puncture (discussed earlier) is performed, usually in the same territory of the fossa as the MitraClip procedure. This approach, by avoiding a thoracic incision, reduces the overall morbidity of the procedure. However, the transseptal approach poses its own unique challenge in maintaining coaxiality while deploying the transcatheter valve. While many cases can be performed with a stiff wire coiled at the LV apex, some cases require the wire to be externalized via a small apical sheath or snared into the distal aorta to provide better coaxial control in the process of transcatheter deployment (Fig. 14.14).

ViR procedures can be performed in a manner similar to ViV procedures with respect of access route and methods of sizing. Appropriate deployment is perhaps more of concern with ViR procedures because device embolization and postprocedure PVL are more likely to occur due to the smaller area of contact between the transcatheter valve and the ring. Excessive oversizing may result in annular reshaping, which could either completely or partially dehisce the annular ring. Undersizing may result in substantial transcatheter PVL or, worse, device embolization.

Another important consideration to be aware of in ViV and ViR procedures is the potential for LV outflow tract (LVOT) obstruction. The overall anterior leaflet length can obstruct the LVOT after transcatheter deployment, resulting in hemodynamically significant and catastrophic functional aortic stenosis. Appropriate sizing and estimation by CT can sometimes help operators predict potential cases where obstruction can occur. In these cases, appropriate positioning, landing, and coaxiality become even more important because a ventricular deployment may certainly result in obstruction. In cases where LVOT obstruction has occurred, transcatheter aortic valve replacements with a self-expanding valve (e.g., Medtronic Corevalve) or alcohol septal ablation have been reported.

Next Generation of Mitral Valve Repair and Replacement Technologies

Unlike the development of transcatheter therapies for aortic valve disease, the development of new transcatheter therapies for MV disease has been much slower. Despite our clinical and pathophysiologic understanding of the mitral apparatus, its components, and pathology, transcatheter MV interventions remain challenging due to the complex anatomy, pathophysiology, and interplay of the MV apparatus and its surrounding structures.

Multiple approaches and technologies are currently under varying stages of development (Table 14.2) for repair of the MV. Most of them are modifications of long-standing surgical techniques in efforts to lower procedural morbidity and mortality with the less invasive approach. While no general classification schema exists, we categorize the pipeline technologies based on the target of repair: leaflet repair, leaflet implant, annuloplasty (direct or indirect), chordal replacement (or implant), LV reshaping, and finally transcatheter MV implantation. For all the unestablished technologies, the clinical data are scarce and limited to either benchtop modeling, preclinical (animal) evaluation, or small case series of first-in-man procedures. Hence the reproducibility and effectiveness of these devices remain to be demonstrated.

The evolution of technology for transcatheter MV implantation has been appealing and interesting. The repair technologies discussed earlier target one specific component of the apparatus, whereas a complete valve implant have led some to argue a "one-device-fits-all" approach to MV disease that would perhaps yield more predictable, durable, and reproducible results. However there remain many challenges before transcatheter MV implantation reaches the clinical echelon of transcatheter aortic valve implantation or MitraClip. First, the mitral annulus is much larger than the aortic valve, asymmetric, highly dynamic, and frequently not calcified. Hence large devices with elaborate anchoring components are required since radial force alone is unlikely to be effective. To date, a total percutaneous approach is not practical because the delivery systems are of large caliber (>32–42F) and inflexible. Also of important consideration are structures in close proximity and at risk for injury or structural deformation after valve implantation: LVOT, left circumflex artery, coronary sinus, and conduction system. And, most importantly, the mitral apparatus and its components have an important interplay with the LV. Disrupting this interplay with a large implant may have deleterious long-term effects of the ventricle that are yet to be uncovered. Multiple devices for transcatheter mitral replacement are in varying stages of preclinical and clinical development (Table 14.2). All prostheses feature self-expanding nitinol frames, triple bovine or porcine leaflets, large delivery systems (32–42F), and mostly transapical access. Each of the valves offers innovative strategies for anchoring and specific designs to fit the complex mitral apparatus. Preliminary data are limited on acceptable implantation success rates and device performance.

Conclusion

Transcatheter MV repair with MitraClip has gained the most traction and clinical data to date. Also at the disposal to operators are potentially beneficial therapies such as ViV and ViR, with transcatheter therapies originally designed for the aortic position. Other therapies in the pipeline, aimed at MV repair or replacement, still have many years to go before they are considered for routine use. Given the different pathophysiologic mechanisms of MR, these devices may be complementary rather than competitive. Careful patient selection and evaluation will be important to delineate the best strategy for an individual patient.

Suggested Readings

Al-Lawati A, Cheung A. Transcatheter mitral valve replacement. *Intervent Cardiol Clin.* 2016;5:109-115.

Athappan G, Raza MQ, Kapadia SR. Mitraclip therapy for mitral regurgitation: primary mitral regurgitation. *Intervent Cardiol Clin.* 2016;5:71-82.

Baim DS. Cardiac ventriculography. In: Baim DS, ed. Grossman's Cardiac Catheterization, Angiography, and Intervention. Philadelphia, PA: Lippincott Williams & Wilkins; 2006:222-233.

Baldus S, Schillinger W, Franzen O, et al. MitraClip therapy in daily clinical practice: initial results from the German transcatheter mitral valve interventions (TRAMI) registry. *Eur J Heart Fail.* 2012;14:1050-1055.

Condado JF, Kaebnick B, Babaliaros V. Transcatheter mitral valve-in-valve therapy. *Intervent Cardiol Clin.* 2016;5:117-123.

Feldman T, Foster E, Glower DD, et al. Percutaneous repair or surgery for mitral regurgitation. *N Engl J Med.* 2011;364:1395-1406.

Feldman T, Franzen O, Low R, et al. Atlas of Percutaneous Edge-to-Edge Mitral Valve Repair. London: Springer; 2013.

Feldman T, Young A. Percutaneous approaches to valve repair for mitral regurgitation. *J Am Coll Cardiol.* 2014;63:2057-2068.

Grossman W. Pressure measurement. In: Baim DS, ed. Grossman's Cardiac Catheterization, Angiography, and Intervention. Philadelphia, PA: Lippincott Williams & Wilkins; 2006:133-147.

Helton TJ, Kapadia SR. Anatomy of Cardiac Valves for the Interventionalist. Structural Heart Disease Interventions. Philadelphia, PA: Lippincott Williams & Wilkins; 2012:27-45.

Lim DS, Reynolds MR, Feldman T, et al. Improved functional status and quality of life in prohibitive surgical risk patients with degenerative mitral regurgitation following transcatheter mitral valve repair. *J Am Coll Cardiol.* 2014;64:182-192.

Maisano F, Alfieri O, Banai S, et al. The future of transcatheter mitral valve interventions: competitive or complementary role of repair vs. replacement? *Eur Heart J.* 2015;36:1651-1659.

Maisano F, La Canna G, Colombo A, et al. The evolution from surgery to percutaneous mitral valve interventions: the role of the edge-to-edge technique. *J Am Coll Cardiol.* 2011;58:2174-2182.

Perpetua E, Levin DB, Reisman M. Anatomy and function of the normal and diseased mitral apparatus: implications for transcatheter therapy. *Intervent Cardiol Clin.* 2016;5:1-16.

Seiffert M, Conradi L, Baldus S, et al. Transcatheter mitral valve-in-valve implantation in patients with degenerated bioprostheses. *J Am Coll Cardiol Interv.* 2012;5:341-349.

Singh GD, Smith TW, Rogers JH. Targeted transseptal access for MitraClip percutaneous mitral valve repair. *Intervent Cardiol Clin.* 2016;5:55-69.

Whitlow PL, Feldman T, Pedersen WR, et al. Acute and 12-month results with catheter-based mitral valve leaflet repair: the EVEREST II (Endovascular Valve Edge-to-Edge Repair) High Risk Study. *J Am Coll Cardiol.* 2012;59:130-139.

Transcatheter Aortic Valve Replacement and Balloon Aortic Valvuloplasty

ANOOP AGRAWAL · JAMES HERMILLER

Introduction

In North America, aortic stenosis (AS) is most commonly a consequence of calcific degeneration of a native trileaflet valve, and moderate to severe AS is more prevalent with advancing age. Bicuspid or unicuspid AS may be present in up to two-thirds of patients with symptomatic AS younger than 70 years of age. Clinical history and physical examination may lead to the diagnosis of AS, but echocardiographic confirmation is obligatory, with high-quality transthoracic echocardiogram (TTE) and Doppler assessment providing most of the necessary information (Table 15.1). Need for invasive hemodynamic assessment is uncommon, except when there is echocardiographic uncertainty.

Severe AS is defined as peak aortic velocity (V_{max}) of 4 m/sec or more, aortic valve area (AVA) of 1.0 cm^2 or less, indexed AVA of less than 0.6 cm^2/m^2, or dimensionless index (ratio of the left ventricular outflow tract [LVOT] to aortic valve velocity time integral) of less than 0.25. Symptomatic severe AS is one of the cardiovascular conditions associated with a marked reduction in life expectancy. Although surgical aortic valve replacement (SAVR) remains the treatment of choice in symptomatic AS and in certain subsets of asymptomatic severe AS, only 50% of such patients are referred for SAVR, and 20% of those do not undergo surgery. Reasons cited for not undergoing SAVR include perceived high perioperative risk, advanced age, lack of symptoms, and patient/family refusal. Prior to the advent of transcatheter aortic valve replacement (TAVR), balloon aortic valvuloplasty (BAV) was traditionally used as a palliative option in patients with symptomatic AS who were considered poor candidates for SAVR. TAVR is now preferred in such patients.

Hemodynamic Assessment of Aortic Stenosis in Catheterization Lab

In current practice, invasive assessment of the pressure gradient across aortic valve (transaortic gradient) is reserved for symptomatic patients with either inconclusive noninvasive evaluation or discrepant clinical findings and for baseline assessment prior to BAV or TAVR.

Procedural Details

Right heart catheterization (RHC) is performed in a standard fashion to determine cardiac output, along with coronary angiography.

Table 15.1

Echocardiographic Assessment for Aortic Stenosis	
Aortic valve morphology	Number of cusps, degree and distribution of calcification, vegetation, or fibrosis; features of prosthetic aortic valve if present
Doppler data	Aortic and LVOT velocity, degree of aortic insufficiency
Measurements	Aortic annulus, LVOT, sinus of Valsalva, ascending aorta
Left ventricle	EF, septal morphology, presence of LV thrombus
Miscellaneous	Any other concomitant valvular pathology or nonvalvular aortic stenosis

EF, ejection fraction; *LVOT,* left ventricular outflow tract.

Supravalvular aortogram to assess degree of aortic insufficiency is not a routine practice but can be done if desired by placing a pigtail catheter a few millimeters above the aortic valve (left anterior oblique [LAO] 20- to 30-degree projection, power injection at 20 cc/sec for 2 seconds). Various preshaped diagnostic catheters can be used to direct a straight wire across the aortic valve. Amplatz left (AL) often provides a coaxial trajectory via femoral access although Amplatz right (AR) or Judkins right (JR) catheters can also be used, particularly for smaller aorta. We have found higher success with AL1 when coming from the left subclavian or left radial and with JR4 for right radial transaortic valve access. For a large root, an AL3 is often required. LAO 10–25 degrees angulation provides optimal visualization of the catheter and aortic jet. With the tip of a stiff-core straight wire (typically 0.038-inch or a straight glidewire) protruding about 1–2 cm, the crossing catheter is directed toward the area of maximum turbulence, which is marked by bouncing of the wire tip. The aortic valve is gently probed by advancing the wire, making short passes until it enters the LVOT. Small clockwise or counterclockwise rotation of the crossing catheter helps to steer the wire as it maps the valve surface. After every 2–3 minutes of an unsuccessful attempt, the wire should be withdrawn and wiped, and the catheter should be flushed to minimize any thrombus formation. Care must be taken not to inadvertently engage the coronaries.

With the wire held securely by left hand once it is through the aortic valve, the crossing catheter is gently advanced a few millimeters into the LVOT. Avoid positioning the crossing catheter deep in the LV cavity because this makes wire exchange difficult while also increasing the risk of ventricular injury. Next, the gantry angle is switched to right anterior oblique (RAO) 30 degrees to visualize the LV long axis. The straight wire is now exchanged for a 260-cm, 0.038-inch J-wire, the tip of which has been gently curved in a broad-based U or "ram's horn" configuration. The size of the loop is approximated to LV cavity size. This curve wraps the LV apex, taking its contour as this wire is gently pushed out of the crossing catheter. The crossing catheter can now be exchanged for a dual-lumen pigtail catheter. Both ports of the dual-lumen pigtail catheter are connected to manifolds, flushed, and zeroed. The proximal port of the dual-lumen catheter needs to be flushed frequently and vigorously because a damped aortic pressure is frequently encountered. Simultaneous LV and central aortic pressure can now be recorded. LV to aortic root (Ao) pullback must be performed after initial hemodynamic assessment to document equal pressures in both the pressure lines. An optimal assessment of the transaortic gradient includes simultaneous recording of LV and central aortic pressure using a dual-lumen pigtail catheter (Langston, Vascular Solutions) or individual catheters placed in the aorta and LV. A transducing femoral arterial waveform in lieu of central aortic pressure, although often employed, can result in either underestimation (peripheral augmentation of pressure waveform and time delay) or overestimation (peripheral arterial disease) of the true aortic gradient. Once the LV and aortic pressures are transduced, the tracings should be inspected for pulse wave contours. While delayed (tardus) and reduced (parvus) aortic upstroke is seen in fixed valvular obstruction, as in AS, dynamic obstruction is associated with a spike-and-dome pattern and can be evaluated further by a slow pullback of the LV catheter from the LV apex all the way to the aortic annulus. An end-hole catheter, such as a multipurpose or Rodriguez catheter with multiple side holes at the distal end, is preferred for intracavitary gradient assessment. Post-PVC (premature ventricular contractions) augmentation of the transaortic gradient can help differentiate a fixed versus dynamic aortic gradient (Fig. 15.1). Once cardiac output and transaortic gradient are acquired, the AVA can be calculated using Gorlin or Hakki equations (Fig. 15.2).

Special Situations and Caveats

1. Crossing the aortic valve is contraindicated in the presence of a mechanical aortic valve or aortic vegetation. If invasive hemodynamic assessment of the aortic valve is required, LV pressure can be obtained via transseptal puncture. Transapical access may be considered in the presence of mechanical aortic and mitral prostheses, although it is rarely required given the availability of TTE or transesophageal echocardiogram (TEE). The presence of thrombus in the LV is an absolute contraindication for hemodynamic assessment of the aortic valve.

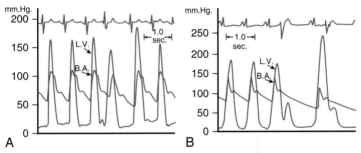

Figure 15.1 Simultaneous left ventricular (LV)-aortic tracing showing change in hemodynamics post-PVC. (A) Rise in LV systolic pressure with little or no change on aortic systolic pressure suggestive of fixed aortic stenosis. (B) Rise in LV systolic pressure with decrease in aortic systolic pressure due to dynamic outflow obstruction. *(From EC Brockenbrough, AG Morrow. A hemodynamic technic for the detection of hypertrophic subaortic stenosis.* Circulation, *1961;***23**:*189–194.)*

Gorlin equation

$$AVA = \frac{CO\ (mL/Min)}{HR * SEP * 44.3 * \sqrt{mean\ aortic\ gradient}}$$

Hakki equation

$$AVA = \frac{CO\ (L/Min)}{\sqrt{peak\ to\ peak\ aortic\ -\ LV\ gradient}}$$

AVA: Aortic valve area in cm^2, CO: Cardiac output, HR: Heart rate in beats per minute, SEP: Systolic ejection period in seconds

Figure 15.2 Equations for calculating aortic valve area.

2. Dobutamine challenge can be performed in the setting of low gradient (mean transaortic gradient <40 mm Hg) with low flow (LV stroke volume index [LVSVI] <35 mL/m^2 and LV ejection fraction [EF] <50%). Dobutamine has a limited diagnostic role in patients with low flow but normal LV EF since further inotropic stimulation will have little impact on stroke volume. In these patients, an increase in aortic valve gradient and a fixed AVA with an intravenous afterload-reducing agent like nitroprusside may facilitate diagnosing true AS. A dimensionless index of less than 0.25 and/or aortic valve calcification may add diagnostic value in some cases.

3. Cardiac output calculated by Fick's or the thermodilution principle systematically underestimates forward flow across the aortic valve if concomitant aortic insufficiency (AI) is present. These phenomenon may lead to an overestimation of AS severity. There are no standardized algorithms to correct for the presence of AI.

Balloon Aortic Valvuloplasty

Introduced for calcific AS in 1986 by Dr. Cribier, BAV causes splitting of fused commissures, cracking of calcific nodules, cuspal tears, and aortic wall expansion at nonfused commissure sites, all leading to improved leaflet mobility. Stand-alone BAV lost favor due to early restenosis, leading to symptom recurrence and lack of mortality benefit. Although the role of BAV had become limited, it saw a resurgence with the advent of TAVR. American College of Cardiology/American Heart Association (ACC/AHA) guidelines recommend BAV as a bridge to SAVR or TAVR in patients with severe symptomatic AS (class IIb indication). Indications of BAV in contemporary practice can be expanded further and are listed in Box 15.1.

Preprocedure Setup

Preprocedure echocardiogram is done to evaluate the severity of AS, degree of AI, annular size, and calcification (Table 15.1). A computed tomography angiography (CTA) of the thoracic/abdominal aorta is not mandatory for BAV but can provide additional anatomic data on the aortic annulus and peripheral vasculature. Patients are pretreated with aspirin unless they are on long-term aspirin therapy. An intra-aortic balloon pump (IABP; Datascope Corp., Fairfield, NJ) or Impella (Abiomed

---

Box 15.1 Indications for Balloon Aortic Valvuloplasty (BAV)

1. Optimization/bridge to future definitive therapy:
   a. Acutely symptomatic or hemodynamically unstable
   b. Bridge to TAVR/SAVR in patients with reversible comorbidities like frailty, renal dysfunction, severe left ventricular (LV) dysfunction, active malignancy etc.
   c. Need for percutaneous coronary revascularization
2. Palliation for symptomatic severe aortic stenosis (AS) patients with poor life expectancy due to noncardiac comorbid conditions who are considered poor candidates for SAVR/TAVR
3. Combined with TAVR, as in balloon-expandable valves
4. Symptomatic patient with upcoming noncardiac surgery that cannot be postponed for SAVR/TAVR
5. Diagnostic BAV: Assess contribution of AS in patients with significant symptoms and concomitant pulmonary pathology
6. Symptomatic severe aortic stenosis in pregnant patient who failed medical therapy
7. Young adults with congenital aortic stenosis

SAVR, surgical aortic valve replacement; *TAVR,* transcatheter aortic valve replacement.

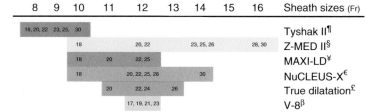

Figure 15.3 Common aortic valvuloplasty balloons and sheath compatibility. Listed numbers within colored boxes represent balloon diameter in mm. Brand names of balloons listed under the heading "Sheath sizes."

Inc., Danvers, MA) should be readily available in case of hemodynamic collapse. TTE equipment should be on standby or available immediately. Defibrillator pads should be attached to the patient's chest in a manner that does not interfere with the fluoroscopic field of view.

Aortic Valvuloplasty Balloon

Commonly used BAV balloons and their properties are depicted in Fig. 15.3. The balloon is sized to annular and LVOT dimensions. Typically minimum or mean axis diameter of the aortic annulus is used as a reference, and a balloon-to-reference ratio of 0.9 : 1.0 is considered ideal. Some operators prefer not to use a balloon diameter greater than LVOT diameter. Undersizing is preferred in patients with eccentric calcification, elderly females, a narrow sinotubular junction, or while using a compliant balloon. Balloon diameters of 20 and 22 mm are most commonly used for adults, with the majority of patients falling in the 18- to 26-mm range. Typically a length of 4–6 cm is chosen regardless of the diameter.

Procedural Details

BAV procedures are currently performed in a retrograde fashion under conscious sedation. Antegrade BAV via transseptal puncture is rarely done. Vascular access defaults to the femoral artery and vein due to a need for large sheath sizes. Both groins should be prepared. Venous access is obtained for right heart cath and temporary pacemaker wire insertion. The common femoral artery is accessed using an anterior wall puncture technique. Ultrasound-guided access has been shown to improve cannulation rates in high bifurcation cases and improve first-pass success along with a reduction in number of attempts, risk of venipuncture, median time to access, and vascular complications. Fig. 15.3 demonstrates sheath size compatibility with common BAV balloons. The arterial access site can be pre-closed with one or two Perclose ProGlide (Abbott Vascular Inc., Redwood City, CA) vascular closure devices. The brachial or axillary artery can be used as an alternative access site in cases of poor peripheral vasculature.

Once arterial and venous accesses are obtained, heparin is administered at 70–90 U/kg for a target activated clotting time (ACT) of 250 seconds or longer. RHC is performed, and cardiac output is calculated. A balloon-tipped bipolar temporary pacemaker catheter is placed at the right ventricular (RV) apex. The pacing threshold is tested, ensuring 1 : 1 capture. Pacemaker rate is set anywhere from 160 to 220 beats per minute, with output typically at 10–20 mAmp. A test pacing is performed at the set rate/output to verify a fall of systolic blood pressure (SBP) below 50 mm Hg. Next, coronary angiography and a supravalvular aortogram are performed if indicated. Moderate AI is not a contraindication, but BAV should be avoided in patients with severe AI. The aortic valve is crossed, and an angled pigtail catheter is placed near the LV apex, as described earlier. A precurved moderate-stiff wire (Table 15.2) is now placed in the LV cavity by gently

Table 15.2

Common 0.035-Inch Stiff Wires and Their Properties			
Name	**Stiffness**	**Tip**	**Special Considerations**
Amplatz Extra Stiff[a]	**	Shapeable	Standard wire for delivery of Edward Sapien valve
Amplatz Super Stiff[b]	***	Shapeable	Delivery of large sheath or transcatheter heart valves
Amplatz Ultra Stiff[a]	***	Shapeable	Stiffer than Amplatz Super Stiff
Confida Becker[c]	***	Pre-curved	Standard wire for delivery of CoreValve, Evolut R, or Portico
Safari2[d]	***	Pre-curved	Standard wire for delivery of lotus valve, multiple curve sizes
Meier[e]	****	Shapeable	Stiff wire for additional support
Lunderquist Extra Stiff[f]	****	Pre-curved	Stiff wire used for delivery of CoreValve/Evolut R in horizontal aorta

[a]Cook Medical Inc., Bloomington, IN.
[b]Boston Scientific Inc., Natick, MA.
[c]Medtronic CoreValve LLC, Santa Ana, CA.
[d]Lake Region Medical, Chaska, MN.
[e]Boston Scientific Inc., Costa Rica.
[f]William Cook Europe ApS, Denmark.

pushing it forward through the pigtail catheter while the catheter itself is pulled back to "unsheath" the wire. We have noticed that although introducing a stiff wire through a pigtail catheter rather than through an end-hole crossing catheter adds an extra step, it decreases the incidence of LV perforation. If needed, the introducer sheath can now be exchanged for a large-bore sheath because the stiff wire provides additional support in navigating through tortuous vasculature. The side-port of the femoral sheath is attached to a pressure manifold for continuous monitoring.

A typical BAV balloon comes in an over-the-wire configuration. The center port is flushed with heparinized saline. The balloon injection port is connected to a 60-cc Luer-Lock syringe partly filled with contrast diluted with saline in a 1:8 proportion. Alternatively a high-pressure three-way stopcock is attached to the balloon injection port; a partly filled 60-cc syringe is attached to one port and a completely filled 10-cc syringe to another. The balloon is prepped by applying negative suction using the 60-cc syringe. The prepped balloon is centered across the aortic valve, rapid pacing is begun at the set rate, and the balloon is inflated rapidly using the 60-cc syringe once systolic pressure falls below 50 mm Hg. Additionally, the three-way stopcock can be turned on toward the 10-cc syringe, which is then used to augment inflation pressure over and above what is achieved by the 60-cc syringe. This step is occasionally required to achieve maximal inflation pressure. The syringe arrangement can be replaced by an indeflator to generate the desired inflation pressure. Typically an assistant inflates the balloon while the operator stabilizes the balloon's position, straddling the aortic valve in the middle. The inflated balloon is kept up for 1–2 seconds and is rapidly deflated thereafter. Rapid pacing is continued until the balloon is completely deflated. Once deflated, the balloon is immediately pulled back into the ascending aorta while maintaining wire position. Additional inflations can be carried out if desired, or the balloon can be exchanged for a dual-lumen pigtail catheter to measure transaortic gradient and LV end-diastolic pressure (LVEDP). After every inflation the SBP should be allowed to recover back to its previous value before repeat inflation is attempted. If the patient's SBP remains below

100 mm Hg, intravenous Neo-Synephrine in doses of 100–200 mcg can be given.

Procedural Success

A residual waist on the inflated balloon indicates incomplete expansion and can be relieved with higher pressure inflation. Successful BAV is often accompanied by resolution of a parvus tardus aortic waveform, improvement in SBP, and resolution of tachycardia. A drop in the mean aortic gradient by greater than 50% and/or an increase in AVA by more than 50% (or an absolute AVA ≥1.0 cm^2) while maintaining cardiac output (CO) signifies successful BAV and can be achieved in most cases. If the results are suboptimal, repeat inflation should be performed using a larger diameter balloon. Following successful BAV, all the wires and catheters are removed and anticoagulation is reversed with intravenous protamine (1 mg per 100 units of heparin). The arterial access site is closed either by cinching the previously placed ProGlide sutures, any other vascular closure device, or manual compression.

Special Considerations

- Due to increased risk of aortic rupture, patients with severe eccentric calcification should have balloon sized to the minor annular dimension and no larger than LVOT diameter.
- Coronary artery disease (CAD) often co-exists with severe AS, particularly in the elderly, and is associated with worse clinical outcome post-TAVR. Transient hypotension during rapid pacing may trigger coronary ischemia and lead to unstable hemodynamic cascade, thus prompting use of hemodynamic support devices, and the use of which is an independent predictor of early and late mortality post-TAVR. Revascularization strategy for patients with significant CAD in the presence of severe AS who are poor surgical candidates is less well defined since most of these patients were excluded from contemporary clinical trials. The short-term safety and efficacy of percutaneous coronary intervention (PCI) in patients with untreated severe AS had been demonstrated in a propensity matched cohort, although patients with an LVEF of 30% or less or a Society of Thoracic Surgery (STS) score of greater than 10 had significantly high mortality. For combined BAV and PCI, a reasonable approach is to intervene on uncomplicated left main stenosis prior to BAV. All other major epicardial stenoses subtending to large myocardial territory can be treated after BAV. High-risk patients with unstable hemodynamics or complex coronary anatomy may benefit from intraprocedural IABP or Impella support during BAV and PCI. Impella can be safely introduced through a severely stenotic valve, helps optimize LV filling pressures pre- and post-BAV, and has been shown to maintain structural integrity up to 3 atm pressure.
- Rapid pacing in the setting of severe LV systolic dysfunction can further compromise cardiovascular status. Care should be taken to minimize pacing duration, inflation time, and total number of balloon inflations.
- Stand-alone BAV in stenotic bioprosthetic valves has no role. These patients should undergo valve-in-valve (ViV) TAVR or SAVR depending on the surgical risk.

Complications

Complications of BAV are listed in Box 15.2. Transient hypotension and bradycardia could be due to vagal response, but persistent hypotension should be promptly evaluated. Acute severe AI is poorly tolerated,

---

Box 15.2 Complications of Balloon Aortic Valvuloplasty (BAV)

1. Persistent hypotension/hemodynamic collapse
   a. Acute severe aortic insufficiency (AI)
   b. Pump failure due to worsened left ventricular (LV) systolic function
   c. Cardiac tamponade due to ventricular rupture
   d. Injury to pulmonary artery (if right heart catheterization was done)
   e. Aortic annular rupture
   f. Vascular injury leading to retroperitoneal bleeding
   g. Respiratory compromise
   h. Rhythm disturbances like high-grade AV block or tachyarrhythmia
   i. Coronary occlusion/dissection leading to ischemia
   j. Air embolism
2. Protamine reaction
3. Seizures
4. Kidney injury
5. Vagal reaction
6. Stroke and other embolic phenomenon
7. Balloon rupture

---

occurs in about 1% of all cases, and is marked by a drop in aortic diastolic pressure and/or increased LVEDP. TTE or aortogram can confirm the diagnosis. Pacing at 100 or more beats per minute may help by decreasing the diastolic filling period. The degree of AI may improve in a few hours due to valve recoil, but persistent hemodynamic compromise requires urgent surgical intervention or TAVR. Rhythm disorders occur in up to 10% of cases and may require drug therapy, cardioversion, or pacing. High-grade AV block requiring a permanent pacemaker is uncommon, occurring in 1% or less. Pericardial effusion causing tamponade occurs in 1% or less, is readily visualized on TTE, and should be drained emergently. Severe vascular complications requiring intervention occur in about 5%–7%. Peripheral angiogram performed antegrade or retrograde can help with both diagnosis and management. Pump failure post-BAV is uncommon, occurring in patients with severe LV dysfunction at baseline. Drug therapy with inotropes or hemodynamic support with IABP or Impella may be required for early stabilization. Aortic annular rupture or injury to the pulmonary artery is rare but catastrophic and requires emergent surgical intervention. Rapid reversal of therapeutic anticoagulation is required in most of the complications mentioned here. Balloon rupture may occur in up to 15% of cases and largely is of no clinical significance unless it is associated with air embolism, which may lead to coronary obstruction and hemodynamic collapse. A ruptured balloon has a much higher crossing profile and may necessitate removing both the balloon and the sheath as a unit while maintaining arterial access with the wire. Rapid pacing, lower profile balloons, and use of vascular closure devices have reduced BAV-related complications with a procedural mortality 0.5%–2.4%, stroke 0.4%–2.0%, and overall serious adverse effects in 15.6% of all cases.

Expected Short- and Long-Term Outcomes

National Heart, Lung, and Blood Institute (NHLBI) registry data demonstrated a drop in mean aortic gradient from 55 mm Hg to 29 mm Hg with an increase in mean AVA from 0.5 cm^2 to 0.8 cm^2. This translated into improved cardiovascular status in more than two-thirds of the patients. New York Heart Association (NYHA) 1–2 functional class improvement is noted in both historical and contemporary data. Increased gradients within 24–48 hours post-BAV are thought to be due to early valve recoil or improved stroke volume. Valve restenosis is related to scar formation and can be seen within weeks post-BAV. Overall, at 6 months, the gradients are between baseline and post-BAV values. In spite of early restenosis, which can occur in up to 50%–70% of patients, symptomatic relief is quite significant and can extend up to 1.5–3 years. The survival curve in this group of high-risk patients is reflective of the underlying disease process, and BAV does not change the natural course of the disease. Repeat BAV is both safe and technically feasible, extends period of hemodynamic relief, and may offer mortality benefit at 3-year follow up. Compared to nonresponders, patients who respond well following "diagnostic" BAV have improved survival, particularly if followed by definitive therapy like TAVR or SAVR. BAV as a bridge to TAVR in selected high-risk patients with NYHA III symptoms, LVEF of less than 30%, pulmonary hypertension, significant mitral regurgitation, and/or significant CAD with indication for PCI may be associated with lower incidence of stroke, death, cardiac tamponade, or conversion to open surgery compared to direct TAVR.

Transcatheter Aortic Valve Replacement

Introduction

The first human implantation of a transcatheter heart valve (THV) was done by Dr. Bonhoeffer in a stenotic RV-to-PA conduit in 2000 and was soon followed by TAVR by Dr. Cribier in 2002. Although TAVR was first performed in an antegrade manner via transseptal puncture, retrograde implantation via the transfemoral (TF) route became favored due to the relative ease of operation and high procedural success and safety profile. Longer sheaths, general anesthesia, larger THV size, improved delivery systems, high-quality cardiovascular imaging, and refined implantation technique led to a greater than 95% procedural success with reduced complications. Decrease in sheath size from 24F to 14F was associated with reduced vascular complications and allowed the majority of the cases to be performed via the TF route. In cases of inadequate iliofemoral access, alternate approaches, including transapical, subclavian, direct aortic, carotid, and caval-aortic, have been successfully utilized. A self-expanding THV, CoreValve (Medtronic CoreValve LLC, Santa Ana, CA), was introduced later, and the next few years saw a rapid growth in TAVR technology with many new designs conceptualized and tested worldwide (Fig. 15.4).

Several important randomized trials led to TAVR procedural acceptance in the United States. The first trial was the Placement of AoRtic TraNscathetER Valve (PARTNER) trial, a randomized multicenter trial that established superiority of TAVR over medical therapy in patients with extreme surgical risk and noninferiority to SAVR in high surgical risk patients, a benefit that persisted at 5 years.

Indications

Symptomatic patients who meet criteria for AVR due to AS should undergo TAVR if they are either at prohibitive surgical risk with expected survival greater than 1 year (class I) or high surgical risk (class IIa). TAVR should not be performed in patients in whom existing comorbidities would preclude the expected benefit from correction of AS.

Patient Selection and Preparation

Patient selection and preparation for TAVR can be summarized in five crucial steps:

- *Establishing diagnosis of severe AS*: Severe AS, if suspected clinically, can be confirmed via TTE, TEE, or invasive hemodynamic assessment as described earlier in the chapter.

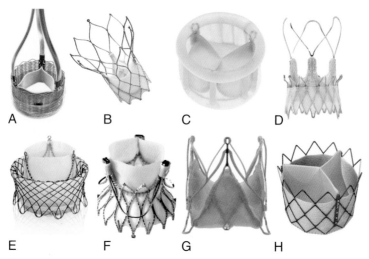

Figure 15.4 Trancatheter aortic valves currently undergoing evaluation or available in other parts of the world. (A) Lotus (Boston Scientific Inc., Natick, MA). (B) Portico (St. Jude Medical Inc., St. Paul, MN). (C) Direct Flow (Direct Flow Medical Inc., Santa Rosa, CA). (D) Acurate valve (Symetis Inc., Ecublens, Switzerland). (E) HLT (Bracco Inc., Princeton, NJ). (F) Engager (Medtronic Inc., Minneapolis, MN). (G) JenaClip (JenaValve Inc., Munich, Germany). (H) Inovare (Braile Biomédica Inc., São José do Rio Preto, Brazil).

- *Presence of symptoms*: Slow indolent disease progression of severe AS is often attributed to "normal aging" by many patients, and clinicians should be vigilant to enquire about new patterns of exercise intolerance. It is reasonable to recommend supervised symptom-limited exercise treadmill testing in patients who have findings suggestive of severe AS but otherwise fail to report any discrete symptoms. While symptoms of severe AS are often underreported, comorbidities like COPD, CAD, and pulmonary hypertension can mimic AS in clinical presentation and must be evaluated. A diagnostic BAV can be performed in selected patients if uncertainty exists about whether AS is causing symptoms.

- *Assessment of surgical risk profile*: Comprehensive surgical risk assessment is an integral part of patient evaluation and can be grouped into four sections. Clinical risk assessment can be done with Society of Thoracic Surgery Predicted Risk of Mortality (STS-PROM) or EuroSCORE. STS-PROM was used in most of the clinical trials and may be a better predictor of surgical mortality in high surgical risk patients undergoing SAVR. Katz Activities of Daily Living and ambulation assessment can be used to assess frailty, which is independently associated with poor long-term outcome. SAVR-specific impediments, such as a porcelain ascending aorta, chest wall deformities, hostile mediastinum, potential for injury due to previous bypass grafts on sternal re-entry, and the like, are not accounted for in traditional risk assessment tools and should be taken into account. Novel risk assessment tools that incorporate many such variables have been suggested. Evaluation by a cardiovascular surgeon with expertise in SAVR is mandatory to establish the surgical risk profile of a patient.

- *Valve type/sizing*: A CTA of the aortic annulus is mandatory for anatomic modeling of aortic annulus, valve, and surrounding structures (Box 15.3) unless poor renal function precludes contrast use, in which case three-dimensional TEE can be done. Measurements derived by two-dimensional TTE/TEE are often

> **Box 15.3** Key Findings and Measurements in Computed Tomography Angiography (CTA)
>
> 1. Aortic annular diameter (minor and major axes, and mean diameter), area, perimeter, mean diameter derived by area/perimeter
> 2. Distribution and extent of annular calcification
> 3. Left ventricular outflow tract (LVOT) diameter, presence of septal bulge
> 4. Height of coronary ostia from annular plane
> 5. Height and diameter of sinuses of Valsalva
> 6. Angle between ascending aorta and LVOT
> 7. Aortic arch anatomy: Presence of dissection, aneurysm, complex atherosclerotic plaque or ulcer
> 8. Vascular anatomy of abdominal aorta and iliofemoral system, including degree of tortuosity, calcification, stenosis, and lumen diameter

inaccurate due to the elliptical shape of the aortic annulus and should not be relied on.

- *Access site*: TF access is the most common site utilized for TAVR, the safety and efficacy of which are well established in large clinical trials. CTA has a key role in preprocedure planning by defining vascular anatomy (Box 15.3). Alternate access sites should be explored in appropriate cases, as mentioned earlier.

The Heart Team Approach

ACC/AHA guidelines recommend an integrated multidisciplinary collaborative management of patients being considered for TAVR. A heart team includes professionals in the fields of general and interventional cardiology, cardiac surgery, cardiac anesthesia, and cardiac imaging working in a collaborative fashion and sharing their expertise in the diagnosis and management of valvular heart disease, particularly TAVR. In addition, a TAVR program should have dedicated care coordinators and nurse practitioners addressing pre- and postprocedure care.

Procedural Details: Initial Setup and Patient Preparation

Preprocedure lab work should include complete blood counts, renal function, and coagulation parameters. The patient is loaded with aspirin 325 mg/day and clopidogrel 300 mg/day prior. Although general anesthesia is still preferred in a majority of the cases, monitored anesthesia care (MAC) is increasingly utilized because it improves lab throughput, enhances cost savings, and decreases length of stay. Also TEE has been used in the setting of MAC without significant issues. Antibiotic prophylaxis is administered per hospital policy. Sites for primary and secondary arterial access are prepped, commonly the bilateral groins, but radial access for the diagnostic pigtail can be employed as well. Alternate access will require site-specific preparations. Internal jugular or subclavian venous access for a temporary pacemaker lead may be considered if the patient is considered high risk for conduction abnormalities.

Vascular Access

The technique for optimal vascular access was described earlier. The right or left femoral artery (based on CTA) is accessed, dilated with a 6–7F dilator, preclosed with two Perclose ProGlide devices deployed at 60–90 degrees to each other (10 and 2 o'clock), and paired sutures are secured by hemostats. Secondary arterial access is obtained (radial or femoral) using a 5F or 6F sheath. Venous access for a temporary pacemaker is obtained contralateral to the THV delivery site or internal jugular vein.

Edwards Sapien 3 THV: Product Information and Technical Details

The Edwards Sapien 3 (S3) is the newest generation of balloon-expandable THV. It is made up of symmetric bovine pericardium leaflets treated with anticalcification substances and mounted on a cobalt-chromium stent scaffold that is manually crimped on a catheter delivery system. It has an outer polyethylene terephthalate (PET) skirt in addition to an inner skirt to minimize paravalvular leakage (PVL), among other design improvements from previous generation valves. An improved Commander Delivery system has a smaller profile and is more flexible. Ascendra+ is the only transapical delivery system commercially available in United States and is compatible with Sapien XT (an older generation Sapien THV). The more ergonomically designed transapical Certitude system for S3 is commercially not available yet.

Arterial and venous accesses are obtained as described earlier. A temporary pacemaker is floated up to the RV apex and pacing threshold and capture is verified. Heparin is given at 80–100 U/kg aiming for an ACT of greater than 300 seconds. A precured Amplatz super-stiff wire is placed in the descending aorta, and the Edwards eSheath (14 or 16F) is inserted over it under fluoroscopic guidance. An angled pigtail catheter is taken up to the right aortic cusp via a secondary arterial access site. A supravalvular aortogram is performed in coplanar or implantation view, making note of annular plane, aortic anatomy, calcification, and coronary filling. The coplanar view, defined by a gantry angle in which all three aortic valve cusps are viewed in the same plane symmetrically, can be approximated using images from previous CTA or coronary angiograms. The aortic valve is crossed using a straight wire as described earlier, which is exchanged for a pigtail catheter, and baseline hemodynamics are recorded. The pigtail catheter is now exchanged for a precured J-tipped Amplatz extra-stiff wire. If not done earlier, an introducer sheath can now be exchanged for the Edwards eSheath over this stiff wire.

The steps of valve preparation are detailed in the product instructions for use (IFU). It should be noted that the crimped valve has about 15 minutes to enter the body. The Edwards Commander Delivery System and its parts are displayed in Fig. 15.5. As the valve is being prepared at the back table, the operator can proceed with the setup for BAV. Typically an Edwards BAV balloon is chosen and is sized 3 mm smaller than the planned valve size. The THV should be fully prepped prior to attempting BAV so that it can be implanted without delay in case BAV causes severe AI.

Threading the delivery system may encounter significant resistance as the THV navigates through the expandable eSheath. Under fluoroscopic guidance, the entire assembly is advanced until the THV exits well beyond distal tip of the eSheath. The THV is aligned to the deployment balloon by disengaging the balloon lock and pulling the balloon catheter until the white warning marker appears, while securing the handle with the left hand. The balloon lock is re-engaged, and a fine adjustment wheel is used to position the balloon such that the THV is positioned midway between the valve alignment markers. The flex wheel is used to gently flex the delivery system as the entire assembly is advanced forward next. Once the S3 is positioned perpendicular to the aortic annulus with its mid-marker at the level of the aortic annulus, it is critical to retract the flex catheter to the center of the triple marker by disengaging the balloon lock and pulling the handle while stabilizing the balloon catheter. After re-engaging the balloon lock, additional fine adjustment to the S3 can be made using the flex wheel and fine adjustment wheel. The sequence of valve deployment

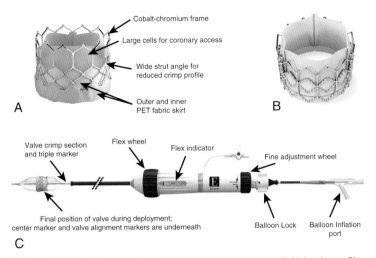

Figure 15.5 The Edwards Commander delivery system. (A) Valve in profile. (B) Earlier version without skirt. (C) Delivery system.

is as follows: breath hold, rapid pace (verify drop in systolic pressure to below 50 mm Hg), cine or fluoroscopy on, supravalvular aortogram via pigtail catheter to verify valve position one last time, pull pigtail catheter out of field as soon as contrast is injected, deploy valve by inflating the balloon, keep inflated balloon in place for 3 seconds and then deflate rapidly, pull balloon out into ascending aorta, and stop rapid pacing. The operator designates roles to each individual of the team so that the process runs smoothly. The deployed valve is functional immediately. TEE, TTE, and/or a supravalvular aortogram can be done now to ensure proper valve function and estimate degree of AI. The delivery system can be taken out by unflexing the catheter and ensuring that the balloon lock is engaged. The eSheath is taken out by cinching the Perclose ProGlide sutures. In difficult cases, a crossover 0.018-inch wire can be placed via contralateral femoral access site so that a peripheral balloon can quickly be deployed for balloon tamponade in case of a failed percutaneous closure or other vascular complication. Open vascular repair is an alternative to percutaneous access and can be used either as a primary method for vascular access/closure or as a bailout strategy.

CoreValve Evolut R (Evolut): Product Information and Technical Details

The Evolut represents the second generation of THV in the CoreValve family. It consists of three valve leaflets made up of porcine pericardium hand-sutured onto a self-expanding nitinol frame and processed with alpha-amino oleic acid. The ventricular aspect of the frame has a skirt made up of porcine pericardium. The device assembly consists of three components: the Evolut, the EnVeo R delivery catheter system (EnVeo), and the EnVeo R loading system (LS) as depicted in Fig. 15.6. Evolut uses a 14F InLine sheath embedded in the delivery system, thus decreasing effective arteriotomy size by 4F. Other major advances of the Evolut system over the CoreValve include better 1:1 response during deployment, self-centering, and ability to fully retrieve a deployed valve. Evolut sizing is better optimized for given annular dimensions, which, combined with optimized radial force, leads to decreased incidence of PVL. BAV is not required prior to placement of the Evolut, although the decision to perform BAV should be taken on a case-by-case basis. We often predilate heavily calcified and/or bicuspid valves. The steps of valve preparation are listed in the product IFU. Once loaded, the Evolut valve should be examined for strut integrity under fluoroscopy because it is difficult to visually evaluate the struts. If signs of misload are detected,

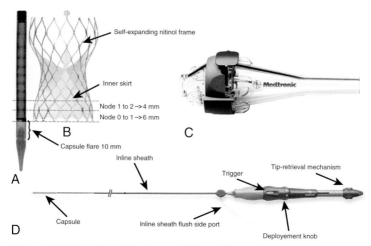

Figure 15.6 The Evolut R valve and EnVeo delivery system. (A) Fluoroscopic view of crimped Evolut R valve. (B) Evolut R valve. (C) EnVeo R Loading System. (D) EnVeo R Catheter.

such as frame deformation, frayed sutures, or valve damage, the Evolut should be unsheathed and examined for structural integrity.

The procedure begins by obtaining arterial and venous accesses as described earlier. An 8F sheath is placed at the primary arterial access site. A straight pigtail catheter is placed in the noncoronary cusp via secondary arterial access, and a supravalvular aortogram is performed in a coplanar view. A curved stiff wire (typically Confida) is placed in the LV apex after the aortic valve is crossed and baseline hemodynamics are obtained. The primary access sheath can now be exchanged for a 14F introducer sheath if BAV is planned or the EnVeo if the valve is being placed without predilatation. It should be noted that the EnVeo system is compatible with 0.035-inch wires and will likely encounter difficulty navigating over an 0.038-inch wire. Care should be taken while advancing the EnVeo through the aortic arch because the capsule may deflect to a greater degree than the shaft, resulting in vascular injury. Finally, the EnVeo is advanced until the distal end of the Evolut (node 0) is about 4 mm below the aortic annular plane. Any parallax of the distal ring, if present, should be removed by adjusting the gantry angle. Deployment begins by rotating the knob in the direction of the arrows, causing the capsule to retract. If ectopy is noted, the RV can be paced at 100–120 beats per minute during deployment to minimize any premature heartbeat that might lead to unpredictable catheter movement. Evolut is deployed in a slow, controlled fashion, with periodic supravalvular angiograms ensuring that the distal end of the stent frame (node 0) is positioned approximately 4 mm below the annular plane. The Evolut can be repositioned during deployment by advancing or withdrawing it until annular contact is not made. Once the Evolut touches the aortic annulus, it can only be withdrawn and should be recaptured if it has to be advanced. The deployment process is paused as the distal radiopaque capsule marker band approaches the distal end of the radiopaque paddle attachment. The Evolut is now fully functional, but still attached to the delivery mechanism in case the operator chooses to recapture it. In addition to visual assessment, the knob provides tactile feedback to indicate this point of no return. An aortogram or echocardiogram is done at this time to evaluate for valve position, degree of AI, and coronary perfusion. Further rotation of the knob releases the Evolut.

After the Evolut is successfully deployed, the EnVeo system is withdrawn until the catheter tip is in the descending aorta. Pulling the handle back as the trigger is pressed and held in position withdraws the catheter tip back toward the capsule. The catheter is withdrawn back until the capsule touches the distal tip of the InLine sheath, at which point the entire system is withdrawn and the vascular access site closed by cinching previously placed Perclose ProGlide sutures or as planned. If postdilatation is required, a 14F introducer sheath can be placed after removing the EnVeo system.

Special Situations

Valve-in-Valve

Use of TAVR in surgical bioprosthetic valve stenosis or in cases of patient–prosthesis mismatch in patients who are at high or prohibitive surgical risk has shown promising results. The transcatheter prosthesis is sized to the type and internal dimensions of the surgical bioprosthesis. Various applications are available to assist in selecting proper THV size. A preprocedure TEE is mandatory to evaluate for the presence of periprosthetic regurgitation, valve thrombosis, endocarditis, and the like, in which, if present, TAVR is unlikely to offer optimal result. ViV is associated with a higher incidence of coronary occlusion (see later discussion), and patients identified as high risk for coronary obstruction should undergo SAVR or a preemptive coronary protection strategy. Although both CoreValve and Sapien XT are approved for use in ViV cases, the supra-annular design of CoreValve has a potential benefit of achieving higher valve area compared to the Sapien XT, particularly in small valves.

Bicuspid/Unicuspid Aortic Valve

With anticipated expansion of TAVR to include lower surgical risk patients, more patients with bicuspid/unicuspid aortic valve (BiAV) pathology will be considered for TAVR. Unique concerns related to TAVR in BiAV include an elliptically shaped annulus and/or asymmetric calcification causing underexpansion and/or noncircular shape of THV, susceptibility of fused commissures to rupture leading to severe AI, or presence of aortopathy with potentially higher risk of dissection or rupture. Major clinical trials excluded these patients, although recent data demonstrate high procedural success. High rates of PVL seen in early case series improved significantly with multidetector CT (MDCT)-guided THV sizing. These patients should be evaluated for aortic pathology that, if present, may favor high-risk surgery over TAVR.

Minimalistic TAVR

Although historically TAVR was done under MAC, challenges with alternate vascular access, need for TEE, and patient comfort led to the majority of procedures being performed in hybrid room under general anesthesia. Technological advancements and technical experience led to TAVR making its way back to the cardiac catheterization lab, where the procedure is performed under MAC with TTE or TEE guidance and selective use of central venous access or invasive hemodynamic monitoring. Percutaneous access of the femoral artery is routinely managed with Perclose ProGlide, and surgical cutdown is reserved for difficult cases. A temporary pacemaker wire is pulled in the catheterization lab itself if no evidence of conduction abnormality is found, or, alternatively, the telemetry floor is equipped to manage transvenous pacemakers. Minimalistic TAVR is a cost-effective strategy for any TAVR program promoting early hospital discharge while providing excellent clinical care.

TAVR Complications

Mortality

Although improvements in technique and technology have led to a drop in procedural mortality to less than 1%, mortality at 1 year following successful TAVR remains high, particularly noncardiovascular deaths. Better patient selection, multidisciplinary management of comorbidities, and addressing TAVR complications are critical in improving outcomes. Patient clinical risk profile seems to be a major determinant of 1-year mortality, as depicted in PARTNER trials where 1-year mortality was 30.7%, 24.2%, and 11.8% in extreme-risk, high-risk, and intermediate-risk cohorts, respectively. Although an STS score of greater than 15, atrial fibrillation, previous coronary artery bypass graft (CABG), previous myocardial infarction, and a creatinine level of greater than 2 have been associated with increased mortality post-TAVR, many of these patients benefit from TAVR. Patients with a life expectancy less than 1 year are poor candidates for TAVR. Major procedural complications like significant AI, major vascular complications, stroke, and the like are associated with increased mortality and should be minimized.

Stroke

Improvements in device technology, better patient selection, and operator experience have led to a decline in clinical stroke, with cumulative incidence at 1 year being less than 5%. New brain lesions on MRI, on the other hand, can be found in 58%–100% of patients. Traditional stroke assessment tools (e.g., the National Institutes of Health Stroke Score [NIHSS]) evaluate only a part of the brain and may not identify all neurologic deficits. The effect of subclinical cerebral embolism on neurocognitive decline remains to be determined, although population-based studies in the pre-TAVR era are suggestive. Cerebral embolic protection devices like TriGuard, Montage, Sentinel (Claret Medical), and Embrella are being evaluated with the aim of reducing cerebral ischemic burden. Although half of all strokes are periprocedural, late strokes are sometimes attributed to new-onset atrial fibrillation or subclinical valve thrombosis. Antithrombotic therapy guidelines (Table 15.3) for post-TAVR patients have mostly been empiric, with ongoing trials to provide evidence-based antithrombotic regimens.

Conduction Abnormalities

Mechanical interaction between atrioventricular conduction tissue and the THV leads to conduction abnormalities seen post-TAVR. New conduction abnormalities occur in about 10%–50% of all patients, are more common with CoreValve, and may be associated with a lack of improvement in LVEF. New pacemaker rates in the TVT registry are noted to be 11% at 1 year. The impact of existing or new pacemakers on 1-year morbidity and mortality due to chronic pacing has been controversial. It is notable that almost 50% of patients who receive a pacemaker upon discharge are not pacemaker-dependent at 6 months follow-up. Clinical variables to predict long-term pacemaker requirement are less well defined, although low implantation depth and previous CABG have been identified as risk factors. The MARE (NCT02153307) study to evaluate incidence and predictors of high-degree atrioventricular block in patients with persistent left bundle branch block (LBBB) at discharge is ongoing.

Perivalvular leak (PVL)

Moderate to severe PVL is associated with poor outcome. Recent trials have reported a significant reduction in PVL at 1 year: 3.4% in the PARTNER IIA trial, 2% in the Sapien 3 registry, and 0% in the REPRISE II trial. This decline in PVL can be attributed to CTA-guided THV sizing; iterative design improvements in THV technology, such as the adaptive seal in the Lotus or external skirt in the S3; routine predilatation of severely calcified and/or BiAV valves, optimal depth of implantation, and the like. An underexpanded valve can be post-dilated with a BAV balloon sized to mean annular diameter. Low implantation of a non-retrievable THV can be treated by placing a second THV.

Table 15.3

Recommendations for Antithrombotic Therapy Following Transcatheter Aortic Valve Replacement (TAVR)

	ACCF/AATS/SCAI/STS Expert Consensus	AHA/ACC Guidelines	CCS Position Statement	ESC/EACTS Guidelines
Long-term antithrombotic treatment	Aspirin 81 mg/day indefinitely	Lifelong aspirin 75–100 mg daily (class 1 class 1b level of evidence: C)	Low-dose aspirin indefinitely	Low-dose aspirin indefinitely
Postprocedural antithrombotic treatment	Aspirin 81 mg/day + clopidogrel 75 mg/day for 3–6 months	Aspirin 75–100 mg/day + clopidogrel 75 mg/day for 6 months	ASA 80 mg/day + thienopyridine for 1–3 months	Low-dose aspirin + a thienopyridine early after TAVI

Valve Durability

Long-term durability data for TAVR do not exist, although 3- to 5-year follow-up data have not shown any structural valve deterioration requiring surgical valve replacement. A certain subset of patients after TAVR do seem to exhibit rapid valve hemodynamic deterioration (VHD), with a 4.5% incidence at 20 months mean echocardiographic follow-up but without increase in death or stroke. Absence of antithrombotic therapy was identified as a major determinant of VHD. Other factors include ViV, THV size of 23 mm or less, and greater body mass index. Incidence of THV thrombosis was reported to be 0.6% from a multicenter experience, with a mean gradient of 41 mm Hg. Exertional dyspnea is the most common clinical presentation, whereas about one-third are asymptomatic. A therapeutic trial of warfarin is reasonable in patients with VHD who are not on antithrombotic therapy even in the absence of visible thrombus. Incidence of subclinical valve leaflet thrombosis has recently been noted to be as high as 40%, with less well-defined clinical implication. The SAVORY registry evaluating the role of four-dimensional CT in subclinical THV thrombosis is ongoing (NCT02426307).

Coronary Obstruction

Coronary obstruction is a result of unfavorable interaction of coronary ostium with the final position of displaced valve leaflets. Coronary obstruction following TAVR is 3–4 times more common in ViV cases where the reported incidence is 2.5%–3.5%. Risk factors include low native or implanted coronary height (distance between coronary ostium and aortic annulus), narrow aortic sinuses, stentless or internally stented bioprosthesis, supra-annular implantation of bioprosthesis, and bulky leaflets of degenerated bioprosthesis. Fluoroscopic risk assessment, for the left main ostium in particular, can be done by supravalvular aortogram in LAO-cranial projection to ensure a coplanar view of the aortic annulus or a view in which the bioprosthetic ring appears as a straight line. CTA provides excellent anatomic modeling that can identify high-risk cases and must be done as part of ViV planning. A virtual THV-to-coronary distance of less than 3 mm is identified as a high-risk feature. Strategies to minimize coronary obstruction may include using a smaller or an underexpanded THV, avoiding high implantation, and use of retrievable THV over nonretrievable THV. Also patients with high-risk features should undergo TAVR under general anesthesia with TEE guidance and hemodynamic support on standby. Active protection of the coronary bed can be considered and includes placing an undeployed stent in the coronary vasculature via a medium-support coronary wire and a guide catheter that does not sit too low in the aortic annulus.

Vascular Complications (VC)

The incidence of major VC has decreased significantly from 15.3% in the TF cohort of the PARTNER trial utilizing 22 and 24F introducer sheaths to 4.2% in the TVT registry. Factors leading to reduced VC include reduced sheath size and sheath-to-artery ratio, improvement in delivery systems, patient selection based on CTA-guided vascular assessment, and increased operator experience. Alternate access sites should be explored in patients with high-risk features for VC.

Other Complications

A stiff wire in the LV or a pacemaker wire in the RV can cause myocardial injury leading to pericardial effusion and tamponade. The incidence is about 1%, and many of those require percutaneous drainage and reversal of anticoagulation as soon as feasible. Device embolization is rare, with an incidence of 0.6%. Contrast-induced nephropathy is seen in 2.2% of patients, with a rare need for hemodialysis. Annular dissection occurs in 0.2% of cases and can lead to rapid hemodynamic deterioration.

Future Directions

The field of TAVR continues to expand with newer technologies and expanded indications. New THV systems are conceptualized and tested worldwide (see Fig. 15.4). Lotus (Boston Scientific Inc., Natick, MA) is a fully repositionable and retrievable THV with an external adaptive seal designed to minimize PVL. Early clinical data showed significant improvement in PVL rates. REPRISE III is a randomized trial ongoing in the United States, the results of which are still awaited. Portico (St. Jude Medical Inc., St. Paul, MN), a fully resheathable and repositionable self-expanding THV, is currently available in Europe for commercial use. PORTICO IDE is an ongoing randomized trial in the United States evaluating the safety and efficacy of Portico in extreme and high surgical risk patients. Expanded indications for TAVR are likely to include patients with intermediate surgical risk, with ongoing studies looking at the role of TAVR in patients with low surgical risk, asymptomatic AS, and moderate AS with concomitant LV dysfunction.

Suggested Reading

Axel Linke SH, Dwyer MG, Mangner N, et al. CLEAN-TAVI: a prospective, randomized trial of cerebral embolic protection in high-risk patients with aortic stenosis undergoing transcatheter aortic valve replacement. Available from: http://www.tctmd.com/show.aspx?id=125256.

Ben-Dor I, et al. Complications and outcome of balloon aortic valvuloplasty in high-risk or inoperable patients. *JACC Cardiovasc Interv.* 2010;3(11):1150-1156.

Ben-Dor I, et al. Balloon aortic valvuloplasty for severe aortic stenosis as a bridge to transcatheter/surgical aortic valve replacement. *Catheter Cardiovasc Interv.* 2013;82(4):632-637.

Brueren G, van den Heuvel A, Tonino P, et al. Investigation of Claret cerebral embolic protection device in preventing cerebral lesions during transcatheter aortic valve replacement (MISTRAL-C). Available from: http://www.tctmd.com/show.aspx?id=132514.

Del Trigo M, et al. Incidence, timing, and predictors of valve hemodynamic deterioration after transcatheter aortic valve replacement: multicenter registry. *J Am Coll Cardiol.* 2016;67(6):644-655.

Dewey TM, et al. Reliability of risk algorithms in predicting early and late operative outcomes in high-risk patients undergoing aortic valve replacement. *J Thorac Cardiovasc Surg.* 2008;135(1):180-187.

Dvir D, et al. Transcatheter aortic valve implantation in failed bioprosthetic surgical valves. *JAMA.* 2014;312(2):162-170.

Dvir D, et al. Coronary obstruction in transcatheter aortic valve-in-valve implantation: preprocedural evaluation, device selection, protection, and treatment. *Circ Cardiovasc Interv.* 2015;8(1).

Goel SS, et al. Percutaneous coronary intervention in patients with severe aortic stenosis: implications for transcatheter aortic valve replacement. *Circulation.* 2012;125(8):1005-1013.

Hermiller JB, et al. Predicting early and late mortality after transcatheter aortic valve replacement. *J Am Coll Cardiol.* 2016;68(24):343-352.

Iung B, Rodes-Cabau J. The optimal management of anti-thrombotic therapy after valve replacement: certainties and uncertainties. *Eur Heart J.* 2014;35(42):2942-2949.

Lansky AJ, et al. A prospective randomized evaluation of the TriGuard HDH embolic DEFLECTion device during transcatheter aortic valve implantation: results from the DEFLECT III trial. *Eur Heart J.* 2015;36(31):2070-2078.

Latib A, et al. Treatment and clinical outcomes of transcatheter heart valve thrombosis. *Circ Cardiovasc Interv.* 2015;8(4).

Leon MB, et al. Transcatheter aortic-valve implantation for aortic stenosis in patients who cannot undergo surgery. *N Engl J Med.* 2010;363(17):1597-1607.

Londono JC, et al. Hemodynamic support with Impella 2.5 during balloon aortic valvuloplasty in high-risk patient. *J Interv Cardiol.* 2011;24(2):193-197.

Mack MJ, et al. 5-year outcomes of transcatheter aortic valve replacement or surgical aortic valve replacement for high surgical risk patients with aortic stenosis (PARTNER 1): a randomised controlled trial. *Lancet.* 2015;385(9986):2477-2484.

Makkar RR, et al. Possible subclinical leaflet thrombosis in bioprosthetic aortic valves. *N Engl J Med.* 2015;373(21):2015-2024.

Mylotte D, et al. Transcatheter aortic valve replacement in bicuspid aortic valve disease. *J Am Coll Cardiol.* 2014;64(22):2330-2339.

Nishimura RA, et al. 2014 AHA/ACC guideline for the management of patients with valvular heart disease: executive summary: a report of the American College of Cardiology/American Heart Association Task Force on Practice Guidelines. *J Am Coll Cardiol.* 2014;63(22):2438-2488.

Otto CM, et al. Three-year outcome after balloon aortic valvuloplasty. Insights into prognosis of valvular aortic stenosis. *Circulation*. 1994;89(2):642-650.

Percutaneous balloon aortic valvuloplasty. Acute and 30-day follow-up results in 674 patients from the NHLBI Balloon Valvuloplasty Registry. *Circulation*. 1991;84(6):2383-2397.

Rodes-Cabau J, et al. Transcatheter aortic valve implantation for the treatment of severe symptomatic aortic stenosis in patients at very high or prohibitive surgical risk: acute and late outcomes of the multicenter Canadian experience. *J Am Coll Cardiol*. 2010;55(11):1080-1090.

Samim M, et al. Embrella embolic deflection device for cerebral protection during transcatheter aortic valve replacement. *J Thorac Cardiovasc Surg*. 2015;149(3):799-805, e1–e2.

Smith CR, et al. Transcatheter versus surgical aortic-valve replacement in high-risk patients. *N Engl J Med*. 2011;364(23):2187-2198.

Valve in Valve phone application. Available from: http://ubqo.com/viv.

van der Boon RM, et al. Pacemaker dependency after transcatheter aortic valve implantation with the self-expanding Medtronic CoreValve System. *Int J Cardiol*. 2013;168(2):1269-1273.

Van Mieghem NM, et al. Incidence and predictors of debris embolizing to the brain during transcatheter aortic valve implantation. *JACC Cardiovasc Interv*. 2015;8(5):718-724.

Webb JG, Dvir D. Transcatheter aortic valve replacement for bioprosthetic aortic valve failure: the valve-in-valve procedure. *Circulation*. 2013;127(25):2542-2550.

Transcatheter Closure of Atrial Septal Defects and Patent Foramen Ovale

WAIL ALKASHKARI · QI LING CAO · ZIYAD M. HIJAZI

An atrial septal defect (ASD) is a communication between the right atrium and left atrium due to an abnormal septation. There are four types of ASDs:

- Primum
- Secundum
- Sinus venosus (superior vena cava [SVC] type and inferior vena cava [IVC] type)
- Coronary sinus septal defect

ASDs are among the most common congenital heart defects (CHD), and they account for one-third of CHD in adults.[1] Significant iatrogenic ASDs also have been described after adopting new modalities of percutaneous transcatheter therapies to the left side of the heart (e.g., Mitraclip for mitral insufficiency).[2] At present, only the secundum type is amenable for transcatheter closure.

Secundum ASD

This is the most common subtype and generally the result of an underdeveloped septum primum and/or excessive resorption of septum primum tissue. The defect is therefore bordered by the limbus of the fossa ovalis or the C-shaped septum secundum. It is twice as common in females as in males. Associated anatomic lesions include mitral valve prolapse, partial anomalous pulmonary venous return, and complex congenital heart defects.

The hemodynamic pathophysiology typically involves a left-to-right shunt at the atrial level. The flow across an ASD or other atrial level shunt occurs mainly in diastole, and its direction depends on the differences in the atrial pressures and compliance rather than on pulmonary vascular resistance (PVR) or systemic vascular resistance (SVR), although these resistances are indirect factors. The compliance of the atria is determined by their respective ventricular compliance, which is dependent on ventricular wall thickness, a function of ventricular pressure and resistance (e.g., PVR for the right ventricle and SVR for the left ventricle). As right ventricular pressure and PVR increase, the wall thickness of the right ventricle increases, leading to a fall in right ventricular and right atrial compliance (i.e., atrial wall becomes stiffer). Normally the mean left atrial (LA) pressure is 6–9 mm Hg and the mean right atrial (RA) pressure is 1–4 mm Hg. This favors a left-to-right shunt.

The pressure in the atria is dependent on the compliance of the ventricles. If the ventricles are poorly compliant or stiff, a higher atrial pressure is required for filling to occur. Unless the communicating defect is small, the amount of flow is dependent on the difference in compliance of the ventricles rather than on the pressure since a large defect will equalize the pressures in the atria. Normally the right ventricular compliance is much higher than that in the left ventricle, resulting in a left-to-right shunt across the ASD, and its magnitude is dependent on the relative difference between the right ventricular and left ventricular compliance.

Left ventricular compliance is relatively stable for the first 20–30 years of life. As aging occurs, the arteriolar elasticity decreases and SVR increases, leading to higher blood pressure. This leads to higher energy expenditure by the left ventricle to overcome increased afterload, and subsequent left ventricular hypertrophy (Laplace's law). The compliance of the left ventricle decreases, with a subsequent elevation in LA pressure and increased left-to-right atrial-level shunt. The shunt results in right-sided volume overload. Thus, the right atrium, right ventricle, pulmonary arteries, and pulmonary vascular bed are enlarged because of the increased volume of the shunt. There is increased flow across an otherwise normal tricuspid and pulmonary valve, leading to increased turbulence or a flow-related gradient across these valves.[3]

Clinical Presentation

Most children with an ASD present with a murmur and are asymptomatic. Occasionally infants may present with breathlessness, recurrent chest infections, and even heart failure. Failure to thrive is an uncommon presentation.

Adults with an ASD typically have a prolonged asymptomatic course. Symptom onset is insidious, most often occurring after the age of 40 or 50. Women may become symptomatic during the physiologic demands of pregnancy or labor, especially if associated with other lesions such as pulmonary stenosis. In adults with an ASD who are less than 40 years of age, there is no correlation between symptoms (New York Heart Association [NYHA] class) and the size of a shunt. Even patients with small (<10 mm) defects can present with significant symptoms. However, the development of symptoms does correlate with age. Major and limiting problems are often experienced after age 65 years.[4]

The clinical course of an unrepaired ASD in adulthood may be significantly affected by hypertension, coronary artery disease, and mitral regurgitation. Patients with unrepaired ASD over 60 years of age often develop atrial fibrillation, an age-related reflection of atrial stretch, which seldom occurs in those younger than 40 years of age.[5]

Symptoms may include the following:
- Reduced exercise tolerance or fatigue
- Exertional dyspnea
- Palpitations (due to supraventricular arrhythmias, frequent atrial fibrillation/atrial flutter in older age) or syncope for sick sinus syndrome
- Atypical chest pain (right ventricular ischemia)
- Frequent respiratory tract infections
- Signs of right-heart failure
- Paradoxical embolism from peripheral venous thrombosis, atrial arrhythmias, unfiltered intravenous infusion, or indwelling venous catheters or pacemaker electrodes.

The physical examination findings depend on the stage of presentation and pathophysiology. For example, cyanosis suggests severe pulmonary hypertension with reversed shunting in the presence of a secundum ASD or superior sinus venosus defect. The physical exam may demonstrate right ventricular impulse. The second heart sound may be widely split, with no respiratory variation. A diastolic murmur at the tricuspid area and/or systolic murmur at the pulmonary area suggests increased blood flow through the tricuspid and pulmonary orifice, respectively, especially if the Qp:Qs ratio is more than 2.5:1 (relative tricuspid and pulmonary stenosis). The clinical findings and auscultation may also be completely unremarkable.

Echocardiography

In the current era of percutaneous device closure of interatrial communications, evaluation with transesophageal echocardiography (TEE), especially if accompanied with real-time three-dimensional imaging or intracardiac echocardiography (ICE) is mandatory prior to consideration of device closure.[6]

Initial screening imaging with transthoracic echocardiography (TTE) may demonstrate a clearly visible defect in the atrial septum, best seen in the apical four-chamber and subcostal long-axis views. However, it is common to see "echo dropout" in the region of the interatrial septum, and this may lead to misdiagnosis. Bubble contrast echocardiography with provocation (e.g., including a sharp nasal sniff, a cough, or the relaxation phase of the Valsalva maneuver) improves diagnostic accuracy. A positive test reveals the rapid transit of bubbles from the right to the left heart within three to five cardiac cycles. The amount of bubbles seen is related to the size of the defect. Late transit (more than five cardiac cycles) of bubbles is associated with intrapulmonary shunting. Intravenous contrast injection in the left arm may diagnose a persistent left SVC with anomalous drainage to the left atrium.

Box 16.1 summarizes the key points regarding TEE evaluation of intracardiac anatomy.

Cardiac catheterization is not usually required for diagnosis. However, in older patients, a diagnostic cardiac catheterization for coronary angiography and hemodynamic assessment may be justified. Patients with high LV end-diastolic pressure (LVEDP) (>14 mm Hg) need medical optimization before closure.[7]

Indications for Percutaneous Closure of Secundum ASD

Large ASDs should be closed to reduce the risk of complications; these may include premature death, atrial arrhythmias, reduced exercise

---

Box 16.1 Transesophageal Echocardiogram Features to Consider for Atrial Septal Defect Closure

1. Demonstration of all four pulmonary veins draining to the left atrium is essential prior to device closure of fossa ovalis defects. Ten percent of secundum atrial septal defects (ASDs) have anomalous pulmonary venous drainage, most commonly of the right upper pulmonary vein.
2. Exclude a superior sinus venosus defect, in the long axis 90-degree view and at 0 degrees rotation.
3. Measure the margins of the atrial septum for suitability for device closure.
4. A detailed mitral valve assessment is mandatory prior to closure because mitral incompetence is a potential complication of device closure. The severity of mitral stenosis and regurgitation are often underestimated in the presence of an ASD.
5. Closure of a defect in the context of significant mitral valve disease will likely worsen symptoms rather than improve them.
6. Exclude intracardiac thrombus.

tolerance, hemodynamically significant regurgitation, right-to-left shunting and embolism during pregnancy, congestive heart failure, or pulmonary vascular disease. Large defects with evidence of right ventricular volume overload on echocardiography may only cause symptoms in the third decade of life or beyond; however, regardless of symptoms, closure is usually indicated to prevent long-term complications.

Symptoms or complications of an ASD are indications for closure regardless of age, including in the elderly. ASD closure will prevent further deterioration and probably will reverse or normalize right ventricular dilation, right ventricular failure, and, to a degree, tricuspid regurgitation (TR).[1] Atrial flutter or fibrillation may be treated before or after defect closure with radiofrequency ablation, depending on the site of origin.[8]

If the patient presents with pulmonary arterial hypertension (PAH), complete assessment of the reversibility of pulmonary vascular disease should be done prior to closure. Closure may be considered in the presence of net left-to-right shunting, pulmonary artery pressure less than two-thirds systemic levels, PVR less than two-thirds SVR, or when PAH is responsive to either vasodilator therapy or test occlusion of the defect. Patients should be treated in conjunction with providers who have expertise in the management of pulmonary hypertensive syndromes.[9]

Closure of an ASD also is reasonable in the presence of paradoxical embolism and documented orthodeoxia-platypnea.[10]

Closure of ASD should be considered in some cases as prophylaxis even if the defect is small. For example, patients who are professional divers or patients undergoing pacemaker implantation will benefit due to a reduced risk of paradoxical embolism.[10]

Pregnancy and delivery are generally well tolerated, even by patients with an unclosed ASD with a significant left-to-right shunt. However, clinical symptoms may emerge during pregnancy or after childbirth. During pregnancy and delivery there is an increased risk of paradoxical embolism, regardless of the defect size.[11] In our practice, we close the defect before planned pregnancy, even if it is hemodynamically insignificant.

Contraindications for Percutaneous Closure of Secundum ASD

Small ASDs with a diameter of less than 5 mm and no evidence of right ventricular volume overload do not impact the natural history of the individual and do not require closure unless associated with paradoxical embolism or at risk of such events.

An absolute contraindication for percutaneous ASD closure is the presence of severe and irreversible PAH with no evidence of a left-to-right shunt.[1] See Box 16.2 for a summary of the indications and contraindications to ASD closure.

Outcomes of ASD Closure

In patients undergoing successful ASD closure before they are 24 years of age, the long-term survival matches that seen in the general population. Significantly shorter survival in patients with pulmonary hypertension (PAP = 40 mm Hg) after age 24 has been reported. Closure in patients over 40 years of age, while reducing mortality, improving symptoms, limiting functional deterioration, and limiting the incidence of heart failure compared with a conservatively managed control group, did not reduce arrhythmias or stroke on long-term follow-up. Independent predictors of mortality include functional NYHA class III–IV, PAP higher than 40 mm Hg, and Qp/Qs of more than 3.5:1.[12]

Box 16.2 Indications and Contraindications to Atrial Septal Defect Closure

Indications

1. Symptoms or complications of an atrial septal defect (ASD)
2. Paradoxical embolism and documented orthodeoxia-platypnea
3. Prophylaxis for professional divers or those undergoing pacemaker implantation
4. Pregnancy and delivery

Contraindications

1. Small ASD (diameter <5 mm) and no evidence of right ventricular volume overload
2. Irreversible pulmonary hypertension
3. Other contraindications include the following:
   - Poor state of the patient with other serious conditions or comorbidities
   - Patients with associated cardiac anomalies requiring cardiac surgery
   - Patients with current systemic or local infection or sepsis within 1 month of device placement
   - Patients with bleeding disorder or with other contraindications to aspirin therapy, unless another antiplatelet drug can be administered for 6 months
   - Presence of intracardiac thrombus
   - Unsuitable defect anatomy including deficient rims, superior/inferior or posterior; deficient anterior rim is not a contraindication for the use of percutaneous closure devices.
   - Patients allergic to nickel may suffer an allergic reaction. This is a relative contraindication. Most nickel allergies are contact reactions. It is unclear if intracardiac devices will mount a similar reaction. A consultation with an allergist may be needed.

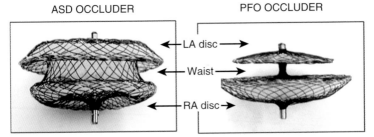

ASD OCCLUDER   PFO OCCLUDER

LA disc — Waist — RA disc

Figure 16.1 Amplatzer atrial septal defect occluder and patent foramen ovale occluder. *LA*, left atrial; *RA*, right atrial.

ASD Closure Devices

Currently there are only two devices approved by the U.S. Food and Drug Administration (FDA) for the percutaneous closure of secundum ASD: the Amplatzer septal occluder (St. Jude Medical, Minneapolis MN) and the Gore Septal (Helex and Cardioform) occluder devices (WL Gore & Associates, Newark, DE). The Gore Helex device has been upgraded to the Gore Septal Occluder (Cardioform). There are several other devices that are not FDA approved but available outside the United States, including the Clamshell, CardioSEAL, Starflex, Biostar (NMT Medical; this family of devices now ceases to exit, but we are mentioning them for historical importance), Cera septal occluder (Lifetech Scientific Corporation), and Occlutech Figulla Flex septal occluder (Occlutech GmbH, Sweden).

The Amplatzer Septal Occluder (ASO)

The Amplatzer septal occluder (ASO) is a self-expandable double disc device made of nitinol (55% nickel, 45% titanium) wire mesh. The ASO is tightly woven into two flat discs (Fig. 16.1). There is a 3- to 4-mm connecting waist between the two discs, corresponding to the thickness of the atrial septum. Nitinol has superelastic properties, with shape memory. This allows the device to be stretched into an almost linear configuration, placed inside a small sheath for delivery, and then return to its original configuration within the heart when not constrained by the sheath. The device size is determined by the diameter of its waist and is constructed in various sizes ranging from 4 to 40 mm (in 1-mm increments up to 20 mm; in 2-mm increments up to the largest device currently available, 40 mm; the 40-mm size is not available in the United States). The two flat discs extend radially beyond the central waist to provide secure anchorage.

The LA disc is larger than the RA disc. For devices 4–10 mm in size, the LA disc is 12 mm and the RA disc is 8 mm larger than the waist. However, for devices larger than 11 mm and up to 32 mm in size, the LA disc is 14 mm and the RA disc is 10 mm larger than the connecting waist. For devices larger than 32 mm, the LA disc is 16 mm larger than the waist and the RA disc is 10 mm larger than the waist. Both discs are angled slightly toward each other to ensure firm contact of the discs to the atrial septum.

A total of three Dacron polyester patches are sewn securely with polyester thread into each disc and the connecting waist to increase the thrombogenicity and endothelialization of the device. A stainless steel sleeve with a female thread is laser-welded to the RA disc. This sleeve is used to screw the delivery cable to the device.

Amplatzer Delivery System

For device deployment, we recommend using appropriately sized sheaths for the device as summarized in Box 16.3. The delivery system is supplied sterilized and separate from the device. It contains all the equipment needed to facilitate device deployment. It consists of the following:

1. Delivery sheath of specified French size and length and appropriate dilator
2. Loading device used to collapse the device and introduce it into the delivery sheath
3. Delivery cable (internal diameter [ID] 0.081 inch): the device is screwed onto its distal end to allow for loading, placement, and retrieval of the device
4. Plastic Pin-vice: this facilitates unscrewing of the delivery cable from the device during device deployment
5. Tuohy Borst valve adapter with a side arm for the sheath, to act as a one-way stop-bleed valve

All delivery sheaths have a 45-degree angled tip. The 6F sheath has a length of 60 cm; the 7F sheath is available in lengths of 60 and 80 cm; and the 8F, 9F, 10F, and 12F sheaths are all 80 cm long.

Amplatzer Exchange (Rescue) System

This is made up of the same components as the Amplatzer delivery system except that the inner lumen and tip of the dilator can

---

Box 16.3 Sheath Delivery System Sizing for Atrial Septal Defect Devices

6F delivery system for devices <10 mm in diameter
7F delivery system for devices 10–15 mm
8F sheath for devices 16–19 mm
9F sheath for devices 20–26 mm
10F sheath for devices 28–34 mm
12F sheath for the 36-mm and 38-mm devices
14F sheath for the 40-mm device

accommodate the delivery cable. It is available in two sizes: 9F (dilator ID 0.087 inch) and 12F (dilator ID 0.113-inch), with a 45-degree curve and 80 cm in length. The distal tip of the delivery cable can screw into the back of another delivery cable. This allows it to become an exchange-length cable. The damaged sheath then can be removed and the rescue sheath with its dilator can be inserted over the cable to recapture the device.

Optional but Recommended Equipment

Amplatzer Sizing Balloon

The Amplatzer sizing balloon is a double-lumen balloon catheter with a 7F shaft size. The balloon is made from nylon and is very compliant, making it ideal for sizing the secundum ASD by flow occlusion ("stop-flow") without overstretching of the defect. The balloon catheter is angled at 45 degrees, and there are radiopaque markers for calibration at 2, 5, and 10 mm. The balloon catheters are available in three sizes: 18 mm (maximum volume is 20 mm and is used for defects up to 20 mm), 24 mm (maximum volume 30 mL and used to size defects up to 22 mm), and 34 mm (maximum volume 90 mL and used to size defects up to 40 mm).

Amplatzer Super-Stiff Guidewire

The 0.035-inch Amplatzer super-stiff exchange guidewire is used to advance the delivery sheath and dilator into the left upper pulmonary vein. Table 16.1 summarizes all the necessary materials for ASD closure.

Step-by-Step Technique: Transcatheter Device Closure of Secundum ASD

Materials and Equipment

1. Single- or bi-plane cardiac catheterization laboratory
2. TEE or ICE
3. Full range of device sizes, delivery and exchange (rescue) systems, sizing balloons
4. A multipurpose catheter to engage the defect and the left upper pulmonary vein
5. Extra-stiff exchange-length wire; for example, a 0.035-inch Amplatzer super stiff exchange length guidewire with a 1-cm floppy tip, but any extra-stiff J-tipped wire may be used

Personnel

1. Interventional cardiologist appropriately proctored to perform device closure

Table 16.1

Materials and Equipment Required for Transcatheter ASD Closure Procedures	
Item	**Size**
Amplatzer Septal Occluder	4–40 mm
Amplatzer PFO Occluder	18, 25, 35 mm
Amplatzer Delivery System	7F–12F
Amplatzer Super-Stiff exchange	0.035-inch, 100-cm-length guidewire
Multipurpose catheter	6F–7F
Amplatzer Sizing Balloon	24, 34 mm
Amplatzer Rescue System	9F, 12F

PFO, patent foramen ovale.

2. Cardiologist (noninvasive) to facilitate TEE or ICE
3. Anesthesiologist if procedure is performed under TEE guidance
4. Nurse certified to administer conscious sedation if procedure is performed under ICE guidance
5. Catheterization laboratory technologists

Method

1. *Preprocedure*: Review all pertinent data relating to the patient and to the defect to be closed and ensure that appropriate devices and delivery systems are available. The procedure and complications should be explained and the opportunity given to ask questions. All preprocedure orders should be given to the patient. Aspirin 81–325 mg should be started 48 hours prior to the procedure. If allergic to aspirin, clopidogrel 75 mg should be used.

2. *Vascular access*: The right femoral vein is accessed using a 7F or 8F short sheath. An arterial monitoring line (e.g., 4F) can be inserted in the right femoral or radial artery, especially if the patient's condition is marginal or if the procedure is performed under TEE and general endotracheal anesthesia. If a subclavian or internal jugular venous approach is used, it is very difficult to maneuver the device deployment, especially with large defects.

   Heparin IV (e.g., 70 U/kg) is given to achieve an activated clotting time (ACT) of more than 250 seconds at the time of device deployment. Antibiotic coverage for the procedure is recommended (e.g., cefazolin 1 g IV), the first dose at the time of procedure and two subsequent doses 6–8 hours apart after the procedure.

3. Routine right heart catheterization should be performed in all cases to ensure presence of normal PVR. The left-to-right shunt can also be calculated.

4. Echocardiographic assessment of the secundum ASD is performed simultaneously using either TEE or ICE. Fig. 16.2 demonstrates full assessment of the defect by ICE.

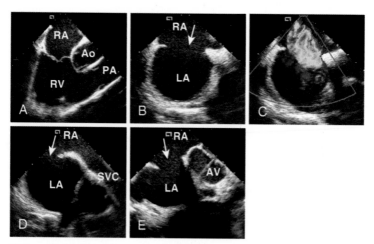

Figure 16.2 Intracardiac echocardiographic images in a patient with a large secundum atrial septal defect (ASD). (A) Home view demonstrating the right atrium (RA), tricuspid valve, right ventricle (RV), aortic root (Ao), and pulmonary artery (PA). (B) Septal view, demonstrating the large ASD (*arrow*), the RA and the left atrium (LA), and the superior and inferior rims. (C) Same view with color Doppler. (D) Caval view demonstrating the entire superior rim and the defect (*arrow*). (E) Short-axis view demonstrating the defect (*arrow*), the Ao, the absent anterior rim and good posterior rim, and both atria. *AV,* aortic valve; *SVC,* superior vena cava.

The important ASD rims to look for are[13]:

- Supero-posterior/SVC rim: Best achieved at the bicaval view
- Infero-posterior/IVC and coronary sinus rim: Best achieved at bicaval view, an important rim to have
- posterior/right upper and lower pulmonary vein rim: Best achieved at short-axis view of aortic valve and apical four-chamber view, respectively
- Supero-anterior/aortic rim: Best achieved at short axis-view of aortic valve; the least important rim; often deficient
- Inferio-anterior/atrioventricular valve rim: Best achieved at apical four-chamber view

   The rims must be sufficient (>5 mm) except for the aortic rim. A deficient aortic rim is not a contraindication to the procedure.

5. *How to cross the ASD*: Use a multipurpose catheter. The MP A2 catheter has the ideal angle. Place the catheter at the junction of the IVC and the right atrium. The IVC angle should guide the catheter to the ASD. Keep a clockwise torque on the catheter while advancing it toward the septum (posterior). If unsuccessful, place the catheter in the SVC and slowly pull it into the right atrium; keep a clockwise posterior torque to orient the catheter along the atrial septum until it crosses the defect. TEE/ICE can be very useful to guide the catheter across difficult defects.

6. Perform a right upper pulmonary vein angiogram (Fig. 16.3A) in the hepatoclavicular projection (35-degree left anterior oblique [LAO]/35-degree cranial). This delineates the anatomy, shape, and length of the septum. This may be helpful when the device is deployed but not released—the operator can position the imaging tube in the same view of the angiogram and compare the position of the device with that obtained during the deployment (Fig. 16.3B and C). Again, this angiogram is optional and not mandatory.

7. *Defect sizing*: Position the multipurpose catheter in the left upper pulmonary vein. Prepare the appropriate size of balloon according to the manufacturer's guidelines. We prefer to use the 34-mm balloon because it is longer, and, during inflation, it sits nicely across the defect. Pass an extra-stiff, floppy/J-tipped 0.035-inch exchange-length guidewire (Fig. 16.4A). This gives the best support within the atrium for the balloon, especially in large defects. Remove the multipurpose catheter and the femoral sheath. We advance the sizing balloon catheter directly over the wire without a venous sheath. Most sizing balloons require an 8F or 9F sheath. The balloon catheter is advanced over the wire and placed across the defect under both fluoroscopic and echocardiographic guidance. The "stop-flow" balloon sizing is performed by inflating the balloon (previously prepared with 1 : 4 diluted contrast) until the left-to-right shunt ceases, as observed by color flow Doppler TEE/ICE. Once the shunt ceases, deflate the balloon slightly until the shunt reappears. This "stop-flow" balloon sizing technique is used to select an ASO device size. The best echo view for measurement is to observe the balloon in its long axis (Fig. 16.4B). In this view the indentation made by the margins of the ASD can be visualized and precise measurement can be made.

8. *Fluoroscopic measurement*: Angulate the x-ray tube so that the beam is perpendicular to the balloon. Various calibration markers can be helpful. Ensure that the markers are separated and discrete. Measure the balloon diameter at the site of the indentation (or at the middle of the balloon) as per the diagnostic function of

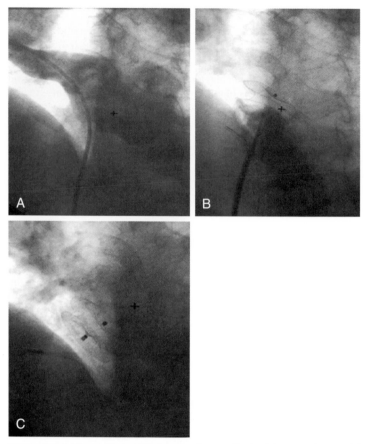

Figure 16.3 Cineangiographic images in a patient with secundum atrial septal defect (ASD). (A) Angiogram in the right upper pulmonary vein in the hepatoclavicular projection (35 degrees left anterior oblique/35 degrees cranial) demonstrating left-to-right shunt. (B) Angiogram in the right atrium in the hepatoclavicular projection prior to release of the device. Correct deployment manifest by opacification of the right atrial disc only, and, on levophase, the left atrial disc only is opacified. (C) Cineangiographic image after the device has been released, demonstrating good device alignment with the septum.

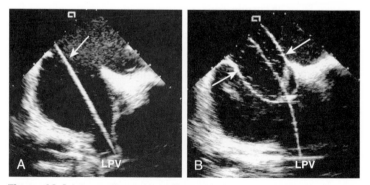

Figure 16.4 Intracardiac echocardiographic images of the patient in Fig. 16.2, showing defect sizing. (A) The exchange wire (*arrow*) across the defect into the left upper pulmonary vein (LUPV). (B) Sizing balloon occluding the defect. This is the stretched diameter (*arrows*) of the defect.

the laboratory (Fig. 16.5). We have found that when a discrepancy exists between the echocardiographic and the fluoroscopic measurements, the echocardiographic measurement is usually more accurate.

Once the size has been determined, deflate the balloon and pull it back into the junction of the right atrium and IVC, leaving the wire in the left upper pulmonary vein. Recheck the ACT and give the first dose of antibiotics.

9. *Device selection:* If the defect has adequate rims (>5 mm), select a device 2 mm or less larger than the "stop-flow" diameter of the balloon. However, if the aortic rim is deficient (<5 mm), we tend to select a device 4 mm larger than the balloon "stop-flow" diameter. In our practice the balloon sizing or fluoroscopic measure is not done routinely. We initially choose a device about 20%–25% larger than the two-dimensional diameter as measured by TEE/ICE. Most of our cases are successful using this approach. However in those patients with complex defects (large ASD >25 mm by TEE/ICE, defects with more than one deficient rim, multiple defects and aneurysmal atrial septum) or in small patients, it is reasonable to plan balloon sizing for device selection.

10. *Device delivery:* Open the appropriate-sized delivery system. Flush the sheath and dilator. The delivery sheath is advanced over the guidewire to the left upper pulmonary vein (Fig. 16.6A). Both dilator and wire are removed, keeping the tip of the sheath inside the left upper pulmonary vein. Use extra care and do not allow air inside the delivery sheath. An alternative technique to minimize air embolism is passage of the sheath with the dilator over the wire up to the IVC, at which point the dilator is removed and the sheath is advanced over the wire into the left atrium while continuously flushing the side arm of the sheath.

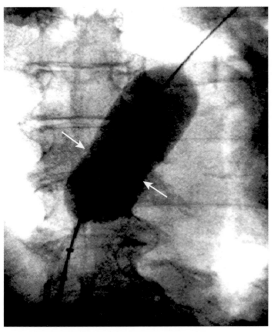

Figure 16.5 Cineangiographic image of the patient in Fig. 16.3 during balloon sizing of the defect, demonstrating the stretched diameter (*arrows*) of the defect.

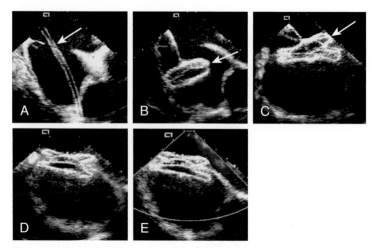

Figure 16.6 Intracardiac echocardiographic images of the patient in Fig. 16.2, showing device delivery and deployment. (A) Delivery sheath (*arrow*) across the defect into the left upper pulmonary vein. (B) The left atrial disc (*arrow*) deployed in the left atrium. (C) The right atrial disc (*arrow*) deployed in the right atrium. (D) The device released, demonstrating good position. (E) Color Doppler demonstrating no residual shunt and patent superior vena cava.

On the back table, the ASO device is then screwed to the tip of the delivery cable, immersed in normal saline to clear air bubbles, and drawn into the loader while under water, injecting saline through the side arm of the loading sheath to expel air bubbles from the system. A Y-connector is applied to the proximal end of the loader to allow flushing with saline. The loader containing the device is attached to the proximal hub of the delivery sheath with a fluid-to-fluid connection. The cable with the ASO device is advanced to the distal tip of the sheath, taking care not to rotate the cable while advancing it in the long sheath to prevent premature unscrewing of the device. Both cable and delivery sheath are pulled back as one unit to the middle of the left atrium. Position of the sheath can be verified using fluoroscopy or TEE/ICE.

11. *Device deployment*: The LA disc is deployed first under fluoroscopic and/or echocardiographic guidance by pulling back the sheath while leaving the disc fixed in the LA away from the LA appendage (Fig. 16.6B). Part of the connecting waist should be deployed in the left atrium, very close (a few millimeters) to the atrial septum (the mechanism of ASD closure using the ASO is stenting of the defect). While applying constant tension on the entire assembly and withdrawing the delivery sheath off the cable, the connecting waist and the RA disc are deployed in the ASD itself and in the right atrium, respectively (Fig. 16.6C).

12. *Device positioning; proper device position can be verified using different techniques*:

    Good device position is evident by the presence of two discs that are parallel to each other and separated from each other by the atrial septum. In the same view the operator can perform the "Minnesota wiggle" (the cable is pushed gently forward and pulled backward). Stable device position manifests by the lack of movement of the device in either direction.

    TEE/ICE: The echocardiographer should make sure that one disc is in each chamber. The long-axis view should be sufficient to evaluate the superior and inferior part of the septum and the short-axis view for the anterior and posterior parts of the disc (Fig. 16.6D and E).

Angiography: is done with the camera in the same projection as for the first angiogram to profile the septum and device using either the side arm of the delivery sheath or a separate angiographic catheter, inserted in the sheath used for ICE or via a separate puncture site. Good device position manifests by opacification of the RA disc alone when the contrast is in the right atrium and opacification of the LA disc alone on pulmonary levophase.

If the position of the device is questionable, the device can be recaptured, entirely or partly, and repositioned following similar steps.

13. *Device release*: Once the device position is verified, the device is released by counterclockwise rotation of the delivery cable using a pin vise. There is often a notable change in the angle of the device as it is released from the slight tension of the delivery cable and it self-centers within the ASD and aligns with the interatrial septum. To assess the results of closure, repeat TEE/ICE, color Doppler, and angiography (optional) in the four-chamber projection. Once the procedure is complete, recheck the ACT and, if appropriate, remove the sheath and achieve hemostasis. If ACT is above 250 seconds, reverse the effect of heparin by using protamine sulfate.

14. *Postprocedure care*: Patients receive a dose of an appropriate antibiotic (commonly cefazolin 1 g) during the catheterization procedure and two further doses at 8-hour intervals. Patients are also asked to take endocarditis prophylaxis when necessary for 6 months after the procedure, as well as aspirin 81–325 mg orally once daily for 6 months. In addition, we have been adding 75 mg clopidogrel for 2–3 months. We have observed that the incidence of postclosure headaches is much less in those patients taking the clopidogrel. The patient is asked not to engage in contact sports for 1 month after the procedure. Full activity, including competitive sports, is usually allowed after 4 weeks of implantation. Magnetic resonance imaging (if required) can be performed any time after implantation.

15. *Postprocedure monitoring*: Patients recover overnight in a telemetry ward. Some patients may experience an increase in atrial ectopic beats. Rarely some patients may have sustained atrial tachycardias. The following day an electrocardiogram (ECG), a chest x-ray (optional) (postero-anterior and lateral), and a TTE with color Doppler should be performed to assess the position of the device and the presence of residual shunt.

Recheck ECG, chest x-ray, and TTE/TEE at 6 months after the procedure to assess everything. If the device position is good with no residual shunt, antibiotic prophylaxis and aspirin can be discontinued. Clinical follow-up can be annually for the first 2 years, then every 3–5 years thereafter. Long-term follow-up of device performance should be assessed and any new information communicated to the patient.

Troubleshooting

Air Embolism

Meticulous technique should be used to prevent air entry. The sheath should be positioned at the mouth of the left upper pulmonary vein. Doing so allows free flow of blood into the sheath. Forceful negative pressure should not be applied to aspirate the sheath. If a large amount of air is introduced on the left side, it will usually pool in the right coronary sinus and right coronary artery. This may manifest with bradycardia, asystole, or profound hypotension. If this occurs, immediately place a right coronary catheter in the right coronary sinus and forcefully inject saline or contrast to displace the air and hence reperfuse the right coronary system.

Cobra-Head Formation

This describes the situation when the left disc maintains a high profile when deployed, mimicking a cobra head. This can occur if the left disc is opened in the pulmonary vein or the LA appendage, or if the left atrium is too small to accommodate the device. It can also occur if the device is defective or has been loaded with unusual strain on it. If this occurs, check the site of deployment; if appropriate, recapture the device and remove and inspect it. If the "cobra head" forms outside the body, use a different device. If the disc forms normally, try deploying the device again. Do not release a device if the left disc has a "cobra-head" appearance.

Device Embolization

If a device embolizes, it must be retrieved, preferably by transcatheter snare and a long sheath; otherwise, by surgery. The transcatheter technique is difficult and should not be performed if the operator is inexperienced in snaring techniques. Furthermore the catheter laboratory should be equipped with large Mullins-type sheaths (12–16F) and also should have various-sized snares. We use the Goose-neck Snare (ev3, Plymouth, MN) or the EN Snare (Merit Medical, Salt Lake City, UT). The device should not be pulled across valves since it may damage the chordae and leaflets. Always use a long sheath to pull the device outside the body. To snare a device, we usually use a sheath that is two French sizes larger than the sheath that was used to deliver the device. On rare occasions, if the LA disc cannot be collapsed inside the sheath, another snare is introduced from the right internal jugular vein to snare the stud of the microscrew of the LA disc and stretch it toward the internal jugular vein while the assistant pulls the device with the snare toward the femoral vein. This allows the device to collapse further and come out of the sheath in the femoral vein.

Prolapse of the Left Disc Across the Defect During Deployment

On occasion, especially in patients with large defects with deficient anterior/superior rims, when the left disc is deployed, it opens perpendicular to the plane of the atrial septum and prolapses through the anterior superior part of the defect. To overcome this problem, use a device that is at least 4 mm larger than the measured "stop-flow" balloon diameter. If this is not possible or it does not work, change the angle of the deployment by placing the sheath either in the left or right upper pulmonary veins rather than mid left atrium. This may change the orientation of the disc. Another potential solution is to use the Hausdorf sheath (Cook Medical, Bloomington, IN), which has two posterior curves at the end. This sine curve can be quite useful in changing the deployment angle.

The use of the dilator technique or balloon-assisted technique is also helpful in preventing prolapse of the LA disc to the right. The dilator technique implies the use of a long dilator from the contralateral femoral vein to hold the LA disc in the left atrium while the assistant/operator deploys the remainder of the device. The balloon-assisted technique is similar to the dilator technique. A guidewire is positioned in the left upper pulmonary vein from the contralateral femoral vein. A balloon is inflated in the right atrium very close to the septum. The device is deployed in the usual fashion. The presence of the balloon will prevent prolapse of the left disc. Once the device has been deployed, the balloon is deflated slowly. After complete deflation, the guidewire is pulled out carefully from the left atrium.

Recapture of the Device

To achieve the smallest sheath size for device delivery, the sheath wall thickness is small, with a resultant decrease in strength. To recapture a device prior to its release, the operator should hold the sheath at the groin with the left hand, and, with the right hand, pull the delivery cable forcefully inside the sheath. If the sheath is damaged or kinked (accordion effect), use the exchange (rescue) system to change the damaged sheath. First, extend the length of the cable by screwing the tip of the rescue cable to the proximal end of the cable attached to the device. Then remove the sheath or, if the sheath is 9F or 12F, introduce the dilator of the rescue system over the cable inside the sheath until it reaches a few centimeters from the tip of the sheath. This dilator will significantly strengthen the sheath, allowing the operator to pull back the cable with the dilator as one unit inside it. Then the operator can decide what to do next (change the entire sheath system or the device).

Release of the Device With a Prominent Eustachian Valve

To avoid the possibility of cable entrapment during release, advance the sheath to the hub of the right disc. Then release the cable and immediately draw back inside the sheath before the position of the sheath is changed.

Closure of Multiple Secundum ASD

If two defects are present and separated by more than 7 mm from each other, cross each defect separately. Size each one, and then leave a delivery system in each defect. Initially deploy the smaller device, then the larger device, and release sequentially, starting with the smaller one.

If there are multiple fenestrations, use the Amplatzer multifenestrated septal occluder–"Cribriform" (these devices are similar in design to the Amplatzer PFO occluder except that the two discs are equal in size). The device should be deployed in the middle of the septum so that it can cover all fenestrations.

Complications

In the U.S. phase II trial comparing device closure to open surgical closure,[14] the incidence of complications was 7.2% for device closure, far less than that encountered when using an open surgical technique (24%). Most complications were related to rhythm disturbances, with very few patients requiring long-term medical therapy. Complications included the following:

1. *Device embolization*: The majority of which were encountered during the early learning curve of the investigators.
2. *Heart block*: Rarely reported. Most likely related to the use of an oversized device.
3. *Atrial arrhythmia*: Significant increase in atrial arrhythmias following device placement, generally resolving by 6 months.
4. *Headaches*: Reported in about 5% of patients following device placement, resolving within 6 months. The use of clopidogrel for 2–3 months after device closure has minimized this complication significantly.

Results

Long-term success is associated with a decrease in RV size, decrease in pulmonary hypertension, inhibition of any shunt and absence of an arrhythmia. Closure rates have been similar to those achieved by open surgical results. However, patients who underwent device closure were somewhat older than those who underwent open surgical closure.

Furthermore the cost of device closure was much less than open surgical closure, and the length of hospital stay was shorter (1 day) for the device group than the surgical group (3.4 days). In a study by Kim and Hijazi,[15] the mean cost for transcatheter closure was $11,541, whereas for surgical closure it was $21,780.

Gore Cardioform Septal Occluder Device

The Gore Cardioform septal occluder device (WL Gore & Associates) is a non–self-centering double-disc device made from five platinum-filled nitinol wires shaped into a right and a left atrial disc, three eyelets, and a locking loop. It is almost completely covered by an expanded polytetrafluoroethylene (ePTFE) membrane (Fig. 16.7). The delivery system consists of a 10F delivery catheter with a 75-cm working length, a control catheter, and a mandrel coupled to a handle that can be easily operated to load, deploy, reposition, and lock the occluder. The occluder is fully retrievable through a retrieval cord. The device is available in sizes from 15 to 30 mm in 5-mm increments. The delivery system fits through an 11F short sheath, and the delivery system can be advanced via monorail over an 0.035-inch wire. Figs. 16.7 and 16.8 demonstrate schematic and real delivery systems of the Gore Cardioform septal occluder.

The device is designed to be flexible and atraumatic, molding itself to the atrial septum and contiguous structures, thus rendering it particularly appealing for use in a growing heart. Similarly the proven low thrombogenicity of ePTFE imparts confidence in delivering devices on the systemic side of the circulation (left atrium). This is of particular relevance in closure of the PFO where there are implications of thrombotic events to the systemic circulation producing transient ischemic

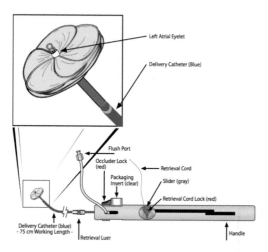

Figure 16.7 Schematic representation of the Gore Cardioform atrial septal defect (ASD) closure device and the delivery system.

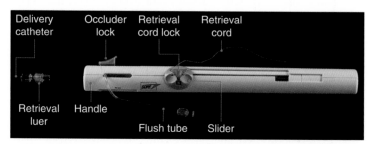

Figure 16.8 The actual delivery system with its various components.

attacks and strokes. ePTFE has been used in various formats as patches and vascular tubes in the growing heart for almost 30 years and thus has proven longevity and biocompatibility with rapid endothelialization characteristics. Studies particular to the Helex device (first generation) have confirmed this excellent biocompatibility.

Patient Selection

The Gore Cardioform Septal Occluder is designed to occlude only the central (secundum) type ASD. The morphology of secundum ASDs is variable, and multiple defects, fenestrated, and aneurysmal ASDs can be closed using this device. A deficient aortic rim, where there is a lack of effacement of the atrial septum at the aorta, can also be accommodated by relative oversizing of the device.

With a non–self-centering device, a device-to-defect diameter ratio of 1.8–2:1 is recommended for ASD closure. With the largest available device being 30 mm, the largest diameter defect that would be closable would be in the range of 15 to 17 mm. In addition, children with large ASDs tend to have a relatively small left atrium. Operators should also be aware that defects measuring more than 15 mm on a standard TTE and with a balloon to size 18 mm or more will be unsuitable for the device.

Technique of Closure

Anesthesia. In children, general anesthesia is required, usually with endotracheal intubation. In adults, conscious sedation can be used if ICE is used; if TEE is planned, general anesthesia is required. In our practice we use ICE exclusively because it has excellent image quality and because endotracheal intubation can be avoided.

Vascular Access. Venous access is established in a manner similar to that described for the ASO device. Heparin 70 U/kg is administered intravenously. A hemodynamic study is performed to assess the shunt and pulmonary artery pressure and resistance. Echocardiography demonstrates the morphology of the ASD with respect to size, margins, proximity to the aorta, and atrioventricular valves. At this stage, multiple defects not apparent on TTE may be imaged, as well as fenestrations and aneurysms of the septum.

The same steps for the ASO are used when placing the Gore Cardioform Septal Occluder device. However, for device size, we use a device size that is 1.8–2:1 the size of the "balloon diameter."

Loading the Device. The Cardioform device is supplied with its own delivery catheter (Fig. 16.8) such that a long Mullins-type sheath is not necessary. The delivery system consists of a 10F delivery catheter with 75 cm working length, a control catheter, and a mandrel. A 0.035-inch guidewire channel is incorporated into the distal end of the delivery catheter; therefore, the delivery system can be tracked in a monorail fashion over this wire.

Loading the Occluder Into the Delivery Catheter
Occluder Preparation and Loading

1. Check the "use by" (expiration date) and the condition of the package.
2. Using aseptic technique, remove the sterile tray from the pouch and remove the packaging tray lid.
3. Remove the device from the package and visually inspect the device for shipping damage. Ensure that the Retrieval Luer is tight.
4. Remove the packaging insert from the handle.
5. Load and flush the occluder:
   a. Submerge the Occluder and catheter tip in a heparinized saline bath during loading to reduce the chance of air entrapment in the delivery system.

    b. Fill a syringe with heparinized saline.

    c. Attach the syringe to a stopcock and the flush port.

6. Flush the device until air no longer exits the tip of the delivery catheter.

7. When the initial flushing is completed, begin loading the Occluder by pushing the slider up to the right until the slider stops.

8. Complete Occluder loading by pushing the slider down and then to the right until it stops.

9. Flush the device again until air no longer exits the tip of the delivery catheter.

10. If additional air removal is desired, it is recommended to deploy the Occluder and repeat steps 6–10 above.

Device Delivery. Load the delivery catheter onto a guidewire through the guidewire port from the luminal surface out; ensure that the occluder is sufficiently withdrawn into the delivery catheter to avoid interference with the guidewire (monorail system). Load the delivery system into the appropriately sized introducer sheath.

Deployment

LA Disc Deployment

1. Under direct fluoroscopic visualization, advance the catheter tip across the ASD until the radiopaque marker at the tip of the delivery catheter is positioned within the middle left atrium. Verify that the tip of the delivery catheter is across the defect and away from the LA appendage using TEE or ICE. Figs. 16.9 and 16.10 demonstrate closure of an atrial septal defect in the same patient under ICE and fluoroscopy guidance.

2. At this stage, the guidewire should be removed before attempting to deploy the occluder.

3. Begin deploying the Occluder left disc by pushing the slider to the left until it stops.

4. Complete Occluder left disc deployment by pushing the slider up and then to the left until a flat left disc has formed. This step may be performed while simultaneously retracting the delivery system to minimize advancement of the Occluder within the left atrial chamber.

5. Gently pull on the handle to bring the left atrial disc onto the surface of the left atrial septum.

6. Deploy the right atrial disc by pushing the slider to the left until it stops and then down. Confirm that the slider has moved completely to the left and down position. Failure to move the slider completely to the left and down position may prevent Occluder locking. Confirm that both left and right discs appear planar and apposed to the septum with septal tissue between the discs.

7. Prior to Occluder locking, assess that the Occluder position and defect closure are acceptable and that the delivery system is not exerting tension on the septum and Occluder.

8. Lock the Occluder by holding the handle in a fixed position to prevent applying tension on the Occluder. Note that excessive compression of the handle may prevent Occluder locking. Next, squeeze and then slide the Occluder lock decisively and with a consistent amount of force to the right. At the completion of Occluder locking, the Occluder is still attached to the delivery system by the retrieval cord. During the Occluder locking step, the delivery catheter moves proximally and may exert minimal tension on the introducer sheath. It is recommended to

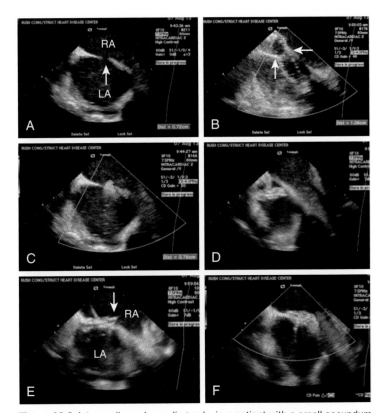

Figure 16.9 Intracardiac echocardiography in a patient with a small secundum atrial septal defect (ASD). (A,C) Septal view, demonstrating the ASD (*arrow*) without and with color Doppler, the right and left atria, and the superior and inferior rims. (B) The left atrial disc (*arrow*) deployed in the left atrium; balloon sizing of the defect, measuring the stop flow diameter, between the two arrows. (D) The left atrial disc is well seen in the left atrium. (E) The right atrial disc (*arrow*) is deployed in the right atrium. (F) After the device has been released, demonstrating good device position and no residual flow by color Doppler.

confirm adequate introducer sheath insertion prior to Occluder locking.

9. If the Occluder position is acceptable, hold the handle in a fixed position, pull up on the red retrieval cord lock, disengage it from the slider, and gently pull the retrieval cord lock until the retrieval cord has been completely removed from the handle.

10. The Occluder is now released from the delivery system, and the delivery system can be removed.

11. Once the retrieval cord is removed, the Occluder cannot be removed using the delivery system.

Device Recapture

1. In the event that the Occluder is malpositioned, embolized, or otherwise requires removal, it may be recaptured with the aid of a loop snare or other suitable means. A long sheath (11F or greater) positioned close to the device is recommended for recapture.

2. Attempt to recapture the device by first snaring the left or right atrial eyelet to facilitate Occluder retraction into the sheath. If necessary, the loop snare may be placed around any portion of the Occluder frame.

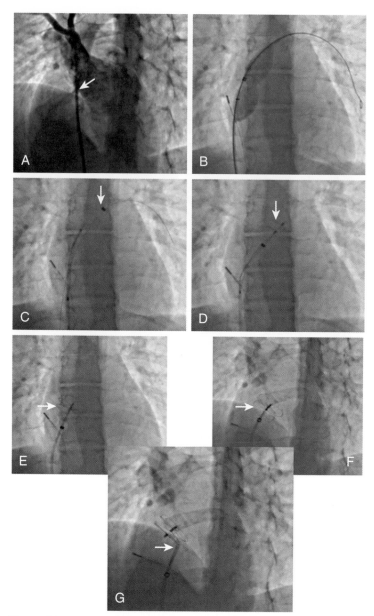

Figure 16.10 Cineangiographic image in the same patient as Fig. 16.9. (A) Angiogram in the right upper pulmonary vein in the four-chamber view, demonstrating the atrial septal defect (*arrow*). (B) Cine fluoroscopy in the straight frontal projection during balloon sizing, demonstrating the constrictions in the balloon. (C) Cine fluoroscopy in the straight frontal projection during passage of the delivery system with its radiopaque tip (*arrow*) over the guidewire in the left upper pulmonary vein. D, cine fluoroscopy in the straight frontal projection after the left atrial disc (*arrow*) has been deployed in the left atrium. (E) Cine fluoroscopy in the straight frontal projection after the right atrial disc (*arrow*) has been deployed. (F) Cine fluoroscopy in the four-chamber view after the right atrial disc (*arrow*) has been deployed and just released from delivery catheter. (G) Final cine fluoroscopy in the four-chamber view after the delivery catheter (*arrow*) has been fully disengaged from the right atrial disc.

3. Pull the Occluder into the long sheath using the snare. If a portion of the Occluder frame cannot be retracted into the long sheath, it may be necessary to remove the Occluder, loop snare, and long sheath as one unit. Do not use excessive force in an attempt to withdraw all of the Occluder into the long sheath. Doing so could result in Occluder damage.

4. Bring the recaptured Occluder into the sheath to avoid pulling the unlocked device across valve tissue.

Complications

Serious complications following Gore Cardioform Septal Occluder closure of an ASD are rare. Embolization occurs, but almost always the device can be retrieved using a snare device and a long 10F sheath. Wire fractures have been seen in a small percentage of patients using the first-generation device (about 5%–6%) and are usually of no clinical consequence because the wire is held secure by the fabric of the device and its comprehensive endothelialization. A wire frame fracture was observed in 9.3% (4/43) of subjects with fluoroscopic evaluation completed at 6 months. No fractures were associated with device instability or clinical sequelae.[16]

Results

Early experience has demonstrated the ease of use of this device, its complete retrievability, and excellent closure of small to moderate ASDs in children. All subjects with an atrial septal aneurysm, multiple fenestrations, or deficient retroaortic rim who received a Gore Cardioform Septal Occluder had complete clinical closure and no serious adverse events at 6 months.[17]

Occlutech Figulla Flex-II Septal Occluder (OFF-II)

The OFF-II is a flexible nitinol mesh that constitutes the left and right discs. The device is very similar to the ASO, but with the absence of the connecting microscrew into the left atrial disc, which improves flexibility and the softness of the device. The ball-and-socket delivery mechanism allows for greater flexibility during deployment, which may be beneficial for large ASDs and deficient rims. Angles are created between the left and right discs that conform to superior alignment after release. These unique features make it an attractive option for complex defects. In a randomized multicenter clinical trial comparing the OFF-II with the ASO, the OFF-II was as successful as the ASO in closing defects.[18] The device required less attempts to align it across the atrial septum compared to the ASO. This may be due to the unique delivery system of the OFF-II device. Furthermore, to date, no case of erosion has been reported with this device. Fig. 16.11 demonstrates the Occlutech Figulla Flex-II device with its delivery system.

Cera Septal Occluder

Cera is a new double-disc ASD occluder. The structure includes a self-expandable nitinol frame covered with bioceramic titanium nitride coating. The left disc is larger than the right, with a short 4-mm connecting waist. A recently published study compared 405 patients who were nonrandomized to Cera ($n = 205$) or the ASO ($n = 200$) for simple and complex ASD closure with a mean follow-up of 13 months. The noninferiority safety and feasibility of the Cera device was demonstrated with a high success in deployment rate (97%) and small residual shunt in both groups (99.5%) at end of follow-up.[19]

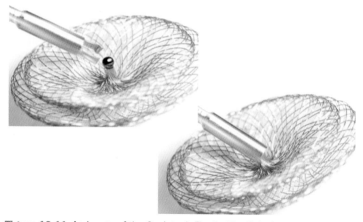

Figure 16.11 An image of the Occlutech Figulla Flex-II device and the delivery system.

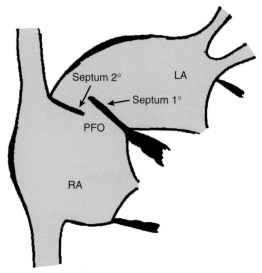

Figure 16.12 Schematic sketch demonstrating the patent foramen ovale (PFO) as a flaplike structure created between septum primum (1°) and septum secundum (2°).

Patent Foramen Ovale

A PFO is part of normal fetal development. Following birth, with an increase in pulmonary blood flow and higher LA relative to RA pressure, the foramen ovale physiologically closes. The foramen is created by the overlap of the septum primum and septum secundum (Fig. 16.12) and fuses closed in later life. This anatomy can behave like a flap valve, opening if the RA pressure exceeds the LA pressure. Pathologic studies have suggested that the foramen ovale may be probe-patent in 25% of the population.

There are three anatomic types: (1) the "flap" type, (2) the tunnel type, and (3) the aneurysmal septum primum with a PFO.

Clinical Significance

A PFO is a potential source for right-to-left intracardiac shunt and can result in paradoxical emboli. Presentation is usually in the third or fourth decade of life and rarely in adolescence.

Cerebrovascular Accident

Paradoxical emboli crossing the PFO, with associated neurologic deficits (or stroke) or other systemic events, are the most easily recognized manifestations of PFO. Cryptogenic stroke (stroke with no identifiable cause) accounts for 40% of strokes in young adults. A PFO was present in 39% of the patients younger than 55 years with cryptogenic stroke compared to 29% in patients with an identifiable cause for the stroke.[10] In addition, certain anatomic features such as large defects (>5 mm), persistent right-to-left shunt at rest, 10 or more microbubbles appearing in the left atrium with a contrast TEE, atrial septal aneurysm (ASA), and presence of a prominent eustachian valve have been associated with a greater risk of paradoxical embolism. ASA is found in approximately 35% of patients with PFO. The other anatomic features were present in 20% of the cryptogenic group versus 9.7% of those patients with an identifiable cause for their stroke.[10]

Risk of Recurrence After a Presumed Cryptogenic Transient Ischemic Attack or Stroke

A recurrence risk of 3%–5% has been reported in most series with medical management of embolic stroke. However, the Warfarin-Aspirin Recurrent Stroke Study (WARSS) yielded a recurrent event or death over a 2-year period of 15% with warfarin and 17% with aspirin when the subset of patients with cryptogenic stroke-only was analyzed.[20] The Mayo Clinic reported a 4.1% recurrence rate of any neurologic event following surgical closure of PFO.[21] It is likely that a percentage of these represent patients in whom the hypothesis that their problem resulted from a paradoxical embolus was incorrect.

There has been inconsistent data on the role of percutaneous closure of PFO in patients with cryptogenic stroke. Recently, three randomized studies have been published (CLOSURE, RESPECT, and PC-trial). None of these demonstrated that percutaneous closure was associated with a decreased incidence of stroke compared to medical treatment with antiplatelet agents or anticoagulants. Nevertheless some subanalyses and meta-analyses of these studies have shown that percutaneous closure of PFO could be beneficial for certain patient groups, especially those with high PFO anatomic features.

However a recent presentation of the extended follow-up of patients who enrolled in the RESPECT trial demonstrated that, with longer follow-up (up to 5.5 years), the trial reached its primary end point of proving that the risk reduction was significant:

1. With device in place, the relative risk reduction is 70% ($p = 0.004$).
2. For patients younger than 60 years, the relative risk reduction for all strokes was 52% ($p = 0.035$).
3. For patients with atrial septal aneurysm and large shunt, the relative risk reduction was 75% ($p = 0.007$).

Based on these data, one can be optimistic that the U.S. FDA will view positively the extended follow-up of patients enrolled in the RESPECT trial.[22]

Systemic Embolization

Patients with a PFO are at risk of systemic embolization, especially in the presence of an indwelling catheter, a pacemaker electrode, or deep vein thrombosis (DVT). Embolization to the coronary artery and peripheral circulation in the presence of these conditions has been reported.[10]

Migraine

Migraine is a chronic neurologic disease characterized by recurrent headache. The condition affects 8%–13% of the adult population and is usually associated with autonomic symptoms or aura. Between 47%

and 48% of patients with migraine have PFO, compared with between 17% and 20% of individuals in the general population.[10]

Platypnea-Orthododeoxia Syndrome

This syndrome is a little-known condition that is hard to diagnose. The main clinical finding is dyspnea or hypoxemia when standing upright. These symptoms typically improve in the decubitus position. The syndrome usually occurs in elderly individuals and has been associated with aortic elongation and other co-morbidities such as pneumonectomy, pulmonary emphysema, and liver cirrhosis which can lead to vena cava displacement when standing. Thus, in patients with PFO, the blood flow is directed toward the vena cava and right-to-left shunt occurs. Diagnosis is made by measuring arterial saturation at different potential shunt locations within the heart. A dynamic echocardiogram can also be recorded to demonstrate PFO. Definitive treatment of platypnea-orthodeoxia syndrome is percutaneous closure of the PFO. Success rates are close to 100%, and the rate of complications is low.[10]

Deep-Sea and Scuba Divers

An interesting group of PFO patients are those who are deep-sea or scuba divers. This population may report decompression sickness with unusual symptoms despite following an appropriate and rigid protocol during a dive ascent. An incidence of neurologic symptoms as high as 61% has been reported. Decompression problems have also led to more brain defects in individuals with PFO than without.[10]

Other conditions that might be related to PFO include high altitude pulmonary edema, obstructive sleep apnea exacerbation, and cerebral white matter lesions.[10]

Transcatheter Closure of PFO

The indications for PFO closure should be tailored according to the clinical presentations. Several devices are currently designed to specifically close a PFO: the Amplatzer PFO occluder (St. Jude Medical, Minneapolis MN), the Figulla Flex PFO occluder (Occlutech GmbH), and the PFO Star devices (NMT Medical). The Gore Cardioform Septal occluder (WL Gore & Associates) was designed for ASD closure; however, it has also been used for PFO closure.

The Amplatzer PFO Occluder

The Amplatzer PFO occluder is a self-expanding, double-disc device made from a nitinol wire mesh (see Fig. 16.1). The nitinol mesh wire is 0.005–0.006 inches in diameter. The two discs are linked together by a connecting waist 2 mm in diameter and 4 mm in length. This thin waist allows free motion of each disc so that the device can conform to the PFO shape as the operator positions the two discs in the plane of the atrial septum. The discs are filled with a polyester fabric sewn securely to each disc by a polyester thread. The polyester increases the closing ability of the device by trapping blood, thus forming the initial plug and promoting the endothelialization of the device.

The devices are available in three sizes—18, 25, and 35 mm—corresponding to the diameter of the right disc. The diameter of the left disc is 18 mm for the 18- and 25-mm devices and 25 mm for the 35-mm device. The connecting waist is the same for both—2 mm in diameter and 4 mm in length. The devices are packaged individually and supplied sterilized and ready for use.

Amplatzer Delivery System

This Amplatzer delivery system is the same as the secundum ASD delivery systems; the PFO occluder devices deploy through a 7–9F sheath. The device is not approved in the United States and is under a clinical trial protocol (the RESPECT trial, which was completed but awaiting FDA decision).

Contraindications

See contraindications for secundum ASD device closure.

Step-by-Step Technique: Transcatheter Closure of PFO

Materials, Equipment, and Personnel. These are the same as for secundum ASD. The preprocedure evaluation is also the same.

Vascular Access. Place a 7F sheath in the right femoral vein. An arterial monitoring line can be useful if the procedure is performed under TEE guidance with general anesthesia. Administer a full heparin dose, and administer antibiotics as for secundum ASD. Perform a right heart hemodynamic study. Perform a TEE/ICE to assess the anatomy of the PFO and to perform a contrast bubble study with and without the Valsalva maneuver.

Some operators determine the septal length and the distance of the surrounding structures, especially the free wall of the atrium. The type of PFO—simple flap, tunnel, or PFO with an aneurysmal septum primum—may influence device selection.

Suggested Measurements With TEE/ICE Images

1. Measure the total septal length and edge of the defect to the mitral valve in the four-chamber view.
2. Measure the distance from SVC to the edge of the defect (long-axis TEE view/caval view by ICE).
3. Measure the distance from the defect to the aorta in short-axis view. Do not implant a device if the distance either from the defect to the SVC or from defect to the aortic root is less than 9 mm.

Device Selection

For defects without an aneurysmal septum primum, use the 18- or 25-mm device, depending on the length of the septum. If there is a significant aneurysm or if the septum primum appears very thin and floppy, use the 35-mm device as long as the distance from the SVC to the edge of the defect and from the edge of the defect to the aortic root is greater than 17.5 mm. If there is an aneurysm and the distance from the edge of the defect to either the SVC or aortic root is between 12.5 and 17.5 mm, the 25-mm device should be used.

Procedure Steps

The procedure is identical to that described for secundum ASD except that balloon sizing is not performed. Prior to device release, careful reassessment of the edge of the device along the free atrial wall by TEE/ICE is needed. Do not release the device if it does not conform to its original configuration or if it appears unstable. In this case, the operator should recapture and redeploy the device. Figs. 16.13, 16.14, 16.15, and 16.16 demonstrate the steps of PFO closure.

Postprocedure follow-up is similar to that for secundum ASD closure except that most investigators maintain 81 to 325 mg/day aspirin for 6 months in combination with an antiplatelet agent, usually clopidogrel 75 mg/day, for 1–6 months. Follow-up echocardiogram at 3–6 months should include assessment for right-to-left atrial level shunt with a venous contrast injection, with Valsalva maneuver.

Complications

RA and Aortic Perforation. A total of two patients in the worldwide data (none in the United States) had this complication. There was one case report by Trepel et al. in a patient who presented with pericardial

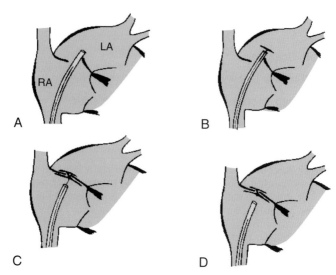

Figure 16.13 Schematic demonstration of patent foramen ovale (PFO) closure using the Amplatzer PFO occluder. (A) Sheath in mid left atrium. (B) Deployment of left atrial disc. (C) Deployment of connecting waist and right atrial disc. (D) Device released.

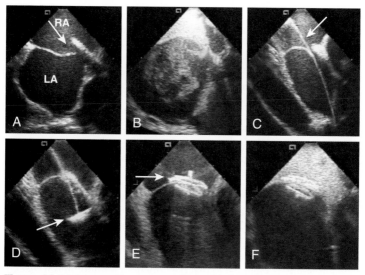

Figure 16.14 Intracardiac echocardiographic images in a young patient who has a patent foramen ovale (PFO), demonstrating the steps of closure. (A) Septal view demonstrating the PFO (*arrow*) and the thin septum primum. (B) Contrast bubble study demonstrating significant right-to-left shunt. (C) Guidewire (*arrow*) positioned through the defect into the left pulmonary vein. (D) Deployment of the left atrial disc (*arrow*). (E) Deployment of the right atrial disc (*arrow*); release of the device. (F) Contrast bubble study repeated after the device has been released, demonstrating successful closure.

tamponade. At surgery, erosion of the RA roof and aortic root was noted. Following this report, the company (St. Jude Medical, St. Paul, MN) introduced the septal measurements, emphasizing the distance of the free RA wall from the defect/device.

Entrapment of Prominent Eustachian Valve on the Delivery Cable. This caused no problems with device delivery and release, but part of the eustachian valve was avulsed. To avoid this, prior to release, advance the sheath to the hub of the right-side disc.

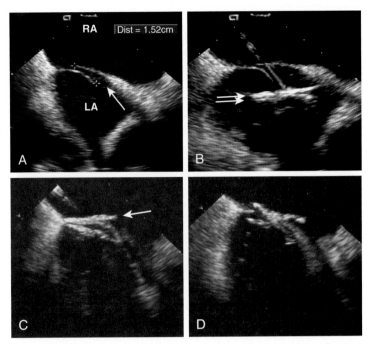

Figure 16.15 Intracardiac echocardiography in a patient with patent foramen ovale (PFO). (A) Septal view, demonstrating the PFO (*arrow*) and the thin septum primum. (B) The left atrial disc (*arrow*) deployed in the left atrium. (C) The right atrial disc (*arrow*) deployed in the right atrium. (D) The device released, demonstrating good position.

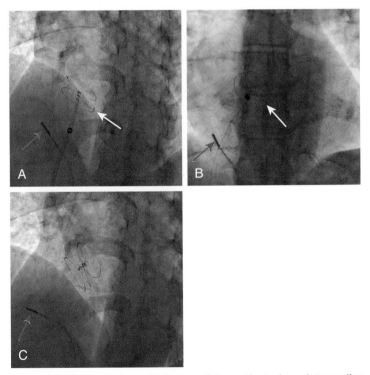

Figure 16.16 Cineangiographic image of the patient whose intracardiac echocardiogram is shown in Fig. 16.14. (A) The left atrial disc (*white arrow*) deployed in the left atrium. (B) The right atrial disc deployed in the right atrium. (C) The device released, demonstrating good position. Red arrow shows position of intracardiac echo transducer.

Results

During phase I of the U.S. clinical Helex trial for ASD, closure rates were in excess of 95% at 3–6 months follow-up. There were no complications related to the device. The length of hospital stay was about 1 day. No episodes of atrial arrhythmias have been reported.

PFO Closure With Helex or With Gore Cardioform Septal Occluder Devices

Both devices are flexible, with low profiles and low thrombogenicity, and both are suitable devices to close the PFO in patients with cryptogenic stroke. The devices are suited to all types of PFO except perhaps those associated with a long flap-like tunnel in excess of 8 mm from the RA to LA aspect. The Helex device is being evaluated in a randomized study (the REDUCE trial) against continued medical therapy for the prevention of stroke recurrence. Closure rates approach 100%, and rates of thrombus formation and recurrent cerebrovascular events have been very low. The enrollment was completed in 2015, and data are being collected for analysis.

Figulla Flex PFO Occluder (FPO)

The FPO occluder comprises two discs made of nitinol wire mesh connected by a 3-mm center waist. Two thin polyethylene terephthalate (PET) patches are integrated into the disc to allow faster sealing of the defect and optimized ingrowth of tissue. A central hub is only located at the RA side of the occluder. The device comes in four sizes: 16/18 mm, 23/25 mm, 27/30 mm, and 31/35 mm for the left and right atrial disc size, respectively. As unique braiding technique, the LA side has a minimal amount of meshwork material, and the entire device is low-profile for easy deliverability. It comes with a single- or double-layered PET patch on the LA side. The double-layer device is specifically designed to provide additional flexibility in patients with challenging anatomy (e.g., tunnel morphology and/or ASA). A self-centering mechanism assists delivery of the system by enabling optimal positioning and repositioning. The delivery system has a locking and retrieval mechanism that allows angulation up to 50 degrees. Sheath size ranges from 7F to 11F.

References

1. Warnes CA, Williams RG, Bashore TM, et al. ACC/AHA 2008 Guidelines for the management of adults with congenital heart disease: executive summary: a report of the American College of Cardiology/American Heart Association task force on practice guidelines. *Circulation*. 2008;118(23):2395-2451.
2. Schueler R1, Öztürk C, Wedekind JA, et al. Persistence of iatrogenic atrial septal defect after interventional mitral valve repair with the MitraClip system: a note of caution. *JACC Cardiovasc Interv*. 2015;8(3):450-459.
3. Sommer RJ, Hijazi ZM, Rhodes JF Jr. Pathophysiology of congenital heart disease in the adult: Part I: shunt lesions. *Circulation*. 2008;117(8):1090-1099.
4. Hossein D, Andrew JB. Percutaneous device closure of secundum atrial septal defect in older adults. *Am J Cardiovasc Dis*. 2012;2(2):133-142.
5. Gatzoulis MA, Rodington AN, Somerville J, et al. Should atrial septal defects in adults be closed? *Ann Thorac Surg*. 1996;61:657-659.
6. Silvestry FE, Cohen MS, Armsby LB, et al. Guidelines for the echocardiographic assessment of atrial septal defect and patent foramen ovale: from the American Society of Echocardiography and Society for Cardiac Angiography and Interventions. *J Am Soc Echocardiogr*. 2015;28(8):910-958.
7. Al-Hindi A, Cao QL, Hijazi ZM. Transcatheter closure of secundum atrial septal defect in the elderly. *J Invasive Cardiol*. 2009;21(2):70-75.
8. Nie JG, Dong JZ, Salim M, et al. Catheter ablation of atrial fibrillation in patients with atrial septal defect: long-term follow-up results. *J Interv Card Electrophysiol*. 2015;42(1):43-49.
9. Balint OH, Samman A, Haberer K, et al. Outcomes in patients with pulmonary hypertension undergoing percutaneous atrial septal closure. *Heart*. 2008;94:1189-1193.

10. Tobis J, Shenoda M. Percutaneous treatment of patent foramen ovale and atrial septal defects. *J Am Coll Cardiol*. 2012;60(18):1722-1732.

11. Zuber M, Gautschi N, Oechslin E, et al. Outcome of pregnancy in women with congenital shunt lesions. *Heart*. 1999;81(3):271-281.

12. Murphy JG, Gersh BJ, McGoon MD, et al. Long-term outcome after surgical repair of isolated atrial septal defect: follow-up at 27 to 32 years. *N Engl J Med*. 1990;323:1645-1650.

13. Amin Z. Transcatheter closure of secundum atrial septal defects. *Catheter Cardiovasc Interv*. 2006;68:778-787.

14. Du ZD, Hijazi ZM, Kleinman CS, et al. Amplatzer investigators. Comparison between transcatheter and surgical closure of secundum atrial septal defect in children and adults. *J Am Coll Cardiol*. 2002;39:1836-1844.

15. Kim JJ, Hijazi ZM. Clinical outcomes and costs of Amplatzer transcatheter closure as compared with surgical closure of ostium secundum atrial septal defects. *Med Sci Monit*. 2002;8(12):787-791.

16. Jones TK, Latson LA, Zahn E, et al. Multicenter pivotal study of the HELEX septal occluder investigators. Results of the U.S. multicenter pivotal study of the HELEX septal occluder for percutaneous closure of secundum atrial septal defects. *J Am Coll Cardiol*. 2007;49:2215-2221.

17. Freixa X, Ibrahim R, Chan J, et al. Initial clinical experience with the GORE septal occluder for the treatment of atrial septal defects and patent foramen ovale. *EurIntervention*. 2013;9(5):629-635.

18. Godart F, Houeijeh A, Recher M, et al. Transcatheter closure of atrial septal defect with the Figulla ASD Occluder: a comparative study with the Amplatzer Septal Occluder. *Arch Cardiovasc Dis*. 2015;108(1):57-63.

19. Astarcioglu MA, Kalcik M, Sen T, et al. Ceraflex versus Amplatzer occluder for secundum atrial septal defect closure. Multicenter clinical experience. *Herz*. 2015;40(suppl 2):146-150.

20. Mohr JP, Thompson JL, Lazar RM, et al. Warfarin-Aspirin Recurrent Stroke Study Group. A comparison of warfarin and aspirin for the prevention of recurrent ischemic stroke. *N Engl J Med*. 2001;345:1444-1451.

21. Hagen PT, Scholz DG, Edwards WD. Incidence and size of patent foramen ovale during the first 10 decades of life: an autopsy study of 965 normal hearts. *Mayo Clin Proc*. 1984;59:17-20.

22. Nietlispach F, Meier B. Percutaneous closure of patent foramen ovale: safe and effective but underutilized. *Expert Rev Cardiovasc Ther*. 2015;13(2):121-123.

17

Pericardiocentesis

PAUL SORAJJA

Cardiac tamponade is a life-threatening disorder that can result from any condition that causes a pericardial effusion. In the cardiac catheterization laboratory, tamponade can result as a complication of any invasive procedure and lead to the rapid demise of the patient due to the swift accumulation of fluid in a poorly compliant pericardial space. Other common causes of tamponade are pericarditis (e.g., viral, uremic, inflammatory, or idiopathic), aortic dissection with disruption of the aortic annulus, malignancy, and ventricular rupture from myocardial infarction. The prompt recognition of the salient hemodynamic features and immediate pericardiocentesis are essential to the successful treatment of cardiac tamponade.

Diagnosis of Cardiac Tamponade

The hemodynamic effects of a pericardial effusion may be acute or gradual, depending on the amount and rate of fluid accumulation. The rate of pericardial fluid accumulation relative to the stiffness of the pericardium determines how quickly the clinical syndrome of tamponade will occur (Fig. 17.1). Normally the pericardial space contains 15–50 mL of fluid with an intrapericardial pressure that approximates intrapleural pressure (–5 to +5 cm H_2O). Fluid accumulation and pericardial restraint lead to rises in intrapericardial pressure. Tamponade occurs when intrapericardial pressure exceeds intracardiac pressure, leading to impaired ventricular filling throughout diastole, increases in pulmonary venous and jugular venous pressures, and reduction in forward stroke volume.

The operator should have a high index of suspicion of tamponade during a procedure whenever hypotension occurs. Tachycardia also is usually present, though may not be evident in patients receiving negative chronotropic agents. Clinical risk factors for tamponade include poor distal positioning of guidewires, oversized stents, use of rotational atherectomy, transseptal puncture, and structural heart interventional procedures (e.g., transcatheter aortic valve replacement, balloon aortic valvuloplasty, mitral valvuloplasty, left atrial appendage closure, etc.). Some proceduralists prefer to have the chest and subxiphoid area sterilized and a periocardiocentesis tray readily available when performing high-risk procedures in order to be able to quickly address tamponade if it occurs.

Echocardiography

Two-dimensional and Doppler echocardiography are commonly used for diagnosing cardiac tamponade. Specific signs of tamponade include collapse of the right atrium and right ventricle, ventricular septal shifting with respiration, and plethora (enlargement) of the inferior vena cava (Fig. 17.2). Respiratory variation in the Doppler mitral inflow is a highly sensitive measure that occurs early in tamponade and may precede

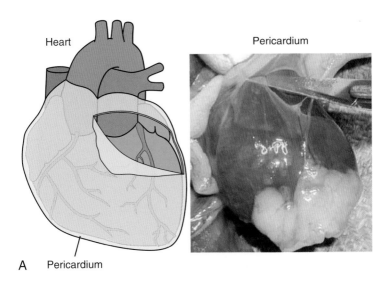

A Pericardium

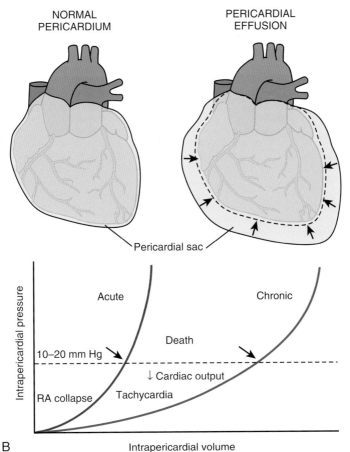

B

Figure 17.1 (A) Pericardium is normally a thin membrane but can thicken with disease and can produce tamponade with a small amount of fluid when not compliant. (B) Illustration of compliance curves and cardiac tamponade. Normal pericardium (A) has steep low-compliance pressure–volume relationship as compared to chronic pericardial effusion with a distensible pericardium (B) producing tamponade only later in its course. *(From Holmes DR, et al. Iatrogenic pericardial effusion and tamponade in the percutaneous intracardiac intervention era JACC Cardiovasc Interv. 2009;2:705–717.)*

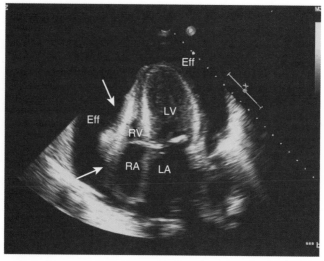

Figure 17.2 Echocardiographic image of pericardial tamponade with right-sided chamber collapse. *LA,* left atrium; *LV,* left ventricle; *RA,* right atrium; *RV,* right ventricle; *Eff* (pericardial) effusion. *(From Holmes DR, et al. Iatrogenic pericardial effusion and tamponade in the percutaneous intracardiac intervention era. JACC Cardiovasc Interv. 2009;2:705–717.)*

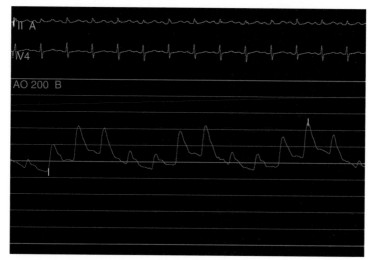

Figure 17.3 Arterial pressure in a patient with dyspnea at rest demonstrating pulsus paradoxus due to cardiac tamponade.

changes in cardiac output, blood pressure, and other echocardiographic findings.

Invasive Hemodynamics

The invasive hemodynamic hallmarks of cardiac tamponade are pulsus paradoxus on the arterial tracing (Fig. 17.3) and prominent *x* descents and blunted *y* descents in the atrial pressure tracings (Fig. 17.4). Preservation of the *x* descent occurs because of the decrease in intracardiac volume during systolic ejection, which leads to a temporary reduction in intrapericardial and right atrial pressures. Elevated intrapericardial pressure impairs ventricular filling during the remainder of the cardiac cycle, resulting in blunting of the *y* descent. Blunting of the ventricular minimum pressures also occurs, corresponding to impairment of filling in early diastole. In patients with cardiac tamponade, the driving

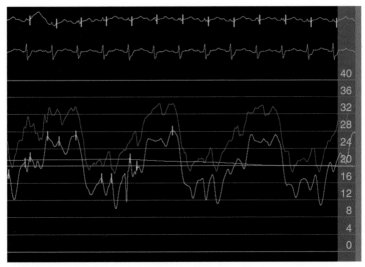

Figure 17.4 Hemodynamics of right atrial (RA) pressure (*red*) and pericardial pressure (*blue*); scale is 0–40 mm Hg. There is matching of phasic waveforms, but RA is higher due to zero offset.

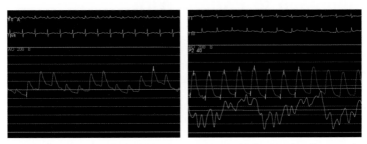

Figure 17.5 Hemodynamics of arterial pressure before pericardiocentesis (*left*) and after pericardiocentesis (*right*). Pericardial pressure is reduced from 24 to 10 mm Hg (*blue*); scale is 0–40 mm Hg.

pressure to fill the left ventricle falls during inspiration. Consequently there is a reduction in left ventricular filling and stroke volume, which manifests as a decrease in aortic pulse pressure during inspiration in a manner analogous to the bedside finding of pulsus paradoxus (see Fig. 17.3).

On relief of pericardial pressure and removal of the effusion, right atrial pressure and pericardial pressure fall usually to normal values if no residual pericardial disease is present (Fig. 17.5). However, in some cases, although pericardiocentesis empties the pericardial space and pericardial pressure falls to near zero, right atrial pressure may be unaffected, signifying the syndrome of effusive-constrictive pericardial disease (Fig. 17.6).

Cardiac tamponade should be suspected in any patient in the cardiac catheterization laboratory with unexplained hypotension, elevated venous pressure, and a compatible history. Unusual manifestations also can occur. Tamponade may occur without elevated jugular venous pressure because of low intracardiac filling pressures (i.e., low-pressure tamponade), such as in dehydrated patients with malignant effusions. Localized tamponade can result from loculated pericardial effusions, such as those that may be present adjacent to the atria in the postoperative setting. Of note pericardiocentesis should not be performed in patients with tamponade and aortic dissection. In such patients, relief of the tamponade will lead to an abrupt increase in systolic blood pressure that may exacerbate the aortic dissection.

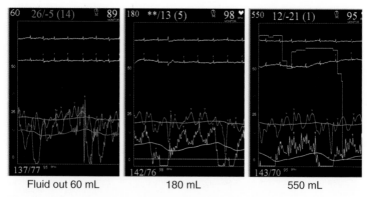

Fluid out 60 mL   180 mL   550 mL

Figure 17.6 Hemodynamics of pericardiocentesis with near normalization of pericardial pressure without change in right atrial (RA) pressure consistent with effusive constrictive pericardial disease.

Careful imaging with transthoracic or transesophageal echocardiography is required to determine the presence of these manifestations of tamponade.

Approach to Patient With Cardiac Tamponade

For all patients, *volume resuscitation* can help provide hemodynamic stability and should be performed in patients with cardiac tamponade. Reversal of anticoagulation and antiplatelet therapy should be performed as clinically permitted. Some proceduralists prefer to defer reversal of anticoagulation until pericardiocentesis has been completed to avoid creation of coagulum, which can complicate aspiration and removal of the pericardial contents. During pericardiocentesis, right heart catheterization with simultaneous measurement of right atrial and pulmonary capillary wedge pressures assist in the diagnosis and for determining the efficacy of the procedure. Pharmacotherapy that increases afterload (vasoconstrictors) or depresses contractility should be avoided because these agents will only exacerbate the impairment in stroke volume that is already present in patients with tamponade.

For most patients, pericardiocentesis is performed with echocardiographic guidance. In some cases, additional use of hemodynamic monitoring through the pericardial needle adds important information during both puncture and after withdrawal of fluid to verify procedural findings. Certainly in emergent situations where echocardiography is not immediately available, pericardiocentesis can be performed in a blind or electrocardiogram (ECG)-guided fashion, usually from the subxiphoid approach. However adjunctive echocardiography plays a significant role in the evaluation of patients with cardiac tamponade and will reduce the incidence of complications related to pericardiocentesis.

Technique for Pericardiocentesis

Box 17.1 lists the equipment commonly used for the pericardiocentesis.

Patient positioning: The patient usually is positioned with head raised approximately 30 degrees to facilitate inferior and apical pooling of the pericardial effusion.

Site of entry: Echocardiography helps to determine the most appropriate site of entry and needle direction (Fig. 17.7). Most frequently the echocardiographic window that is closest to the effusion is selected. Common portals of entry are subxiphoid and apical, but other locations

> **Box 17.1** Equipment for Pericardiocentesis
>
> Sterile gloves, mask, and gown
> Povidone-iodine solution or other skin antiseptic
> Sterile transparent plastic drape
> 20- or 25-gauge needle for local anesthesia administration
> Local anesthesia (e.g., 1% lidocaine)
> 18-gauge polytef-sheathed venous needles of varying lengths (5–8 cm)
> Syringes (10 mL, 20 mL, and 50 mL)
> 0.035-inch J-tipped guidewire
> Scalpel (no. 11 blade)
> 5F or 6F introducer sheath
> 5F or 6F 65-cm pigtail catheter with multiple side holes
> 4 × 4 inch gauze for dressing and ointment
> 1-liter vacuum bottle or comparable fluid receptacle
> Labels for specimen collection
> Sterile isotonic saline (for catheter flush)

have included axillary and left or right parasternal (see Fig. 17.7). Advantages of the subxiphoid approach are lower risks of pneumothorax and laceration of internal mammary or intercostal arteries. For the subxiphoid approach, the needle must be angled and move freely below the bottom rib as it attaches to the inferolateral surface above the xiphoid process (typically one fingerbreadth inferior and lateral to the edge of the xiphoid). Punctures that are too high and near the junction of the xiphoid angle can pose challenges to delivering the needle under the rib. When using a parasternal approach, the needle should pass 1 cm lateral to the sternum to avoid injury to the internal mammary artery; the risk of pneumothorax increases with further lateral positioning. For intercostal approaches the needle should pass superior to the rib margins to reduce the risk of injury to the neurovascular bundle. The angle of entry and direction should be transfixed in the operator's mind. The site of entry can be marked with an indelible pen. The precordial or subxiphoid area is sterilized with antiseptic solution and covered with a sterile drape.

Needle insertion: Following local anesthesia, an 18-gauge, thin-walled polytef-sheathed needle is inserted at the entry site using the predetermined angulation. The needle is advanced with gentle aspiration into the pericardial space. Aggressive aspiration may cause tissue occlusion of the needle and inhibit detection of pericardial fluid. Once fluid has been obtained, the needle is advanced slightly further (~2 mm) to ensure placement of the sheath into the pericardial space. Once the needle is in the pericardial space, the polytef sheath then is advanced over the needle, followed by withdrawal of the needle. The needle should not be readvanced once it has been removed from the sheath. Alternately, a needle and sheath system (e.g., micropuncture kit) can be used. Fig. 17.8 shows a pericardial needle and stopcock arrangement designed to check pericardial pressure, then aspirate pericardial fluid and discharge the fluid into a pericardial drainage bag.

Confirmation of location: Agitated saline is injected into the sheath via a three-way stopcock with echocardiographic imaging, usually with the imaging performed from a position separate from the needle site (e.g., apical imaging during subxiphoid access for puncture) (Fig. 17.9). If the agitated saline does not enhance the pericardial space, then repositioning of the needle by either withdrawal or another needle passage is performed. Radiographic contrast can also be administered under fluoroscopy. Small test injections should be given initially to exclude myocardial positioning, which is seen as myocardial staining. Contrast swirling will indicate a ventricular location, whereas pooling suggests intrapericardial positioning. Alternatively the needle (before it is withdrawn) or the sheath can be connected to tubing connectors for pressure transduction. Intrapericardial pressure will be similar to

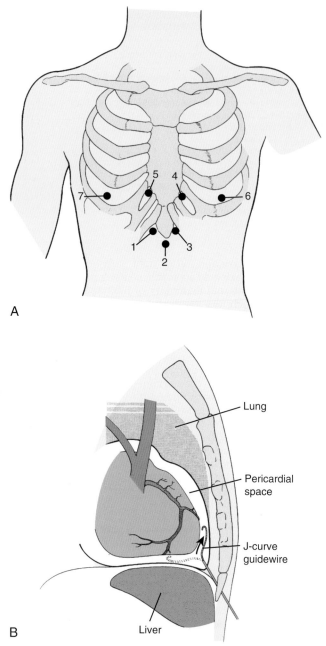

Figure 17.7 (A) Locations for pericardiocentesis. (*1, 2, 3*) Xiphoid approaches, (*4*) fifth left intercostal space at sternal border, (*5*) fifth right intercostal space at the sternal border, (*6*) apical approach, (*7*) approach for major fluid accumulation on the right side. (B) Passing a flexible J-curve guidewire through pericardial needle into the pericardial space. *(A is modified from Spodick DH. Acute pericarditis. New York: Grune & Stratton, 1959; B is from Tilkian AG, Daily EK. Cardiovascular procedures: diagnostic techniques and therapeutic procedures. St. Louis, MO: Mosby, 1986.)*

the atrial pressure, whereas ventricular systolic pressure waveforms can immediately alert the operator to inadvertent ventricular perforation. For operators using an ECG-guided approach, the needle is connected to an alligator-tipped electrode. With myocardial contact, ST-segment elevation (i.e., injury current) will be detected that may not appear on other electrocardiographic leads (Fig. 17.10).

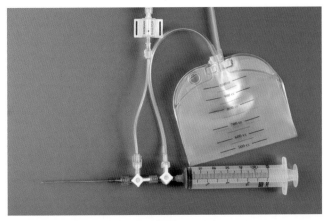

Figure 17.8 Pericardial needle attached to stopcocks which connect to pressure line and drainage bag. *(Courtesy of Merit Medical, Inc.)*

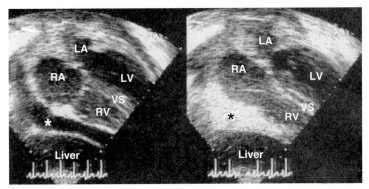

Figure 17.9 Use of agitated saline contrast medium for confirmation of sheath position in pericardial space. Pericardial effusion was visualized by imaging from subcostal position remote from entry site on chest wall before injection of agitated saline contrast medium *(left)*. Injection of agitated saline contrast medium provides dense opacification of pericardial space, confirming sheath position *(right)*. *LA,* left atrium; *LV,* left ventricle; *RA,* right atrium; *RV,* right ventricle; *VS,* ventricular septum; *,* pericardial space. *(From Tsang TS, Freeman WK, Sinak LJ, et al. Echocardiographically guided pericardiocentesis: evolution and state-of-the-art technique. Mayo Clin Proc. 1998;73:647–652.)*

Catheter placement: Following confirmation of position, a J-tipped guidewire is inserted through the polytef sheath into the pericardial space. On fluoroscopy, the wire can be seen passing along the pericardial reflection. A small skin incision with a scalpel is made, followed by exchange for a 5F or 6F introducer sheath and removal of the dilator. A multihole pigtail catheter is then inserted, followed by removal of the introducer sheath, leaving only the smooth-walled pigtail catheter in place. Positioning of the pigtail catheter can be reconfirmed using either echocardiography or pressure measurement.

Aspiration: Manual techniques or a vacuum bottle can be used to remove the pericardial effusion. For patients with tamponade due to cardiac perforation, care should be taken to remove as much pericardial fluid as possible because this will facilitate sealing of the perforated site. For patients with other causes of pericardial effusion, complete apposition of the parietal and visceral layers also will reduce risk of recurrence. Inability to aspirate despite a persistent pericardial effusion on echocardiography should lead to repositioning of the pigtail catheter. Occasionally, puncture of a tense pericardium will lead to discharge of pericardial contents into a pleural space, resulting in less than expected removal via aspiration. Normalization of atrial pressures

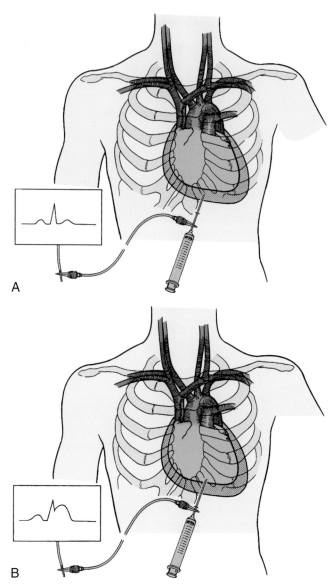

Figure 17.10 (A) Electrocardiographic monitoring of pericardial needle tip. Note normal ST segment while tip is not touching the epicardium. (B) When needle tip touches epicardium, current of injury ("contact" current) with elevated ST segment is seen. *(From Tilkian AG, Daily EK. Cardiovascular procedures: diagnostic techniques and therapeutic procedures. St. Louis, MO: Mosby, 1986.)*

documented with simultaneous right heart catheterization helps to ensure successful removal of the pericardial effusion and relief of cardiac tamponade. For patients with large volume removal due to acute hemorrhage, cell savers often are used to minimize blood loss.

Post-pericardiocentesis management: The pigtail catheter is sutured to the chest wall, connected to a stopcock, and flushed every 4–6 hours with heparinized saline to maintain patency. Standard indwelling catheter care with complete dressing changes every 72 hours is recommended. When drainage becomes minimal (<25 mL/day) and echocardiography shows no recurrent effusion, the pigtail catheter can be removed. For completely drained pericardial effusions, the risk of recurrence is low (<10%) with the exception of certain etiologies (e.g., bacterial infection, malignancy). Samples of pericardial fluid should be sent for appropriate chemistries, cultures, and cellular analysis.

Complications

When pericardiocentesis is performed by experienced operators, complications are infrequent (<1.5% of patients). The most serious complication is laceration of a coronary artery. Perforation of either the right or left ventricle also may occur, but this is rarely of clinical significance. Bleeding and tamponade from coronary or ventricular perforation can be detected by continuous monitoring of atrial pressure, which will increase in the event of these complications. Acute left ventricular failure with pulmonary edema has been reported as a complication of pericardiocentesis, but the cause of this phenomenon is not known.

While most pericardial effusions can be treated percutaneously, a surgical approach may still be required. Loculated effusions, posterior effusions, or pericardial clot formation from recent hemorrhage may be difficult to remove percutaneously. A large volume of surgical drainage often is required for effusions due to bacterial infection. For patients with refractory pericardial effusions (e.g., due to malignancy), balloon pericardiotomy to allow drainage into the pleural or peritoneal space may be a therapeutic option.

Suggested Readings

Hermany PL, Zack C, Cohen HA, et al. Comparative outcomes of pericardiocentesis in the United States by hospital procedure volumes. *J Am Coll Cardiol*. 2013;61.

Holmes DR, Nishimura R, Fountain R, et al. Iatrogenic pericardial effusion and tamponade in the percutaneous intracardiac intervention Era. *JACC Cardiovasc Interv*. 2009;2:705-717.

Le RJ, Clain J, Sinak L. Cardiac tamponade or something more: when hemodynamics don't improve with pericardiocentesis. *J Am Coll Cardiol*. 2016;67(13_S):1044.

Little WC, Freeman GL. Pericardial disease. *Circulation*. 2006;113:1622-1632.

Maisch B, Seferovic PM, Ristic AD, et al. Guidelines on the diagnosis and management of pericardial diseases executive summary: the task force on the diagnosis and management of pericardial diseases of the European Society of Cardiology. *Eur Heart J*. 2004;25:587-610.

Meltser H, Kalaria VG. Cardiac tamponade. *Catheter Cardiovasc Interv*. 2005;64:245-255.

Tsang TS, Enriquez-Sarano M, Freeman WK, et al. Consecutive 1127 therapeutic echo-cardiographically guided pericardiocenteses: clinical profile, practice patterns, and outcomes spanning 21 years. *Mayo Clin Proc*. 2002;77:429-436.

Tsang TSM. Echocardiography-guided pericardiocentesis for effusions in patients with cancer revisited. *J Am Coll Cardiol*. 2015;66(10):1129-1131.

18

Septal Ablation for Hypertrophic Obstructive Cardiomyopathy

PAUL SORAJJA

Introduction

Dynamic left ventricular outflow tract (LVOT) obstruction affects approximately three-fourths of patients with hypertrophic cardiomyopathy (HCM) and can lead to debilitating cardiac symptoms. For appropriate candidates with drug-refractory symptoms and suitable anatomy, alcohol septal ablation is now an established therapy. Due to the complexities in the evaluation and treatment of HCM patients, alcohol septal ablation should be performed in centers with expertise in the comprehensive, longitudinal care of these patients. This chapter discusses patient evaluation, selection, and performance of alcohol septal ablation in HCM.

HCM is an inheritable cardiac disorder with a prevalence of 1 in 500 persons. Of these, approximately three-fourths will have dynamic LVOT obstruction. While many patients are only minimally affected, LVOT obstruction in HCM can lead to symptoms of heart failure, angina, and syncope; in some reports, its presence has been associated with an increased risk of death. Negative inotropic agents, such as beta-receptor antagonists, disopyramide, or calcium-channel blockers (i.e., verapamil, diltiazem), represent the cornerstone of drug therapy for symptomatic LVOT obstruction. When severe symptoms persist despite pharmacotherapy, definitive septal reduction therapy should be considered.

Surgical myectomy, in which a surgeon uses a transaortic approach to resect ventricular septal hypertrophy, has been the time-honored standard for septal reduction therapy. In 1995, Ulrich Sigwart first described percutaneous alcohol septal ablation as an alternative therapy for the relief of LVOT obstruction in patients with HCM. The aim of alcohol septal ablation is to induce a localized, controlled myocardial infarction (MI) at the site of hypertrophy that is associated with the onset of LVOT obstruction. The effect of alcohol septal ablation is reduction or elimination of systolic thickening of the basal ventricular septum, thereby preventing systolic excursion into the LVOT. Ventricular remodeling and thinning of the basal ventricular septum from the procedure also may occur.

Patient Evaluation

Although the techniques of alcohol septal ablation share similarities with percutaneous coronary intervention, patients with HCM are

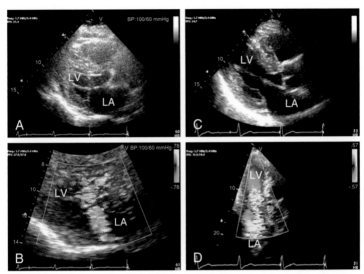

Figure 18.1 Patient selection for septal ablation. (A,B) Appropriate patient for septal ablation. There is septal hypertrophy, systolic anterior motion of the mitral valve, and posteriorly directed mitral regurgitation that is secondary to the outflow obstruction. (C,D) This patient has obstructive hypertrophic cardiomyopathy, but the mitral regurgitation is secondary to a flail mitral leaflet. Note the anterior course of the mitral regurgitant jet, which is not typical for that due to outflow obstruction. *LA,* left atrium; *LV,* left ventricle.

inherently complex due to the heterogeneity of the disease. Thus the evaluation for septal reduction therapy, as well as the performance of these procedures, should be accomplished in a center with established expertise in HCM (class I recommendation). A comprehensive clinical evaluation and echocardiogram should be performed in all patients and include consideration of symptoms, family history, and risk factors for sudden cardiac death, as well as candidacy for the different modes of septal reduction therapy. Informed consent for the procedure should be obtained through a shared decision-making process, with a detailed discussion of the comparative outcomes of surgical myectomy and alcohol septal ablation. Informed consent requires a full understanding of the limited data on long-term survival after the procedure, the risk of pacemaker dependency, the relatively lower success rate due to its dependence on coronary anatomy, and potential complications related to cardiac catheterization and instrumentation of the coronary arteries.

Principal goals of the echocardiogram are to (1) characterize the morphology of the ventricular septum (e.g., asymmetric vs. concentric hypertrophy, ventricular septal thickness), (2) determine the association of the ventricular hypertrophy with dynamic LVOT obstruction, (3) evaluate the severity of LVOT obstruction with calculation of the gradient, (4) examine the mitral valve anatomy and regurgitation, and (5) exclude other indications for cardiac surgery (e.g., valvular aortic stenosis, subaortic membrane) (Fig. 18.1). Transthoracic echocardiography with two-dimensional and Doppler imaging suffices in nearly all patients. In some patients, the achievement of these goals requires further evaluation with either cardiac magnetic resonance imaging and/or invasive hemodynamic catheterization.

An accurate determination of the severity of LVOT obstruction is of paramount importance in the evaluation of HCM patients. Characteristically LVOT obstruction in HCM is dynamic and exquisitely sensitive to ventricular loading conditions and contractility. The operator should be cognizant of this sensitivity when examining hemodynamic data from both the echocardiogram and invasive catheterization. Careful attention must be given not only to the initial LVOT gradient observed at rest but also to all dynamic and provocable gradients observed during the evaluation. For patients without significant LVOT obstruction at rest, provocative maneuvers should be performed. These maneuvers can include Valsalva strain, variation with respiration, post-premature ventricular contraction accentuation, amyl nitrate inhalation, exercise, and isoproterenol administration. Dobutamine, which can elicit LVOT gradients in persons with normal hearts, should not be used due to its lack of specificity.

For HCM patients undergoing cardiac catheterization, the most accurate method for the invasive evaluation of LVOT obstruction in HCM entails a transseptal approach with positioning of a balloon-tipped catheter (e.g., a 7F Berman catheter; Arrow International Inc., Reading, PA) at the left ventricular inflow region and a pigtail catheter placed retrograde in the ascending aorta for simultaneous measurement of the LVOT gradient. The transseptal approach helps to avoid catheter entrapment, which can be difficult to distinguish from changes in left ventricular pressure that occur due to the dynamic nature of LVOT obstruction. Use of an 8F Mullins sheath for transseptal access also enables recording of left atrial pressure via the side arm for assessment for concomitant diastolic dysfunction.

Alternatively left ventricular pressure can be assessed with a 5F or 6F catheter placed retrograde across the aortic valve. In this technique, a catheter with shaft side holes should not be used because some or all of the holes will be positioned above the level of subaortic obstruction, thus leading to erroneous measurements of left ventricular pressure and the LVOT gradient. Catheters that may be used for this purpose are a multipurpose or a Halo pigtail catheter. Absence of catheter entrapment should be confirmed with hand contrast injections or demonstration of pulsatile flow from the catheter with disconnection from the extenders used for pressure transduction.

Patient Selection

Proper patient selection is critical to the success of septal ablation. Criteria for septal ablation include:

1. Severe, drug-refractory cardiac symptoms (New York Heart Association functional class III/IV dyspnea or Canadian Cardiac Society angina class III/IV) due to obstructive HCM
2. Dynamic LVOT obstruction (gradient ≥30 mm Hg at rest or ≥50 mm Hg with provocation) that is due to septal hypertrophy and systolic anterior motion of the mitral valve
3. Ventricular septal thickness of 15 mm or greater; patients with markedly severe hypertrophy, especially 30 mm or greater, should be avoided
4. Absence of significant intrinsic mitral valve disease
5. Absence of the need for concomitant cardiac surgical procedure (e.g., bypass grafting, valve replacement)
6. Informed patient consent

Although younger age has not been an absolute contraindication to the procedure, septal ablation generally has been reserved for older adult patients due to the limited data on long-term survival of the procedure. In national guidelines, septal ablation is discouraged for those younger than 40 years, and performance of the procedure in the very young (<21 years) is explicitly not advised (class III recommendation). Alcohol septal ablation should be performed only by operators with expertise and as part of a longitudinal, multidisciplinary program dedicated to the care of patients with HCM (class I recommendation).

Procedural Technique for Alcohol Septal Ablation

Patient Comfort

Alcohol septal ablation typically is performed with conscious sedation using standard arterial access (6F or 7F). Either radial or femoral artery access can be utilized, with the priority being patient comfort during the procedure to avoid patient movement. Patient movement that leads to malpositioning of the catheters can have highly adverse consequences for alcohol ablation. For example, balloon sealing may be disrupted and lead to alcohol spillage and an excessive MI. Moreover, pacemaker dislodgement can lead to cardiac arrest during the procedure. Maintaining patient comfort, including adequate levels of anesthesia to treat the effects of the alcohol-induced infarction, is a key component of septal ablation.

Temporary Pacemaker Placement

The risk of pacemaker dependency from septal ablation varies according to the baseline electrocardiographic abnormalities. Septal ablation frequently results in right bundle branch block (approximately 50% of cases). Thus, for those patients with left bundle branch block, severe left axis deviation, or a very wide QRS complex, the rate of pacemaker dependency approaches 50%. However permanent pacemaker dependency from complete atrioventricular block still occurs in 10%–15% of patients with a normal electrocardiogram.

For those without a previously placed permanent device, internal jugular venous access is utilized for temporary pacemaker placement because this site allows upright patient positioning with the catheter in place during the postprocedural observation period. Conventional 5F or 6F temporary pacemakers or balloon-tipped catheters have been utilized for alcohol septal ablation. Of note, these temporary pacemaker catheters can become easily dislodged. The long indwelling time for these catheters postprocedure (24–72 hours) also has been associated with cardiac perforation. In our practice, we have observed no cardiac perforations with the use of a low-profile, less traumatic temporary pacemaker (2F Medtronic 6416-140) that is actively fixed. In all cases, the temporary pacemaker should be placed distal or away from the target site of ablation to ensure continuous capture during induction of the septal infarction. For cases where electrical capture is lost without lead dislodgement, one should suspect myocardial edema or infarction at the site of pacemaker placement.

Coronary Angiography

The primary goal of coronary angiography is to determine the most appropriate septal artery for the procedure. Both arteries should be evaluated because basal septal branches occasionally arise from the proximal right coronary artery. With a right anterior oblique angulation of the left coronary artery, straight and caudal views facilitate examination of the angulation of the origin of the septal artery, whereas cranial projections can assist with the length of the vessel. Left anterior oblique projections should be used to demonstrate the course of the artery in the ventricular septum.

When using transthoracic echocardiography, it is important to choose the most proximal septal artery available first for selected contrast injections. Otherwise acoustic shadowing of the ventricular basal septum during the contrast injection can occur and prevent the operator from appropriately identifying the target area for alcohol ablation.

Alcohol Ablation

Conventional 6F or 7F guide catheters are used to engage the left coronary artery with standard procedural anticoagulation (e.g., heparin 70–100 U/kg). A relatively large guide catheter is needed to be able to fully inject contrast and opacify the coronary artery while containing the balloon catheter. Both a small primary and a large secondary bend should be placed on the tip of a 0.014-inch guidewire to facilitate entry into the candidate septal artery. The guidewire needs to be placed as distal as possible to secure support for placement of the balloon catheter; in many instances, the guidewire can be advanced through septal branches that are not visible on angiography, akin to techniques used for percutaneous revascularization of chronic total occlusions via septal-septal collaterals.

Next, a slightly oversized, short-length, over-the-wire balloon (1.5–2.5 mm × 8–10 mm length) is placed entirely into the septal artery using standard catheter techniques. Oversizing of the balloon allows occlusion of the septal artery at low pressures (3–4 atm), which permits injection of material through the balloon lumen of the catheter. Following inflation of the balloon catheter, the guidewire is carefully withdrawn. Angiography of the left coronary then is performed to demonstrate no communication between the septal artery and left anterior descending and also to confirm the course of the target vessel through the ventricular septum on fluoroscopy.

Next septal angiography and echocardiographic localization of contrast is performed. Many operators solely use angiographic contrast (full-strength, 1–2 mL) for this interrogation, while others follow the septal angiogram with an injection of echocardiographic contrast (e.g., Definity, 0.5–1 mL). It is important to note that, during septal ablation, all injections of the septal artery through the balloon catheter should be performed gently to avoid opening of septal-septal collaterals. The septal angiogram confirms patency of the vessel for ablation and localization (i.e., no untoward collateralization or dissection). Simultaneous two-dimensional echocardiography identifies the perfusion bed (Fig. 18.2). Multiple echocardiographic views must be used to confirm enhancement of the septal hypertrophy intimately related to LVOT obstruction but no targeting of undesirable locations, such as the right ventricle, free walls, or papillary muscles.

After delineation of the targeted myocardium, desiccated ethanol is infused slowly over a period of 3–5 minutes followed by slow flush of normal saline. There are no firm definitions of appropriate alcohol dose, though a general guideline of 0.8–1 mL per 10 mm thickness of the ventricular septum can be considered. The total dose should be minimized as much as possible and not exceed 3 mL. Notably, in series demonstrating favorable survival after alcohol ablation, the average dose of alcohol was 1.9 mL. The use of alcohol is preferred because this agent immediately results in a discrete MI. In other percutaneous methods (e.g., vascular coiling, covered stent placement), septal infarction may not result due to septal collateralization that is either pre-existing or develops during follow-up. Hemodynamics are monitored during alcohol instillation.

The balloon should be left inflated following saline flush for 5–10 minutes to reduce the likelihood of alcohol extravasation. For patient comfort, intravenous analgesia (e.g., fentanyl 25 mg) frequently is given prophylactically or intermittently as needed. For patients without significant reduction of either the resting or provoked LVOT gradient, other septal perforator arteries can be targeted and treated in similar fashion. Repeat coronary angiography should be performed to demonstrate patency of the left anterior descending, its major branches, and ablation of the septal artery(ies).

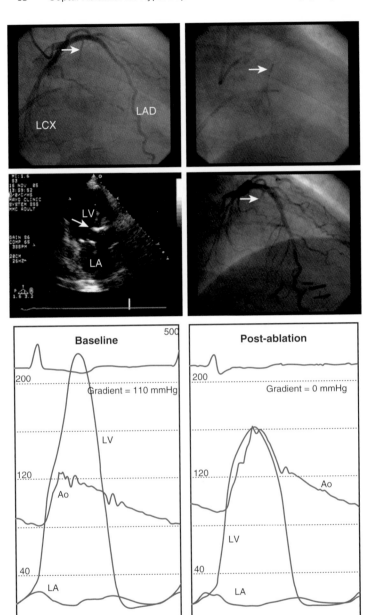

Figure 18.2 Percutaneous septal alcohol ablation. *Top left*: Baseline angiogram of the left coronary artery showing the septal perforator artery (*arrow*) to be used for ablation. *Top right*: An over-the-wire balloon (*arrow*) is inflated in the perforator artery followed by contrast injection through the balloon. *Middle left*: Echocardiographic contrast is injected through the balloon and visualized with simultaneous echocardiography. *Middle right*: Following injection of alcohol, the septal artery (*arrow*) is obliterated. *Bottom left*: Before septal ablation, the left ventricular outflow tract gradient is 110 mm Hg. *Bottom right*: Following septal ablation, there is no left ventricular outflow tract gradient. *Ao*, ascending aorta; *LA*, left atrium; *LAD*, left anterior descending; *LCX*, left circumflex; *LV*, left ventricle. *(From Sorajja P, Nishimura RA. Myocardial and pericardial disease. In CathSap version 3, by permission from American College of Cardiology Foundation.)*

Clinical Outcomes

Acute Procedural Success

In published series, the magnitude of LVOT gradient reduction with septal ablation has ranged from 55% to 75%. Acute procedural success, when defined as a 50% or greater reduction in the peak resting or provoked LVOT gradient with a final residual resting gradient of less than 20 mm Hg, occurs in 80%–85% of patients. In addition to proper patient selection, factors associated with a higher likelihood of acute hemodynamic success include relatively less septal hypertrophy, lower LVOT gradients, and operator experience (Fig. 18.3). Further reduction in the LVOT gradient over 3–6 months after the procedure also occurs due to ventricular remodeling and basal septal thinning. Regression of myocardium both at the site of LVOT obstruction and remote from the ventricular septum has been demonstrated using cardiac magnetic resonance imaging.

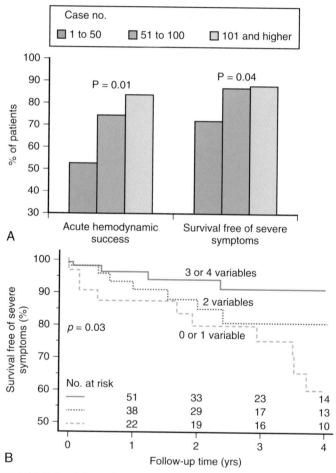

Figure 18.3 Predictors of procedural success with alcohol septal ablation. *Top:* Case volume and clinical outcome. *Bottom:* Survival free of severe symptoms (New York Heart Association functional class ≥III, Canadian Cardiac Society Angina class ≥III, or need for myectomy) in the overall population (*top*) and according to the number of favorable clinical variables present (*bottom*). Factors were age ≥65 years, left ventricular outflow tract gradients <100 mm Hg, left anterior descending diameter <4.0 mm, and basal ventricular septal ≤18 mm. *(From Sorajja P, et al. Predictors of an optimal clinical outcome with alcohol septal ablation for obstructive hypertrophic cardiomyopathy. Catheter Cardiovasc Interv. 2013;81:E58–E67.)*

The major limitation to higher success rates is the lack of an appropriate septal artery, which may be absent in up to 20% of patients. The most common complication of septal ablation is temporary or complete atrioventricular block. Other potential complications are cardiac tamponade, dissection of the left anterior descending artery, ventricular tachycardia or fibrillation, and free wall MI. For these reasons, patients are observed in an intensive care setting for at least 3 days after the procedure. Overall, the published periprocedural mortality rates are 1%–2%.

Symptom Improvement

Septal ablation leads to significant clinical improvement, as measured by both subjective functional class and objective testing, such as treadmill exercise time and peak myocardial oxygen consumption. The clinical efficacy of septal ablation is related to the degree of reduction in severity of the LVOT gradient. Overall, septal ablation typically results in a 20%–30% increase in objective measures of functional capacity.

Several studies have shown these clinical improvements to be sustained in follow-up of more than 1 year, with several reports showing

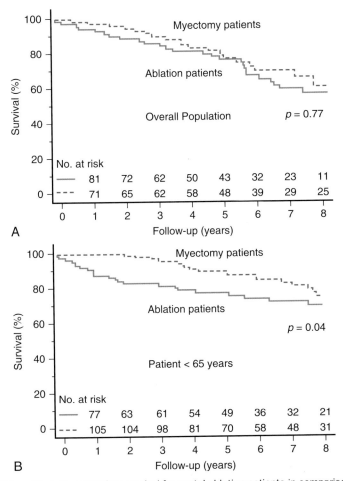

Figure 18.4 Symptom-free survival for septal ablation patients in comparison to surgical myectomy. Survival free of severe symptoms and death was comparable in the overall population (A), but was inferior among patients <65 years (B). *(From Sorajja P, et al. Survival after alcohol septal ablation for obstructive hypertrophic cardiomyopathy. Circulation. 2012;126:2374–2380.)*

effects comparable to that of surgical myectomy. Nonetheless, in younger patients (age <65), symptom relief may be greater with surgical myectomy (Fig. 18.4). The reasons for this observation are not clear but may be related to the residual gradients present after ablation (typically 10–20 mm Hg) that are higher than those after surgical myectomy (typically <10 mm Hg). Younger, more active individuals may less tolerate these relatively higher residual gradients. Residual gradients after alcohol septal ablation are importantly related to long-term survival and relief of symptoms (Fig. 18.5).

Survival

Several published studies have compared the results of septal ablation to surgical myectomy with follow-up ranging from 3 months to 8 years. Overall survival has largely been comparable to that of surgical myectomy, although discrepant results have been reported. In a single-center study of 177 patients treated by experienced operators, 8-year survival free of all-cause mortality (including appropriate defibrillator discharge) after septal ablation was 79.0% and was similar to a matched general population of individuals as well as patients who underwent surgical myectomy (Fig. 18.6). The combined annual rate of sudden cardiac

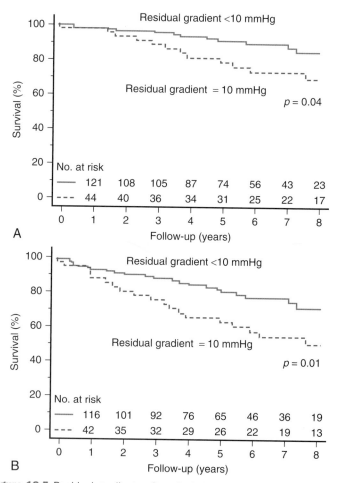

Figure 18.5 Residual gradients after alcohol septal ablation and survival. (A) Survival free of all-cause mortality. (B) Survival free of death or severe symptoms. *(From Sorajja P, et al. Survival after alcohol septal ablation for obstructive hypertrophic cardiomyopathy. Circulation. 2012;126:2374–2380.)*

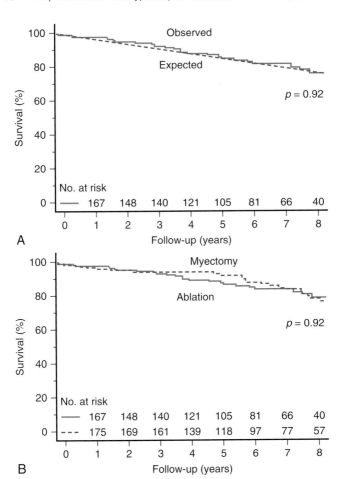

Figure 18.6 Comparison of survival after septal ablation to a matched cohort of surgical myectomy patients. (A) The 8-year mortality (including defibrillator discharge for lethal arrhythmia) for septal ablation patients was similar to the published mortality rates for a comparable U.S. general population. (B) The overall survival (including defibrillator discharge for lethal arrhythmia) for septal ablation patients also was comparable to age- and sex-matched patients who underwent isolated surgical myectomy. *(From Sorajja P, et al. Survival after alcohol septal ablation for obstructive hypertrophic cardiomyopathy. Circulation. 2012;126:2374–2380.)*

death and unexplained death for ablation patients was 1.51% (95% confidence interval, 0.75%–2.67%). Conversely in a study of 91 patients treated at a different institution, sudden cardiac death occurred in 20% of ablation patients over a follow-up period of 5.8 years. The different outcomes in these studies cannot be completely reconciled, although it is important to note that alcohol dose was considerably higher in the latter study (3.5 mL among all patients; 4.5 mL in the first 25 patients) than in the multiple other reports (1.8–2.0 mL). Several studies have demonstrated similar efficacy with low and high alcohol doses. Thus the dose of alcohol should be minimized while performing alcohol septal ablation. Further study on the long-term effects and risk of sudden death with alcohol septal ablation is still required.

Suggested Readings

Agarwal S, Tuzcu EM, Desai MY, et al. Updated meta-analysis of septal alcohol ablation versus myectomy for hypertrophic cardiomyopathy. *J Am Coll Cardiol.* 2010;55:823-834.
Elesber A, Nishimura RA, Rihal CS, et al. Utility of isoproterenol to provoke outflow tract gradients in patients with hypertrophic cardiomyopathy. *Am J Cardiol.* 2008;101:516-520.

Fernandes VL, Nielsen C, Nagueh SF, et al. Follow-up of alcohol septal ablation for symptomatic hypertrophic obstructive cardiomyopathy: the Baylor and Medical University of South Carolina experience 1996 to 2007. *JACC Cardiovasc Interv*. 2008;1:561-570.

Gersh BJ, Maron BJ, Bonow RO, et al. 2011 ACCF/AHA guideline for the diagnosis and treatment of hypertrophic cardiomyopathy: a report of the American College of Cardiology Foundation/American Heart Association Task Force on practice guidelines. *J Am Coll Cardiol*. 2011;58:e212-e260.

Jensen MK, Almaas VM, Jaobsson L, et al. Long-term outcome of percutaneous transluminal septal myocardial ablation in hypertrophic obstructive cardiomyopathy: a Scandinavian multicenter study. *Circ Cardiovasc Interv*. 2011;4:256-265.

Leonardi RA, Kransdorf EP, Simel DL, et al. Meta-analyses of septal reduction therapies for obstructive hypertrophic cardiomyopathy: comparative rates of overall mortality and sudden cardiac death after treatment. *Circ Cardiovasc Interv*. 2010;3:97-104.

Ommen SR, Maron BJ, Olivotto I, et al. Long-term effects of surgical septal myectomy on survival in patients with obstructive hypertrophic cardiomyopathy. *J Am Coll Cardiol*. 2005;46:470-476.

Sigwart U. Non-surgical myocardial reduction for hypertrophic obstructive cardiomyopathy. *Lancet*. 1995;346:211-214.

Sorajja P, Ommen SR, Holmes DR Jr, et al. Survival after alcohol septal ablation for obstructive hypertrophic cardiomyopathy. *Circulation*. 2012;126:2374-2380.

ten Cate FJ, Soliman OII, Michels M, et al. Long-term outcome of alcohol septal ablation in patients with obstructive hypertrophic cardiomyopathy: a word of caution. *Circ Heart Fail*. 2010;3:362-369.

Percutaneous Repair of Paravalvular Prosthetic Regurgitation

PAUL SORAJJA

Introduction

Paravalvular regurgitation is common, occurring in 5%–10% of surgical prostheses and 40%–70% of patients who have transcatheter valve replacement. The majority of affected patients are asymptomatic and live without significant morbidity. In a subset of patients, however, paravalvular prosthetic regurgitation can cause debilitating symptoms of heart failure or hemolytic anemia.

For symptomatic patients, it is important to note that open surgical treatment always necessitates reoperation and that these patients frequently have severe morbidities that can significantly increase the surgical risk. Moreover, open surgery also may not be successful due to tissue characteristics that heralded the development of the paravalvular regurgitation. Percutaneous methods for repair have now been developed and represent a safe and effective therapy for paravalvular prosthetic regurgitation when performed by experienced operators. Percutaneous therapy is inherently attractive as a relatively less invasive option for paravalvular prosthetic regurgitation and now is typically considered to be primary therapy for eligible patients.

Clinical Evaluation

The evaluation of patients with paravalvular prosthetic regurgitation is comprehensive and multidisciplinary. The clinical criteria for percutaneous repair of paravalvular regurgitation is provided in Table 19.1. A history and physical examination must include a search for endocarditis and hemolytic anemia, even when there are not findings suspicious for these disorders. Active endocarditis is a contraindication to the procedure. The presence of hemolytic anemia necessitates a higher degree of procedural success (i.e., no residual regurgitation), which should be discussed when obtaining informed consent.

The primary imaging modality for the evaluation of paravalvular prosthetic regurgitation is echocardiography. The primary goals of the echocardiographic study are to determine the severity and location of the paravalvular regurgitation (including size and distance from the valular ring of the defect from the prosthesis annulus), the degree of ventricular compensation, and the presence of central valvular regurgitation and to exclude concomitant indications for open surgery. It is important to note that echocardiography can be limited by acoustic shadowing. Thus detailed studies with multiple echocardiographic windows and, if needed, multiple modalities (i.e., transesophageal,

Table 19.1

Clinical Criteria for Percutaneous Repair of Paravalvular Regurgitation

- Symptomatic paravalvular regurgitation; if asymptomatic, evidence of left ventricular decompensation needed
- Operators and imaging specialists skilled in the procedure
- Absence of all of the following:
  - active endocarditis
  - instability of the prosthesis
  - significant prosthetic valvular regurgitation
  - other indications for cardiac surgery

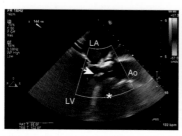 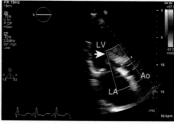

Figure 19.1 Echocardiography of paravalvular prosthetic regurgitation. Acoustic shadowing can limit the ability of echocardiography to detect paravalvular regurgitation. *Left*: Transesophageal echocardiography immediately after transcatheter implantation of a 26-mm Sapien valve shows minimal central regurgitation (*arrowhead*). Acoustic shadowing (*asterisk*) is present and does not allow visualization of the anterior area of the Sapien valve. *Right*: Significant anterior paravalvular regurgitation is evident on apical long-axis view using transthoracic echocardiography (*arrowhead*). *Ao*, aorta; *LA*, left atrium; *LV*, left ventricle.

intracardiac, transthoracic) should be employed. As examples, anterior defects may be difficult to visualize with transesophageal imaging, while posterior lesions can be challenging to assess with transthoracic imaging (Fig. 19.1).

Two-dimensional and Doppler echocardiography is utilized as the initial screening tool. In addition, for patients with mitral defects, three-dimensional studies with color imaging are particularly useful in providing detailed morphology to plan and guide percutaneous repair and also are less susceptible to interobserver variability for quantitation. Notably, although quantitation of native valvular regurgitation with echocardiographic techniques has been well established, the criteria for determining severity of paravalvular prosthetic regurgitation are less well studied. Cardiac magnetic resonance imaging may be considered because its incremental utility over echocardiography for quantitation of regurgitation has been demonstrated, with less susceptibility to interobserver variability.

Because noninvasive imaging studies can present challenges, there should be a high degree of suspicion for clinically significant paravalvular defects in patients with heart failure or hemolytic anemia. For those patients with inconclusive noninvasive imaging studies, an evaluation in the cardiac catheterization laboratory with a detailed hemodynamic assessment and angiography should be performed (Fig. 19.2).

For all patients, clinical judgment regarding severity and the likelihood of associated symptoms must be exercised. Defects that are not classically severe can still be hemodynamically significant and may benefit from therapy, but the decision to pursue such treatment should be individualized. In this regard invasive hemodynamic studies with direct examination of ventricular filling pressures at rest and exercise may be helpful in the evaluation.

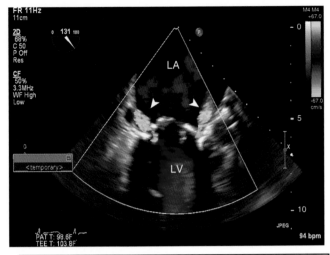

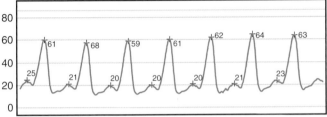

Figure 19.2 Hemodynamic evaluation of paravalvular regurgitation. Paravalvular prosthetic regurgitation with two defects surrounding a mitral bioprosthetic valve (*top, arrowheads*). The degree of regurgitation appears mild to moderate on transesophageal echocardiography. However, invasive hemodynamic evaluation with direct measurement of left atrial pressure shows a tall V wave and a mean pressure of 38 mm Hg (*bottom*).

Patient Selection

In national guidelines on valvular heart disease, percutaneous repair of paravalvular prosthetic regurgitation is recommended for patients with severe symptoms or hemolysis, who are at high risk of surgery, and who have suitable anatomic features (class IIa recommendation). In addition, many specialists also consider percutaneous treatment for asymptomatic patients with ventricular decompensation and for patients who are not at high risk of open surgery. Percutaneous repair can be considered to be the initial approach because procedural failure, with recognition of the known invasive risks, does not preclude further surgical therapy. Due to its considerable technical challenges, percutaneous repair should not be performed in centers without expertise in the procedure (Table 19.2). Other contraindications are active endocarditis, a rocking prosthesis, or significant valvular regurgitation. Patients with either bioprosthetic or mechanical prostheses can be treated. The risk of leaflet impingement is relatively higher for those with mechanical prostheses but can occur in all patients (see the section on "Procedural Techniques").

Computed Tomography Studies for Procedural Guidance

Cardiac computed tomography (CT) is highly accurate for examining the orientation of paravalvular leaks and surrounding calcification. These imaging studies provide detailed information regarding camera

Table 19.2

Equipment for Percutaneous Repair of Paravalvular Regurgitation

Aortic Lesions

- Two 6F arterial access sheaths
- 12F Gore Dryseal sheath
- 260-cm, extra-stiff 0.035-inch Glidewire; 0.018-inch may be necessary in some cases
- 0.032-inch extra-stiff Amplatz wires, exchange-length is preferred
- 6F diagnostic coronary catheters: 6F AL-1, AL-2, multipurpose
- 15- or 20-mm gooseneck snare
- 4F to 8F Cook Flexor shuttle sheaths, 90 cm in length; alternatively, glidehead catheters
- AVP-2 and AVP-4 device occluders, 6- to 14-mm diameter; ADO-2, VSD also optional

Mitral Lesions

- 6F venous and arterial access sheaths
- Standard transseptal puncture equipment according to operator preference
- 20F Gore Dryseal sheath
- 260-cm, extra-stiff 0.035-inch Glidewire; 0.018-inch may be necessary in some cases
- 0.032-inch extra-stiff Amplatz wires, exchange-length is preferred
- 8.5F, small- or medium-curve Agilis sheaths (St. Jude Medical)
- 5F multipurpose diagnostic coronary catheters, 6F multipurpose guide catheters; 6F Judkins right coronary catheter
- 15- or 20-mm gooseneck snare
- 4F to 8F Cook Flexor shuttle sheaths, 90 cm in length; alternatively, glidehead catheters
- AVP-2 and AVP-4 device occluders, 6- to 14-mm diameter; ADO-2, VSD also optional

setup in the catheterization laboratory and thus help facilitate the success of percutaneous closure. Imaging is performed with contrast and electrocardiographic (ECG) gating; a slice thickness of 0.6 mm or less is needed for maximal spatial resolution. Using information from echocardiography, the CT scan is reconstructed with views of the exit point of the regurgitant jet whose paravalvular continuity can then be examined (Fig. 19.3). CT imaging can also be used to examine the leaflet morphology (i.e., pannus) to determine the valvular contribution to regurgitation. This incremental utility may be of particular clinical benefit when there is significant acoustic shadowing on echocardiography. In some laboratories fusion CT imaging can be used to facilitate percutaneous closure. In this technique CT data are co-registered to cardiac structures (i.e., chambers, valves, coronary arteries), thus enabling overlay onto the fluoroscopy screen. Fusion CT imaging is then used to guide access (transseptal antegrade vs. retrograde apical) and to assist with defect wiring and device placement.

Device Occluders

The most commonly used device occluders for percutaneous repair of paravalvular regurgitation are the Amplatzer vascular plugs (St. Jude Medical, Fridley, MN). These devices are made of self-expanding nitinol, are deliverable through small-caliber catheters (e.g., 4F) with or without rails, and have retention disks to help reduce the risk of embolization after deployment. While the AVP-2 and AVP-4 devices are available in the United States, the AVP-3 is available only in Europe. A device occluder specifically designed for treatment of paravalvular regurgitation is the Occlutech PLD, which also is available only in Europe. Other commonly used devices include the Amplatzer muscular ventricular

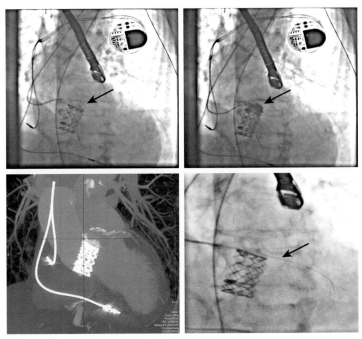

Figure 19.3 Computed tomography guidance for percutaneous repair of paravalvular prosthetic regurgitation. *Top left*: During retrograde attempt, the wire (*arrow*) cannot be passed across the defect because it cannot be maneuvered between the native leaflets and the Sapien prosthesis. *Top right*: Selective cusp angiogram demonstrates catheter placement exterior to native leaflets (*arrow*). *Bottom left*: Computed tomography imaging aligns the prosthesis with the defect immediately exterior to the prosthesis and provides the camera angles to the operator. *Bottom right*: The operator places the image intensifier in the same position and then wires the defect (*arrow*).

septal defect (VSD) and ductal occluders (ADO and ADO-2) (St. Jude Medical, Fridley, MN). The VSD and ADO occluders require relatively larger sheaths for delivery but have been successfully employed in select cases. The ADO-2 is a newer occluder, but has a maximal waist size of only 6 mm (disc size = 12 mm).

It is important to note that catheter accommodation for the various device occluders is not described well in the manufacturers' labeling. Several guidelines, which have arisen from trial and error, are noteworthy: (1) a 6F multipurpose guide catheter (Cordis Co, Bridgewater, NJ) will accommodate a 12-mm AVP-2 plug; (2) a 4F diagnostic multipurpose catheter or Glidecath (Terumo Medical Co, Somerset, NJ) will accommodate a 4-mm AVP-4; (3) a 4F Cook Flexor Shuttle sheath (Cook Medical, Bloomington, IN) will accommodate an 8-mm AVP-2; and (4) a 6F Cook Flexor Shuttle will accommodate a 12-mm AVP-2 and a 0.035-inch extra-stiff Amplatz wire simultaneously or two 0.032-inch extra-stiff Amplatz wires together.

Selection of the device occluder for percutaneous repair is largely empiric; sizing balloons are not recommended. A general guideline is a device waist that is 2 times that of the largest diameter measured on echocardiography. Due to the serpiginous nature of paravalvular defects, multiple, small-size occluders frequently are used rather than a single large device.

Aortic Paravalvular Regurgitation

The most common approach for percutaneous repair of aortic para-valvular regurgitation is retrograde via the femoral artery (Fig. 19.4).

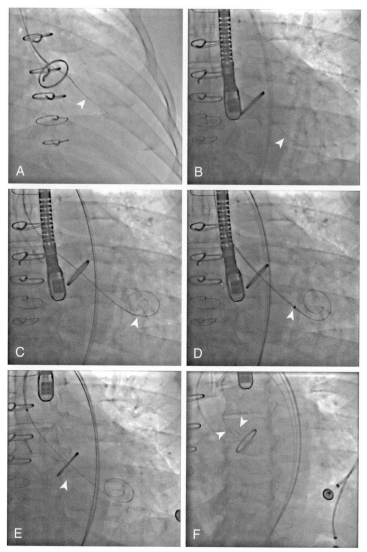

Figure 19.4 Percutaneous repair of paravalvular aortic prosthetic regurgitation. (A) A multipurpose, 6F diagnostic catheter (*arrowhead*) is steered toward a posterior defect, which is then crossed with a 260-cm, angle-tipped, extra-stiff Glidewire. (B) The multipurpose catheter (*arrowhead*) is advanced into the left ventricle. (C) A 260-cm Safari wire is placed across the defect using the multipurpose catheter (*arrowhead*). (D) Over the stiff Safari wire, an 8F Cook Flexor Shuttle (*arrowhead*) is passed into the left ventricle, followed by placement of two 0.032-inch extra-stiff Amplatz wires. (E) With the stiff wire left in place in an anchor technique, the dilator is removed and a 12-mm AVP-2 (*arrowhead*) is deployed across the defect. (F) The Flexor sheath is removed and then reinserted only over the stiff wire. A second 12-mm AVP-2 plug is then advanced and deployed alongside the first device occluder. Simultaneous echocardiography and aortography demonstrates safe, complete treatment of the regurgitation, including no leaflet impingement. The devices are then released.

These procedures can be performed with either conscious sedation or general anesthesia, depending on the echocardiographic modality to be used. Different echocardiographic modalities for procedural guidance are possible, but the choice depends on the location of the lesion and the need to minimize acoustic shadowing of the regurgitant jet (e.g., transesophageal for posterior defects; transthoracic for anterior ones). Intracardiac echocardiography also can be used. In some cases, the catheter for intracardiac echocardiography can be manipulated into the right ventricular outflow tract to provide imaging details that may not be seen with transesophageal or transthoracic echocardiography.

Steps for Percutaneous Repair of Aortic Paravalvular Prosthetic Regurgitation

1. Bilateral femoral artery access (one 12F Gore Dryseal sheath and one 6F standard sheath). The large access site should be preclosed with two sutures.
2. Placement of a steerable 5F or 6F coronary catheter (e.g., multipurpose for posterior defects; Amplatz left for anterior ones) in the ascending aorta.
3. The image intensifier is oriented to remove any overlap of the defect and the prosthesis. Without accurate positioning of the imaging intensifier, it is difficult to determine if the guidewire is being passed into the defect external to the prosthesis. This positioning can be approximated (e.g., left anterior oblique cranial for posterior defects; right anterior oblique caudal for anterior defects) or accurately determined from CT imaging. If biplane imaging is available, the second image intensifier is used to show the prosthesis *en face* where possible, to help demonstrate external placement of the wire.
4. Crossing of the defect with angled-tip, exchange length 0.035-inch Glidewire (Terumo), which is advanced into the left ventricle. With care to avoid entanglement in the mitral valve apparatus, the wire can be advanced out the aortic prosthesis. Operators should also take care to avoid entry into the coronary arteries, whose avoidance is easily demonstrated in the left anterior oblique projection.
5. A 4F to 8F 90-cm Cook Flexor sheath is advanced over the Glidewire into the left ventricle.
6. The device occluder is advanced through the Flexor sheath. The distal segment is placed in the left ventricle. The device occluder is extruded with retention disks positioned on the ventricular and aortic sides of the defect or, as frequently with AVP-4 plugs, wholly within the defect.

Alternatively, once the Glidewire is across the defect, the coronary catheter can be advanced into the left ventricle and be used to exchange a 0.032-inch Amplatz extra-stiff wire to enable placement of a delivery catheter. In all cases, selection of the delivery catheter is dependent on (1) the size and number of device occluders that are needed, (2) difficulty encountered in passing the catheter across the defect, and (3) need for an anchor wire or rail (see the "Techniques" section).

The final assessment must include evaluation for prosthetic leaflet impingement and residual regurgitation. Angiography is also recommended to exclude arterial occlusion for patients who require large or multiple device occluders and those with small aortic sinuses, low coronary height, or defects located near the coronary ostia. Once the final assessment is satisfactory, the device occluders are decoupled through counterclockwise rotation of the delivery cables.

Mitral Paravalvular Regurgitation

For patients with mitral paravalvular regurgitation, percutaneous repair is performed with general anesthesia and transesophageal echocardiography (TEE). The most commonly used approach is femoral venous access with transseptal puncture and antegrade cannulation of the defects from the left atrium (Figs. 19.5 and 19.6). Alternatively direct

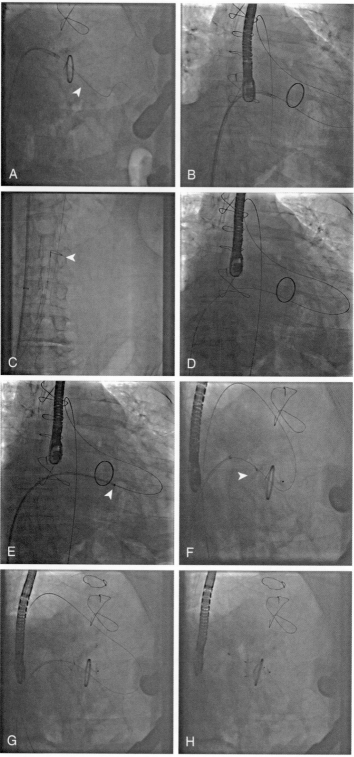

Figure 19.5 Percutaneous repair of paravalvular mitral prosthetic regurgitation (A) A steerable 8.5F Agilis sheath is placed in the left atrium, followed by advancement of a Glidewire (*arrowhead*) across the defect. (B) The guidewire is advanced across the aortic valve and into the descending aorta. (C) A 15-mm gooseneck (*arrowhead*) is used to snare the wire. (D) The guidewire is exteriorized out the contralateral femoral artery. (E) Over the guidewire, an 8F Cook Flexor Shuttle sheath (*arrowhead*) is advanced across the defect into the left ventricle. (F) A 12-mm AVP-2 is advanced across the defect with the rail in place. (G) The same Flexor sheath is removed and then reinserted over only the guidewire, followed by placement of a second 12-mm AVP-2. (H) Following confirmation of normal leaflet function and no residual regurgitation on echocardiography (see Fig. 19.6), the two AVP-2 device occluders are released.

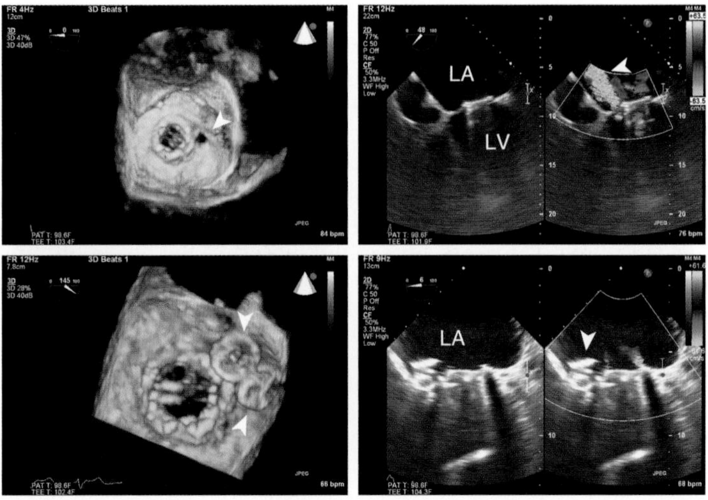

Figure 19.6 Echocardiography of percutaneous repair of paravalvular mitral prosthetic regurgitation. These images are from the procedure illustrated in Fig. 19.5. *Top left*: Three-dimensional transesophageal echocardiography showing a large medial paravalvular leak (*arrowhead*). *Top right*: Color-compare view showing significant paravalvular regurgitation (*arrowhead*). *Bottom left*: Two 12-mm AVP-2 device occluders are placed (*arrowheads*). *Bottom right*: Following treatment, there is no residual paravalvular regurgitation (*arrowhead*). *LA*, left atrium; *LV*, left ventricle.

transapical puncture or a retrograde approach (via the femoral artery) with retrograde cannulation from the left ventricle also can be successful.

Steps for Percutaneous Repair of Mitral Paravalvular Prosthetic Regurgitation

1. Right femoral venous access is obtained with standard techniques followed by placement of a 20F Gore Dryseal sheath. The site can be preclosed for hemostasis after procedural completion.

2. Standard transseptal puncture with guidance from fluoroscopy and echocardiography is used to access the left atrium. In patients with posterior-medial defects, a posterior puncture to gain height on the mitral valve is needed. This helps to avoid the acute angulation to the defect that can pose challenges for catheter engagement.

3. A steerable 8.5F guide (Agilis catheter, St. Jude, Fridley, MN) is loaded with a telescoped catheter system consisting of a 6F 100-cm multipurpose guide and a 5F 125-cm multipurpose diagnostic catheter. The steerable guide can be small- or medium-curved; small-curved guides are particularly helpful for medial defects.

4. Using echocardiography and fluoroscopy, the system is steered toward the defect, which is crossed with an exchange-length, 0.035-inch angle-tipped Glidewire (Terumo). Three-dimensional echocardiography is very useful for guiding the position of the catheters relative to the mitral prosthesis. Fluoroscopy should demonstrate positioning of the steerable guide and guidewires external to the prosthesis ring.

5. The two multipurpose catheters are placed sequentially into the left ventricle, followed by removal of the diagnostic catheter.

6. A device occluder can be passed through the 6F guide, which can accommodate a 12-mm AVP-2. Alternatively the guide can be exchanged over a 0.032-inch extra-stiff Amplatz wire for a

larger catheter (e.g., 90 cm, 6F to 8F Cook Flexor Shuttle) that enables either multiple device placements or anchor wiring.

7. Similar to treatment of aortic defects, the distal retention disk of the occluder is extruded from the guide into the left ventricle, followed by straddling of the defect with the retention disks on both sides.

8. Once leaflet impingement has been excluded on both echocardiography and fluoroscopy, the device occluder is released.

Guidance from TEE is essential to the success of the procedure. The echocardiographer and operator should communicate freely with regards to the location of the defect and its cannulation. While a clock-face method has been proposed for this communication, this approach can be challenging due to the opposite viewpoints of fluoroscopy versus the traditional left atrial surgical view obtained by TEE. Our preferred method relies on anatomically correct terminology (anterior vs. posterior, lateral vs. medial) and triangulation between the aortic valve (i.e., anterior), left atrial appendage (i.e., anterolateral), and atrial septum (i.e., medial). For patients with mechanical valves, the location of the prosthetic commissures also can assist with orientation.

An alternative approach to these defects is retrograde from the femoral artery, where a coronary catheter (e.g., Judkins right, Amplatz left or right, or internal mammary) is placed into the left ventricle and oriented posterior toward the defect. This technique may be particularly useful when the defect is located medially and cannot be crossed from the left atrium. The defect can be crossed with relatively softer wires, such as 0.014-inch or 0.018-inch coronary guidewires if the Glidewire proves to be too stiff for passage. In the transapical technique, defect cannulation and device placement is similar to the antegrade approach. CT guidance with fusion imaging has been demonstrated to be beneficial when performing the apical puncture and for steering toward the paravalvular defect.

Transcatheter Rails

Paravalvular defects can be serpiginous and calcific and thus be difficult to cross with delivery catheters. Transcatheter rails can be used to gain support for catheter crossing in these instances, as well as to avoid repeat wire crossing of the defects.

Transcatheter rails were originally described for the treatment of congenital heart lesions. These rails are created by snaring of a guidewire that has been placed across the paravalvular defect followed by exteriorization to provide the operator with both ends of the wire (see Figs. 19.4 and 19.5). Typically a steerable gooseneck snare (15 or 20 mm) can be used. The location of the snaring is easiest in smaller caliber vessels (descending aorta instead of the ascending aorta), and thus the guidewire needs to be advanced as far as possible once it has been used to cross the paravalvular defect. The transcatheter rail can be placed left atrial-ventricular-aortic or left atrial-ventricular-apical for mitral paravalvular defects. For aortic paravalvular defects, the rail can easily be placed aortic-ventricular-aortic or, in select cases, aortic-ventricular-apical or left atrial-ventricular-aortic. Once the rail has been created, the operator can advance a guide catheter with support from an assistant who provides tension on both ends of the wire. Importantly, if an appropriately sized delivery catheter is chosen (e.g., 8F, 90-cm Flexor shuttle), device occluders can be inserted alongside the rail. Maintaining the rail across the lesion thus allows the operator to try various device occluders for the effect of reducing regurgitation, as well as the placement of multiple occluders simultaneously (see anchor technique discussed later). As an example, an 8F Flexor shuttle will accommodate a 12-mm AVP-2 and an 0.035-inch Glidewire simultaneously.

When creating transcatheter rails, it is important to note that injury to surrounding structures can easily occur from guidewire tension. Harm can result from damage to the prosthetic or native leaflets, myocardial injury, severe bradycardia from atrioventricular node pressure, and disruption of the mitral valve apparatus from chordal entanglement. Thus transcatheter heart rails should only be performed with careful hemodynamic monitoring and simultaneous echocardiography.

Multiple Device Placement and Anchor Wiring

Paravalvular defects frequently are eccentric and may sit close to the surgical sewing ring. In these instances, device overhang can result in leaflet impingement of the valve, particularly with mechanical prostheses. To help avoid leaflet impingement, as well as to achieve greater reduction in regurgitation, multiple, smaller device occluders can be utilized through use of an anchor wire.

In this technique, a large-bore guide catheter (e.g., ≥6F, 90-cm Cook Flexor Shuttle) is placed into the left ventricle once the defect is crossed with a hydrophilic guidewire. This guide catheter can accommodate multiple, extra-stiff guidewires, which can then be used to place the delivery catheters either simultaneously or sequentially. In the simultaneous technique, two extra-stiff wires are extruded through the guide catheter followed by placement of two separate guides (each typically 6F multipurpose). The device occluders are then placed through these guide catheters for simultaneous deployment across the paravalvular defect.

In the sequential technique using an anchor wire, a device occluder is placed alongside the guidewire, which remains within the guide. The guidewire may be curled in the left ventricle or be snared to create an exterior rail. Once the device occluder is placed in the paravalvular defect, the guide catheter is removed and reinserted over only the guidewire, leaving the delivery cable attached to the occluder and exterior to the guide catheter. The process of placing additional device occluders can then be repeated as the operator sees necessary. Once the final position of the device occluders is satisfactory, the cables are decoupled.

The anchor wire technique is also useful for maintaining a position across the paravalvular defect in the event that an occluder needs to be exchanged for different or multiple other devices. If anchor wiring is used, large-bore sheaths are required to accommodate the multiple delivery catheters and wires. The DrySeal sheath (W.L. Gore, Flagstaff, AZ), with its inflatable cuff, is uniquely suitable for maintaining hemostasis for this purpose.

Clinical Outcomes

Procedural success for percutaneous repair of paravalvular prosthetic regurgitation, using a strict definition of reduction to mild regurgitation or less and no major adverse events, occurs in approximately 80% of patients (~90% for moderate residual regurgitation or less). Complications are relatively infrequent, with a 30-day rate of adverse events of 2.6% for stroke, 1.7% for sudden or unexplained death, 0.9% for emergency surgery, 5.2% for periprocedural bleeding, and 0.5% for death. Periprocedural bleeding can arise from cardiac perforation, apical puncture, and use of large vascular access sheaths, and during bridging anticoagulation. Closure of apical puncture sites with surgical glue or vascular plugs has been utilized to help promote hemostasis.

The most common reasons for procedural failure are prosthetic leaflet impingement or inability to cross the defects with either a wire or delivery catheter. Prosthetic leaflet impingement (~5% of cases) can occur with any prosthesis but is more common in mechanical valves. Particular care must be taken to ensure proper leaflet function for both bioprosthetic and mechanical valves, with both imaging and hemodynamic assessments to be performed (i.e., gradient calculation). Release of tension on the system after device release can lead to repositioning of the occluder; thus, the possibility of leaflet impingement should be re-examined after final deployment. With use of smaller devices to minimize leaflet impingement, it is important to be certain of the stability of the device prior to release. Overall, the rate of device embolization during these procedures is approximately 2.5%.

The degree of residual regurgitation directly relates to relief of symptoms and better survival. In a 3-year study, 3-year survival was 64%, and New York Heart Association (NYHA) functional class improved only in those patients with residual regurgitation of mild or less (Fig. 19.7). Patients with hemolytic anemia require near complete or complete closure for symptomatic relief. Operator experience with the adoption of recently evolved techniques (e.g., anchor wire, three-dimensional imaging, transcatheter rails) is an important predictor of success with the therapy (Fig. 19.8).

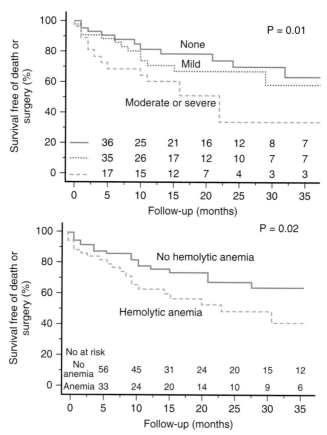

Figure 19.7 Survival after percutaneous repair of paravalvular prosthetic regurgitation. *Top:* Survival free of death or need for cardiac surgery according to residual regurgitation after paravalvular repair. *Bottom:* Survival free of death or need for cardiac surgery according to the presence of hemolytic anemia as an indication for the procedure. *(From Sorajja et al. Long-term follow-up of percutaneous repair of paravalvular prosthetic regurgitation. J Am Coll Cardiol. 2011;58:2218–2224.)*

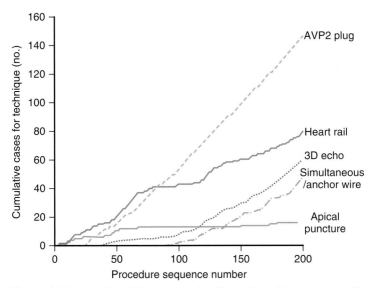

Figure 19.8 Adoption of imaging and catheter-based techniques with increasing operator experience in percutaneous repair of paravalvular prosthetic regurgitation. The graph shows the cumulative number of times a technique was used over an experience of 200 patients. *(From Sorajja et al. The learning curve in percutaneous repair of paravalvular prosthetic regurgitation: an analysis of 200 cases.* JACC Cardiovasc Interv. *2014;7:521–529.)*

Suggested Readings

Adams DH, Popma JJ, Reardon MJ, et al. Transcatheter aortic-valve replacement with a self-expanding prosthesis. *N Engl J Med.* 2014;370:1790-1798.

Altiok E, Frick M, Meyer CG, et al. Comparison of two- and three-dimensional transthoracic echocardiography to cardiac magnetic resonance imaging for assessment of paravalvular regurgitation after transcatheter aortic valve implantation. *Am J Cardiol.* 2014;113:1859-1866.

Davila-Roman VG, Waggoner AD, Kennard ED, et al. Prevalence and severity of paravalvular regurgitation in the Artificial Valve Endocarditis Reduction Trial (AVERT) echocardiography study. *J Am Coll Cardiol.* 2004;44:1467-1472.

Hamilton-Craig C, Boga T, Platts D, et al. The role of 3D transesophageal echocardiography during percutaneous closure of paravalvular mitral regurgitation. *JACC Cardiovasc Imaging.* 2009;2:771-773.

Jelnin V, Dudly Y, Einhorn BN, et al. Clinical experience with percutaneous left ventricular transapical access for interventions in structural heart defects a safe access and secure exit. *JACC Cardiovasc Interv.* 2011;4:868-874.

Kappetein AP, Head SJ, Genereux P, et al. Updated standardized endpoint definitions for transcatheter aortic valve implantation: the Valve Academic Research Consortium-2 consensus document. *J Am Coll Cardiol.* 2012;60:1438-1454.

Kodali SK, Williams MR, Smith CR, et al. Two-year outcomes after transcatheter or surgical aortic-valve replacement. *N Engl J Med.* 2012;366:1686-1695.

Kumar R, Jelnin V, Kliger C, et al. Percutaneous paravalvular leak closure. *Cardiol Clin.* 2013;31:431-440.

Luciani N, Nasso G, Anselmi A, et al. Repeat valvular operations: bench optimization of conventional surgery. *Ann Thorac Surg.* 2006;81:1279-1283.

Maganti M, Rao V, Armstrong S, et al. Redo valvular surgery in elderly patients. *Ann Thorac Surg.* 2009;87:521-525.

Momplaisir T, Matthews RV. Paravalvular mitral regurgitation treated with an Amplatzer septal occluder device: a case report and review of the literature. *J Invasive Cardiol.* 2007;19:E46-E50.

Nishimura RA, Otto CM, Bonow RO, et al. 2014 AHA/ACC guideline for the management of patients with valvular heart disease: a report of the American College of Cardiology/American Heart Association Task Force on Practice Guidelines. *J Am Coll Cardiol.* 2014;63:e57-e185.

Rubino AS, Santarpino G, De Praetere H, et al. Early and intermediate outcome after aortic valve replacement with a sutureless bioprosthesis: results of a multicenter study. *J Thorac Cardiovasc Surg.* 2014;148:865-871.

Ruiz CE, Jelnin V, Kronzon I, et al. Clinical outcomes in patients undergoing percutaneous closure of periprosthetic paravalvular leaks. *J Am Coll Cardiol.* 2011;58:2210-2217.

Sorajja P, Cabalka AK, Hagler DJ, et al. Long-term follow-up of percutaneous repair of paravalvular prosthetic regurgitation. *J Am Coll Cardiol.* 2011;58:2218-2224.

Sorajja P, Cabalka AK, Hagler DJ, et al. Percutaneous repair of paravalvular prosthetic regurgitation: acute and 30-day outcomes in 115 patients. *Circ Cardiovasc Interv.* 2011;4:314-321.

Sorajja P, Cabalka AK, Hagler DJ, et al. The learning curve in percutaneous repair of paravalvular prosthetic regurgitation: an analysis of 200 cases. *JACC Cardiovasc Interv.* 2014;7:521-529.

Spoon DB, Malouf JF, Spoon JN, et al. Mitral paravalvular leak: description and assessment of a novel anatomical method of localization. *JACC Cardiovasc Imaging.* 2013;6:1212-1214.

Zogbhi WA, Chambers JB, Dumesnil JG, et al. Recommendations for evaluation of prosthetic valves with echocardiography and Doppler ultrasound. *J Am Soc Echocardiogr.* 2009;22:975-1014.

Left Atrial Appendage Therapies

MATTHEW J. PRICE

Atrial fibrillation (AF) is the most common sustained arrhythmia and is increasing in prevalence due to the aging population. It is associated with a 4- to 5-fold increased risk of stroke and systemic embolism. Chronic therapy with oral anticoagulation (OAC) is underutilized, and long-term, safe, and consistent treatment can be difficult. Transcatheter closure of the left atrial appendage (LAA) represents a nonpharmacologic, mechanical approach to stroke prevention. This chapter summarizes the rationale for therapy, describes appropriate patient selection, and outlines the procedure steps to achieve successful outcomes.

Rationale for Transcatheter Closure

The LAA appears to be the dominant source of thromboembolism in AF. It is a multilobed, trabeculated, broad-shaped structure with a narrow neck, predisposing to stagnation and thrombosis. The morphology of the LAA is variable and can be generally classified in one of the following categories: windsock, cactus, cauliflower, and chicken wing (Fig. 20.1). OAC with warfarin reduces the risk of ischemic stroke by approximately two-thirds compared with placebo. However, successful treatment with warfarin is difficult due to a narrow therapeutic window, numerous food and drug interactions, and bleeding. The non–vitamin-K antagonist oral anticoagulants (NOACs) are noninferior or superior to warfarin for the prevention of stroke and systemic embolism and are more convenient because they do not require monitoring. The efficacy of the NOACs compared with warfarin is driven primarily by reduced hemorrhagic stroke. OACs are underutilized among indicated patients due to real or perceived contraindications predominantly related to bleeding risk. A local, nonpharmacologic approach to stroke prevention reduces the risk of stroke while eliminating the ongoing risk of bleeding associated with OACs.

Thromboembolic and Bleeding Risk Assessment

Assessments of thromboembolic and bleeding risks are essential components for patient selection. The $CHADS_2$ and CHA_2DS_2VASc scores are well-validated risk schemes based on a particular individual's comorbidities that can estimate a yearly risk of thromboembolic events and identify patients who may derive clinical benefit from OAC (Tables 20.1 and 20.2). The 2014 American Heart Association/American College of Cardiology/Heart Rhythm Society (AHA/ACC/HRS) Guideline for the Management of Patients with Atrial Fibrillation recommend the use of OACs in patients with CHA_2DS_2VASc scores of 2 or higher (class I, level of evidence: A); European Society of Cardiology (ESC) guidelines

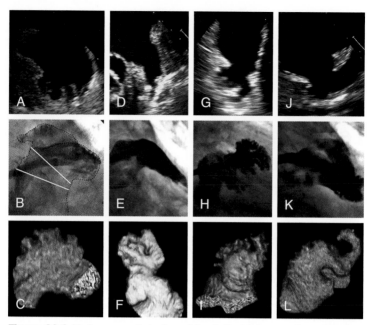

Figure 20.1 Various morphologies of the left atrial appendage. The four proposed classifications of left atrial appendage (LAA) morphologies as shown by transesophageal echocardiography (*top*), cine angiography (*middle*), and three-dimensional computed tomography (*bottom*). (A–C): cauliflower; (D–F): windsock; (G–I): cactus; (J–L): chicken wing. *(From Biegel R, et al. The left atrial appendage: anatomy, function, and noninvasive evaluation. JACC Cardiovasc Imaging. 2014;7(12):1251–1265)*

Table 20.1

Thromboembolic Risk Scores for Patient Selection Prior to Left Atrial Appendage (LAA) Closure	
$CHADS_2$	
Characteristic	**Points**
Congestive heart failure	1
Hypertension	1
Age ≥75 years	1
Diabetes mellitus	1
Stroke, transient ischemic attack, or thromboembolism	2
Maximum score	6
CHA_2DS_2VASc	
Characteristic	**Points**
Congestive heart failure	1
Hypertension	1
Age ≥75 years	2
Diabetes mellitus	1
Stroke, transient ischemic attack, or thromboembolism	2
Vascular disease (prior MI, PAD, or aortic plaque)	1
Age 65–74 years	1
Sex category = female	1
Maximum score	9

MI, myocardial infarction; *PAD*, peripheral arterial disease.
From January CT, et al. 2014 AHA/ACC/HRS guideline for the management of patients with atrial fibrillation: a report of the American College of Cardiology/ American Heart Association Task Force on Practice Guidelines and the Heart Rhythm Society. *J Am Coll Cardiol.* 2014;64(21):e1–e76.

Table 20.2

HAS-BLED Bleeding Risk Score	
Characteristic	Points
Hypertension (uncontrolled systolic blood pressure >160 mm Hg)	1
Abnormal liver or renal function[a]	1 each, maximum 2
Stroke (previous history)	1
Bleeding history or disposition (e.g., anemia)	1
Labile INR (i.e., time in therapeutic range <60%)	1
Elderly age (>65 years)	1
Drugs that promote bleeding or excess alcohol consumption (>7 units per week)	1 each, maximum 2
Maximum score	9

[a]Abnormal liver function was defined as cirrhosis or biochemical evidence of significant hepatic derangement; abnormal renal function was defined as serum creatinine >200 µmol/L (2.26 mg/dL).
From Pisters R, et al. A novel user-friendly score (HAS-BLED) to assess 1-year risk of major bleeding in patients with atrial fibrillation: the Euro Heart Survey. *Chest.* 2010;138(5):1093–1100.

also recommend OAC in patients with CHA_2DS_2VASc scores of 2 or higher (class I, level of evidence A), and state that OAC should be considered in patients with CHA_2DS_2VASc scores of 1 (class IIa, level of evidence A). The HAS-BLED score (Table 20.2) provides better predictive capacity for bleeding events in OAC-treated patients compared with other scores and highlights risk factors that can be actively managed to reduce bleeding risk.

Indications for Closure

Patients should not have other reasons to be treated with long-term OAC (e.g., mechanical prosthesis, mobile aortic atheroma, recurrent deep venous thrombosis); patients with mitral stenosis should also be avoided because this condition is associated with left atrial thrombus not involving the LAA. At present, the Watchman occluder (Boston Scientific, Natick, MA) is the only LAA closure device approved by the U.S. Food and Drug Administration (FDA) for stroke prevention (Fig. 20.2). The FDA indications for use (Box 20.1) and the Centers for Medicare and Medicaid Services (CMS) national coverage decision (Box 20.2) serve as the framework for appropriate patient selection.

Anatomic Evaluation for Feasibility

Assessment of LAA size and shape is required to determine the feasibility of Watchman closure: LAA ostial width must be adequate to provide appropriate device compression (8%–20%) while at the same time allowing sufficient depth to accommodate it (the device length is roughly the same as its diameter). Transesophageal echocardiography (TEE) is the standard screening imaging technique. The following features should be identified by preprocedural TEE:

- Any LAA thrombus (if present LAA closure is contraindicated)
- Presence and magnitude of pericardial effusion, if any, to serve as baseline reference after device implantation
- LAA shape (in particular, chicken wing)
- Maximum diameter of the LAA ostium
- Maximum LAA depth

The LAA is measured in a systematic fashion from the midesophageal view at 0, 45, 90, and 135 degrees. The LAA ostium is formed *superiorly* by the left upper pulmonary vein (LUPV) limbus and

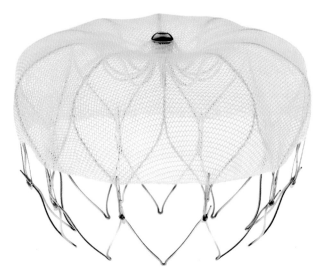

Figure 20.2 Watchman left atrial appendage (LAA) occluder. The device is made of a self-expanding nitinol frame with a polyethylene terephthalate fabric 160-µm mesh cap. The device size corresponds to the width of the device at its proximal shoulders; available sizes are 21 mm, 24 mm, 27 mm, 30 mm, and 33 mm. Device length is approximately equal to its diameter. Distal fixation anchors secure the device within the LAA trabeculae. It attaches to the delivery cable at a central threaded insert.

Box 20.1 U.S. Food and Drug Administration (FDA) Indications for Use for the Watchman Left Atrial Appendage (LAA) Occluder

The Watchman is indicated to reduce the risk of thromboembolism from the LAA in patients with nonvalvular atrial fibrillation (AF) who:
- are at an increased risk stroke and systemic embolism based on $CHADS_2$ or CHA_2DS_2VASc scores and are recommended for oral anticoagulation (OAC)
- are deemed by their physicians to be suitable for warfarin; and
- have an appropriate rationale to seek a nonpharmacologic alternative to warfarin, taking into account the safety and effectiveness of the device compared to warfarin.

Appropriate rationales for seeking an alternative to warfarin include:
- a history of major bleeding while taking therapeutic anticoagulation therapy
- the patient's prior experience with OAC (if applicable)
- a medical condition, occupation, or lifestyle placing the patient at high risk of major bleeding secondary to trauma

---

inferiorly by the area adjacent to the mitral valve annulus and above the left atrioventricular groove, which contains the left circumflex artery (Fig. 20.3). The ostial diameter is defined as the distance from a point just distal to the left circumflex artery to approximately 1–2 cm from the tip of the LUPV limbus. Alternatively, the LAA ostium can be measured by drawing a line from the mitral valve annulus across to the LUPV perpendicular to the planned axis of the delivery ("access") sheath. Depth is defined as the distance from the midpoint of the line that defines the ostium to the deepest point within the LAA, preferably at the apex of the anterior-most lobe (Fig. 20.4). The maximal width and maximal depth may be identified at different planes on TEE. The starting point for the smallest acceptable device is a size at least 10%–20% greater than the *maximum* width; once the operator engages the LAA with the access sheath during the procedure, a larger device may be selected if sufficient depth can be achieved. The patient may

> **Box 20.2** Summary of Centers for Medicare & Medicaid Services National Coverage Decision for Left Atrial Appendage (LAA) Closure
>
> (1) The device must have received U.S. Food and Drug Administration (FDA) approval
> (2) The patient must have:
> - A CHADS$_2$ score ≥ 2 or a CHA$_2$DS$_2$VASc score ≥ 3
> - A formal shared decision-making interaction with an independent physician using an evidence-based tool on oral anticoagulation (OAC) in patients with atrial fibrillation (AF) prior to LAA closure
> - A suitability for short-term warfarin but deemed unable to take long-term OAC
> (3) The patient is enrolled in, and the hospital must participate in, a prospective, national, audited registry (i.e., the American College of Cardiology National Cardiovascular Data Registry left atrial appendage occlusion [LAAO] registry)
> (4) The operator has performed ≥ 25 interventional cardiac procedures that involve transseptal puncture through an intact septum

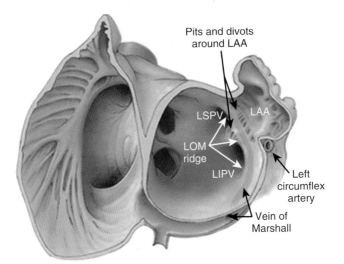

Figure 20.3 Anatomy of the left atrial appendage and its surrounding structures. *LAA*, left atrial appendage; *LOM*, ligament of Marshall; *LSPV*, left superior pulmonary vein; *LIPV*, left inferior pulmonary vein. *(From DeSimone CV, et al. A Review of the Relevant Embryology, Pathohistology, and Anatomy of the Left Atrial Appendage for the Invasive Cardiac Electrophysiologist. J Atr Fibrillation. 2015;8(2):81–87.)*

not be a candidate for closure if the maximal LAA depth on TEE is not sufficient for the smallest acceptable device based on the maximal LAA width (i.e., the LAA is shallow and wide). Cardiac computed tomography (CT) may be useful in cases where the LAA anatomy is unclear or of borderline feasibility according to TEE.

Procedure

Procedure Room Setup

Suggested procedure room equipment is listed in Table 20.3. The procedure can be performed in a standard cardiac catheterization laboratory. Key participants include an anesthesiologist, an imager (which in some cases may be the anesthesiologist), and the implanter. General sedation is used for patient comfort, to protect the airway in

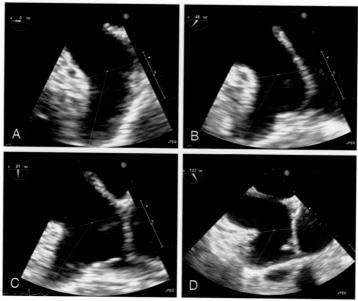

Figure 20.4 Preprocedural transesophageal echocardiography (TEE) assessment of the left atrial appendage (LAA) for Watchman occluder implantation. TEE is performed prior to the procedure to exclude the presence of LAA thrombus and to confirm LAA anatomy is feasible for occlusion. The diameter and depth of the LAA are measured at 0, 45, 90, and 135 degrees (Panels A, B, C, and D, respectively). The diameter of the LAA is defined as the distance from a point just distal to the left circumflex artery to roughly 1–2 cm from tip of the left upper pulmonary vein (LUPV) limbus. An initial device size is selected to be approximately 10%–20% greater than the maximal width, provided there is sufficient depth; the decision on device size may be adjusted after fluoroscopic landmarks are obtained once the access sheath is advanced deep within the LAA. In this case, the LAA has a modest anterior "chicken wing" morphology, which may increase procedural complexity but did not preclude procedural success. *(From Price MJ. Left atrial appendage occlusion with the WATCHMAN™ for stroke prevention in atrial fibrillation. Rev Cardiovasc Med. 2014;15(2):142–151.)*

the setting of prolonged TEE imaging, and to avoid sudden movements by the patient when the operator is manipulating equipment deep in the LAA, which might result in cardiac perforation. The fluoroscopy C-arm is rotated so that it is just to the left of the operator thereby allowing more freedom of movement for the echocardiographer, who is sitting at the head table. Appropriate radiation shielding is placed in front of the echocardiographer and anesthesiologist. The ultrasound machine is slaved to the boom so that the operator can see TEE images in real-time.

Anticoagulation

Unfractionated heparin (UFH) is used during the procedure, with a goal activated clotting time (ACT) between 250 and 300 seconds. Many operators administer a half-dose of UFH after placement of the sheaths and prior to transseptal puncture (TSP) and the remainder after left atrial access has been successfully accomplished. An ACT should be obtained frequently throughout the procedure to ensure appropriate anticoagulation is maintained for the duration of the procedure. Reversal of therapeutic warfarin is not required for the procedure, but this depends on operator preference and comfort; NOACs should generally be held according to their respective instructions for use.

Table 20.3

Procedure Room Equipment for Transcatheter Left Atrial Appendage (LAA) Closure	
Item	**Use**
8F sheath	Initial venous access
5F sheath	"Bailout" sheath in other vein (no need for neck line)
8.5F transseptal (TS) sheath	TS access
Transseptal needle[a]	TS access
12F dilator	To aid introduction of access sheath into venotomy
16F sheath	In case of venous tortuosity or challenging sheath manipulation
Extra-stiff Amplatz wire, 0.35-inch	Exchange of TS sheath for access sheath
Inouye (ProTrack) wire 0.25-inch	For difficult access sheath exchanges
6F straight pigtail	To advance access sheath deep into LAA
PTA Balloon: 5.0 mm × 40 mm	To dilate interatrial septum (IAS) when access sheath cannot cross
Perclose Proglide	For preclosure of venous access
Pericardiocentesis kit	To treat tamponade
Cook 18F sheath xx-mm	For embolized device retrieval
Gooseneck or other snares	For embolized device retrieval

[a]Commonly used curves include the BRK (St. Jude Medical) or CO (Baylis Medical).

Venous Access

At the start of the procedure, right femoral venous (RFV) access is established with a standard introducer sheath, typically 8F. The vein can be pre-closed with a single Perclose device (Abbott Vascular, Santa Clara, CA); alternatively, a "figure-of-eight" stitch at the end of the procedure can be used, obviating the need and cost of a closure device. Once the Perclose has been deployed, an 8.5F transseptal sheath is advanced over a 0.32-inch wire into the superior vena cava (SVC) in preparation for transseptal puncture (TSP). A 16F introducer sheath in the RFV is helpful in situations where the pelvic veins are highly tortuous, the subcutaneous tissue scarred due to prior procedures, or when there is significant obesity. The transseptal sheath is directly introduced through this larger introducer, and TSP performed, followed by introduction of the 14F delivery sheath. A second, lower profile (e.g., 5F) sheath is placed in the left femoral vein (or adjacent to the initial puncture in the right femoral vein) in order to draw blood for measurement of ACTs and to serve as central venous access in case of hemodynamic compromise and/or tamponade. This second sheath also eliminates the need for venous access in the neck, which improves patient comfort postprocedure and minimizes anesthesia setup time.

Transseptal Puncture

The TSP procedure can be divided into the following steps:
- Tenting of the interatrial septum (IAS) with the transseptal sheath dilator
- Advancement of the transseptal needle through the IAS
- Passage of the transeptal sheath dilator and sheath into the left atrium
- Removal of the dilator and flushing of the transseptal sheath

For LAA closure, the TSP site should be located inferior and posteriorly because this orients the access sheath co-axially with the LAA (Fig. 20.5). Potential complications of TSP are listed in Box 20.3.

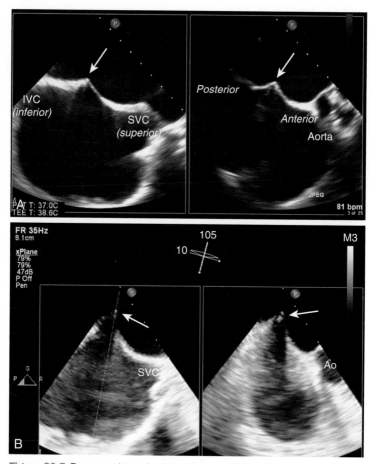

Figure 20.5 Transesophageal echocardiogram (TEE) guidance of transseptal puncture for left atrial appendage (LAA) occlusion. The location of the transseptal puncture is visualized by multiplanar imaging of the bicaval and aortic short axis planes. *Clockwise* rotation of the transseptal system by the operator will direct the system more posteriorly, away from the aorta (visualized in the aortic short axis plane), while withdrawal of the system will bring the puncture inferior (visualized in the bicaval plane). (A) Anatomic orientation of the multiplanar image of the interatrial septum (IAS). The transseptal needle is tenting the mid-portion of the interatrial septum. (B) For LAA occlusion, an inferior-posterior puncture should be made because this provides a coaxial approach for equipment to be introduced into the LAA. *Ao*, Aorta; *IAS*, interatrial septum, *SVC*, superior vena cava; *arrows*, tenting of interatrial septum by transseptal needle.

Box 20.3 Potential Complications of Transseptal Puncture
Pericardial effusion and subsequent cardiac tamponade
Stroke
Myocardial ischemia/ST-T changes in the inferior leads
Persistence of atrial septal defect
Aortic root puncture
Puncture or tearing of right or left atrial free wall
Death

From Early MJ. How to Perform a Transseptal Puncture. *Heart.* 2009;95:85–92.

Once the TSP sheath is introduced into the LA, pressure should be measured. A mean LA pressure of 10 mm Hg or higher is recommended before device deployment so that LAA size is not underestimated. Boluses of normal saline should be administered until the goal LA pressure is achieved. The sheath is then exchanged for the 14F access sheath over an 0.35-inch extra-stiff Amplatz wire in the LUPV. Entry of the wire into the LAA should be fastidiously avoided because this can result in cardiac perforation, particularly during the exchange maneuver. A 0.25-inch Inouye wire (ProTrack Pigtail, Baylis Medical, Montreal, Canada) can be used for catheter exchange if the LUPV cannot be wired easily: the Inouye wire has a flexible spiral tip with a supportive body, which facilitates catheter exchanges by maintaining left atrial access and reducing the risk of perforation.

Delivery Sheath Selection

The Watchman delivery ("access") sheath comes in three different shapes: double, single, and anterior curve (Fig. 20.6). The double-curve sheath is sufficient to provide depth and coaxial orientation within the LAA in the majority of cases. The single-curve sheath may be advantageous when there is a single (or dominant) posterior lobe. The anterior-curve sheath is helpful to achieve a coaxial position when the LAA has a markedly anterior orientation.

Advancement of Delivery Sheath Into LAA

The access sheath and dilator are advanced over the stiff wire anchored within the LUPV (or the Inouye-type wire). The side port of the access sheath should be oriented at approximately 3 o'clock as the sheath and dilator cross the septum. Once the dilator tip has reached the middle of the left atrium, the dilator is fixed and the access sheath advanced over it. Simultaneous TEE imaging of the basal short axis of the IAS is helpful to monitor the sheath as it crosses the septum: persistent tenting of the IAS can occur if the sheath or dilator cannot fully cross. In this case, balloon septostomy with a 5.0 × 40-mm PTA balloon is required to dilate the IAS sufficiently for sheath advancement.

The sheath should be carefully flushed with saline after the dilator and wire are removed. The operator must be meticulous in preventing the introduction of air within the sheath and subsequently the left atrium because this is the primary cause of procedure-related stroke. A 6F straight pigtail catheter is introduced into the sheath, advanced

Double-curve access sheath	Single-curve access sheath	Anterior-curve access sheath

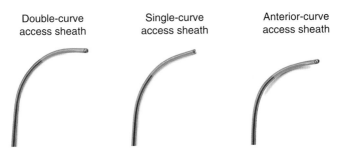

Figure 20.6 There are three currently available delivery sheaths for use with the Watchman system, depicted here. The double-curve access sheath (*left*), single-curve access sheath (*middle*), and anterior-curve access sheath (*right*) all have slightly different configurations that allow the operator the ability to successfully implant a Watchman device in a wide array of patients, regardless of the anatomy. Careful preplanning of the procedure, with experience concerning the angulation of the major lobe of the appendage and the orientation of the system from the septum to the opening of the appendage will facilitate choosing one sheath over another.

into the left atrium, and connected to the manifold for contrast injections. The operator then intubates the LAA with the pigtail catheter; this is often facilitated by gentle counterclockwise (anterior) rotation of the sheath under TEE guidance.

LAA angiography is performed with a hand-injection of contrast through the pigtail catheter in a right anterior oblique (RAO)-caudal (30 degrees/30 degrees) projection. This projection is the fluoroscopic equivalent of the TEE 135-degree view, laying out the LAA in short axis so that the ostium is clearly defined. Calcification of the left coronary artery or a prior left circumflex coronary stent, if present, can also aid in identifying the fluoroscopic location of the LAA ostium.

The pigtail catheter should be advanced deeply into the lobe that will provide the coaxial deployment of the occluder; this is generally—but not always—the most anterior lobe. The operator then advances the access sheath carefully over the pigtail until adequate depth is obtained for the planned device size. Gentle counterclockwise (anterior) rotation of the sheath may facilitate this maneuver. When the sheath cannot be advanced deeply into the LAA because it is not sufficiently coaxial, options for the operator include an alternately shaped sheath or to re-perform the TSP in a more favorable location (usually lower and/or more posteriorly) (Fig. 20.7). A 16F sheath in the right femoral vein should be used if it is difficult to torque the access sheath or tactile feel is lost due to excessive venous tortuosity or scarring of subcutaneous tissue. Rarely the access sheath may kink at the IAS; in this situation, the sheath should be removed over a wire, a balloon septostomy performed, and a new access sheath advanced into the LAA for device deployment.

Fluoroscopic Assessment of Delivery Sheath Depth and Device Size Selection

Three radiopaque markers on the access sheath act as landmarks for estimating the proximal landing site of the occluder device (Fig. 20.8). The more distal marker signifies the estimated landing site of a 21-mm device; the middle marker, a 27-mm device; and the proximal marker, a 33-mm device. For example, if the goal is to implant a 27-mm device (based on TEE measurements), the sheath must be advanced deeply enough into the LAA so that the middle marker is at or just distal to the LAA ostium (Fig. 20.9).

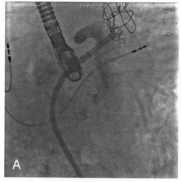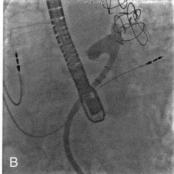

Figure 20.7 Influence of transseptal puncture location on sheath delivery into left atrial appendage (LAA). (A) The double-curve access sheath cannot be positioned deep within the LAA because it is not coaxial with the LAA ostium, even after substantial counterclockwise rotation. (B) An anterior curve sheath is optimally positioned after performing another transseptal puncture more inferiorly than the first, allowing successful deployment of a Watchman 24-mm device.

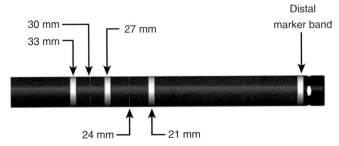

Figure 20.8 Watchman device size relative to access sheath marker bands.

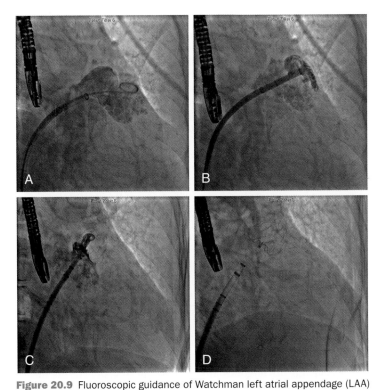

Figure 20.9 Fluoroscopic guidance of Watchman left atrial appendage (LAA) closure. Baseline transesophageal echocardiogram (TEE) demonstrated a maximal LAA ostium width of 25 mm; therefore a 30-mm occluder represents the smallest acceptable device size to provide the minimum allowable compression (at least 8%). (A) LAA angiography is performed in the right anterior oblique-caudal projection through a 6F diagnostic pigtail catheter that has been advanced through the dedicated 14F access sheath. The distal-most marker delineates the tip of the access sheath, which is at the LAA ostium. (B) The access sheath is advanced deeply into the LAA over the pigtail catheter while applying counterclockwise rotation to orient the sheath coaxially with the LAA ostium. The first (most proximal) and second markers are nearly straddling the plane of the LAA ostium (*arrows*), consistent with sufficient depth for a 30-mm device. (C) LAA after device deployment. Contrast can enter the LAA through the perforated cap of the device, which endothelializes in the weeks following implantation. The proximal shoulders of the device (*arrows*) rest at the level of the LAA predicted by the fluoroscopic markers prior to delivery. According to TEE, the widest diameter of the device was 25.6 mm, consistent with adequate compression (14.7%). (D) Fluoroscopy of the device after release from the delivery cable. *(From Price MJ, Holmes DR. Mechanical closure devices for atrial fibrillation.* Trends Cardiovasc Med. *2014;24(6):225–231.)*

Device Deployment

The manifold is connected to the flush port of the delivery system, ventilation is held, and the pigtail catheter removed. The delivery system, which contains the preloaded device, is flushed, introduced into the access sheath, and advanced until the radiopaque marker of the distal end of the delivery system is aligned with the distal marker of the access sheath. Filling the access sheath with contrast after introducing the delivery system can help delineate the distal end of the sheath and its relationship to the backwall of the LAA. Once the markers are aligned, the operator stabilizes the proximal end of the delivery system and retracts the access sheath so that it snaps into the delivery system, creating a single assembly. The operator loosens the valve on the delivery system, holds the deployment knob stable, and retracts the access sheath/delivery system assembly to unsheathe and deploy the self-expanding device. It is imperative that the distal end of the device (the "feet") remain fixed in position and not move forward because this could cause tearing of the friable LAA wall, nor should the feet fall back because this will cause the device to be deployed proximally. This can be accomplished by gentle counterforce on the deployment knob as the sheath/delivery system assembly is retracted. Angiography is performed to assess device position. The optimal angle to delineate the relationship between the device and the LAA ostium, including whether all lobes are covered, is the RAO-caudal projection. Cranial and anterior-posterior (AP)-caudal projections can be used to examine the relationship between the device and the anterior and posterior aspects of the LAA, respectively.

Release Criteria

TEE is performed at 0, 45, 90, and 135 degrees. Residual flow around the device, if any, should be identified. The width of the device (shoulder-to-shoulder in the plane where the threaded insert is visualized) should be measured at each angle (Fig. 20.10). The following "PASS" criteria must be met prior to releasing the device. The device is released by rotating the deployment knob counterclockwise 3–5 full turns.

- *Position*: The proximal shoulders of the device are at or just distal to and spans the entire LAA ostium
- *Anchor*: Gently pull back and release the deployment knob to visualize movement of device and LAA together
- *Size*: The maximum diameter of device by TEE is consistent with adequate device compression (see Table 20.4)
- *Seal*: Ensure all lobes are distal to the shoulders of the device and sealed (≤5 mm jet on TEE)

Device Retrieval

If the device is too distal, it can be partially recaptured and redeployed by fixing the deployment knob and advancing the access sheath/delivery system over the shoulders of the device up to but not past the distal fixation anchors. Once the shoulders have collapsed into the sheath, the entire system is withdrawn to the desired location and the device redeployed as described previously. If the device is too proximal, full retrieval of the device is required. The delivery system is then withdrawn from the sheath, the sheath flushed, and the pigtail catheter reinserted to reposition the access sheath into the LAA.

Complications

Major complications during and after transcatheter LAA closure include pericardial effusion, procedure-related stroke, device embolization, and vascular access site issues (Table 20.5).

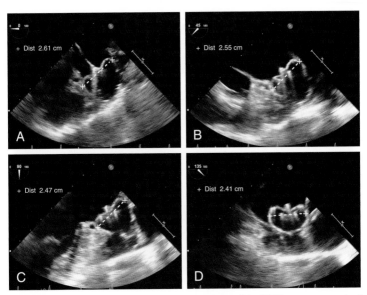

Figure 20.10 Transesophageal echocardiographic (TEE) assessment of Watchman device implantation. After deployment of a Watchman 30-mm device, the left atrial appendage (LAA) is assessed at 0, 45, 90, and 135 degrees (Panels A, B, C, and D, respectively). Compression is determined by measuring the distance across the shoulders of the device in the plane of the threaded insert. In this case, the device diameter ranges from 24.1 mm to 26.1 mm (13%–20% compression), is well-positioned, there is no color flow around the device into the LAA, and the LAA moved with the device as a unit when the delivery cable was tugged gently. Therefore the device was released from the cable with successful LAA occlusion. *(From Price MJ. Rev Cardiovasc Med. 2014;15:142–151.)*

Table 20.4

Compression Table for Watchman Devices	
Device Size (mm)	Deployed Diameter (mm)
21	16.8–19.3
24	19.2–22.1
27	21.6–24.8
30	24.0–27.6
33	26.4–30.4

Management of Pericardial Effusion

Since it is the most common complication associated with LAA closure, a thorough understanding and plan for the management of a significant pericardial effusion is critical for all operators performing the procedure. Evaluation of any baseline pericardial effusion and constant communication between the echocardiographer and the operator regarding the status of the pericardial space can identify issues before frank tamponade occurs. Patients should be closely monitored in the postprocedure recovery area for at least the first hour postprocedure; any hypotension should be considered tamponade unless proven otherwise. For slow-growing effusions, pericardiocentesis followed by placement of a pericardial drain and reversal of heparin anticoagulation (if equipment is no longer in the left atrium) is usually adequate. Small LAA tears, lacerations, and perforations will often close spontaneously if blood is aggressively removed from the pericardium. A second femoral venous sheath placed at the beginning of the procedure can serve as a "bailout" in case of hemodynamic compromise, unless the anesthesiologist has placed a jugular venous line. This second venous access is used for fluid administration or for autotransfusion in the setting of massive pericardial hemorrhage.

Table 20.5

Major Procedural Complications of Transcatheter Left Atrial Appendage (LAA) Closure and Potential Preventative Strategies		
Complication	**Cause**	**Preventative Strategy**
Pericardial effusion	Initial transseptal puncture	Transesophageal echocardiogram (TEE) guidance (e.g., X-plane) Avoid severe tenting of interatrial septum (IAS)
	Guidewire or catheter into LAA or through atrial wall after initial transseptal puncture	Advance dilator into LAA under fluoroscopy over 0.32-inch wire with distal curve, pigtail wire, or coronary wire
	Manipulation of delivery sheath/system into and within LAA	Advance delivery sheath into LAA over pigtail catheter rather than guidewire
	Device deployment and retrieval	Maintain delivery sheath position; minimize retrievals and reimplantations if possible
Procedural stroke	Pre-existing thrombus in LAA	Careful baseline TEE
	Insufficient anticoagulation	Monitor anticoagulation, if possible; consider anticoagulation prior to transseptal puncture
	Air embolus from delivery sheath/system	Flush sheath only after entering LAA and after device exchange, if performed
Device embolization	Inappropriate size	Tug-test; confirm device compression or appropriate fluoroscopic appearance
	Inappropriate position	Confirm device position and seal by TEE and fluoroscopy
Vascular (hematoma, arteriovenous fistula, pseudoaneurysm, bleeding)	Venous access	Careful technique; consider ultrasound guidance

From Price MJ. Prevention and management of complications of left atrial appendage closure devices. *Interv Cardiol Clin.* 2014;3:301–311.

Autotransfusion

Autotransfusion of blood aspirated from the pericardium enables the operator to maintain hemodynamic stability (until surgery can be performed) and attempt to seal the cardiac perforation despite substantial and persistent fluid accumulation. Autotransfusion is accomplished using the following steps:

- Place a pericardial drain or an 8F or 9F sheath in the pericardium
- Place a 5F–8F sheath into the femoral vein (or was already placed at the start of the procedure as a "bailout"). Alternatively, a large-bore sheath in the neck can be used.

- Connect the drain to the sheath with a stopcock and male-to-male tubing (or an appropriate adapter if male-to-female tubing is used)
- Aspirate blood from the drain using a large syringe, and then push it back into the venous system
- Use a cell saver system, if available

This can be continued for a several minutes until the pericardium is dry, which often stops the leak by allowing the perforation to seal. Never reintroduce blood into the left atrium (i.e., through the delivery sheath) or the arterial system.

Postprocedure Management

Adjunctive Pharmacology

- Discharge: Aspirin 81 mg/day and warfarin, adjusted to achieve an international normalized ratio (INR) of 2.0–3.0 until 45-day visit.
- Bridging with low-molecular-weight heparin until INR is therapeutic was not part of the trial protocols and is not required or recommended.
  - 45 days: Discontinue warfarin if 45-day TEE shows LAA seal (peri-device flow, if present, ≤5 mm), continue aspirin, start clopidogrel 75 mg/day
  - 6 months: Discontinue clopidogrel, continue aspirin monotherapy

Follow-up Imaging

A TEE should be performed at 45-day and 1-year follow-up, assessing the device at 0, 45, 90, and 135 degrees.

Suggested Readings

Camm AJ, Lip GY, De Caterina R, et al. Guidelines ESCCfP. 2012 focused update of the ESC guidelines for the management of atrial fibrillation: an update of the 2010 ESC guidelines for the management of atrial fibrillation. Developed with the special contribution of the European Heart Rhythm Association. *Eur Heart J.* 2012;33:2719-2747.

Holmes DR Jr, Doshi SK, Kar S, et al. Left atrial appendage closure as an alternative to warfarin for stroke prevention in atrial fibrillation: a patient-level meta-analysis. *J Am Coll Cardiol.* 2015;65:2614-2623.

Holmes DR Jr, Kar S, Price MJ, et al. Prospective randomized evaluation of the Watchman Left Atrial Appendage Closure device in patients with atrial fibrillation versus long-term warfarin therapy: the PREVAIL trial. *J Am Coll Cardiol.* 2014;64:1-12.

January CT, Wann LS, Alpert JS, et al. 2014 AHA/ACC/HRS guideline for the management of patients with atrial fibrillation: a report of the American College of Cardiology/American Heart Association Task Force on Practice Guidelines and the Heart Rhythm Society. *J Am Coll Cardiol.* 2014;64:e1-e76.

Price MJ, Valderrabano M. Left atrial appendage closure to prevent stroke in patients with atrial fibrillation. *Circulation.* 2014;130:202-212.

Price MJ, Reddy VY, Valderrabano M, et al. Bleeding outcomes after left atrial appendage closure compared with long-term warfarin: a pooled, patient-level analysis of the WATCHMAN randomized trial experience. *JACC Cardiovasc Interv.* 2015;8:1925-1932.

Price MJ. Prevention and management of complications of left atrial appendage closure devices. *Interv Cardiol Clin.* 2014;3:301-311.

Reddy VY, Sievert H, Halperin J, et al. Percutaneous left atrial appendage closure vs warfarin for atrial fibrillation: a randomized clinical trial. *JAMA.* 2014;312:1988-1998.

Index

Note: Pages followed by *b*, *t*, or *f* refer to boxes, tables, or figures, respectively.